The HOSKEN REPORT

GENITAL AND SEXUAL MUTILATION OF FEMALES

Fourth Revised Edition

FRAN P. HOSKEN

PUBLISHED BY WOMEN'S INTERNATIONAL NETWORK NEWS

ISBN 0-942096-09-6

TO THE READER

Since the subject of this report may be not at all familiar, some suggestions are made on how to deal with so much new information that has been entirely ignored by the health field and the international press. Despite some recent media attention, the facts published by the press often are wrong, distorted, taken out of context and even exploited and sensationalized including for personal gain. Good questions to ask always are: Will this information help stop the mutilations in Africa? Will this in any way improve the situation of the still quite helpless anonymous girl children and young women in Africa? And, most of all: What does this information accomplish to improve health services and health education for women?

This report was written to document the health facts in order to improve the health of women through more and better health services. Most of all, health education by and for women is needed to enable them to help themselves and their children. This has to be done with international support as it is an international problem. The Oral Rehydration Program by WHO and UNICEF and joined by many other international organizations works on the grass-roots level all over the developing world: it serves as an example that this can be done, that women and familiescan be reached in rural areas.

This report provides many hundreds of footnotes and is developed as a reference work. It is based on the previous three editions of the report but has been entirely rewritten and new information covering the more than 10 years since the last edition has been added. Since the subject is very controversial, everything has been documented with published references in many publications in English, French and German that are available in or with the help of major university or medical libraries. The documentation eventually will be made available through an archive in the Special Collection: Women of Northwestern University in Evanston, Illinois.

This report also will be followed by an abbreviated popular version incorporating key chapters and which will feature personal stories by African women to give the issue a human face, which some may claim this academic report lacks.

HOW TO READ THIS REPORT:

The key chapter that should be read first is **The Health Facts and Overview**. This chapter also should be used as reference throughout, as it provides an essential map and statistics and contains the factual and biological background of everything discussed in this report, including the politics.

The chapter on **The World Health Organization Seminar** provides the essential background to all other chapters and is referred to throughout the Country Reports and the Politics.

The Country Studies are the substance of the report, documenting the diversity and imagination with which patriarchal societies mutilate their female children to assert absolute male control.

The chapter on **Politics** documents that unfortunately the attitudes toward women that form the basis for FGM in Africa have support in the male dominated institutions everyhere in the world and especially in the international patriarchal health and population control systems as well as the United Nations.

Women and Health is new in this edition. It documents what positive initiatives there are in Africa and around the world to eradicate FGM. It is clear that FGM is based on attitudes and ideas about women that must be fundamentally changed everywhere if these practices are to be permanently eradicated. Positive initiatives that have produced any measurable beneficial results are still very limited; the money and effort spent on them will have to be greatly increased, given the extent of the problem.

TABLE OF CONTENTS

FOURTH REVISED AND UPDATED EDITION: January 1994

Published by:
WOMEN'S INTERNATIONAL NETWORK NEWS, 187 Grant Street, Lexington, MA 02420 USA

ISBN 0-942096-09-6

PREFACE TO THE FOURTH EDITION

This fourth, revised and updated edition for the first time has something positive to report. The objective of this edition, as all previous ones of this report, is to provide a comprehensive record of female genital mutilation (FGM) from a global perspective. The first edition of this report I published the end of 1978, or before the World Health Organization Seminar in February 1979 in Khartoum on Traditional Practices Affecting the Health of Women and Children, which opened the issue of FGM for international action. The second and third editions followed in 1980 and 1982 adding more information. But it took until 1984 before any preventive actions were started in Africa. This edition is different because it finally can describe some positive actions and FGM prevention programs in Africa: There has been a major change in attitude in Africa under the leadership of African women as recorded in the chapter on Women and Health.

There also has been some very limited change by a few international organizations concerned with health and development: But the majority of those working in Africa, especially in the population field, are more concerned with upholding the status quo. There are a few remarkable exceptions of organizations that have taken the lead such as Population Action International (PAI) and several Scandinavian development groups. But it is essential that major changes concerning priorities for prevention and participation by women be introduced in all health and population programs in Africa if any headway to eradicate FGM is to be made. (See The Politics of FGM.)

The previous or third edition of this report was published in December 1982 with a postscript added in spring of 1983, after my return from yet another research trip to East and West Africa. Since then much has happened which fortunately includes some consciousness raising about FGM and the status of women. But this awareness only began to have some impact on the media in the US quite recently, which predictably sensationalize FGM instead of supporting the women in Africa who are really working for change. The Inter-African Committee on Traditional Practices Affecting the Health of Women and Children (IAC), founded in 1984 with its many affiliates all over Africa has real potential to reach the people in Africa who must be persuaded to put their leadership behind this cause. And without restoring the health of so many millions of women in Africa, this continent, I fear, has no chance to develop or become productive to support its burgeoning population.

The other great problem affecting African health is AIDS. Both FGM and AIDS are interrelated - as even a cursory examination shows. Both not only reinforce the fundamental problems Africa faces about custom and tradition and the status of the majority of its population - women and children - but these problems together attack the very survival of a large part of its population who still have little control over their lives.

It is shocking to learn the new estimates - very carefully tabulated - of the number of women and girls affected by FGM in continental Africa (excluding several countries of the Arab Peninsula and Asia). This estimate of about 110 million is very conservative and includes mostly countries where at least half or a substantial number of people are involved. Since FGM is an ethnic practice, it is not related to political boundaries and is of course brought along by the many refugees of the escalating civil wars all over Africa to wherever they go. And with this, the modernization and medicalization of FGM, which is going on now in all urban areas in Africa are also spreading, including to the Western world. (See Health Facts and Overview.)

Despite the statement published by the World Health Organization in 1982 - or three years after the ground-breaking Khartoum Seminar, for a variety of reasons and pushed by economic greed, the introduction of FGM into medical and health practice as an elective "fee for service" surgery is spreading (see The Western World, The WHO Seminar and The Politics of FGM).

The health care systems all over the world and especially international health services have always been dominated by patriarchal attitudes that ignore women's needs, as extensively documented only recently in the US for example regarding breast cancer. In developing countries the overwhelming numbers of women dying or permanently maimed due to childbirth have been entirely ignored until quite recently.

How is it possible to ignore some 500,000 annual deaths of women, most of them preventable, due to pregnancy-related causes? Belatedly the international medical establishment has taken note; but it is astonishing that though the maternal mortality rates in sub-Saharan Africa are the highest in the world in the areas where FGM is practiced, the Safe Motherhood initiative - as this international campaign for safe childbirth is called - is refusing to acknowledge the existence of FGM. This damaging attitude of denial must be protested and FGM prevention included in the campaign in affected areas.

It is unconscionable to deliberately ignore the truth for patriarchal reasons by supporting male domination in Africa at the price of women's torture and lives. For the same reasons the silence surrounding FGM is still maintained by all international organizations working in population control in Africa. The budgets for population control for instance for the US Agency for International Development have been between $250-300 million annually; but not a cent for prevention of FGM is included. Family planning education programs in Africa still pretend FGM does not exist, thus contributing to the introduction of the mutilations into the health care systems all over Africa.

This I have also stated and documented in my Congressional testimonies since 1980, most recently in June 1993 before the Foreign Operations Subcommittee of the Appropriations Committee. (See Women and Health - Political Action to Stop FGM.) Investigation shows that our taxes support the medicalization of FGM throughout Africa, because internationally funded family planning and health programs in Africa do nothing to prevent FGM and deliberately ignore the ongoing mutilations. As a result the new equipment, training and tools these programs bring along are used to do the operations which also are increasingly introduced into the health care system. That prevention can be effectively organized on the basis of family planning - as the same people and health care institutions are involved - has been demonstrated by the Cairo Family Planning Association, which has organized and run for years an effective anti-FGM education campaign in Egypt (see Case History: Egypt and Women and Health).

The spread of FGM all over the world is supported by the failure of international programs to stop the mutilations in Africa. The same people in Africa who have contact with international activities are the ones most likely to seek asylum in Europe or America in case of revolution or civil war. They are led to believe that FGM is accepted everywhere, as the international family planning and health programs in Africa do not discourage FGM. Indeed the mutilations are practiced in refugee camps in Africa with the knowledge of UNHCR (United Nations High Commission for Refugees) who are responsible for the camps and the health teams that work there, as documented in this report.

In Canada and Europe including Sweden and the Netherlands, wherever health services are provided by the government, immigrant families from Africa, recently mostly from Somalia, have come to clinics asking to have their small daughters excised and/or infibulated the modern and medical way. Apparently such services are available from hospitals in African towns, as is also documented by the FGM prevention program in Kenya. (See Women and Health Strategies, Kenya.)

The time has come, as outlined in the chapter on Women and Health, to demand that all government supported international health and population programs in Africa integrate preventive education as part of all their programs in the field in all countries where FGM is practiced. Such preventive education must be coordinated with all parts of the programs and into all program activities and not as separate initiative. This can be done immediately and at no extra cost.

It is much easier to replace a damaging tradition with a new and more rewarding activity, rather than to prohibit it outright. Replacing FGM with family planning since both are concerned with reproduction, is a viable strategy which I have proposed for a long time. Surely this could be done readily by any international family planning organization working in Africa in FGM-affected areas, provided they are interested in women's health. And health must be the priority. Women in developing countries have recently raised the question about health and international population control in **the Women's Declaration on Population Policies,** which will be further discussed at the 1994 UN Conference on Population and Development scheduled for Cairo. (See Politics of Population Control.)

A convincing argument can be made about the cost of FGM to each African government in terms of increasing health care costs and services required by mutilated women, as pointed out in the cost analysis in Health Facts and Overview. Health care costs are also discussed as reason to support change by the program to eradicate FGM in Sierra Leone by Dr. Koso-Thomas (see Women and Health Strategies). African governments pay for all hospitals and health services as well as for the time lost from work due to illness as a result of FGM by their female employees. The health and hospital costs due to FGM were already pointed out by the Somali delegation at the Seminar in Khartoum in 1979.

It is very encouraging to see that African women living in Africa are beginning to speak up and demand to be heard on their own behalf and for change in Africa. It is quite misleading to think that anything can be changed in Africa by TV or film shows in the US, or columnists creating controversies or other kinds of media hype, that mainly benefit the promoters who use the issue to attract attention to themselves. This sort of thing is here today and gone tomorrow as soon as something new and more exciting comes along.

All useful action takes place in Africa, where the real work for change must be done, especially in rural areas. To work for change is not glamorous but often very frustrating and time-consuming, as the musical media groups who have ventured there to teach about AIDS evidently learned. One hears no more about African-American entertainers who recently went to Uganda and elsewhere to promote prevention of AIDS.

To be sure, money is urgently needed where women's health is concerned. Without sufficient and continuing financial support, nothing in Africa or the rest of the developing world can succeed. But the international methods used by development programs of introducing a new activity that is funded for a few years with the expectation that it will be continued locally, have proved to be an illusion. There is no one who can afford to continue any programs in Africa or elsewhere in developing countries, no matter how worthwhile. FGM will not stop after a few years of teaching; such an effort requires continuous support and motivation, working with people for a long time to change attitudes and to make change rewarding for those who are willing to take risks.

In the section on Women and Health a variety of programs in Africa are outlined, but these are mostly pilot projects or recently established with no long term experience. Many of them follow the familiar model of other development programs. The **Childbirth Picture Books (CBPB)** which teach reproductive health with pictures, published by **WIN NEWS** take quite a different approach. They simply provide information in accessible form, leaving the teaching to the people themselves and to absorb new ideas at their own pace. More than 50,000 books are in use in Africa in four languages distributed for the past ten years. Of course I believe that by much larger distribution of the **CBPBs** a great deal can be accomplished at very modest costs. I hope to have a chance to try this out in future in different environments, including testing results.

The programs to stop FGM outlined in this report all lack the continuing funding needed for long-range education; and they lack international support by the health and development communities including the UN and its agencies. Not even the national eradication program the Burkina Faso government started more than 4 years ago and which has a comprehensive national plan, has any substantial international support. The IAC network, which needs regular continuing support for its unique task of holding together so many activities in different countries, is constantly struggling for funds.

Unfortunately it is necessary to deflate some of the optimism created by the array of positive initiatives described in Women and Health. Given the number of people involved, the huge regions we are talking about and considering that the vast majority of the populations concerned are illiterate, it is essential to greatly increase all actions.

Yet compared to ten years ago when the third edition of this report was published, everything has changed. At last it is possible to talk about FGM without getting a blank stare or being attacked as a racist, as I have been so many times. "Political correctness" is one of the real obstacles for change or a rational approach in the interest of the people most affected - women and girls. And "political correctness" though this term was invented recently in the US, very much dominates all international activities and the UN, which is the most patriarchal system with an overriding interest to preserve the status quo.

All the efforts of setting up programs to stop FGM, of promoting women's health and supporting African women who have the courage to speak up and support change are being undone by the destructive policies of the World Bank. Structural adjustment has been especially damaging in Africa, forcing countries to shrink their economies in order to pay back past loans. The lack of capital creates ever more poverty especially among women who face the responsibility for supporting their children. The forced repayment has syphoned off funding from the health systems of most African countries. The results are devastating, especially for women's health and maternity services.

In most of sub-Saharan Africa maternity hospitals have always been poor and over-crowded as I reported in **WIN NEWS** after every trip to East and West Africa visiting hospitals. Despite the pronatalist attitudes, the men who run African governments utterly neglect the most basic health needs of women where childbirth is concerned. Over the years the maternity sections of hospitals I revisited were ever more depleted and over-crowded, lacking the most essential medicines and tools.

Under threat of cutting off all future credit, governments in Africa are forced to pay back loans to the World Bank. The money is taken from essential services including health and education. In turn maternities are cut back most because men make the decisions and they are not effected themselves. But though WHO and UNICEF know the situation and UNICEF even noted an increase in infant mortality in recent annual reports especially in Africa, they say nothing at all about the cause - the policies of the World Bank.

It is unconscionable for the World Bank to pretend to be concerned about maternal mortality by funding a few research grants while taking away the most essential services for women in African hospitals. In African countries where FGM is widely practiced and where women need real help in childbirth, the World Bank policies have killed more childbearing women than anywhere else. But those who know the facts are mute, and no one is interested in this ongoing destruction of women's health and lives.

The organizations I contacted for help after my most recent trip to East and West Africa were not interested and the articles I wrote about these problems were ignored. The so-called Safe Motherhood initiative which was started with a conference in 1987 in Nairobi by the World Bank, WHO and UNFPA have ignored not only FGM but the conditions in African hospital maternities which contribute to the staggering maternal mortality.

No one can tell African governments what to do is the politically correct answer by international and UN agencies and "respect for culture" is the misogynist slogan by these men who run them that protects the torture and murder of thousands of helpless little girls every year. Viable programs to prevent FGM need first of all a health care system that serves women's needs; in pronatalist Africa this means reliable services for childbirth and reproductive health especially maternity services and most of all childbirth education.

Prevention should be the priority, especially prevention of damaging traditional practices. Prevention is much more cost-effective than curative care, yet it is exclusively curative care that has been introduced in Africa by WHO and all other international health programs. What health care there is, for instance, in Francophone countries in West Africa is limited to the capitals or a few large cities. Therefore, health education and preventive care are even more important if there is a concern for women's health. And prevention is the basic issue when it comes to FGM.

A health education corps of young people, modeled after the Peace Corps - as suggested in the section on health strategies - is one option. The Chinese barefoot doctor system which trained thousands of community health workers to deal with basic health problems in the villages and prevent infections, is all but forgotten now: it is an effective way to teach preventive care on the grassroots level. But this is something Africans must be encouraged to develop themselves; yet for a start it needs to be internationally funded and promoted. For instance funding could be provided to train an African women's health corps to teach in rural areas about reproductive health, nutrition and prevention of FGM.

Finally the issue of violence must be examined. FGM is nothing so much as a culturally approved form of violence against women, quite aside from culturally approved wife beating which is practiced by most African men. Such family violence must be taken seriously and stopped if we are concerned about peace and human rights.

Family violence has been ignored at our peril as the escalating civil wars all over Africa show, quite aside from growing local ethnic and tribal conflicts and widespread politically motivated attacks. Sub-Saharan Africa at present is the region with the most refugees in the world.

Tribal warfare was always widely practiced all over Africa as historical accounts document; these conflicts could do only limited damage given traditional arms. But with modern weapon systems, introduced by Western powers, the whole situation and the nature of the violence have vastly changed.

Riane Eisler's work, examining the causes of conflict, domination and violence in the public sphere is quoted in the introduction. She shows how socialization in the family or private sphere affects behaviour in the public domain of the male leadership and she challenges the tolerance of family violence. "Today more and more people are challenging force-backed domination in the private sphere and long-ignored traditions of violence against women and children are for the first time in history, being brought out in the open." In the Chapter on "The Politics of FGM" this correlation is detailed with the example of Somalia. And Eisler points out that young people accustomed to see violence and domination, beatings and torture in daily family life, view this as normal and become insensitive to inflicting pain.

African boys who grow up in families where girls are routinely mutilated, where women are beaten and violated and treated like slaves accept such behavior as normal. They continue this behaviour when they form families and use violence without restraint in public as a way of life and to get what they want. The TV broadcasts in 1992 from Somalia showed women and children starving while well-fed boys and men brandishing automatic weapons visibly enjoyed their power derived from withholding food from their own mothers, sisters and daughters by violence.

FGM is a training ground for male violence. It is used to assert absolute male domination over women not only in Somalia but all over Africa. Decision makers concerned with international affairs ignore these violent family customs at the cost of international peace. The costs of peace keeping are rapidly escalating in sub-Saharan Africa which is the most violent region of the world with men on a senseless rampage for power while millions of African refugees - mostly women and children - wander over their destroyed lands.

This question must be asked about African men: Where do they stand? Why are there so few African leaders who not only say stop the mutilations - as President Moi of Kenya has done - but who back this up by educating their people and supporting real change. While many other African leaders have paid lip service and have made public statements about abandoning damaging traditions, one looks in vain, except for Burkina Faso, for any male leadership to put the statements into practice. A few physicians have joined the IAC or speak against FGM, but neither the male dominated medical profession in Africa nor any of the male political leaders or other men of influence have had the courage or the conviction to face this issue and address its cause.

One needs to ask again and again all African men and challenge their silence: By remaining mute they support the continuation of FGM. By speaking for African tradition without opposing FGM, they condemn millions of girls to unspeakable suffering. How can an educated African man today deny his responsibility for FGM which is on his shoulders as long as he remains silent and which diminishes not only him but all other African men. The time to remain silent is long since gone; those who say nothing now must be held responsible.

It has taken more than a year of persistent effort to rewrite and update this report. But I am trying to describe a moving landscape full of changing people. In February 1994 another IAC regional conference is scheduled in West Africa which will bring together people - women and men - from all over Africa, deeply concerned about changing their African customs. They are putting their abilities on the line to work for change in their own societies. These women and men and the leadership of the IAC not only need our good wishes and moral support, but also need real and tangible financial support and help of every kind to carry out and carry on their tasks. And they need many more to join them in their pioneering work to change their own societies, one family at a time.

Finally a personal note: given the topic of this report and the fact that this information has been gathered and researched for more than 20 years, I shall refrain from citing any names. But I want to thank here the many, especially in Africa, who have shared their knowledge with me; their information is reflected in this work. But I am especially grateful to the few whose help, essential support and encouragement have made my travels in Africa my research and this work possible.

I have been asked again and again ever since I started writing and publishing about FGM in 1975: How did you find out about FGM, which was so carefully concealed especially from Western women, and why are you still persuing this? I heard about FGM quite by accident the first time I traveled all over Africa in 1973, but it was next to impossible at that time to get any facts. As a journalist and working for women's rights and development I was determined to learn the reason for all the secrecy.

The second question why did I get involved and after 20 years why am I still persuing it? The answer is how could I not? How could I turn away from such needless suffering, which by my silence and by doing nothing I would condone. As founder and publisher of an international journal on women and development - **Women's International Network- WIN NEWS** - I cannot ignore the deliberate mutilation of millions of girls and women without trying to do anything about it. And I am convinced human beings are able to change.

I have always believed that it is possible to eradicate these terribly damaging customs in less than a lifetime. They are not only a violation of human rights but I believe they violate the dignity and worth of every woman, indeed every human being, in a direct and personal way. I believe all people all over the world, women and men, girls and boys have the right to control their own bodies and lives and must by enabled to do so. These mutilations are inflicted on young children for no other reason than that they are female, with the purpose to interfere in their normal, natural functions and personality. How can one work for justice, for human and women's rights, for equality and democracy while ignoring these senseless violent attacks on millions of defenseless children with the objective of controlling their behavior and to establish male superiority.

I also believe that all of us who have access to information and knowledge of the biological and sexual facts about reproduction must share this information with those who do not . Because this information is essential to lead a healthy and productive life and no one has the right to withhold, distort or otherwise manipulate the biological facts which make us free to lead responsible lives. For that reason I have started the information campaign with the **Chilbirth Picture Books** which are designed to distribute this essential knowledge everywhere in the world.

When I started my investigation I was all alone, there was nobody I could ask about anything. First of all I had to establish the facts about FGM and develop the epidemiology, which was essential before anything else could be done. When I started to research FGM, there were practically no publications available and the few medical articles were scattered in several languages throughout the medical literature. If you looked under circumcision in a medical library - as I did - there were dozens of articles on male circumcision and nothing on women.

The term FGM which I established later was unknown and unused and totally rejected in Africa. The extent of the operations was entirely unknown and unrecorded; nothing at all was published in West Africa and only in Kenya and Sudan some medical surveys existed including the most comprehensive study by Dr. Abu el Futu Shandall of Khartoum, which is still the most comprehensive clinical study ever made (see Case History: Sudan).

It took years before I was able to put together some reliable facts, sending out many hundreds of questionnaires all over Africa and visiting the maternity sections of hospitals in East and West Africa including Sudan, Kenya, Egypt, Ethiopia, Somalia, Nigeria, Burkina Faso, Cote d'Ivoire, Mali, Senegal, and Sierra Leone. Many of the basic facts reported here are from the midwives whom I met there. I also made it a point to write to the authors of all medical publications on FGM I could find for more information.

When I began to publish some of the facts, WHO cautioned all its staff to stop replying to my inquiries. UNICEF simply stated that FGM is a cultural practice in which the agency would not interfere (see The Politics of FGM).

Gradually I developed an extensive network which was mainly concerned with communication. First of all I collected information to establish the truth and publish what had been deliberately concealed as a shared conspiracy of silence by all international agencies operating under the same patriarchal rules. Those concerned with international health including WHO were only interested in continuing to conceal the facts to hide their complicity - especially after I started publishing. No African networks existed, and with a few exceptions such as Sudan, no African had ever done any research let alone publish any information on FGM.

At first all newspapers and magazines which I approached as a journalist simply refused, stating this topic was not "suitable" - literally every well-known paper refused to publish "such things". I finally succeeded to publish one article in a small academic magazine. A year later a research article on FGM and fertility in Africa I wrote was published in a journal on women's health, which was later also translated and published in Germany Italiy and France. This article I sent to **the Tropical Doctor** in the UK because that well known international medical magazine had published on FGM before: the editor invited me to submit an article describing the information I had gathered visiting African maternity hospitals. My article on **The Epidemiology of FGM** - the first time this term was used officially - persuaded the WHO to call the Khartoum Seminar on Traditional Practices Affecting the Health of Women and Children. They could no longer deny the facts or evade their responsibility - which they had done for years - by maintaining the silence.

After the WHO Seminar in Khartoum - to which I was invited to present a global review of FGM and participate as member of the seminar secretariat - opened the issue for international action, nothing happened for five years. The issue was entirely ignored again by all international organizations including by WHO itself. In 1983 after I traveled again all over East and West Africa introducing the **Childbirth Picture Books** with the **Additions on Excision and Infibulation** to midwifery schools and health departments, FGM was once more forgotten I found. These books were designed to help implement the WHO Seminar Recommendations. But as I stated in the Appendix to the third edition of the **Hosken Report** written in spring of 1983 after my return from Africa, the recommendations I found were all but ignored.

In **WIN NEWS** I continued to report on FGM in every issue and **WIN NEWS** is the only journal that has maintained a continuing section on FGM reporting new information four times a year. The entire history of FGM is recorded as it happened in **WIN NEWS**. But it was obvious all along that an effective action program would have to be started in Africa and by Africans.

The IAC organized in 1984 at a conference in Dakar and based on the WHO recommendations of 1979, which they expanded, by now has established an Africa-wide network with affiliates all over East and West Africa. It is important especially now to support this network, the only regional African women's network for the eradication of FGM that exists. It is based on exchange of information and mutual technical support, raising funds for all affiliates. A plan of action for the coming years is decided at each regional conference which is held in Africa every few years.

In 1994 the IAC and their affiliates are celebrating the l0th Anniversary of the organization of the IAC. To gain international support and attention for FGM the IAC as an African organization working with and for African women is unique and has accomplished more than anyone connected with this issue could hope for - given the problems. There are of course other local or national initiatives, but there are also many local and national problems. And there is the constant threat of civil war - such as the one that destroyed Somalia and everything that had been so carefully developed there to stop FGM (see Women and Health).

At the IAC conference in February 1994 new plans will be made for the coming years by the IAC network members from all African countries that have developed action plans - or are planning to do so. This and all new developments will continue to be reported in **WIN NEWS**.

Fran P. Hosken, December 1993.
Lexington, Massachussetts, USA.

INTRODUCTION

Mutilation, Morality and Facts // Initiatives for Change // Family Planning in Africa
The Absence of Women in Development and International Affairs
Somalia: Family, Tradition and Violence // Culture, Custom and Tradition
Women Speak: Beginning of Change
The Failure of Effective International Support for Prevention of FGM
Women's Rights are Human Rights // Outlook and Reality

Genital and sexual mutilation of women and girls has been practiced by the male dominated tribal societies of Africa and the Middle East for many centuries. It was first recorded in Egypt 2000 years ago, as documented in the chapter on history. For the first time this Report brings together all the known facts on female genital mutilation which have been concealed all over the world, especially from women.

Due to population growth, which is still increasing in Africa despite international support of family planning in most countries affected by FGM (Female Genital Mutilation) more female children than ever before are mutilated every year - including thousands of infants. Secrecy not only protects these operations and perpetuates them, but secrecy mystifies the devastating health and psychological results from the victims who are unable to relate cause and effect as the biological facts of reproduction are concealed.

The traditional rituals are being abandoned under the impact of modernization; but the physical operations continue, and they are done to ever younger children even where FGM traditionally was a puberty rite. The mutilations are practiced in all cities, even where they did not exist before, for instance in Accra, Ghana, and Alexandria, Egypt, due to increasing mobility. African immigrants also continue the mutilations abroad, wherever they go in Europe or America. The many refugees from the continuing African civil wars bring their customs along. The mutilations are now done on newborn girls, as newspaper reports and criminal cases confirm, for instance in France.

African health personnel and physicians trained in Western health care perform the operations for a fee on the children of the well-to-do all over Africa and the Middle East, under the dubious excuse that to mutilate little girls in sanitary ways is an improvement. Tools, training and antibiotics contributed under international health assistance programs are used to mutilate ever more little girls. The operations are "modernized" with the knowledge of Western physicians and health teams working in Africa and the Middle East. FGM is deliberately ignored by all internationally financed health and family planning programs, introduced with the assistance from United Nations agencies and from the US, Europe and other Western countries. None of them have included prevention of FGM in their programs - which shows their criminal contempt for women's health.

According to the World Health Organization (WHO), Africa has the highest AIDS infection rates in the world, due to African sexual customs and traditions, but the fact that FGM is one of the major causes of infection is also ignored. Recently many "Safe Motherhood" Programs have been started in sub-Saharan Africa - where the maternal mortality is the highest in the world - but all of them ignore the existence of FGM!

Though I have repeatedly testified in Congress, including before the decision-making Congressional committees that provide funding for health and family planning programs, the administrators of the Agency for International Development (US AID) have yet to officially acknowledge the Khartoum Seminar Recommendations of the WHO, which urge preventive education (see The World Health Organization). To integrate preventive teaching - providing basic information about the biological facts of reproduction and showing graphically the damage done by FGM - would be an easy and effective way to curtail FGM, improve health and increase the acceptance of family planning.

The work of the IAC - the Inter African Committee on Traditional Practices Affecting the Health of Women and Children [1] was acknowledged when its director Berhane Ras Work visited US AID in Washington in the summer of 1988, but none of the AID missions in Africa have provided support to IAC affiliates (see Women and Health). A cable sent by Washington headquarters at that time to all the missions in Africa was ignored.

What is documented in this report casts doubts on all the achievements for human rights, for human dignity, and for a better life that have been praised all over the world. Human rights are indivisible; they apply to every society and culture and continent. We cannot differentiate between black and white, rich and poor, male and female, or between North and South, the industrialized or developing countries, if the concept of human rights is to mean anything at all. And we cannot allow a female child to be brutally mutilated because she is black or brown claiming this is her "culture and tradition", a mutilation and violation of her integrity that we absolutely reject for a white child.

FGM as discussed here is a gross violation of human rights. FGM not only violates the human right to health of the victims directly affected, but these mutilations also represent a violation of the very essence and spirit of femaleness everywhere by mutilating the female natural potential, to ensure submission to male exploitation and demands.

The United Nations Human Rights Office in Geneva has recognized FGM: A special Rapporteur has been appointed who has produced research reports and held meetings. But no action for change has been initiated, nor was support provided for local activities. **The Country Reports on Human Rights Practices,** published annually by the United States Department of State, [2] have for the past five years included FGM, citing every country where it is recorded. For the past two years, violence against women and wife abuse have also been cited as human rights violations, in an official recognition of women's human rights. But no country has followed up. These Country Reports are submitted to the US Congress to make documented information available to Congressional committees that fund international assistance programs. Congress can stop international assistance and agreements where human rights violations persist.

The first step for change in countries where FGM is practiced is to include preventive education in all existing health and family planning programs, for instance those funded by US AID and implemented by all its contractors, as I pointed out in my recent Congressional Testimony for the Subcommittee on International Operations of the Appropriations Committee, which funds all US AID activities.[3] This can be done immediately at no additional cost and could affect millions of people all over Africa.

The Universal Childbirth Picture Book/Program (CBPB) [4] was developed by Women's International Network and published by **WIN NEWS** [5] following the Khartoum WHO Seminar of 1979. It is designed to support implementation of the Seminar Recommendations and has Additions to Prevent Excision and Infibulation in English, French and Arabic; a Somali translation has recently been added. * The **CBPBs** have proved immensely useful on the grass-roots level, as they are easy to understand regardless of language or literacy and dont need health experts to introduce them (see Women and Health).

This report is designed not only to provide the facts on FGM but also to support the eradication of all forms of these mutilations wherever practiced. Our ever-smaller world makes us all responsible for what we do, as well as what we fail to do. There is no place to hide. We also must examine and confront all other forms of female mutilation; the crippling of women in a much broader sense, both physical and psychological. Such mutilations go on in every society today and in many different forms all over the world. The contempt for the female of the species, which is the basic cause of all mutilations, discrimination and abuse by men must be challenged and dealt with everywhere and at its source. We shall never succeed to change behavior unless we confront its cause.

The fact that today many thousands of helpless girl-children from newborn babies to teenagers continue to be subjected to these cruel operations is due to another kind of mutilation, or crippling of the human spirit. Though these operations damage the health of more than 110 million women in continental Africa, as the latest estimate tabulated in this report shows, they are still concealed by their own families and communities as well as by those responsible for health in each country. International organizations of all kinds are also involved in this cover-up, including United Nations agencies, especially those concerned with health and development - UNICEF, WHO, UNFPA and UNDP.

---

* The **CBPB** is also available in Spanish and is printed in six Indian languages by CHETNA in India, and also published in Nepal. Please contact **WIN NEWS** for more information.

The unwillingness by men to come forward and confront FGM as criminal child abuse - despite the recently formulated international Children's Rights Convention - as well as a human rights violation is not limited to Africa. However, since the last edition of this report 10 years ago, much has changed. Many private organizations have worked hard to support local programs in Africa and the Middle East and developed many viable initiatives together with African women. The IAC, organized in 1984, has established an extensive framework for action with its affiliates in most African countries where the mutilations exist. But there is no leadership by the UN agencies who have the resources and the support system to act on the necessary scale. (See The Politics of FGM.)

The latest statistics show that there are now more mutilated girls and women in Africa than ever before due to population growth. In an age of instant communication, this simply is intolerable because it could be stopped if any of the international agencies had the will to do so - especially UNICEF, WHO and UNFPA: They have all the necessary local facilities in the field, the infrastructure and the contacts.

UNICEF has a global mandate to protect children, especially their health. Women all over the world are contributing to UNICEF and supporting this agency. Why then is Mr. James Grant, the director of UNICEF, an American, so utterly failing to provide leadership even now? FGM by now is not only known but has created an uproar in many European countries, as African immigrants continue to practice the mutilations where they settle (see: The Western World). The denial of help and health to many millions of children because they are female and regarded by African men who support FGM as their property can no longer be tolerated. The right of a woman to control her own body, her sexuality and reproductive organs is the most basic of all human rights. These mutilations have been called catastrophic from a medical point of view. But any form of mutilation of the female body to diminish a woman's normal sexuality must be categorically rejected, just as any operation on the male to cripple his sexuality is condemned.

Mutilation, Morality and Facts.

At the end of the 20th century we are, I believe, sufficiently mature to discard medieval sexual assaults on the female children as a means to prove male sexual superiority; yet this is the basic reason for these mutilations and why they are not stopped by men. Irrational fear of female sexuality has always been a dark and damaging undercurrent and cause of vicious persecution and violence against women, perpetrated under the cloak of morality in many societies. The witch hunts in medieval Europe and Colonial America, organized by the Catholic Church and other Christians, are one example of patriarchal morality for which thousands of women were tortured to death. Today we have the means to instantly communicate the facts on reproduction and sexuality that families, especially the young in Africa and the Middle East, so desperately need to reject the terrible fears and dangerous myths that ruin their health and lives (see The Politics of FGM). The **Childbirth Picture Books** were designed to show one way and have proved themselves on the grass-roots level. There are many other actions and local initiatives that need to be organized now, for instance those linked with teaching family planning.

It is evident that female genital mutilation can be abolished and permanently wiped out if we really make the effort. By now the issue is discussed quite openly in the cities of many African countries. Preventive actions have been started in many affected areas. We are able to teach those who cling to distorted beliefs some better ways to cope with themselves, reproduction and sexuality: everyone has the capacity to learn. Information about the basic human biological facts that every person needs to know can and must be made available to everyone. In the preface of their book, Masters and Johnson ask:

> "How can biologists, behaviorists, theologians, and educators insist in good conscience upon the continued existence of a massive state of ignorance of human sexual response, to the detriment of the well-being of millions of individuals? Why must the basics of human sexual physiology create such high levels of personal discomfort among the very men and women who are responsible for guiding our culture? There is no man or woman who does not face in his or her lifetime the concerns of sexual tensions. Can that one facet of our lives, affecting more people in more ways than any other physiologic response. . . be allowed to continue without benefit of objective, scientific analysis?" [6]

There is no excuse, given the present state of communication technology, for tolerating the confusion, the terrible harm, the disruption and the destruction created by ignorance about sex. In no other area has the fight against freedom of information been waged more destructively than in the area of human reproduction and sexuality, led by the male religious and political "moral" leadership of each country. Yet, sexuality and reproduction are of prime importance to everyone's life.

Now that the truth about human sexuality has been established by Kinsey, [7] by Masters and Johnson, and by the Hite Reports, [8] why are the facts not taught in every school and especially in the developing world? Why do government health and education departments still fail to protect the children from often lifelong damage to their health by failing to teach the biological facts and respect for their bodies that everyone, especially girls - who will bear and raise the children, the future of each country - need to know?

Why don't health professionals in each government make it a priority to teach all the people the basic biological facts about their own bodies and how children are conceived and born - what everyone most urgently needs to know, especially in African countries where fertility is so highly prized? The confusion about reproduction, about male and especially female sexuality not only creates personal misery and terrible health problems but greatly increases each government's health expenditures due to unnecessary emergencies. In all African countries health services are paid by the government. With sexually transmitted diseases at an all time high and AIDS decimating African populations -Africa has the highest AIDS infection rate in the world according to WHO - it is essential to teach about reproduction and sexuality by any and all means.

Initiatives for Change

The technical and communication tools are available everywhere to organize health information programs that also reach the rural areas and teach what every family needs to know including nutrition and family planning, quite aside from essential facts about personal hygiene, reproduction and sexuality. While modern communication tools have been used for political purposes for years, they have not been used on a similiar scale for public health. And that is what needs to be done.

That people all over Africa on the grass roots level are interested in straightforward information on how their bodies function I have learned from the distribution of our **Childbirth Picture Books (CBPBs)** with the Additions to Prevent Excision and Infibulation and the thousands of letters received by **WIN NEWS,** with more coming every week. * These letters from men and women in summary state: Now that we have learned what happens as a result of the operations we shall not have our daughters operated.

Instead of developing education and information programs and materials to teach prevention of FGM as the WHO Seminar Recommendations propose (see the World Health Organization), there is more and more money spent on "research". While it should be applauded that the silence has been lifted, these publications are of no practical use to the victims of FGM. Indeed such research is often used as an excuse for doing nothing by organizations working in health and development, claiming they need more information before they can develop any action programs - except that the actions never materialize. Still, the organizations claim at international meetings or when challenged that they are working on research.

Another approach used by family planning programs is for trained researchers to ask carefully devised opinon questions of selected target groups which are then computerized and tabulated in different ways to extract a remarkable profusion of statistical results. Such investigations can only be carried out in very small areas on a limited number of people of specific ethnic groups. But FGM is spread over huge regions of the whole continent of Africa and parts of the Middle East and is practiced by a diversity of ethnic groups; most of them do not even know that FGM exists anywhere else. What is more, rural Africans are very friendly and try to please: They will tell a researcher whatever they think he/she wants to hear in order to please.

---

* Excerpts of these letters are printed in **WIN NEWS** in the section on Genital and Sexual Mutilation, which is included in every issue and continuously reports on FGM.

But all these very different people, ethnic groups and societies involved in FGM - indeed, every human being everywhere - share the same biological process of reproduction, of conceiving and bearing children, no matter how this process is warped, misused, exploited and terribly damaged by cultural practices and damaging traditions. And this biological, physical basis of the human body which every human being shares can and must be explained because the human body is quite complicated.

What we need to ask is if such detailed gathering and tabulating of data in a few areas in Africa are really useful in organizing programs to stop FGM. Is it not much more productive to teach people something positive they need to know and are most eager to learn about as the experience with the **CBPB**s shows - that is, how their own bodies' function, about reproduction and sexuality? Experience shows that explaining the biological facts about reproduction in a form that can be understood by everyone usually is quite convincing if it is presented in a straightforward way. Letters received from many areas in Africa confirm that people - both men and women - when presented with the graphic facts of the damage done by the mutilations - reject them for their daughters.

Almost everyone in areas where FGM is practiced knows of girls who have died or is aware of women who have had trouble in childbirth. Therefore, the biological facts when presented - especially in graphic form - provide people with explanations for their own problems and experiences regarding FGM.The wide acceptance and success of the **Childbirth Picture Books** confirm my conviction that people everywhere in the world are able to understand what is to their advantage and they are able to use the message of these books to stop mutilating their children.

Of course, it would be possible to make specific tests of the **CBPBs**, designing a testing program to collect opinions of the people in a given area before and after handing out the books. There are international consulting firms who for many thousands of dollars could carry out such tests in different areas of Africa and provide computerized results.

I have always felt that our limited money is better spent on printing and distributing more books in Africa rather than paying for such investigations. I trust the people who write me from many different countries of Africa - and I shall be glad to share the letters with anyone interested. Of course if someone wants to spend the money on tests, as described above, I shall accept gladly. But given our very limited funds it would be irresponsible to pay for tests rather than for printing and distributing more books.

Family Planning in Africa

Family planning programs by now have reached practically all countries of Africa though tto few rural areas. But the success of family planning programs has been quite limited in terms of numbers. Despite all the millions of dollars spent and despite famines and droughts and civil wars, the population of most African countries is rapidly growing - more than in Asia or in any other developing region, although AIDS may soon have an impact on that. But what is astonishing is that family planning programs have had so little positive influence on women's health and none that is known in preventing FGM.

For instance, large family planning programs in Kenya, sponsored by the World Bank and by US AID which are implemented by many contractors (mostly headed by men) and by the Kenyan Government, have been active for at least 10 years. None of them have bothered to investigate the spread of FGM. One would think that, out of basic human concern for the women for whom the family planning programs are designed, the program planners would include some preventive measures. The mutilations practiced in many rural areas of Kenya are quite drastic, besides the many ethnic Somalis who live in northern Kenya all practice infibulation. There is a permanent waiting list of many hundreds of women at the Kenyatta hospital, the largest hospital of Kenya in Nairobi, for fistula operations. Fistulas, causing incontinence, are internal injuries due to obstructed labor which most often is the result of FGM (see: Health Facts and Overview))

But family planning programs in Kenya, as well as elsewhere in Africa, are not interested in women's health; they are concerned with population control. Family planning programs in Africa have deliberately ignored FGM, though they conduct detailed research on all aspects of fertility, what people know about contraception quite aside from how many children they want and much more.

In 1988 I visited the planning office in Abidjan, Cote d'Ivoire, of a very large regional family planning program funded by US AID that had started to conduct detailed research into fertility, maternal mortality and other health aspects of the different target populations. I asked one of the African physicians in charge about FGM, which is practiced thoughout the program area and is one of the major causes of maternal mortality. The doctor looked at me with obvious disapproval and said, "This is a sacred rite in our country - we never talk about that."

Though it is obvious from a woman's view that health is the priority where family planning is concerned and that family planning education programs have an obligation to teach about health including prevention of genital mutilation and other damaging traditional practices, this is not done anywhere in Africa including by the family planning groups affiliated with IPPF - the International Planned Parenthood Federation the largest and most influential private association with affiliates all over the world: but IPPF headquarters in London provide no information or guidelines on preventing FGM (see the Politics of FGM). Family planning programs in Africa pretend FGM does not exist and women's reproductive health is not their concern.

Family planning is, of course, urgently needed by African women - more than 80 percent of mothers suffer from anemia due to too-frequent pregnancies; but the priority of those who plan and design the programs - mostly men - is population control: There is little concern for women's health and none about FGM. This misdirection of these programs which are supported to the tune of many of millions of dollars annually, makes it all the more important for women to be heard and for women professionals to have an equal voice in the planning and direction of these activities so that women's health needs are attended to. Damaging traditional practices related to childbearing, including FGM, must be dealt with rather than ignored (see The Politics of FGM).

Part of my recent testimony in Congress before the Appropriations Committee, Subcommittee on Foreign Operations dealt with the failure of both UN agencies and US AID-funded programs to include prevention of FGM in health and family planning programs. This Congressional Subcommittee oversees the US AID budget and also all US contributions to UN agencies.

The Absence of Women in International Development and International Affairs

In my testimony I also pointed out that equal employment rules are not effectively implemented at United Nations agencies - to which the US contributes - as they lack an independent structure to adjudicate complaints. Equal employment rules have been implemented many years ago throughout the US government, European and many other governments. Unless more women are in decision-making positions in UN agencies concerned with development and especially in family planning, women's needs and women's health will continue to be ignored. At present there are only 3.4 percent women in decision-making jobs in the UN and UN agencies according to their own statistics.

It is no secret that most family planning programs in Africa are failing and many development programs as well, despite huge sums spent - money which in many cases is borrowed from the World Bank. Family planning and other development programs are planned and designed by technical experts at the World Bank. Their high-salaried international staff of advisors - all men - can be found in luxury hotels all over Africa. But these men are never held responsible if a program fails. Still the money must be repaid.

The World Bank has forced economic austerity and severe cutbacks on many African countries which borrowed huge amounts in the 1980s. The forced repayment has created great hardship especially for women who never were consulted about the loans nor were they beneficiaries. Not only have women lost their jobs, but all services, especiallly in health, have been drastically cut - which affects women most of all due to frequent childbearing. Few African women are involved in planning or implementation of development programs and even fewer are in decision-making positions in governments. The Decade for Women declared by the United Nations and highlighted by three World Conferences (1975 in Mexico, 1980 in Copenhagen and 1985 in Nairobi), had little impact on the number of women in decision-making positions in the UN system. Women continue to be excluded, indeed women are still entirely outside of all international affairs.

The absence of women has a major influence on the design and priorities of development programs as the neglect of women's health in family programs and the total disregard for FGM show. While the number of women in most professional occupations has dramatically increased in the past 20 years, there still are very few women in international affairs and even fewer in the UN and its agencies. While all governments that make financial contributions to the UN system have long since instituted effective equal employment rules, the UN agencies have no such rules nor has its Secretariat. And even if such rules exist on paper, there is no independent judicial body to oversee them - as **WIN NEWS** has reported many times over the years. [9]

Discrimination against women by the UN and in international development has a major influence on the quality and most of all the priorities of the decisions - as shown above with the example of family planning. If there were more women in WHO and UNICEF offices in Africa, it would not have been possible to conceal FGM almost completely until 1979 and to ignore the permanent health damage inflicted on millions of women.

The peacekeeping activities of the UN are failing. The male-dominated UN system is led by an Egyptian, Mr. Boutros Boutros-Ghali, who was a high-placed government official in his country where polygamy is legal and where even now more than half of the female children are subjected to excision, while in southern Egypt infibulation is practiced as well. In Yugoslavia and in Somalia, the UN is ineffective, paralyzed, ignored or ridiculed and attacked. And there are many other conflicts, for instance in Sudan, Liberia or Angola, where the UN peacekeeping has failed to stop the continuing slaughter.

It should be apparent to everyone by now that different skills and attitudes from those characteristically displayed by men in power are needed for peacekeeping activities: Women's talents in negotiating should at the very least be tried. But most of all it is becoming increasingly clear that the whole UN system set up 45 years ago is obsolete and does not serve present needs. How can the UN serve its mandate of keeping peace when it quite obviously excludes and discriminates against half of the world - all women? How can the UN pretend to promote democratic principles when it is based on highly visible discrimination throughout this entire male-dominated autocratic system? The UN needs to be fundamentally reorganized and changed, giving women an equal voice.

At present, in the summer of 1993, the UN peacekeeping activities in Somalia are deterioriating into warfare and publicly displayed contempt for the UN on the part of Somali warlords. All respect for the UN is vanishing due to its ineffective discriminatory male leadership which does not serve present-day needs.

Somalia: Family, Tradition and Violence.

In Somalia, what little order had been achieved in past months is breaking down: It is increasingly clear that the Somali men (women in that traditional country are not consulted) are unable to govern themselves or keep peace - yet much of the Somali population continues to depend on international food distribution. Somalia also is the country where FGM is practiced in the most brutal form - infibulation - and no female child is allowed to escape from this savage torture or live a normal life.

The time has come to look at this situation from a woman's view to analyze cause and effect. There are lessons to be learned from what is happening in Somalia that apply to the rest of Africa - wherever FGM is practiced. In June 1988, the government of Siad Barre organized an international conference in Mogadishu to draw attention to its national program to eradicate infibulation throughout Somalia - with Italian help. [10] But much more support was needed for such a truly revolutionary effort that also could set an example for the rest of Africa - hence the international conference. (See Case History: Somalia.)

It is astonishing, that although the entire diplomatic corps and all the UN agency representatives came to the opening and closing ceremonies in the Parliament and praised this remarkable effort which also attracted international press attention, nothing has ever been said about it anywhere since. The remarkable courage and leadership of Somalian women and the considerable efforts of the Somalian government to support this essential social change should be praised. everywhere. The objective was to free the people from these terrible traditions which undermine the health of the entire female population and all family life, as well as damage national and economic development.

But these efforts to stop FGM have been ignored ever since, as if the social conditions of a country did not matter. Yet it is precisely the social conditions of each country that make the difference between productiveness and poverty, between cooperation and rule by force, between mutual support and exploitation, and, finally, between peace and war.

When the US troops were first sent to Somalia in December 1992, it was important to provide some background for all the horrors shown on TV - especially since I had visited Somalia three times and was one of the invited speakers at the 1988 Conference on Strategies to Eradicate Infibulation. Though Somalia was in the news almost every day in 1992, none of the media ever reported about the mutilations and violence that is traditionally practiced against all female children and how this affects the entire society. Here is some of the press release sent out at that time:

> "For many months now the terrible, senseless violence and civil war in Somalia has been shown on TV: dying, shrunken children held by emaciated desperate women in rags often too famished to eat when they are finally reached by some international rescue teams. These pictures of human suffering and degradation are followed by those of healthy young Somali men and boys, well-fed and laughing, brandishing their automatic weapons and visibly enjoying the violence.
>
> These young Somali men, some barely teenagers, with their weapons . . . are preventing food from reaching those dying from hunger: their own mothers, sisters and young children. But none of the TV commentators have ever talked about the gender of the victims they show every day . . . Women and children are most of the victims of the horrendous civil war made by power-hungry men.
>
> The truth must finally be told: The young Somali men with guns have grown up in families where all girls and women are infibulated - no Somalian girl is allowed to escape these 'traditions' enforced by men who hold all the power in each family. At an early age, when a girl is still too young to resist or escape, she has her clitoris cut out and all external genitalia carved away by force. Then the bleeding sides of the large lips are sewn up or held together by thorns and a paste and the girl with her legs tied up is left lying on a mat for several weeks. If the girl survives and the wound has healed, the entrance to the vagina is closed except for a tiny opening created by inserting a splinter of wood or reed.
>
> Why are Somalian girls so terribly mutilated - there is no ceremony attached to this. Because men require a closed bride as price for marriage and marriage is compulsory in Somali Moslem society. These mutilations go on in each family and have been practiced as long as anyone knows. Men make all the decisions in each family as well as in Somali society, as one can see now on TV.
>
> A boy who has grown up exposed to such brutality practiced in his own family on all girls and women is accustomed to abusing every female at will, and has no restraint or compassion for human suffering. He sees girls and women being purchased by men - polygamy is the rule - who inspect them to see if they are properly closed. Only then do they pay the bride-price, negotiated between men, before they are allowed to cut the bride open for intercourse. And intercourse has to be frequent to keep the wound from closing again. But the most terrible problems that result from the mutilations happen in childbirth.
>
> These are the traditions in Somalia - practiced by all including the leaders . . . As long as we shut our eyes and ignore such horrendous violence in the name of tradition there is no stopping Somali men who have learned violence from early childhood on in their own families: and the civil war will go on and on. A society where men traditionally use their power to mutilate their own female children is not viable in our world. Men who practice such brutality in their own families know no restraint: Somalia is reaping the results of its own traditions. The victims once again are women and their young children. But no one speaks for them!" [11]

I believe that these lessons must finally be learned and understood not only in Africa but everywhere else in the world and by all of us who wish Africans well. What we learn in our own families affects our whole life our future and our communities.

Africa is the most violent continent demonstrating the direct relationship between family violence and civil or tribal warfare. What are called "cultural traditions" in reality are practices that support the ritual abuse of women, systematically damaging women's health and strength to make sure of their subordination to men. The traditional adversary relationship between women and men can be observed throughout rural Africa even today. The subservience of women is confirmed by traditional polygamous marriage arrangements which make women into wholly owned property of men. The traditional exclusion of women from landownership, the principal resource in every agricultural society, assures their dependence on men while the fruits of their labors in the fields as well as their children are owned by men. African traditions deprive women of all personal rights and make them into wholly owned resources of men.

It is essential to make this issue clear in order to work for change. These African traditions, so eloquently described and praised by President Kenyatta's book **Facing Mount Kenya**, are human rights violations in today's world: Slavery in any form is no longer acceptable. From an economic view these traditions greatly damage development as the enormous economic problems in almost every African country confirm. Change- guaranteeing civil and human rights to women - is in the interest of every government.

Routinely performed mutilations of all female children, wife abuse sanctified as a custom which Kenyan parliamentarians recently defended as their traditional family right, the selling by fathers of their barely teenage daughters to the highest bidder, and rape practiced in many African societies to prove manhood are all "traditions".

After the rapes and murders in July 1991 in St. Kizito - a Catholic boarding school in Meru, Kenya - were reported around the world, the male-dominated government did literally nothing to change the conditions in the schools. Seventy-one teenage school girls were brutally raped and nineteen killed in a weekend mass attack by their own male schoolmates with whom they lived and learned every day. The response of the principal of the school was "the boys never meant any harm against the girls; they just wanted to rape." [12] None of the responsible school officials were punished. But what was nowhere reported is that Meru is an area where FGM is practiced on every girl even today, though they go to school. The Catholic Priests who run the schools do nothing; they never have even tried to prevent the mutilation of the girls in their own schools.

Recently a similar assault took place in another girls' school in Kenya staged by a group of boys - also internationally reported. In Kenyan newspapers rapes of schoolgirls are reported regularly. Rape and violence against women go on all over Africa, but Kenyan newspapers are more alert and less censored. Condoning such traditions by young boys is an education for lifelong violence as the continuous civil wars all over Africa confirm.

Though violence against women in all kinds of vicious ways goes on all over the world there is one difference: For African men to subject their own small daughters to FGM in order to sell them for a good bride-price shows such total lack of human compassion and such vicious greed that it is hard to comprehend. But what needs to be examined is what influence do such customs have on the character formation of boys who learn such behaviour from their fathers. If we want peace in Africa, this kind of socialization for violence of the young must stop.

This question must be asked: What is the relationship between the constant civil wars in Africa carried on with unmatched brutality and the mutilation of female children as a celebrated traditional practice in each family, quite aside from continuous family violence? It is quite irresponsible for the international press to omit all information on family customs, for instance when reporting on Somalia. Family customs educate young boys for a life of violence or peace, for using force or negotiation, for rape and murder or for compassion and respect of human life.

The male political leadership of Africa must be challenged to stop the terribly damaging customs of family violence including FGM by setting an example with their own families. The results of these violent customs can be seen today all over Africa's ongoing tribal and civil wars. The time has come for international agencies, anthropologists and international organizations to stop protecting violence against women and FGM as "cultural traditons" as UNICEF, WHO and many others still do (see The Politics of FGM).

Culture, Custom and Tradition

In her classic book on **Female Sexual Slavery,** [13] Kathleen Barry put it this way:

> "Across cultures the family is the basic unit of individual male power. Whether in the tribal hut, rural cottage, city apartment, or government mansion - each man's home is his castle. And each man's home is private. It is in that privacy that female sexual slavery flourishes. . .
>
> In addition to being cautioned against the invasion of man's privacy, arguments of cultural relativism are used to discourage examination of the similarities in female sexual slavery as it is practiced through the family across cultures. Cultural relativism asserts that the practices within any specific culture are unique to the values, systems, and practices within that culture. For the cultural relativist there are no universal standards and the morality and values of one national culture cannot be compared to that of any other.
>
> Cultural relativism dominates social, political and academic thought today and it serves as a justification of many inhuman social practices. . . There is nothing unique across cultures in the practices of the enslavement of women except perhaps the diversity in the strategies men employ to carry them out. . ." [14]

Claims of ethnocentricity are constantly leveled against all who speak for women's rights, though such claims fly in the face of all human rights initiatives and especially the Universal Declaration of Human Rights. The claims of cultural relativism also are entirely incompatible with the **Convention on the Elimination of all Forms of Discrimination Against Women**, which formally came into force in September 1981. It is the most important human rights document for women, expanding the Universal Declaration of Human Rights. It was fashioned by women in a remarkable consensus on their rights, totally discrediting the claims of cultural and political relativism made by men in all patriarchal societies.

Quite similar claims of cultural relativism were made at the World Conference on Human Rights in Vienna, Austria, held June 14-25, 1993, where some Asian countries led by China and Indonesia claimed that human rights standards of justice should be modified by cultural and traditional factors, virtually compromising the objectives of this world meeting. Anthropologists in the name of culture and tradition have defended FGM continuously and many still do - they are regularly consulted by development planners especially regarding health and family planning programs.

But it is outrageous that FGM is practiced in refugee camps in Africa with the full knowledge of UNHCR, the UN High Commission for Refugees, who are responsible for refugee camps worldwide, and with the consent of those who run each camp. This fact has been reported from Sudan where UNHCR had camps for Ethiopian refugees and in Somalia. In a research paper presented at the 1984 Conference by the National Council for International Health in Washington DC, Dr. Sandra Gove who had worked in camps of Somalian refugees documented that infibulation continued to be practiced with the knowledge of the health team and the camp administrators. It was claimed that the "culture" of the refugees was already under assault and therefore the health team would not stop the refugees: instead the lives of helpless refugee girls were sacrificed. [15]

The "culture and tradition" label is so often used that it must be analyzed. Why are women singled out as "keepers of tradition"? Tradition is stressed when it comes to keeping women "in their place" - in Africa and all over the world - that is, without education or resources, dependent, ignorant, illiterate, and isolated. How often have we heard a politician or a religious leader address a group of women and then praise them as "keepers of tradition," encouraging them "to uphold the cherished values of the past, the family and home". The hidden message of the man on the podium is: Stay out of politics - we don't want women here; get back to the past where women had no voice and no vote. Go back into the kitchen and serve your husband, the head of the family.

Culture, custom and tradition: why are they made out to be beneficial for women, when mostly just the opposite is true? Everywhere "culture and tradition" is used to keep women backward and in the past, a past where no one dared to challenge male authority and where women were excluded from all political and public life by man-made laws.

The patriarchal family structure vests all decisions in the male head of the family and is supported by men everywhere as their primary and most important power base. This universal, hierarchal structure is used worldwide to socialize all female children into a submissive, inferior position, while boys are socialized for violence and war. This "order" is upheld by men everywhere by any and all means: even at the price of women's lives.

FGM, polygamy, the seclusion of women, and the bride-price are all cultural practices that are still claimed to be an important part of African and Middle Eastern culture. Slavery, it must be remembered, also is a "tradition"; so is cannibalism, footbinding in China, and widow burning in India. Those who speak for the importance of keeping all traditions, by implication speak for slavery which was widely practiced world-wide, for instance by the much admired cultures of Greece and Rome and until quite recently all over Africa and the Middle East.

Finally, this must be asked: who profits from tradition? The answer is men, as a group and in all societies, because tradition enforces rules made by those in control - men - to keep their power. Most traditional practices share these: they victimize females and support patriarchal rule; they enhance the power of men and they specifically support the control of the male head of the family.

Unfortunately the exploitation of women under the label of "culture and tradition" continues today. It is used by all religious leaders from the Pope to the Moslem leaders to the fundamentalist Christian preachers on TV who all propagate the same view of women as submissive servants of men. Anthropologists speak for them and all those who claim to conserve our valuable heritage. While there are of course many wonderful and joyful cultural traditions specifically for women including clothes, food, dancing and festivals, the other side of this coin is a slippery slope for many unsuspecting young women and girls, especially if they do not realize that this path may lead to loss of control over their independence and rights and even their lives.

Tradition is the reason most often given in Africa and the Middle East for practicing excision and infibulation on children, who are subjected to these operations by force. Yet the goal of all African countries is national development, using modern methods and tools. Therefore abolishing damaging traditional practices that are responsible for countless painful deaths, and that damage women's health, thus increasing health care costs, surely must be a priority. Why inflict permanent health damage on a young girl who will suffer for the rest of her life because of "tradition" when modernization and development are the national goal?

The term "tradition" according to Webster, means to deliver or hand down a doctrine, a belief, or custom from the past. Tradition is a contradiction of the goals of development loudly proclaimed by every African and Middle Eastern government. Tradition supports the continuation of the past, the refusal to change or accept anything new.

Tradition in rural Africa means the subordination of females to males, the individual to the family group ruled by a man who makes all decisions. Tradition demands the subordination of families to the collective village life, where all decisions are made by the elders and chiefs, who with a few exceptions are always men. The hierarchical structure of rural life does not tolerate individual accomplishment or change.

Modernization and development are the goals of all African and Middle Eastern governments today and of all programs of international development agencies, as well as of countless private as well as charitable organizations working all over Africa. There is no African or Middle Eastern political leader who has not embraced the Western life-style for himself and his family, including cars, TV, air conditioning, jets, Western clothes and food, and most of all, Western health and medical care. Every African government is organized along imported administrative and legislative systems, using imported technology and imported training. Clearly, modernization and change are the policies of all African governments today, and rightly so.

Modernization and development foster individual growth, education and achievement. Each person is responsible for his or her own actions and life. Personal initiative is rewarded; education and self-improvement are desired by all. By definition the goals of tradition and development are incompatible.

Women speak : Beginning of Change

Women all over the world are beginning to speak for their rights and against their abuse by cultural traditions that are incompatible with human rights and women's dignity. At the World Conference on Human Rights in June 1993 in Vienna, Austria, women from all regions of the world jointly organized a tribunal documenting women's human rights violations and presented a global list of human rights demands that were officially recognized and incorporated in the conference documents. [16]

The formation in 1984 of the Inter African Committee (IAC) [17] on Traditional Practices Affecting the Health of Women and Children in Dakar, following up on the recommendations made at the WHO Seminar in Khartoum in 1979, was an all-important first step for women in Africa speaking against traditions that violate their integrity. It also was an important step for women's human rights all over the world. By now the IAC has affiliates in most African countries where FGM is practiced as well as in Egypt. The IAC has held two regional conferences to gather support and make its work known; a third one is scheduled for 1994. Most of all they accomplished that African rulers and governments in the countries where FGM is practiced have officially rejected the mutilations.

For instance the Kenyan government for many years supported FGM under the leadership of its greatly admired president Kenyatta, who personally had supported FGM as an all important tradition and had made the institutionalization of FGM one of the causes of independence around which he gathered the support of Kenyan men. And Kenyatta had a great deal of influence all over Africa where his support for the mutilations was admired. It was therefore remarkable, when, in 1982, Kenyatta's successor - President arap Moi - only a few years after Kenyatta's death, prohibited FGM by decree; but there was no educational campaign. However, in neighboring Somalia a national governmental campaign against the mutilations was organized in the mid 80s and run by the Somali women's organization (See Case History: Kenya and Case History: Somalia.)

Besides the Somalian government before it collapsed, the government of Burkina Faso in 1988 began to organize a countrywide initiative to abolish FGM, which is practiced often in severe forms all over that country and region. The leadership recognized that the mutilation of girls, resulting in lifelong damage to women's health, is incompatible with the goals for national development and represents an enormous financial burden in terms of health care costs (see Case History: Burkina Faso).

Unfortunately Burkina Faso, a very poor landlocked country, does not have the kind of support from France (which formerly administered Burkina Faso and large areas of West Africa) which Somalia got from Italy, the former colonial power in southern Somalia. France never paid any attention to FGM or to the needs of women and still does not provide any assistance for prevention of the mutilations. Instead, the criminal courts in Paris where many West Africans go to get work, convict Africans (so far only women) who continue the practice on their children in France. But in Africa, where the French government has much influence due to its large financial contributions to its former colonies, France continues to close its eyes to the practice.

The progress made since the last edition of this report is enormous. At the end of 1982, when the third edition was published there was virtually no activity anywhere in Africa to stop FGM. The WHO Seminar and its recommendations, which still serve as guidelines today, were forgotten as I learned when I visited again all the East and West African countries and their maternity hospitals in early 1983 to introduce the **Childbirth Picture Books** in English and French with the **Additions to Prevent Excision and Infibulation.**

In the Postscript of the third edition to the **Hosken Report** I reviewed country by country what I had found: It was very discouraging that so little had changed. WHO and UNICEF, despite their claims that they were offering assistance which they publicized at the 1980 UN "Mid-Decade" Women's Conference in Copenhagen, had done nothing at all anywhere. Their representatives in East and West Africa whom I visited on that trip knew nothing about the promises the agencies had made on paper, and the WHO recommendations were quite ignored. Some of the West African women's groups on their own organized conferences where FGM and other damaging traditions were discussed, but they did not get any international help. (See section on FGM in every issue of **WIN NEWS.**)

The politics of UNICEF - which is run by men especially their offices in Africa - are to pacify women with all kinds of promises, as they did at the 1980 UN Women's Conference. The organization depends on women's donations and support by the public. Every industrialized country has UNICEF fund-raising committees assisted mostly by women volunteers. But despite their internationally made promises, the UNICEF office in Cairo refused to support the first major community education program to stop FGM proposed to them in 1980. However, the Cairo Family Planning Association under the leadership of Aziza Hussein developed a groundbreaking initiative which has continued for more than ten years, organized and carried out by women. (See Country Report: Egypt.) But women who support UNICEF must demand control as this agency utterly fails its mission today.

The real challenge is to reach the people in the rural areas of this huge and very diverse continent which is still predominantly agricultural and where many people continue to live a nomadic way of life that has not changed for centuries. But the environmental conditions have changed due to the recurring droughts especially in the Sahel region in West Africa and have virtually wiped out the economic subsistence base of nomadic life. It is known that most nomadic people in Africa practice infibulation or excision wherever they live. Due to their way of life it is very difficult to provide them with modern health services or education; often they shun all contacts with the rest of the world.

Among the positive developments that have taken place in recent years are preventive actions, information and training programs, local conferences and meetings held in many African cities and the extensive work of the IAC ever since 1984. Especially in Nigeria (see Women and Health and Case History: Nigeria) the national IAC program has developed and implemented many positive information and training initiatives. [18] The conspiracy of silence has been broken in most African countries, and it is no longer possible to exclude the issue from international conferences or exclude all reports on FGM from newspapers as a subject "unfit for discussion" as many editors stated in the past when I sent them reports from my African trips.

The arrival in Europe, the United States and Canada of more and more refugees from Africa, due to the many civil wars, especially recently from Somalia, has resulted in public discussion of the issue in countries where health services are paid by the government. Some immigrant families bring their daughters to the clinics asking to have them excised or infibulated. Evidently such services are available in African hospitals - as also documented in this report. (See Case History: Somalia and Case History: Mali).

European health ministries and Canada had to deal with such requests, informing hospitals and health personnel about FGM, that such mutilations are illegal and criminal child abuse. In the US where health services are privately paid no policy is implemented at present but legislation has been introduced. The decision what to do is left to each physician. There are many rumors, but to date it has been impossible to document any medical case histories of mutilations performed in the US. (See Women and Health.)

The Failure of Effective International Support for Prevention of FGM

Despite many recent positive developments in Africa - and this is where preventive actions must be focused most of all - it would be a serious mistake not to face reality. The reality is that all major internationally funded health and family planning programs in Africa still continue to ignore FGM in their programs, though their workers in the field are no longer able to deny that the mutilations exist.

The US Agency for International Development (USAID) is financing family planning programs in Africa and Egypt but they still don't acknowledge the existence of FGM. (See The Politics of FGM.) The US provides funding for more family planning activities than any other country. It is essential that family planning activities in Africa incorporate preventive education in all their training and family planning education programs if any real headway is to be made. Experience shows, that this only can be achieved by using the political route; hence my Congressional testimonies on the subject.

While African countries have recently shown their willingness to support preventive programs it is clear that international funding is needed to make any real progress especially in terms of reducing the numbers of mutilated girls.

As a result of rapid population growth especially in sub-Saharan Africa the total number of mutilated women is constantly increasing. Many more very young girls are excised today. In urban areas often small infants are operated on as parents claim they dont remember the pain. But these mutilations have lifelong damaging health effects and can never be reversed. The tabulated estimates and statistics show an increase in numbers correlated with the increase in population as preventive programs so far have not reached enough families to make a measurable difference. (See Health Facts and Overview.) And these numbers will continue to grow unless some comprehensive, internationally supported regional actions are organized.

But there are already internationally funded family planning programs established in practically all countries where FGM is practiced, as well as health programs including many by WHO and UNICEF. USAID provides the funding for extensive family planning programs, planned and implemented by many different private contractors working in different African countries often involving many millions of dollars and projected for years. Family planning programs by now are accepted all over sub-Saharan Africa and since they are concerned with reproduction it is logical that they should integrate prevention of FGM in all their teaching and educational activities.

To organize a separate multimillion dollar effort to prevent FGM, which is what it would cost to effectively eradicate these practices, would be enormously difficult. It is much more efficient and cost-effective to integrate prevention in all ongoing family planning and health programs. This can be done at not much extra cost by the same people who can be trained to incorporate preventive teaching to stop FGM in the ongoing programs that already exist or are being organized.

The groundbreaking work of the IAC to show the way needs to continue. But separate progams, going it alone, and in many different countries will not be able to reach the very large populations involved in FGM, especially in rural areas. The experience of the IAC can also be useful to teach family planning program contractors how to integrate prevention of FGM in all their field work. The experience of AIDoS - the Italian Association for Women in Development, [19.] who worked in Somalia on the national eradication campaign and are now working with the IAC in several African countries, similarly could teach the family planning program providers how to integrate prevention of FGM.

But so far all attempts to raise the consciousness of the USAID contractors who run the family planning programs have failed: They simply do not want to know about FGM even if it is practiced in their program areas. The directives for change must come from USAID who provide the program guidelines. The contractors are accountable to the USAID administrators and to Congress, who approves funding for all major programs (see Women and Health and The Politics of FGM). To raise the consciousness of the new administration of USAID needs political action from many women and organizations; yet my testimony in Congress is still the only one.

As a result of the Safe Motherhood Conference in 1987 in Nairobi, sponsored by the World Bank and cosponsored by WHO and UNFPA, [20.] many local and regional conferences and publicity for safe motherhood have been initiated worldwide, including in Africa, with all health ministries participating. Though obstructed labor was one of the problems discussed as a major cause of death in childbirth, which is the highest in the world per capita in sub-Saharan Africa, FGM was never mentioned, though it is the cause. In Kenya, where the initial conference was held, the majority of women and girls are mutilated. To date no preventive action has been taken by the health ministry nor by the multimillion dollar family planning programs sponsored by USAID and the World Bank in Kenya or anywhere else, though by now all the facts about FGM are evident..

Safe motherhood conferences and activities are organized worldwide, including in Africa and the Middle East by Family Care International, [21.] who also publish a great deal of literature. Though of course they have the facts on FGM and I sent them repeatedly all the information as well as **Chilbirth Picture Books,** the women in New York who run the organization pretend FGM does not exist and have never responded: It is unconscionable to deliberately ignore one of the major causes of childbirth complications and death in Africa while claiming to work for safe motherhood.

It is, of course, of great importance to women that the preventable childbirth problems in developing countries at long last are internationally addressed. Half a million women around the world die every year from pregnancy related causes, most of them in developing countries, so WHO estimates, and most deaths could be prevented. A "Mother Care Project" has been funded by USAID "to improve pregnancy outcomes for mothers and children." It consists of a five year technical assistance contract to John Snow, Inc., [22] a US corporation working in development. A large number of reports and papers have been published as well as a newsletter "Mother Care Matters". But any information or even mention of FGM and the terrible problems it causes in childbirth are entirely ignored though in continental Africa more than 110 million women are mutilated.

The safe motherhood initiatives are designed to raise the consciousness of decision makers in health ministries and also to stimulate international action. WHO publishes a newsletter **Safe Motherhood** [23] on the worldwide activities on this subject providing contacts, resources, as well as reporting on actions. But one looks in vain among all this information for any mention of FGM.

Yet WHO in 1979 had sponsored and organized the seminar on "Traditional Practices affecting the Health of Women and Children" in Khartoum where FGM was for the first time openly discussed from a health view by health ministry delegations from nine African and Middle Eastern countries and where specific recommendations were drawn up which have served as guidelines ever since. (See World Health Organization Seminar.) But ironically, they are now ignored by WHO.

The question is why? Why do internationally sponsored programs concerned with women's health and especially motherhood fail to acknowledge the existence of FGM, let alone act on this major public health problem? One reason is that no one wants to start talking about the subject - neither the African professionals concerned with health, nor the international sponsors. For instance when a major health program - to develop the first country-wide health delivery system in Somalia - was planned, neither the health ministry representatives nor the USAID sponsored international health team ever mentioned the fact that every woman in Somalia was infibulated and that all hospitals in Mogadishu were always full of victims suffering severe health problems due to FGM.

After reading the Somalian health program proposal, I sent fact sheets, medical articles, selected literature on FGM and the WHO Seminar recommendations to USAID to distribute to the program developers. As a result, FGM was at last discussed. According to the final program, after the subject was brought up, the health ministry representatives introduced the USAID team to a group of experts who had been working for some time on a program to eradicate infibulation - right in the ministry. But neither the Somalis nor the US team - most of them men - wanted to be the first ones to discuss FGM as a health issue, though FGM affects literally the entire female population. FGM was and is ignored by all USAID health programs in Africa. All of them have failed as the record shows - including the program in Somalia. The reason: their failure to deal with reality.

But by now FGM is openly discussed all over Africa and around the world, and factual information is readily available to anyone interested and certainly to everyone concerned with women's health, childbirth and family planning. To refuse to acknowledge FGM and the terrible lifelong health problems that result for whatever reason is inexcusable - and those who do so must be held personally responsible for participating in the mutilation of the helpless African girl-children, much as the person who drives the getaway car shares the responsibility for the crime.

From an international viewpoint, it is no longer feasible to deny that FGM exists or the damage which results. Health and family planning and especially safe motherhood programs will have to acknowledge not only the existence of FGM but the loss of life and the mounting health costs that the continuation of these practices entails. Instead of treating the eradication of FGM as a separate isolated activity, it is logical as well as far less costly and much more effective to integrate the prevention of FGM into all family planning, health and safe motherhood programs. It is obvious to anyone who knows the terrible effects of FGM on childbirth that to seriously work for the reduction of maternal deaths in areas where FGM is practiced, preventive education to stop the mutilations must be integrated into all educational efforts or the whole activity must be called a farce.

From all points of view, it is in everyone's interest to work for the eradication of FGM. There are many thousands of female babies who must be protected now to save them from the mutilations and the future problems they would face, especially in childbirth. There are thousands of girls being mutilated continuously; many require immediate help in hospitals or clinics and/or transfusions, as the research published by Dr. Koso Thomas in Sierra Leone has established. [24] But in rural areas, transfusions are not available, so the girls bleed to death. Due to the hardened scars from the mutilations, women often cannot dilate and give birth normally. Without trained help, they die or the vagina ruptures resulting in incontinence. All childbirth statistics, for instance those published by WHO, confirm that the per capita death in childbirth in Africa is the highest in the world. The reason is FGM.

From an economic point of view, it is persuasive for each health ministry to stop FGM as hospitals have to deal with FGM injuries and pay for the health care costs which are funded by each government. Furthermore the cost of work time lost is also paid by the government since it is the largest employer. And finally the death of so many women and girls is an irreparable loss for each family and country. Dr. Koso Thomas computed these costs for Sierra Leone and compared them to the costs of a national eradication program. She found that the entire program could be amortized in 20 years from savings in hospitalization and work time lost - and pay for rehabilitation of mutilated women. [25]

If teaching prevention of FGM is made a part of every health and family planning program, the costs to each one would be very small; they would reinforce each other, accomplishing much more than separate programs. Collaboration in preventive teaching should be organized by all family planning and health programs in African and Middle Eastern countries where FGM is practiced. The teaching experience of the IAC and the Cairo Family Planning Association certainly can show how. (See Women and Health.)

As the experience with the **Childbirth Picture Books (CBPB)** shows, people on the grass roots level are ready for change, which the hundreds of letters from Africa I receive continuously from users of the **CBPBs** confirm. These letters also show great interest in reproduction: Fertility is very important to every family. Any threat to fertility raises concern. FGM is such a threat, as the **CBPBs** show and teach, but this has not been understood by most people in Africa: They practice FGM to enhance fertility!

Medicalization, that is, the introduction of FGM into the modern health care system, must not only be rejected but it should be discussed openly as it is going on throughout Africa and especially in Egypt, which has an extensive health care system. The failure to integrate prevention and to discuss FGM by family planning and health programs, promotes the introduction of FGM into the modern sector, with the claim "it is better to do it in the hospital." Physicians and trained health workers - many of them trained by international programs - make money from the mutilations, quite aside from traditional birth attendants who have always practiced FGM. (See Case Histories.)

Because of the silence on FGM by those in charge of international health programs many African health care workers use antibiotics, training and tools provided from abroad to mutilate little girls for a fee. WHO in 1982 released a statement unequivocally condemming the medicalization of FGM in all health care settings. [26] The misguided idea that it is an improvement to mutilate a child under sanitary conditions must be finally shown for what it is: criminal child abuse, as it is done for money by those who know the results. A mutilation done under sanitary conditions is still a mutilation, and medicalizing the procedure often leads to even more problems in childbirth as the experience in Somalia and elsewhere confirms. (See Health Facts and Overview.)

The fact that immigrants and refugees bring with them their customs including FGM is well-known. The countries where they are accepted temporarily or permanently have alerted their health providers, clinics and hospitals; they also should educate immigrants as Canada is doing, after accepting thousands of Somali refugees. Organized medicine must face its responsibilities as the College of Physicians and Surgeons in Canada did by prohibiting the operations by its professional members and issuing directions to physicians on how to assist mutilated women in childbirth. [27] All Canadian health care is paid for by the government. According to Canadian law FGM violates several existing provisions and would result in a criminal charge of assault for causing bodily harm.

France always ignored FGM in Africa and did nothing for many years, though FGM was practiced among West African immigrants and workers, for instance in the Paris region. G.A.M.S., a private women's group, was formed to teach the wives of immigrants from Francophone West Africa - many of whom are illiterate - to stop mutilating their children in France. [28] After three girls died, the French government began to prosecute parents and excisors, as the mutilations are criminal infractions of the French legal code. Therefore West African families now send their daughters back home to be mutilated.

In Britain, where FGM is prohibited by a special law passed in 1985, the Foundation for Women's Health, Research and Development - FORWARD - was funded to educate immigrants. [29] Since health care all over Europe is paid for by the respective governments, warnings have been sent to all hospitals about the mutilations. (See The Western World.) But the real work to stop FGM must be done in Africa and by Africans.

AIDS, that is the HIV/AIDS epidemic, is spreading rapidly especially in Africa, where the infection of young women is as high as that of men. WHO estimates that more than 8 million people in sub-Saharan Africa are infected - by far the largest number of any region in the world and the death toll is rapidly increasing . [30] There is no doubt that FGM greatly contributes to the infections - though this is never discussed anywhere in the extensive literature. The conditions under which the mutilations are performed - usually on a group of girls with the same tools, sterilization is unknown - provide the perfect opportunity for infection. The first sexual intercourse with a mutilated woman entails lacerations and often cuts providing many opportunities for infection. The sexual customs by African men, polygamy, widely practiced rape often of children, prostitution and child marriage quite aside from sexual violence result in the present epidemic of sexually transmitted diseases including the proliferation of AIDS.

But international programs, including family planning, are failing to spell out the truth that African customs and traditions must change, starting with the sexual relations between women and men in each family. AIDS is beginning to decimate whole regions and deaths will steadily increase: The time to change male sexual customs is overdue.

Women's Rights are Human Rights

FGM is a human rights violation. This was officially recognized by the UN Human Rights Office in Geneva by appointing a Human Rights Rapporteur already in the 1980s under the title of "Traditional Practices Affecting the Health of Women and Children". The Rapporteur collects information and all official papers on FGM. In the spring of 1991, a seminar on Traditional Practices Affecting the Health of Women and Children was hosted by Burkina Faso, organized by the UN Human Rights Office in Geneva. [31] Representatives from fifteen East and West African countries came to the meeting. A series of recommendations was made, as is customary at such intergovernmental meetings, most of them addressed to other UN Agencies and governments, generating a lot of papers. But there is no way to persuade the participants to follow any recommendations. UNICEF did not even bother to send a representative.

The seminar recommended again that the term "female genital mutilation" should be used in place of "female circumcision" as the latter "did not reflect the gravity of such practices." A similar recommendation was made half a year earlier at the November 1990 IAC regional conference in Addis Ababa. Besides FGM, other damaging traditional practices were discussed such as nutritional tabus for women, damaging traditional birth practices, son preference and more. The Special Rapporteur of the UN Human Rights Center also visited the Sudan and Djibouti to discuss FGM and other damaging traditional practices with pertinent Governement officials. [32] It is a fact, unfortunately, that this effort, as well as many others concerning Human Rights have been entirely ignored by politicians.

The Human Rights Conference held in Vienna June 14-25 1993, recommended that the UN Human Rights Office be given higher status in the UN hierarchy. The Final Recommendations of the Working Group on Women's Human Rights at the conference were adopted by the official conference and incorporated into the official papers. The opening of the women's statement underlines the facts that "in all regions it has been found that the UN and governments have by and large failed to promote and protect women's human rights, whether civil and political, economic and social or cultural. . ."

Recommendation 9 states:

> "The World Conference should reaffirm the right of women to the enjoyment throughout their life span of the highest standard of physical and mental health as affirmed in the Women's Convention. This requires governments to respect women's fundamental rights to accessible quality care, reproductive health, health education and to ensure that motherhood results from a free and informed decision by each woman. . ." [33]

Finally it is recommended that "systematic crimes against women are crimes against humanity - the failure of governments to prosecute those responsible for such crimes implies complicity." Gender specific abuses are especially cited: FGM certainly is such a gender specific abuse.

FGM is a violation of the UN **Convention on Elimination of All Forms of Discrimination Against Women - CEDAW,** also called the Women's Convention, and specifically of several paragraphs in this important document for women's rights.

Besides the United Nations the US government has also cited FGM as a human rights violation in the **Country Reports on Human Rights Practices** prepared annually by the State Department. For a number of years citations of FGM have been included in all country reports where it is practiced under the section "Discrimination Based on Race, Sex, Religion, Language and Social Status". Recently also reports on Family Violence against women have been included. These Country Reports have the purpose to inform Congress about Human Rights violations. Congress is empowered to cut all support programs, for instance USAID assistance or other privileges such as special trade agreements with countries cited for repeated human rights violations.

Quite aside from formal documentation, agreements or any human rights reports, it is self-evident that any deliberate physical mutilation especially of the female genital organs is a violation of this person's integrity and her human right to health much as the mutilation of male genital organs is. The excision of the penis which is the equivalent of excision of the clitoris is instantly recognized as a severe physical genital mutilation with permanent consequences and is a criminal offense. The same is true of what is done to female children resulting in permanent health and psychological trauma. Both are human rights violations. (See Health Facts and Overview.)

In 1976 **WIN NEWS** began to collect signatures worldwide on a letter and statement addressed to the Secretary General of the United Nations and the Office of Human Rights concluding with this statement .

> "the mutilation of the genital organs of the female body for any reason whatsoever is a fundamental offense against the human rights of all women in general and specifically against the female children and women who are mutilated."

Despite the many thousands of signatures from women and men all over the world sent to the UN Human Rights Office for action and despite a visit to Geneva to their offices, the matter has been and continues to be entirely ignored by their annual meetings of governments on human rights. But though nongovernmental organizations are entitled to speak at these meetings, none of them have ever addressed human rights violations of women. Political and civil rights of men are all that is ever discussed. The right to health or women's rights have never been mentioned by anyone.

Amnesty International (AI) over the years and despite many contacts with their international office in London has refused to concern itself with FGM or provide any assistance, claiming that this issue is strictly "outside their mandate". This despite efforts by their national groups to get the organization involved. To the present time the AI leadership states that FGM is not a concern they can adopt.

Experience shows that in order to achieve any positive results, it is necessary to work on the grass-oots level where it really matters and where change affects real people and lives. The above cited human rights recommendations have to be translated into political action by women. Experience shows that when women have trusted men to implement change, women have lost out. There must be a large enough number of women (at least 40 percent) in all decision making areas and especially where funding is allocated, or all resolutions and recommendations for women remain just paper.

The Outlook and Reality.

Men have never acted when it comes to women's rights and especially where reproduction is concerned because it is in their self-interest to keep women under their control. Controlling women's reproduction is a direct means to that end: FGM directly supports that goal. This report confirms that even now African and Middle Eastern men as a group support FGM; but these practices could not continue today without the support of men all over the world, who do nothing to stop them, not even the men who work in international health, as is documented here.

Men in influential positions, including the men in decision-making positions at WHO, UNICEF, UNFPA and in health ministries, as well as political leaders in Africa and around the world, are silent. By their failure to act they are directly supporting the continuation of FGM. That must be challenged by women everywhere. Though it is always stressed by men that women do the operations on the children, the fact is, that as long as men make FGM a requirement for marriage, women have no alternative in societies where there is no option but marriage and where women have no choice. If men rejected mutilated brides, the operations would stop instantly everywhere.

These facts demonstrate that it is essential for women to acquire political power in order to effect real change - and the eradication of FGM is such a change. Unless this is accomplished, women will never be able to achieve equality anywhere. The systematic practice of violence against women by men is what keeps inequality in place everywhere and keeps women out of decision-making positions.

A remarkable, just-published Canadian report **Changing the Landscape: Ending Violence - Achieving Equality,** sponsored by the Ministry for the Status of Women [33] documents with hundreds of examples the connection between male violence against women and persisting inequality, how violence by men in the family reinforces institutionalized discrimination and inequality, which in turn is supported by male dominated governments. The title of the report is significant - we must change the landscape, that is, the entire environment; to change one area will not accomplish what needs to be done. The same is true of FGM, which is a form of institutionalized male violence. The failure to act forcibly against the mutilations assures the continuation of the practice. It simply is not true - as is often said, that FGM will stop on its own. Rather it is now being medicalized.

It is essential for women to work for political control to assure change - for instance control of government health departments, of WHO and of UNICEF- institutions that are discriminating against women in many different ways. Because health is the most important issue for women, therefore health is tightly controlled by men. How could little girls continue to bleed to death from being brutally mutilated if male dominated institutions would not be involved in the violence by tolerating it? It is a sad commentary for the status of men that there is no group of men today - including health professionals - who work effectively against FGM. When it comes to FGM the issues are clear and it is here that we must draw the line: this cannot be allowed to continue; there is no more excuse; the facts are all known; it is time to demand that institutions stop the violence now!

In the US, where women supposedly enjoy all rights, it was recently found that the men who make the essential decisions about health, ignored women's health needs in favor of men. All major health research studies by the government have been concerned with the health status of men while ignoring breast cancer which kills thousands of women every year, spending the money instead on researching diseases that affect mostly men.

In international affairs the discrimination practiced at the UN and its agencies - as cited above - has and is terribly damaging to women in developing countries. The US today is a major contributor in terms of funding international activities and development. All European countries, also Australia, New Zealand and Japan, contribute to UN agencies, besides funding their own international programs, including those in health; they are also members of WHO. That means women who pay taxes in all countries that contribute funds to development have a right to demand that women's needs are taken care of equally. To achieve equal representation, only women should be hired by UN agencies until parity is achieved. Only then will development priorities change, women will have a voice and institutionalized violence against women will decrease. Women in developing countries are ready to take over and run the international programs - better than men.

Aside from the UN and other international governmental programs, many direct initiatives to stop FGM can be organized. For instance setting up peer groups of health professionals to collaborate across countries and cultures to stop FGM. There are international professional organizations in many health occupations that could make the eradication of the mutilations a professional goal. Communication technology can reach literally everywhere and can also communicate on a very basic personal level: for instance with inexpensive tape recordings it is possible to reach people's consciences, hearts and minds everywhere. That it is possible to change people's ideas the huge advertising industry around the world has certainly shown.

On the grass-roots level modern versions of "coming of age" rites could be promoted in place of the mutilations. For instance celebrating such accomplishments as getting school diplomas, learning to read and write or performing specific community tasks in education and health, or digging wells, laying pipelines - to show maturity and responsibility. Such accomplishments could be cited at a community festival, welcoming the achiever as mature citizen for her or his contributions. (See: Women and Health.)

To introduce change requires local leadership. And change is what the future is all about. To be able to cope with the ever-accelerating changes of our physical, intellectual and technical environment is a constant challenge. It is essential for a successful life to learn to cope with change and to change our own lives and attitudes. Especially as women we must take responsibility for changing ourselves and our own future and that of our children. We can rely only on ourselves in order to gain control over our bodies and our lives. In the final analysis that is what it is all about: to take control of our own future

Women's needs are ignored and neglected by male decision makers and male dominated governments and institutions: Women continue to be excluded from the all-important decisions over peace and war, life and death, with terrible results. No one has defined the issues of the necessary global revolution for social change more succinctly than Riane Eisler in her defining work for a partnership society - breaking away from the viscious cycle of male domination and violence that has distorted all human institutions, our human relationships and lives. Violence against women has become accepted as "custom and tradition" all over the world - FGM is one terrible manifestation of this in one region of the world: It could not continue today unless men everywhere shared the underlying attitudes of contempt for femaleness. Eisler's work documents this with hundreds of examples from all over the world and proposes change:

> "The link between cruelty and violence in the private sphere of the family and the cruelty and violence of authoritarianism and other forms of oppression and domination in the political sphere is all too real. Today, as never before in human history, the world stands at a crossroad. On the one side the well trodden path of violence and domination - of man over woman, parent over child, race over race, nation over nation, and man over nature. On the other side lies a very different path: the road to a world where our basic civil, political and economic rights - including protection from domination and violence - will at long last be respected." [34.]

Many years ago, when I first learned the truth about FGM, like many other women I was unwilling to believe, let alone face the truth. Nothing in my experience and life in Europe and the US or in my many travels all over the world had prepared me for such revelations: They forced me to re-think and re-examine everything I had believed and I had learned. From all my travels in Africa and my many conversations with women from all different countries and backgrounds, what the midwives in the city hospital in Bamako told me years ago, after describing the problems of FGM in their society, has stayed with me ever since: Change cannot be effective partially - everything must change; our whole society must be reorganized until women take their rightful place.

We must take our rightful place everywhere in the world: No one will give it to us least of all those who enjoy all the privileges of their domination and control. In the worldwide revolution by women to gain control over our own bodies, our own reproduction and sexuality, and thus our own lives, the eradication of sexual mutilations is an imperative; it is both a symbol as well as a cornerstone. In the battle for freedom of choice, the issue of female genital mutilation is a fundamental and pivotal political concern.

FOOTNOTES

1. Inter African Committee on Traditional Practices Affecting the Health of Women and Children (IAC), 147, rue de Lausanne, CH-1202 Geneva, Switzerland; c/o Economic Commission for Africa, ATRCW, P.O. Box 3001, Addis Ababa, Ethiopia.
2. **The Country Reports on Human Rights Practices** are submitted every year in February to the Committee on Foreign Relations, US Senate and the Committee on Foreign Affairs, US House of Representatives by the Department of State. The Reports are available from the US Government Printing Office, Washington, DC 20402. See **WIN NEWS** Spring issues 1993/'92/'91, etc. section on Human Rights.
3. Hosken, Fran P. **Testimony Submitted to the Foreign Operations Subcommittee, Committee on Appropriations**, U.S. Senate, Senator Patrick Leahy, Chair, June 15, 1993.
4. Hosken, Fran P. **The Childbirth Picture Book/Program** - "A picture story of reproduction from a woman's view" - pictures by Marcia L. Williams. Published since 1980 by Women's International Network News. Books, flipcharts, color slides in English, French, Spanish, Arabic and Somali (also printed in India in six languages, in Nepal and the Marshall Islands). Additions to prevent exicision and infibulation in English, French and Arabic. Nutrition supplements in English, French and Spanish. For community health workers and families worldwide.
5. Women's International Network - **WIN NEWS**, "an open participatory quarterly journal by, for and about women" started publication in 1975 and reports on women's development from all regions of the world. Editor/publisher Fran P. Hosken, 187 Grant St., Lexington, MA 02173 USA. **WIN NEWS** has featured a section on FGM in every issue since summer 1975, (third issue).
6. Masters and Johnson. **Human Sexual Response**. Little, Brown & Co., Boston, 1966, Preface, pp. vi, vii.
7. Kinsey, Alfred C., and Staff of the Institute for Sex Research of Indiana University. **Sexual Behavior in the Human Male**, 1948; **Sexual Behavior in the Human Female**, 1953; W.B. Saunders Co., Philadelphia.
8. Hite, Shere. **The Hite Report on Female Sexuality**. Dell Publishing Co., Inc., New York, 1976. **The Hite Report on Male Sexuality**, Alfred A. Knopf, New York, 1981.
9. See **WIN NEWS**, Vol. 19, No. 1, Winter 1993, p.6 "Sexual Harassment at the UN," and Editorial. See also **The New York Times**, December 20, 1992, p. 37. See also **WIN NEWS** Vol. 19, No. 3, Summer 1993, Editorial and pp. 6-7. From: Testimony Submitted to the US Congress, Foreign Operations Subcommittee, Committtee on Appropriations, June 15, 1993:

   "We urge this Committee to attach binding requirements for Equal Employment of Women and protection from sexual harassment - including an independent board to adjudicate disputes and complaints - to all funds contributed/donated to United Nations bodies and international institutions, including and especially the World Bank/IMF, the UN Secretariat, WHO, UNICEF, FAO, etc. They should be required to develop affirmative action plans with specific timetables and goals."
10. Conference Report: **Female Circumcision Strategies to Bring About Change**. Proceedings of the International Seminar on Female Circumcision 13-16 June 1988, Mogadisho, Somalia. See also **WIN NEWS**, Vol. 13, No. 4, Autumn 1987, pp. 19-21 and **WIN NEWS** Vol. 14, No. 3, Summer 1988, pp. 24-35.
11. Hosken, Fran P., Women's International Network News, 187 Grant Street, Lexington, MA 02173. Press Release: **Somalian Women: The Facts We Need to Know**, Dec. 1992. This press release was printed by several newspapers in the US.
12. See **WIN NEWS**, Vol. 17, No. 4, Autumn 1991, pp. 37-39, "Rape and Murder at Kenyan Catholic Boarding School in Meru", excerpts from **The New York Times**, July 29 and August 4, 1991. **WIN NEWS** features a regular section on Women and Violence, which reports from all over the world.

FOOTNOTES (continued)

13. Barry , Kathleen. **Female Sexual Slavery**. Prentice-Hall, Inc., Englewood Cliffs, NJ , 1979.
14. Ibid., pp. 139-140.
15. Gove, Sandra, M.D., M.P.H., and Diamondstone, Laura, R.N., P:H.N. **Medical Team Interaction with Female Circumcision in a Refugee Camp, Bo', Somalia**. Medical Volunteers International, a nonprofit group based in San Francisco, 2546 Great Highway, San Francisco, California USA 94116. (See **WIN NEWS** Vol. 10, No. 3, Summer 1984, pp. 38-40).
16. World Conference on Human Rights, Vienna, Austria, June 14-25, 1993. Centre for Human Rights, United Nations, CH-1211 Geneva 10, Switzerland; Centre for Human Rights, New York Office, Room S-2914, United Nations, New York, NY 10017 USA See **WIN NEWS** Vol. 19, No. 3, Summer 1993, pp. 9-13.
17. IAC, see Footnote No. 1.
18. IAC - Nigeria, IAC Office: Mandilas Motors Complex 9-13, Atitebi St., (Off Apapa Rd.) Ebute - Metta, Nigeria. P.O. Box 6051, Lagos, Nigeria; President IAC - Nigeria: Dr. Irene Modupeola Thomas. A newsletter "Your Task" is being published.
19. AIDoS (Italian Association for Women in Development), via dei Giubbonari, 30 int. 6. 00186 Rome, ITALY. AIDoS developed a complete teaching programs including video tapes and training manuals for Somalia with the SWDO (Somali Women's Democratic Organization) which they recently adapted for several other African countries including Ethiopian and the Gambia. They could be readily adapted for integration in and use with family planning programs.
20. Safe Motherhood Conference, Nairobi, 10-13 February 1987. Sponsored by World Bank, 1818 H St., N.W., Washington, DC 20433. Cosponsors: World Health Organization (WHO) and United Nations Fund for Population Activities (UNFPA). See **WIN NEWS,** Vol. 13, No. 2 Spring 1987, pp. 23-26).
21. Family Care International (FCI), 588 Broadway, Suite 503, New York, NY 10612. Newsletter and other publications are available.
22. John Snow, Mother Care, 1616 Fort Myer Drive, 11th Floor, Arlington, VA 22209. "Mothercare aims to improve pregnancy outcomes for women and newborns, through a household and community-based approach." A large number of publications are available.
23. "Safe Motherhood" is a newsletter published by WHO three times a year in French and English by the Maternal Health and Safe Motherhood Programme, Division of Family Health, World Health Organization, 1211 Geneva 27, Switzerland.
24. Koso-Thomas, Olayinka, M.D. **The Circumcision of Women: A Strategy for Eradication**. Published by ZED Books Ltd., 57 Caledonian Road, London N1 9BU, England. See **WIN NEWS,** Vol. 13, No. 3, Summer 1987, p. 34.
25. Master of Public Health (MPH) Thesis by Dr. Koso-Thomas. From the Abstract: "A 20-year program is proposed for appropriate intervention activities to eradicate the practice in one African country, Sierra Leone. It is anticipated that at the end of the plan period, the mental and physical well-being of the 70 percent of the population who are now at risk will be restored. . . The proposal has two main areas of impact: **Health Education**, to increase knowledge of the dangers of circumcision and to correct wrong religious doctrines, and **Health Care**, to provide early diagnosis, treatment, and complete rehabilitation of the victims of circumcision. . . A Budget has been included which outlines the cost to the Nation. . ." See **WIN NEWS** Vol. 8, No. 3 Summer 1982, p. 45-48.

FOOTNOTES (continued)

26. World Health Organization (WHO) Statement of WHO Position and Activities regarding the Medicalization of Female Genital Mutilation: "WHO has consistently and unequivocally advised that female circumcision should not be practiced by any health professionals in any setting - including hospitals or other health establishments. . ." Submitted to the UN Sub-Commission on Prevention of Discrimination and Protection of Minorities. Working Group on Slavery. June 1982. See **WIN NEWS** Vol. 18, No. 4, Autumn 1992, p. 30. WHO, 1211 Geneva 27, Switzerland.
27. "College of Physicians and Surgeons of Ontario, Canada Prohibits FGM", Press Release; 80 College St., Toronto M5G 2E2, Canada. See **WIN NEWS** Vol. 18, No. 2 Spring 1992, p. 46.
28. Groupe Femmes pour l'Abolition des Mutilations Sexuelles (G.A.M.S.), Maison des Femmes, 8 Cite Prost, 75011 Paris, France.
29. Foundation for Women's Health Research and Development (FORWARD), Africa Centre, 38 King St., Covent Garden, London WC2E 8JT, United Kingdom. Training guides and information materials are available as well as a newsletter. The First Study Conference on Genital Mutilation of Girls in Europe was held July 6-8, 1992. See **WIN NEWS** Vol. 18, No. 4, Autumn 1992, p. 37.
30. Reid, Elizabeth. **Young Women and the HIV/AIDS Epidemic & Development**. United Nations Development Programme (UNDP), One United Nations Plaza, New York, NY 10017 (see **WIN NEWS** Vol. 19, No. 1, Winter 1993, pp. 24-25). Berer, Marge and Ray, Sunanda. **Women and HIV/AIDS - An International Resource Book**. Pandora Press, 77-85 Fulham Palace Rd., Hammersmith, London W6 8JB, England. See **WIN NEWS** Vol. 19, No. 3, Summer 1993, p. 30. Mann, Jonathan M., M.D., General Editor; Tarantola, Daniel, J.M., M.D., Scientific Editor. **AIDS In The World - The Global AIDS Policy Coalition**. Harvard University Press, Cambridge, Massachusetts. See **WIN NEWS** Vol. 19, No. 3, Summer 1993, pp. 28-29.
31. United Nations Human Rights Center Seminar on: Traditional Practices Affecting the Health of Women and Children, April 29-May 3, 1991, Ouagadougou, Burkina Faso. United Nations Center for Human Rights, CH-1211, Geneva 10, Switzerland; (HR/SEM.1/1991/1). See **WIN NEWS** Vol. 17, No. 3, Summer 1991, p. 31. See also **WIN NEWS** Vol. 18, No. 4, Autumn 1992, p. 34.
32. Study: **Traditional Practices Affecting the Health of Women and Children**, Final Report by the Special Rapporteur, Mrs. Halima Embarek Warzazi. Commission on Human Rights, Sub-Commission on Prevention of Discrimination and Protection of Minorities, Forty-third Session, Item 4 of the provisional agenda (E/CN.4/Sub.2/1991/6), United Nations Center for Human Rights, CH-1211, Geneva 10, Switzerland: Visits to the Sudan and Djibouti and Organization of Regional Seminars (excerpts). (See **WIN NEWS** Vol. 18, No. 2, Spring 1992, p. 42).
33. World Conference on Human Rights: Vienna, Austria, June 14-25, 1993. **The Equal Status and Human Rights of Women** - from the "Vienna Declaration and Programme of Action". (HR/VIE/42. 25 June 1993.) Centre for Human Rights, United Nations, CH-1211, Geneva 10. Switzerland. See **WIN NEWS**, Vol. 19, No. 3, Summer 1993, pp. 9-13.
34. Report: **Changing the Landscape: Ending Violence - Achieving Equality.** Canadian Panel on Violence Against Women. Pat Freeman Marshall, Cochair. Marthe Asselin Vaillancourt, Cochair. To: the Minister responsible for the Status of Women, Canada.
35. Eisler, Riane. "The Challenge of Human Rights for All: What We Can Do." From **The Years Ahead**, published by The World Future Society, Bethesda, Maryland , USA. See **WIN NEWS** Vol. 19-4, Autumn 1993, Editorial. Riane Eisler is the author of **The Chalice and the Blade: Our History, Our Future**, Harper & Row, San Francisco, CA.

PART ONE
HEALTH FACTS AND OVERVIEW

This summary of the health facts of female genital mutilation (FGM) provides an overview: It should be read first as it gives essential information which must be clearly understood when reading the rest of this report and especially the country case histories, where field investigations in Africa and research are brought together. This report documents that female genital mutilation is a major public health problem that damages the health and lives of more than 100 million girls and women in Africa and the Middle East. It adversely affects development in more than twenty-six countries in a vast area from the Persian Gulf and the Red Sea to the Atlantic Coast. The mutilations are also practiced in a less damaging form by some Moslem groups in Malaysia and Indonesia.

Recently it has been found that African and Middle Eastern immigrants to Europe and North America and other regions continue to practice these mutilations on their children nomatter where they go to live.(see below).

This Report was published first in 1979 - this is the fourth revised and updated edition. It documented for the first time all the facts about genital mutilation and established the epidemiology or how very widespread these mutilations are, which were hidden for two thousand years; more recently they were deliberately ignored by all those concerned with development (see chapter on "Politics"). With its publication all excuses of ignorance have been removed. But knowledge involves responsibility - what is reported here requires us to act. In Women's International Network - **WIN NEWS**[1] new information on Female Genital Mutilation (FGM) is reported in every issue. This quarterly journal , which I have published since 1975, also reports on our grass roots initiative of distributing our **Childbirth Picture Books**[2] with their Additions to prevent Excision and Infibulation to local community health and midwifery groups all over Africa and the Middle East. These graphic teaching materials produced in many languages are accesible to people with limited reading skills and are readily understood regardless of language or literacy according to the hundreds of letters we receive from all over Africa and worldwide.

What is documented in this report is presented from a woman's view which must come first. This does not exclude, however, the fact that these traditional practices do very real damage to the development and economy of each society and country - see below - as is also shown in the case study of Sierra Leone. Economic studies should be made in all countries where FGM is practiced to show decision makers what these damaging traditions really cost in terms of each national budget.

But the **terrible suffering and severe psychologial trauma** that FGM imposes on female children and women at an early age and throughout life can never be measured in economic terms. They must be understood for what they are: a social burden of sexual violence imposed by the patriarchal system on those least able to protect themselves to keep them in servitude to men. To defend such practices on cultural grounds, as is done too often, is a distortion of the meaning of culture.

It also has been recently documented that FGM contributes to the spread of AIDS (Acquired Immune Deficiency Syndrome) , which is rapidly growing throughout Africa: In no other continent are so many women infected and they transmit the infections to their children often before they are born.

Young girls and children who are subjected to these mutilations are never asked and do not know what is done to them. They and their mothers have no choice and are not only ignorant of the health dangers involved and the lifelong suffering they cause, but they are also unaware that these mutilations are not practiced in most of the world. Women believe that these practices are "necessary" and have to be done - with all kinds of myths and stories told by different ethnic groups why - or they will be outcasts of their family and society and will not be able to have children. And children are essential in Africa.

Those of us who know the truth must face our responsibility to make the health facts and information about reproduction and sexuality known and available everywhere and especially to the victims of these damaging practices so their daughters will be spared. In our age of electronic communication where information can reach instantly all over the world, why are the most basic facts about human biology and reproduction still concealed?

"Female Circumcision" is the popular, but medically incorrect, name still used in Africa for a variety of mutilating genital operations to which female children and young women are subjected. At the 1990 conference in Addis Ababa by the **IAC - the Inter African Committee on "Traditional Practices Affecting the Health of Women and Children"** [3] the delegations from more than twenty African countries unanimously voted that "Genital Mutilation" was the term they and all others concerned with this issue should use.

From a biological and health view the operations on girls are not a counterpart to male circumcision - though both operations are often done as puberty rites. But what is done to girls has a different purpose and results: A healthy and most sensitive organ is removed. From a biological viewpoint the genital mutilations performed on females are the equivalent of the amputation of part or all of the penis - with very similar physical and sexual results (see comparison below) and quite different from what is done to boys. With boys the foreskin is cut, though both operations may result in deadly infections.

For Moslems the removal of the foreskin is an absolute religious requirement demanded by the Koran and it is also a requirement for "manhood" throughout tribal Africa. But there is no mention of female circumcision anywhere in the Koran as all Moslem religious authorities have confirmed including El Azhar University in Egypt, the leader of Moslem scholarship. Nevertheless some local Moslem sheiks and leaders preach that "female circumcision is a religious requirement". The women who can neither read nor write have no choice but to accept what these men of religion claim. Indeed who would dare to question them? (see "Case History: Sudan").

Since some African and Arab traditionalists still object to calling these female genital operations a "mutilation", the definition of the word should be examined. According to Webster, to mutilate (from "mutilus" - maimed) means "to cripple, to injure, to damage, or otherwise make imperfect, especially by removing an essential part or parts". The term "mutilation" quite correctly describes what is done by the operations - which remove the most sensitive organ of the female body - and irrevocably injure and damage the female person.

The female genitalia that are created "perfect" are deliberately crippled and altered according to custom. It is men who determine what becomes a custom and finally a tradition in each society. The objective, which is quite openly stated by African and Middle Eastern men, is to deprive women of sexual pleasure and to keep women under male control. In Moslem countries women are told that they are unable to control their sexuality; therefore they must be excised. In different ethnic groups, the genital operations take different forms and are performed on girls of different ages, with a variety of different reasons given (see below). The purpose and medical results, however, are the same.

It should be noted here that men in all societies so far have failed to organize effective actions to stop female genital mutilation though the facts are known by now to health professionals. All over the world men have formed organizaions to stop health abuses of every kind. But no organization to date exists to prevent men from having their daughters mutilated despite the fact that the real reason the mutilations continue today is that men refuse to marry women who are not "done" (that is, excised or infibulated - according to the local practice).

In Africa and the Middle East fathers arrange the marriages of their daughters and they collect the bride-price: therefore they see to it that their daughters are mutilated - as otherwise they dont get paid; the money and gifts involved often are considerable, so the girls are often sold while still children. Since women have no alternative but marriage, the mutilations continue. Men claim the operations are"women's affairs", refusing to take responsibility. But if men rejected marriage with mutilated women, the practice would stop immediately. **Where is the leadership of men?**

DEFINITIONS OF THE OPERATIONS

Three kinds of operations, popularly called female circumcision in Africa and the Middle East, are described in the medical literature.These definitions by gynecologists are derived from observations and case histories, that is, after the fact, rather than by the operators who have no knowledge of anatomy. All the operations are performed without anesthetic, often on struggling children held down by force, frequently on the ground under highly septic conditions, using a variety of tools. These definitions are summarized from descriptions given throughout the medical literature. (See footnotes: Verzin, Shandall, Cook.)

1. **Sunna Circumcision (Sunna means "tradition" in Arabic)**
   Removal of the prepuce and the tip of the clitoris (mildest form). This delicate operation is rarely performed in Africa and the Middle East, given the lack of anatomical knowledge of the operators, the crude tools used and the environmental conditions (operations are done on the ground, in dark huts, under trees, etc.)
2. **Excision/Clitoridectomy**
   Removal of the clitoris and also often adjacent parts including the labia minora and sometimes all exterior genitalia. In some areas, additional cuts into the vagina are added (to make childbirth easier, the opposite is true). Excision is the most frequent operation.
3. **Infibulation (Pharaonic Circumcision)**
   After the removal of the clitoris and labia minora as well as parts of the labia majora, the two sides of the vulva are closed over the vagina. This is done by fastening together the bleeding sides of the labia majora with thorns or catgut or some sticky paste. A small opening is created by inserting a splinter of wood to allow for elimination of urine and later menstrual blood. The legs of the child are then tied together, immobilizing her for several weeks or until the wound is healed

The mortality of girls and women due to all these operations no doubt is high; but no records are kept. Primary fatalities are not recorded; death in childbirth, due to obstructed labor caused by the mutilations, is never related to genital operations anywhere.

The term Excision/Clitoridectomy, popularly called "Female Circumcision" is used in Africa to describe all kinds of genital operations, the extent of which can only be determined by gynecological examination. The damage done, or the severity of the operation, depends on local customs, on the operator's skill and on the tools used. Traditionally, sharp stones or special knives are used; recently, mostly razor blades. The more traditional the population group, the more drastic the operation; that is, the more flesh is removed.

Old women who are sometimes called "midwives," though they have no health training, perform the operations traditionally in most of Africa and the Middle East: in some areas excision is an inherited trade and special "excisors" go from village to village. Sometimes male operators are involved; for instance, in northern Nigeria and Egypt barbers do the operations in urban areas. Physicians now perform the operations on the children of the wealthy for a fee (for instance, in the Sudan, Nigeria, Egypt, Somalia, etc.) They are also often done by trained midwives as a way to make money.

Infibulation is known as "Pharaonic Circumcision" because it always has been practiced in Upper Egypt and was known to the ancient Egyptians. The term "infibulation" goes back to the Romans. Fibula means clasp or pin in Latin. A fibula was used to hold together the toga, the loose garment worn by Roman men. To prevent sexual intercourse, the Romans fastened a fibula through the large lips of women and a ring or fibula through the foreskin of men - usually slaves.[4] Infibulated female slaves from Upper Egypt and Sudan fetched a higher price on the slave markets of Cairo up to the 19th century, as childbearing hampers work.

Infibulation may also occur spontaneously by adherence of the wounded sides of the labia, especially where extensive excision operations are performed, for instance, in Senegal, Burkina Faso and Mali,

The objective of infibulation is to make sexual intercourse impossible. At present infibulation is practiced as a rule chiefly by Moslems, according to all available sources, because of the importance and value Moslems attach to virginity. Infibualtion is performed to guarantee that a bride is intact - the smaller her opening, the higher the bride-price. A girl is often inspected by the female relatives of the husband-to-be before the bride-price is paid.

Women who are infibulated have to be cut open to allow penetration - and more cuts are needed for delivery of a child. Wives, traditionally, are re-infibulated for instance, in the Sudan and Somalia after the baby is born; and when the child is weaned, they are opened again for intercourse. During her reproductive life, a woman used to go through this process with each child; and in some areas it still continues today. The decision rests with the husband, who has several wives. For instance, the Somali men who came to the Benadir hospital - the largest hospital for women and children in Mogadishu - demanded that their wives be re-infibulated after delivery, so the head nurse told me. And the same demand was made by Somali refugees in Canada.

For instance, in the Sudan, it has been reported that women often demand re-infibulation after delivery to make intercourse more pleasurable for the husband. A woman must please sexually, or she may be divorced, which means loss of her children, loss of all economic support,and disgrace for her and her family. It also was the custom for men to have their wives re-infibulated when they left home for extended periods of time.

In West Africa infibulation is usually not done by sewing or other fastening devices: by tying the legs of the girl together after the operation in a crossed position, the same results are achieved. If an excision operation is drastic, the scars at times obliterate the bodily openings, as is reported in the medical literature - when girls bloated from retention of urine or menstrual blood come to the hospital.

On a visit to Ouagadougou, Burkina Faso, in 1977, while I was in the maternity hospital, a woman in labor with her first child was brought in: she could not deliver as she was almost completely closed. There was nothing at all left of her external genitalia. She had evidently conceived through a tiny opening - as is also reported in the medical litereratu re.

Excision and infibulation are performed on the ground, under septic conditions, with the same knife or tool used on all the girls of a group operation. In cases of fatalities, most often the result of cutting a blood vessel, neither the operator nor the operation is ever blamed. The conditions under which the mutilations are done provide the perfect opportunity for the transmission of AIDS - which is higher in Africa than anywhere in the world with more women infected.

The locations for the operations vary: under a special tree, in designated woods, inside huts, in the backyards of houses, sometimes furtively at dawn. In the Sudan, the operation takes place in the house or a walled yard in the presence of many women, strictly segregated: Men may not attend the gathering, or "celebration," though young boys do. In many ethnic groups in Central and West Africa, men participate in the village celebrations but are not allowed to be present at the cutting. Everywhere, the fathers of the girls pay the fees for the operations. The male village elders in sub-Saharan Africa decide when the operations are to be done, while the fathers present their children.

The health sector worldwide is controlled by men, internationally as well as in each country. The World Health Organization (WHO) issued in June of 1982 a position statement: "Female cicumcision is a traditional practice which can have serious health consequences and is of concern to the World Health Organization. WHO has consistently and unequivocally advised that female circumcision should not be practiced by any health professionals in any settings - including hospitals or other health establishments." (See Appendix). This recommendation is strongly supported by the IAC - the Inter African Committee - and its affiliates in more than 22 African countries (see above).

Nevertheless it is a fact that trained health workers and physicians in Africa use the mutilations to make money. In several African countries the mutilations were and are being done on very young girl children by health workers trained by internationally supported programs often using donated equipment and drugs. (See country reports on Somalia, Mali, Nigeria.).

Traditionally the operations are performed at various ages, from newborn babies (for example, in Ethiopia and among the Yoruba in Nigeria) to puberty. The Masai in Kenya and Tanzania are said to perform the operations on the wedding night. In Mali, the midwives in the Gabriel Toure Hospital in Bamako state that in some ethnic groups a woman is excised after her first child in order to keep her faithful to her husband, who has several wives.

In most of sub-Saharan Africa the operations traditionally were performed as a puberty or coming-of-age rite on girls twelve to fifteen years old or just before menstruation. Recently, the age at which excisions are performed has become much younger in the towns, also in some rural areas and the procedure has been stripped of all "traditions"- only the cutting continues. (See "Case History: Kenya")

Infibulation traditionally is practiced on children six to eight and sometimes younger. Recently the age at which infibulation is performed has also been reduced to as young as three or less in the urban areas, for instance, in Sudan or Somalia. Awa Thiam in **Parole aux Negresses**, [5] tells the story of a young woman from Mali who only discovered that she was infibulated when she was to be married. She had no memory of the operation and was kept in ignorance about her condition as well as reproduction until her father had arranged her marriage.

Many of the traditional ceremonies surrounding the operations have been greatly simplified or quite abandoned under the impact of modernization, especially in urban areas. However, the mutilations continue to be performed on ever-younger children, as the parents are afraid that girls, once they know what is in store for them, will refuse. Girls living in towns are sometimes brought back to their villages and forcibly subjected to FGM. The grandmothers and older women of the family see to it that all the girls are operated on. However, the decisions in each family are made by men, who also pay for the operations and negotiate the marriage. In many ethnic groups, girls who are not mutilated are considered unfit for marriage: That means the father cannot collect the bride-price, therefore, he has his daughters mutilated. In turn, a father will not pay for a bride for his son nor will a man buy a wife who is not excised. Thus, the operations continue. Marriage is obligatory for all throughout Africa and the Middle East, and it is strongly advocated by the Koran.

The operations are now performed in the modern health sector of many African cities, for instance, in Mali, Somalia, Nigeria, Sudan, Egypt and more. The operation may be done in a hospital or an infirmary or at the private office of a physician depending on what the father is willing to pay. If the daughter dies from the operation, the father loses the bride-price. Thus, the incentive is to use modern health practices for this purpose - that is imported tools and antibiotics as well as surgical techniques. But of course only wealthy men can pay a doctor or a midwife.

Many village girls who have learned something about the pain of the operation try to run away - the only place to go is to the nearest town or the capital. Since they have no skills and are illiterate, the only way they can survive and earn a living is through prostitution. African towns and cities are overflowing with prostitutes - many of them infected with AIDS. The mutilations and the violent sexual customs of men as well as rape which is widely practiced traditionally - resulting in lacerations - are some reasons why AIDS is overwhelming Africa.

Almost every family in West Africa has lost at least one daughter due to FGM - which is one reason why the mutilations are now practiced on ever younger children - so the midwives in the Gabriel Toure Hospital told me. They now have excisors right in the hospital to mutilate the newborn babies so they are not infected and there is help available if a blood vessel is cut.

In recent years more and more immigrants and refugees are coming to **Europe** and **North America** from Africa and the Middle East and they bring their customs with them. In most European countries where health services are paid for by their governments health ministries alerted all hospitals and practitioners that these mutilations are prohibited. In Britain special legislation was passed in 1985 after it was reported that a physician had done the operation in his office in London on the wife of a wealthy African who demanded it as "cure against her infertility".

In **France,** large numbers of immigrants from West Africa live and work around Paris, After ignoring FGM for many years, the French government had to take action when three little girls born to Malian immigrants living in the Paris area died as result of the mutilation - they bled to death. Now the matter is in the criminal courts (see "The Western World"). In **Australia** the issue was extensively discussed in the press repeatedly, but no one was able to produce any documented cases of mutilations done in Australia.

In **Canada,** which recently had a large influx of Somalian refugees (all women in Somalia are infibulated), the College of Physicians and Surgeons of Ontario warned all their members against performing the mutilations and provided specific information how to take care of infibulated women [6]. By contrast in the **Netherlands** physicians were discussing the introduction of legislation in the summer of 1992 to "legalize" the mutilations so they can be done in hospitals, paid for by the government . Many Somalian refugees are coming to this liberal country. Under the pretext that immigrants cannot be robbed of their "traditions", some physicians proposed to operate on the small daughters of immigrants - doing a permanent mutilation that they would categorically reject for their own children. This is the ultimate form of racism and greed. Unfortunately the physicians in the Netherlands are not unique. (See "The Western World")

In the **United States** the facts regarding FGM done by immigrants on their daughters have never been documented, though no doubt the mutilations are practiced. The physician/ patient privacy rules are protecting the practice, and since health care is not paid for by the government, physicians can do whatever they want or get paid for. [7] At this writing not a single case of FGM done in the **United States** has been medically documented.

However, in 1980, a United States Sunday newspaper supplement, **The National Black Monitor** which is distributed all over the country and published by a consortium of publishers of black community papers - all men - distributed an editorial in one of their supplements advocating the importation of FGM "as a social safeguard". They proposed this African tradition should be introduced in the United States to prevent "teen sex and parenthood" and to"control the sexual waywardness in girls". These self appointed male leaders of US Afro-American communities advocated "hygienic experimentation with female circumcision" - showing some drawings of African men and women in surgical gowns and rubber gloves surrounded by medical equipment. After a letter writing campaign organized by **WIN NEWS** the **Black Monitor** editors had to explain the truth about FGM to their readers and apoligize to women. (See "The Western World")

FGM has been cited as **a Human Rights violation** in the Country Reports on Human Rights Practices, issued every year by the United States Department of State based on legislation. (See **WIN NEWS** Spring issues 1990, '91 and '92.) The United Nations Commission on Human Rights also has recognized FGM as a human rights violation. In the spring of 1991, a seminar on "Traditional Practices Affecting the Health of Women and Children" was held in Burkina Faso, sponsored by the United Nations Center for Human Rights with fifteen countries participating, most of them from West Africa. FGM was the main topic of the agenda. [8] The participation of so many West African governments in this conference is remarkable, considering that only a few years ago the subject of FGM could not be discussed in any meeting in Africa, as United Nations Agencies claimed "only a few isolated people in remote areas practice this" and "we cannot interfere in culture and tradition."

Up to the World Health Organization (WHO) Seminar in Khartoum in 1979 (see: "WHO Seminar") African and Middle Eastern leaders silenced every attempt to discuss FGM. Indeed President Kenyatta made FGM a requirement among his followers in Kenya and he influenced the leaders all over Africa. (See "Case History: Kenya") It was therefore especially important that his successor, President Daniel arap Moi, categorically prohibited FGM throughout Kenya in 1982 and repeated this interdiction since. But neither Kenya nor most other African countries have initiated effective education or other follow-up programs, except for Somalia, now totally destroyed by civil war, and Burkina Faso, which hosted the Human Rights Conference cited above and organized a national campaign. Almost all initiatives to stop FGM are supported from abroad. All health care and especially maternity services have been drastically cut back due to World Bank/IMF (International Monetary Fund) "Structural Adjustment" rules that have fuerther devastated the ailing African economies. (See "Women and Health: Actions for Change".)

DAMAGE TO HEALTH

The health facts given here are summarized from the medical literature and from direct information from midwives and physicians in Africa.

The most important clinical study is a survey of 4,024 women, published in the **Sudan Medical Journal,** by Dr. Ahmed Abu-El Futuh Shandall.[9] This study of actual case histories observed by the author in the Khartoum Hospital over a period of many years also lists the types of operations encountered and tabulates the statistics of health problems resulting from genital operations. Dr. Shandall goes beyond citing the medical facts and health statistics and makes important suggestions for abolishing the mutilations.

The most comprehensive summary made of the medical literature concerning damage to physical health resulting from infibulation (Pharaonic Circumcision) was edited by Dr. R. Cook when he worked in the Eastern Mediterranean Regional Office of theWorld Health Organization.[10] This paper covers medical publications on female genital operations from 1931 to 1976, providing an overview of the realities of the health problems of women subjected to these operations.

In the British medical journal **Tropical Doctor**, Dr. J. A. Verzin published an article, "Sequelae of Female Circumcision",[11] which provides a thorough survey of the immediate and long-range health problems resulting from genital mutilation from evidence encountered in medical practice.

In the above named publications and in other medical literature on FGM the following health problems are recorded:

Immediate Results: primary fatalities resulting from hemorrhage (uncontrolled bleeding); shock due to blood loss and pain (no anesthetic is given); septicemia (blood poisoning); infections of the wound, including tetanus, which is fatal; retention of urine immediately following the operation due to occlusion or because of pain when urinating; trauma (injury) to adjacent tissues - the rectum, the urethra; failure of the wound to heal and spreading of the infections as tools are never sterilized.

In some areas, especially in West Africa, the operators throw dirt on the wound to stop the bleeding; ashes, pulverized animal feces are also used, resulting in fatal infections. Many traditional treatments applied to the wounds increase the damage and danger of the operations. Excision by cauterization (burning) is also reported in the literature, resulting in extensive infections and scars.

Long-Range Results: urinary problems due to chronic infection, which also may lead to infertility; difficulty in passing urine as well as menstrual blood and painful menstruation; malformations, including cysts. Keloid formation (hardening of the scars) is especially prevalent among Negroid peoples causing obstructed labor which may result in death in childbirth.

Many coital difficulties are reported, especially where infibulation is practiced. Often the bride must be cut open before penetration can take place, which causes injury and more infections. Excision can also result in an almost complete closing of the vagina by adherence of the excision wound, which is reported in West Africa and elsewhere in areas where excision is extreme.

Lack of orgasm is reported where studies on this subject were made. Women in many societies are not aware that intercourse can be pleasurable for them. Painful coitus is the most frequent result of the operations and sexual intercourse often recalls the pain of the mutilation.

Many difficulties in childbirth are reported due to the excision scars which prevent dilation: tears, hemmorhage and infections often result. Delay in labor and prolonged second-stage labor as well as uterine inertia are reported; obstructed labor is a frequent result; sometimes brain damage or death of the baby due to lack of oxygen occurs, especially with the first child. The highest maternal and infant mortality rates in the world are recorded in the regions where genital mutilation is practiced. But the recently organized (1987) "Safe Motherhood Campaign" by WHO and the World Bank and other governmental and private agencies is ignoring FGM - despite the African statistics on FGM and despite conferences held by the campaign in Africa.

In case of infibulation, unassisted childbirth is impossible; if there is no one to cut the infibulation, both mother and baby often die.The formation of vesico/vaginal (or recto/vaginal) fistulae (rupturing of the vaginal wall) are reported due to obstructed labor, resulting in incontinence. This makes the women outcasts of their families and communities, as they are continuously dribbling urine and feces. The Kenyatta Hospital in Nairobi, for instance, always has a waiting list of hundreds of women for fistula operations, which are difficult procedures that often fail.

Women with fistualae can be found in many African hospitals in all areas where genital mutilation is practiced, though only a few hospitals can perform these difficult operations which require special aftercare for several weeks. In Addis Ababa a unique privately organized Fistula Clinic is run by a husband and wife physician team from Australia and New Zealand. They have the highest success rate and are teaching doctors how to do these difficult operations (see "Case History: Ethiopia").

Psychological Results and Background: The effects of sex trauma, of fear and the extreme pain of the operations as well as the prolonged suffering afterward, have never been conclusively investigated. Only one study exists at present by Dr. T. A. Baasher, which analyzes the responses of seventy women to a questionnaire about their opinions concerning circumcision. [12] But this study does not deal with the lifelong psychological effects on the mentality of mutilated women. The permanent psychological damage of this torture to which often very young girls are subjected by their own families, those they love and trust, has to date been quite ignored.

The debilitating pain of menstruation (as a result of the operation), the agony of the first intercourse, especially for the infibulated, the prolonged suffering in childbirth, no doubt create deep psychological wounds as well as physical ones. No clinical investigation exists on the subject. At the present time, most women and young girls who are subjected to these operations are unaware that any alternatives exist or that these mutilations are not practiced in most of the world. Up to 80 percent of the women in rural areas of many African countries where FGM continues to be practiced are still illiterate.

The effects of sexual castration (which these operations actually are) on the personality development of a girl have also been quite ignored. Yet it is clear that the permanent deprivation of a human being's most powerful instinct has deeply depressing psychological results, especially since in Africa and the Middle East a female's purpose in life is to serve the sexual satisfaction of her husband, to bear "his" children and tto provide food.

No inquiry has even been suggested by WHO or others concerned with health to investigate the psychological results on children and women of the sexual violence that is practiced routinely by African men under the label of "cultural practices" (see country reports). The medical literature reports on the physical damage sustained by girls and young women - their genitalia torn apart due to the brutal sexual attacks by men including their husbands - for instance, in Ethiopia and Nigeria. In every hospital maternity ward such information is available, but no one cares. The psychological results are entirely ignored in the medical literature. Suicides by young women, unable to cope with the sexual ordeals to which they are subjected by men and due to the torture of repeated childbirth, are reported, for instance, in Burkina Faso.

Genital mutilation can only be understood in the context of the psychological climate created by the all-pervasive, male sexual violence that forms the unseen background of African and Middle Eastern family life. Women in the West have only recently started to speak about male family violence - in Africa it is still a mute subject. African men claim - for instance, the members of the Kenyan Parliament - that wife abuse is a hallowed African tradition they want confirmed in their new family legislation.

The dreadful physical injuries that can be seen in hospitals are only the tip of the iceberg. The apathy and fatalism that can be observed among many African and Middle Eastern women are their psychological defenses against the traditional sexual violence, torture and trauma they suffer from men of their own families from which they are unable to escape. These violent sexual practices by men, are sanctioned and validated by anthropologists as "important traditions that must be preserved". They are also the reason why AIDS is overwhelming Africa and why Africa is the continent where more women are infected than anywhere else - according to all statistics published by WHO.

The feudal village social order, which still prevails in most rural areas is characterized by group behavior that does not recognize individual responsibility by men for violence against women. The bride-price, which is still the rule in almost all African ethnic and social groups as well as in most of the Middle East, is nothing more than a sale price of women which is negotiated between men. If a woman does not produce offspring in a given time, she is returned and the bride-price has to be returned as well. Polygamy is practiced throughout Africa and the Middle East, though most men are unable to support even one wife and her children. Polygamy also contributes to the spread of AIDS.

Traditionally hunting and warfare were the predominant occupation of African men. The latter continues up to the present - no other area in the world has as many civil wars and continuous bloody conflicts (for example Liberia, Somalia, Sudan, Mozambique, Uganda, Rwanda, Angola, Nigeria, Congo, South Africa, and more,) quite aside from constant local ethnic conflicts that are not reported by the international press. No other continent has as many refugees: Predictably women and children are the vast majority of the victims of this constant warfare and violence by men.

Unfortunately these traditional attitudes and practices are never discussed by anthropologists, most of whom praise "culture and tradition" no matter how damaging to women and children - the majority of each society - and even though many traditional practices are human rights violations recognized by the very conservative Human Rights Commission of the United Nations. The horrendous reality of the most brutal civil and tribal warfare by men in Somalia has been daily shown on TV for many months. But no one seems to comment that all the Somali men and boys with guns seem well fed and healthy, while the women and children are starving, and sick. The time has come to point out the truth - that the attitudes and customs of men must change if African society is to survive and flourish on this huge, most beautiful and richly endowed continent.

While the recurring African droughts can be dealt with by temporary organized efforts from outside, the rapidly declining agricultural production all over Africa requires a complete re-orientation of customs and traditions that must include first of all a change of attitudes and habits of men. African traditions of tribal warfare and sexual violence are not compatible with contemporary life in our interconnected world and are devastating for the majority of the population of Africa, that is women and children who are victimized by the utterly senseless aggression of men. Yet women produce most of the food that Africa needs to survive.

Change in attitude by men has to start within each family by recognizing the equality and dignity of women and their children who are and always have been the productive members of African society and who are ruthlessly exploited, violated and abused by African men as this report documents with irrefutable facts. The time to change African customs and traditions is long overdue as the proliferation of AIDS and the ever growing number of refugees as well as the ever increasing local warfare, misery and poverty vividly demonstrates - which we all now can see on TV.

REASONS GIVEN

Many colorful myths are related all over Africa as reasons for the operations. Though all the myths are still believed by the ethnic groups involved especially in the rural areas, many of the reasons are contradictory and none of them are compatible with biological facts.

Most Africans who practice these mutilations believe that these customs are decreed by the ancestors and, therefore, must be complied with. But the decisive factor is that men refuse to marry women who are not excised. Since marriage is still the only career for a woman in most of Africa and the Middle East, the operations continue. "No proper Kikuyu would dream of marrying a girl who has not been circumcised" is the often cited statement by Jomo Kenyatta, the revered leader of Kenya, from his book, which was written in the 1930s and continues to be published.[13] It explains the customs of the Kikuyu, the dominant population group of Kenya, who still control Kenya's political life. As President of Kenya for life, Kenyatta had great influence on Africans well beyond the borders of Kenya, and his much quoted pronouncement is responsible for the mutilation of many thousands of helpless little girls and untold suffering and deaths all over Africa.

Excision, cutting out the most sensitive organ of a woman's body, extinguishes sexual sensitivity and response to touch: That this is recognized in Africa and the Middle East is confirmed by the reason most frequently given for the operations, which is "to keep moral behavior of women in society" and "to assure the faithfulness of women to their husbands" - who usually have several wives. In sub-Saharan Africa the operation traditionally is performed just before marriage as a puberty rite: It is claimed that a woman can be accepted into adult society and get married only after she is excised.

In the Sudan and the Middle East and in Moslem societies, it is said that a woman is incapable of controlling her sexuality - hence she must be excised or infibulated, or she will disgrace her family. A woman who is not mutilated is risking her and her family's status in society and is considered to be a prostitute. Infibulation is practiced mostly in devout Moslem areas to guarantee chastity visibly. The honor of the family is involved; and the smaller the opening of a girl, the higher the bride-price. This, however, does not prevent frequent divorces. Women are objects of trade between men. After divorce a woman is re-infibulated by her family and sold again to another man. Infibulation, it is believed, assures the husband that the children of the woman he purchased really are his own (see "Case History: Somalia").

Infibulation is traditionally performed on much younger children than excision or long before puberty on girls four to eight years old. In most ethnic groups excision traditionally was and is a coming-of-age rite, performed at puberty on girls twelve to fourteen or just before menstruation and marriage, except at the Masai where the operation is done after marriage, so some reports state. Child marriage is still practiced in much of Africa. Traditionally groups of girls are excised together in a secluded location outside the village under a special tree or in a special secret bush that no one is allowed to enter (see "Case History: Sierra Leone"). The village chief decides which is a good day and time for the excision procedure- after consulting the "spirits". Traditionally the girls are kept in seclusion for several weeks or longer and are instructed in the "duties" of a wife. If a girl dies, it is blamed on her, or it is said that the ritual was not properly performed - never on the operator or the mutilation.

Initiations involving excision and clitoridectomy are also practiced by Christian converts of all denominations. While in the past, some of the Protestant missionaries, for instance, the Scottish Church Missionary Society in Kenya in the 1920s, strongly opposed these operations, but little or nothing is said against them now. The Roman Catholics always condoned genital mutilation and never objected to any of these torturous operations on helpless female children under the pretext that men refuse to marry girls who are not mutilated and so the Catholic community would diminish.

Excision is also perceived as a way to increase fertility. It was widely believed that a woman who is not excised is unable to have children; the wish of most women is to have as many children as possible, especially sons, on which their status in society depends. Infertility is a tragedy for an African woman whose status depends on the number of children she bears. The biological facts about reproduction are unknown or ignored. In Kenya and elsewhere it was widely believed that excision is essential for fertility.

It is widely believed, for instance, in Mali, Burkina Faso and all over West Africa, that the clitoris connotes maleness while the prepuce of the penis represents femaleness. Hence, both have to be removed before a person can be accepted as an adult in his/her sex and mature society. The clitoris also is viewed as a dangerous organ - for instance in Burkina Faso and much of Francophone Africa. It will kill the baby during childbirth therefore it has to be removed. Another widely told myth is that the clitoris will damage the husband's genitalia during intercourse and injure him or make him infertile. The Bambara in West Africa claim the clitoris is the equivalent of the penis and therefore must be removed before childbearing is possible.

It is also believed, for instance in Ethiopia, that a girl who is not excised will run wild and disgrace her family. It is said that FGM needs to be done to "calm" a girl and make her quiet. In Egypt, aesthetic reasons are sometimes cited for the operation, and this is occasionally said in other areas of Africa as well. It is claimed that a woman's external genitalia are ugly and must be removed to make her acceptable to a man.

Hypertrophy of the clitoris - by which is meant an unusual enlargement of that organ which will, it is claimed, protrude between a woman's legs if not cut off - is cited as reason for excision in Ethiopia and also in parts of Nigeria. The Catholic Church sanctioned the mutilation of all female children of its converts on those grounds (see "Case History: Ethiopia").

Health reasons are often cited, especially in urban areas where the traditional myths are forgotten. Cleanliness is the reason given also by middle class families in areas as far apart as Cairo and Bamako. In Sudan, also, traditionally the operation is connected with cleanliness and is called "Tahur", which in Arabic means purity. A woman is considered dirty and polluted unless she is mutilated. The same is also often said in Somalia.

Many of the reasons given by local populations are quite similar, though they have been arrived at quite independently as no connection or communication exists between the population groups involved. Most myths about female sexuality in Africa and all over the world are promoted by men, which documents the amazing worldwide similarity of male attitudes concerning female sexuality. Obviously, all of the myths are designed to justify and continue the operations, from which men derive power and control over women as a group. This is, of course, the real reason why these operations continue today and why they are being rapidly introduced into the modern sector throughout the African continent with the collusion of Western men led by anthropologists who claim that Africans cannot be "deprived of their traditions" and especially the male-dominated health system which makes money from FGM: The social rites and ceremonies are forgotten but the surgery continues.

Many different, fanciful stories are told about FGM in the ethnographic literature. One tale citing why clitoridectomy is practiced is related by Jacques Lantier as told to him by a witch doctor, which has amazing contemporary relevance:

> "The great Spirit has created a woman in such a way that he alone can create life in her at the moment of conception. The Spirit has never made anything without good reason. A woman has two different and separate areas where she experiences desire and excitement: the clitoris and the vagina. The vagina is closed and can't be opened until the husband, chosen by the ancestors, breaks and the closure and thus makes a passage for the Spirit to enter and to continue the family. The Spirit decrees that this part of her body must not be soiled and he alone wants to give the woman the greatest possible pleasure. The Spirit has given woman a clitoris so she can enjoy it before marriage and still remain pure. The pleasure she experiences will create in her a desire for marriage. One does not cut off the clitoris in small girls because they use it to masturbate. Only when they are ready to procreate is it removed; and once it is, they feel deprived. Their desire then is concentrated in one place only, and they promptly get married. The couple experiences great happiness as the Spirit said it should be." [14]

This story and similar ones are told by different African ethnic groups. But what is astonishing is that it propagates the very same male myth as the one prevalent among male medical professionals, and especially by Freud. Freud's misconceptions were accepted throughout the male-dominated educated Western world with the same reverence as the ultimate wisdom of the African witch doctor. Obviously, neither Freud nor the African witch doctor was aware that they both were enthralled by the same self-serving male misconception - that of vaginal orgasm. In both cases, women were made to pay the price- in Africa, often with their lives.

The operations are now performed on much younger children especially in the towns, as it is feared by men that the girls will resist once they go to school or find out what really is done to them. Some run away - usually to the nearest towns. One Malian girl in 1991 came all the way to Paris as she had a friend in Bamako who was a stewardess for an airline. Her family threw her out when she refused to undergo excision prior to marriage as required traditionally in her village. She now is trying to get permission to stay in France as a refugee. But her mother paid the price - her husband banned her from her home and village and he took away all her children. She is treated as an outcast by her family and community.

In areas where traditionally the operations were a coming-of-age custom, they are now done on very young children, sometimes a few years old or even shortly after birth. The stated purpose of the operation in most of sub-Saharan Africa - introduction to adult life - has disappeared. Nevertheless, the mutilations continue to be practiced even in families of government officials and political leaders where many of the men have been to European or Western universities. The reason given by these men is African tradition - yet the men have rejected all other traditions for their own Westernized personal lives.

For instance, a few years ago a Somali delegate to a United Nations conference when I questioned him said yes, he had all his daughters infibulated. I asked him why: "It is the custom - everyone does it." This after he had delivered a speech on the efforts of the Somalian government to modernize their country and to abolish all traditions! (See "Case History: Somalia".)

It would be interesting to make a survey among African and Middle Eastern ambassadors and United Nations delegates - many of them polygamists - to learn if they have their daughters excised and infibulated and why. Many of these leaders of their societies have studied at European or American universities and have adopted for themselves a completely Western life- style, clothes, cars, planes, TVs and Western tools. Why then, do they continue to subject their daughters to sexual mutilation without a thought of the terrible suffering involved? How dare they use tradition as an excuse to mutilate their own children and worst of all why does the international diplomatic community permit these men to continue what is regarded all over the world as criminal child abuse?

In France poor immigrant families are in criminal court for mutilating their children and all over the world FGM is prohibited as child abuse. Yet the African diplomats and leaders of their countries - for instance, delegates at the United Nations in New York- are free to mutilate their own children, though it is a human rights violation according to the United Nations. Not one has ever publicly renounced the practice as they should as leaders of their communities and countries. But nobody has ever questioned the personal behavior of African and Middle Eastern leaders or how they treat their families.

GEOGRAPHIC DISTRIBUTION

Excision is practiced in a broad area all across Africa parallel to the Equator: from Egypt, Ethiopia, Somalia, Kenya and Tanzania in East Africa to the West African coast, from Sierra Leone to Mauritania and in all countries inbetween, including Nigeria, the most populous one. Excision is also documented in the southern part of the Arab Peninsula and around the Persian Gulf, including Yemen, Oman, the Arab Emirates and Bahrain - where the operations are reported to be decreasing. The map shows the areas affected according to definite documentation. FGM is an ethnic traditional practice and has nothing to do with the political borders of Africa, which were drawn in the 19th century. A less damaging form of genital operation is traditionally practiced on Moslem girl-children in Malaysia and parts of Indonesia.

In more than twenty-six countries of the African continent, FGM is practiced today by some ethnic groups - most often by a majority of the inhabitants. However, there are exceptions: For instance, the Luo, the second largest ethnic group of Kenya, the political rivals of the dominant Kikuyu, do not operate on their girls or their boys - though they are surrounded by ethnic groups who do.

Infibulation is practiced on all females, almost without exception, in all of Somalia and wherever ethnic Somalis live (Ethiopia, Kenya and Djibouti). The operation is traditionally performed on much younger children than excision, usually on four- to eight- year- old girls, long before puberty, with no ritual. Infibulation is also performed throughtout the upper Nile Valley, including southern Egypt, in Eritrea, in parts of Ethiopia and all along the Red Sea coast.

Practically all Moslem Sudanese subject their girls to the operations; only the non-Moslem inhabitants of the southern provinces, who are from different ethnic groups, do not practice any kind of female genital mutilation. But at present with Moslemization spreading in the south of Sudan due to the civil war, infibulation is also being propagated with Moslem domination.

In West Africa, infibulation is documented at the present time in Mali among some Moslem population groups. It is also practiced in northern Nigeria (Moslem area), according to a medical source, and is said to be practiced by some traditional groups living along the river in Senegal. No doubt infibulation is also practiced in other remote areas of West Africa. It sometimes occurs spontaneously as a result of extensive mutilation. This is reported in the medical literature from West Africa, including Cote d'Ivoire and Burkina Faso, where the operations are done in radical ways. A worldwide survey on FGM was prepared by me for the World Health Organization seminar in 1979 on "Traditional Practices Affecting the Health of Women and Children" and published in the second volume of the seminar report. This survey is based on an extensive literature search and field work all over Africa. An updated version of this research was published a year later in my article, "Female Genital Mutilation in the World Today: A Global Review".[15]

EXCISION AND INFIBULATION IN AFRICA

1 ETHIOPIA AND ERITREA
2 SUDAN
3 SOMALIA
4 KENYA
5 EGYPT
6 UGANDA
7 TANZANIA
8 DJIBOUTI
9 CENTRAL AFRICA
10 NIGERIA
11 GHANA
12 BURKINA FASO
13 COTE D'IVOIRE
14 MALI
15 GUINEA
16 SIERRA LEONE
17 SENEGAL
18 THE GAMBIA
19 MAURITANIA
20 LIBERIA
21 TOGO
22 BENIN
23 CAMEROON
24 CONGO
25 GABON
26 ZAIRE
27 CHAD
28 NIGER
29 LIBYA
30 ALGERIA
31 YEMEN
32 SAUDI ARABIA
33 ANGOLA
34 ZAMBIA
35 MOZAMBIQUE
36 SAHARA
37 MOROCCO
38 RWANDA
39 BURUNDI
40 MALAWI
41 OMAN

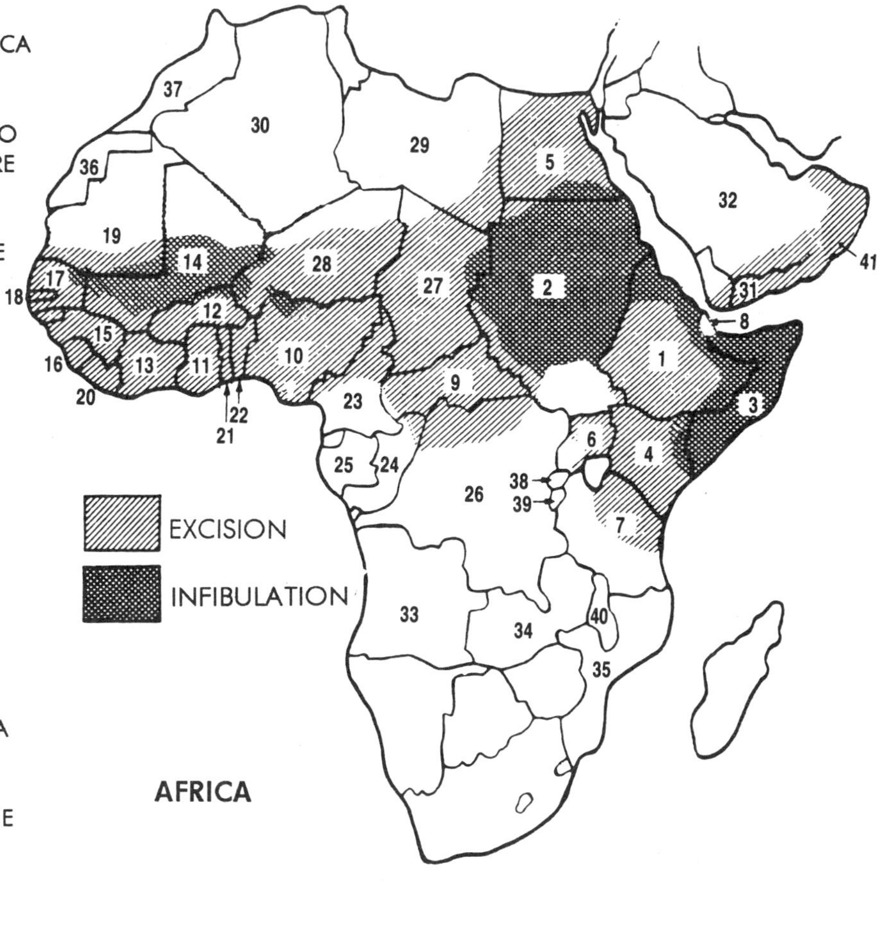

The most detailed national study was conducted in the Sudan by Dr. Asma el Dareer of the Medical Faculty of theUniversity of Khartoum.[16] In Nigeria, a national survey was made by the Federal Ministry of Health, Department of Medical Statistics, that showed that FGM is practiced in most Nigerian states.[17] (See "Case History: Nigeria") Partial surveys have been made in other countries. In Sierra Leone, a study by Dr. Koso-Thomas established that the operations are practiced throughout the country. (See "Case History: Sierra Leone".) Due to population growth, urban immigration, civil wars and greater mobility FGM is spreading to ever more and larger areas.

ESTIMATE: TOTAL NUMBER OF GIRLS AND WOMEN MUTILATED IN AFRICA

Countries with Large % Mutilated	Total Population in Millions	Number of Women (50% of Total)	Percent Mutilated Women	Estimate Total in Millions
EAST AFRICA				
Egypt	54.7	27.35	50%	13.675
Sudan	25.2	12.6	80%	10.080
Somalia	8.4	4.2	98%	4.116
Djibouti	0.4	0.2	98%	0.196
Ethiopia	51.7	25.85	90%	23.265
Kenya	24.6	12.3	50%	6.150
	165.0	82.50		57.482 (Mill.)
WEST AND CENTRAL AFRICA				
Nigeria	118.8	59.4	50%	29.700
Mali	8.1	4.05	75%	3.037
Burkina Faso	9.1	4.55	70%	3.185
Senegal	7.4	3.7	50%	1.850
Cote d'Ivoire	12.6	6.3	60%	3.780
Sierre Leone	4.2	2.1	80%	1.680
Guinea	7.3	3.65	60%	2.190
Liberia	2.6	1.3	60%	0.780
Togo	3.7	1.85	50%	0.925
Benin	4.7	2.35	50%	1.175
Chad	5.0	2.5	60%	1.500
Gambia	0.9	0.45	60%	0.27
Central Africa	2.9	1.45	50%	0.725
Ghana	15.0	7.5	30%	2.25
	202.3	101.15		53.047 (Mill.)
Estimated Total Number of Mutilated Women and Girls in East, West, and Central Africa in Millions				**110.529 (Mill.)**

There are a number of other African countries adjoining those cited above where a small percentage of the population practices FGM. These include Cameroon, Congo, Zaire, Mauritania, Tanzania and Uganda. The total number of mutilated girls and women in these countries is estimated to be between 2 and 3 million. This number should therefore be added to the total above.

In addition, the mutilations are practiced on the Arab peninsula in Yemen, Oman and the United Arab Emirates.

A less damaging form of FGM is practiced in some areas of Malaysia and Indonesia by devout Moslems. The mutilations in Asia are not indigenous but were imported with Moslemization. There are sporadic occurrences of FGM in other Moslem areas, for instance, on the Indian subcontinent.

The estimates above of the percentages of mutilated women / girls are low and may be higher in many areas / countries. They are based on the ethnic groups known to practice FGM living in each country. The figures cited here must be continuously updated as population growth in most African countries is very high (between 2 and 3 percent) - in some areas, much more (Kenya, more than 4 percent). AIDS is beginning to affect an increasing number of people in Africa and more women - therefore also children - are infected than in any other region of the world. There is no doubt that FGM contributes to AIDS.

Female Genital Mutilation Outside of Africa and the Middle East

No reliable documentation exists that in the past or traditionally FGM was practiced outside of Africa and the Middle East - the areas shown on the map above - except by some Moslem groups in Malaysia and parts of Indonesia. In Asia, the operations were imported with Moslemization in the 14th century; therefore they are only practiced by devout Moslem families and never by any other ethnic group. The operations in Asia seem to be less damaging and quite limited compared with African and Middle Eastern customs and do not remove the clitoris or impede childbearing as in Africa; but they can cause infections and blood poisoning. Infibulation is unknown.

At the 1988 International Conference in Mogadishu on "Circumcision: Strategies to Bring About Change", a physician from Indonesia and a member of the medical faculty of Gadjah Mada University at Jogjakarta presented his research on this subject with the conclusion that at present the operations are carried out mostly as symbolic ceremonies and any surgical intervention "involves a light puncture of the tip of the clitoris." [18] But what is done in the villages by traditional midwives who do the circumcision of girls is not known though it certainly does not compare to what is practiced in Africa and the Middle East and has no adverse effects on childbirth according to physicians. However, the very idea that the genitalia of a girl must be cut, manipulated or altered to make her acceptable to society and a husband seems an aberration no matter what the pretext or religious justification. (See "Asia: Indonesia and Malaysia").

While there are records when the operations were brought to Asia, in Africa and the Middle East they are indigenous and practiced long before conversion to Islam. Some documentation exist that FGM was already practiced in ancient Egypt. (See "History")

A clear distinction must also be made between sporadic and isolated occurrences of the operations and the systematic subjection of all female children belonging to an ethnic group, as is the case in Africa. Recently a researcher in Bombay, India, has found that some members of a Moslem sect in western India, the Bohras, practice the sunna type of FGM- shrouded in strict secrecy. Apparently this group was converted to Islam by missionaries from Egypt who introduced this practice which is said to consist in nicking the clitoris, allegedly to curb female sexuality. [19]

In the medical literature, several sporadic occurrences of genital operations are cited outside of Africa or the Middle East. These citations are all from more than hundred years ago with no medical case histories to back them up and are based on traveler's reports related as anecdotes in the anthropological literature. For instance, an operation called introcision (cuts into the vagina) is said to have been practiced in the 19th century among the indigenous population of Australia; no medical case histories exist and reports from hospitals in the area confirm that the operations are not practiced now and have not been seen for many decades.

Another frequent citation in the medical literature concerns a small group of orthodox monks in Czarist Russia called Skoptsi, who are said to have practiced self-castration of both men and women; this reference goes back to the first edition of the anthropological study by Ploss, [20] which was published in 1885 and has no social significance. But, unfortunately, it has been picked up in the medical literature and is cited over and over, creating a great deal of confusion.

It is possible that some isolated cases of female genital operations can be found among some isolated populations, though this cannot be compared with what is practiced in Africa and the Middle East today, where thousands of girls every year are systematically forced to undergo these mutilating operations with terrible lifelong results for their health. In Africa and the Middle East, female genital mutilations are a major public health concern that must be dealt with as a governmental responsibility and on a regional level, as the operations affect most of the female population in many countries and greatly increase maternal and infant mortality. The highest infant and maternal death rates (due to childbirth) in the world today are recorded in the regions where female genital mutilation is practiced in Africa.

The number of girls and women subjected to FGM outside of Africa is difficult to estimate. How many female children continue to be subjected to these operations in Malaysia or Indonesia, where they are reported with only some ethnic groups, cannot be established without field work: That means visiting Moslem hospitals, village dispensaries and family planning clinics. It would be necessary to talk to local midwives as they do the procedures in the villages on small girls and of course infections are always a danger where cutting is involved.

At present, it is also difficult to estimate the number of women and girls mutilated in the southern part of the Arab Peninsula and along the Persian Gulf, and it is unknown if the operations are practiced anywhere in Saudi Arabia or other Middle Eastern countries as mostly nomadic groups are involved who do not use hospitals and refuse all modern health care.

The mutilations, as stated before, now are also brought along by African and Middle Eastern immigrants especially to Europe and North America, though in a new environment, all surrounding rituals and the pretext that this is an important tradition are gone, only the surgery remains. This is discussed in the chapter on "The Western World".

EXCISION/INFIBULATION: EFFECT ON SEXUAL RESPONSE

At the Fifth Obstetrical-Gynaecological Congress in Khartoum, Sudan, in 1977. Dr. Salah Abu Bakr showed a series of slides of the cell structure of specimens from the clitoris and labia minora of several children, made from the parts cut off at an excision operation.[21] The greatly enlarged specimens, seen through a microscope, showed an abundance of nerve endings which could be clearly seen, darkened by special dyes used in the preparation of medical slides.

Dr. Bakr also showed similarly prepared slides made from the scar tissues of several adult women which were removed during repair operations: the few nerve endings that remained were encapsulated in sheets of fibrous tissue which renders them functionless. Dr. Bakr explained, "excision and infibulation results in destruction of the nerve supply of the vulva; consequently, sexual arousal cannot take place."

Touch organs (Pacinian corpuscles), Dr. Bakr stated, are removed by the operation, making the genital area insensitive to touch. Thus, it is physically impossible for an operated woman to be sexually stimulated by intercourse or respond to touch in the genital area.

Alternatively, some of the nerves may be accidentally bundled together by the cuts made during the operation and trapped in the scar tissue. As a result, touching such an area may become very painful, making sexual intercourse an ordeal.

This study by Dr. Bakr should finally lay to rest the claims made (often by male anthropologists) that the operations do not affect female sexual response. Without nerve endings, one cannot feel; much like without eyes, one cannot see. To ask women in Sudan who have undergone FGM about their sexual experiences as some researchers claim to have done seems an exercise in futility and worse: how can one explain orgasm to someone who has been mutilated as a child and associates the genital area with pain! As the groundbreaking study of Dr. Shandall at the Khartoum Hospital established, sexual intercourse is frequently painful for women who have undergone infibulation, quite aside from the terrible ordeal of childbirth. [22] In view of these studies, claims made that excision and infibulation do not damage sexual response - allegedly based on interviews with Sudanese women - are obviously absurd. What is more, Sudanese women never talk about sexuality with strangers from abroad.

A FEMALE/MALE COMPARISON

The equivalent of excision/clitoridectomy is the excision of part or all of the penis. The equivalent of removing the tip of the clitoris (Sunna Circumcision) is the same as the removal of the glans of the penis - both are most sensitive and full of nerve endings.

From the point of view of anatomy, the clitoris and the penis are parallel organs, which is also confirmed by their embryonic development.

Fertility is not impaired by either excision of the clitoris or excision of the penis; production of semen by a man continues. Conception and pregnancy of a woman proceeds much the same in excised as in normal women. Excision of the penis does not affect the production of sperm and semen, anymore than excision of the clitoris affects ovulation. Children can be conceived by artificial insemination, which can be accomplished with simple tools, for instance, a spoon.

Orgasm for men who have had penisectomies clearly is not possible, nor is it possible for women who have had clitoridectomies.

Penisectomy does not affect elimination of urine of the male, anymore than clitoridectomy affects urination of the female, as soon as the wound is healed. But, while a man whose penis has been cut off experiences no other health problems after the wound has healed, the scars created by the female operation often result in terrible problems at childbirth. The tissues that must greatly stretch to let the baby come out are scarred and have lost their elasticity. Obstructed labor, as a result of genital operations, costs many women and babies their lives after causing terrible suffering and agony.

It is claimed frequently in the literature written by men that Sunna Circumcision (cutting off the tip of the clitoris), does no harm. Sunna circumcision is the same operation as cutting off the tip or glans of the penis: would men claim this does no harm ? How would a man who claims that female circumcision does no harm like to have the most sensitive part of his body cut off?

A discussion of male excision as an alternative to operating on females will make the issue quite clear. The option of introducing the female operation into modern health care was discussed in the International Seminar of the World Health Organization in Khartoum in February 1979 by Sudanese physicians "to prevent worse harm." This option is also, proposed repeatedly by Western male physicians as is documented in this report (see "The Western World") and was again suggested in 1992 by physicians in the Netherlands who want to mutilate the infant daughters of Somalian refugees - at taxpayers expense in government hospitals under the pretext to prevent "worse harm."

The (former) Director of the Population Program of the United States Agency for International Development, Dr. Ravenholt, claimed that genital operations on females are "nothing but a traditional method of birth control." It must be pointed out that male excision would be much more effective.

Men in much of Africa and the Middle East claim that there is a "need" for excising females as a means of controlling their sexuality. It is clear that the "need" for sexual control of males is very much greater; rape and sexual assault are increasing all over the world; male excision certainly would take care of that. Furthermore, male excision would quite eliminate the "need" for female excision and would also greatly reduce the spread of AIDS.

Female sexual satisfaction is not dependent on penetration by the male penis: on the contrary, as has been documented some time ago by Drs. Masters and Johnson[23] and in **The Hite Report**.[24] Female sexual satisfaction and orgasm are achieved by clitoral stimulation. Therefore, female orgasm is quite independent of males and is not affected by excision of the penis. However, rape and sexual assault of women would be eliminated by penisectomies - which would be a very great benefit to all societies.

Before the introduction of clitoridectomy into modern medical practice is further discussed, male excision should be considered as an alternative. In Khartoum, at the WHO Seminar, the proposal to "modernize" genital mutilation by performing the operations in a hospital setting was voted down by all the women present; however, it has come up repeatedly since, always proposed by men. Therefore, a comparative research study sponsored by WHO of the biological and health facts involved should be made to clarify the situation. A cost benefit analysis of male excision (penisectomy) versus female clitoridectomy will clearly show the advantages of penisectomy. No doubt such a study will also raise the consciousness of men and should be presented to all politicians in Africa and the Middle East as well as to all physicians so keen to introduce FGM into hospital practice.

COST ANALYSIS

The terrible human costs of the operations cannot be measured and are paid first of all by the young female children and women of Africa and the Middle East, sometimes with their lives.

The costs to governments, however, can be accounted for in monetary terms. By implication, the costs must be also faced by international agencies including those of the United Nations and the international development agencies in each country.*

There are four principal areas of costs involved:

1. The costs due to loss of life of female children and young women who are dying as the direct result of the operations. They represent an irretrievable loss to their own families, communities and each country.
2. The costs of injuries, infections and of making childbirth more hazardous as well as costs of lifelong health problems. With more women seeking help in the hospitals, the costs of health assistance are growing for each government. According to the regional office of WHO in Alexandria it was estimated that during one year (July 1977-July 1978) in a single hospital of that region, 1967 days of hospitalization were needed to care for those seeking help as a result of complications due to genital operations. "The costs are obviously high - especially in a developing country whose health resources are generally scarce."[25]
3. The costs of work time lost due to illness, including the recurring menstrual problems caused by the operations that have to be borne by each employer. The largest employer in each African/Middle Eastern country is the government. When health insurance and social security arrangements are instituted, the costs of genital mutilations will have to be directly paid in health care costs by each insurer and by each government. These costs directly affect the development budget and the costs of development plans.
4. The costs of introducing the operations into hospitals in Africa/Middle East, including the necessary drugs and care, would be well beyond the budget of any African/Middle Eastern country, especially since this means a continuously growing expense. By comparison, a national health education campaign to abolish these damaging practices would be a one-time expense. Such a budget is available for Sierra Leone (see "Case History: Sierra Leone") showing that it costs less to organize and run such a campaign over a twenty-year period than the health costs involved in caring for the injured girls and women. The campaign furthermore would eliminate all future costs due to FGM.

From this accounting, it is obvious that the costs faced now by organizing nationally and internationally supported local health education and prevention campaigns against female genital mutilations will represent a very large net savings of direct expenses over the coming years. The emphasis should be on positive health and especially preventive health care. This is ever more urgent due to the growing disaster of AIDS to which FGM greatly contributes.

The objective is to eliminate genital mutilation by putting in its place positive mother and child care practices through education in reproductive health, childbirth, child spacing, personal hygiene, nutrition, and more. Health education campaigns in family health directed to the whole family and especially women will immeasurably improve the health and well-being of each country and community. Such campaigns will result in better health for the younger generation, and they will add up to a net reduction in health and medical budgets. The **Universal Childbirth Picture Book/Program,** organized by Women's International Network, has proved to be a very effective teaching tool regardless of language or literacy, on the grass roots level. These Books with Additions to prevent Excision and Infibulation are used successfully all over Africa. (See Women and Health).

---

* Development assistance is financed by taxes, which in turn are paid by you and me. Therefore, we have a right to speak on how this money should be spent and make our wishes known to the governmental agencies involved. In the United States write to the Chief Administrator, US/AID, Department of State, Washington, DC 20523.

FROM AN ADDRESS BY MS. EDNA ADAN ISMAIL, WHO REPRESENTATIVE AT DJIBOUTI, AND FORMER DIRECTOR OF TRAINING, HEALTH MINISTRY OF SOMALIA

> "I thank you for having given me the opportunitiy to bring your attention to the subject of female genital mutilation. In various modifications, the operations rank high in the list of preventable health hazards and affect almost all of the female population of Djibouti, Somalia and Moslem Sudan and millions of women in other countries in Africa.
>
> It may be appropriate here for me to describe more fully the mental and physical injuries and complications suffered by such a large number of our sisters and daughters. Female circumcision - the traditional name used in most of Africa - can be described as the partial or total excision of the female genitalia. . ."

After outlining the different types of operations (see above), Ms. Ismail described the situation from her own experience working for many years as the Director of Midwifery and Nurses Training in the Health Ministry of Somalia. First a description of the operation:

> "The operations are carried out by women who earn their living by the performance of such operations, including the opening up, after marriage, of the bride; these women are also often the village midwives. Such women have no knowledge of asepsis or anatomy and use no form of anesthesia.
>
> The operations may also be done by paramedical personnel in their spare time; such people use local anesthesia, sterile instruments and have some knowledge of the importance of asepsis. However, because of the local anesthesia, the child struggles less and more tissues may be cut away.
>
> In Somalia, the operations are done on young girls between the ages of five and eight, and may be done on individuals or groups of girls, either related or neighbors. The child is made to squat on a stool or mat with a strong woman pinning back her arms and shoulders. Two more women each hold one of her legs and stop her from struggling.
>
> The operator sits in front of the child and with a razor blade or other sharp instrument, excises the clitoris, labia minora and the inner walls of the labia majora. Using thorns which she has preselected, she inserts three or four on opposite sides of the labia majora, winds a string or a strip of cloth around the thorns in order to hold them together, very similar to how boots are laced. She then sprinkles the wound with a powder mixed from sugar, gum and myrrh. This forms a glue and sticks to the cloth, thorns and blood and forms a crust which stops the bleeding. The child is then bound from the waist to her toes and is made to lie on her side on a mat.
>
> Aftercare depends on the type of operations performed. In Somalia it may consist of the cauterization of the wound, the application of herbs which are believed to have haemostatic properties and enhance healing. The girls' diet is restricted in order to prevent frequent bowel movements and her drinking is also limited to a few sips of water at a time. Fumigations are frequent in order to dispel any undesirable odors and evil spirits."

Next Ms. Ismail reviews the many health problems including the resulting mental trauma based on her own experience as a trained midwife and teacher of midwifery:

> "As you can imagine, there are many complications; shock from fear, pain and hemorrhage. Extensive lacerations may be sustained which may involve the vaginal and urethral openings, as well as sometimes the rectum. The hemorrhages may be so severe that quite a few children are brought into the hospital for suturing of deep lacerations and for blood transfusions.
>
> Within the first ten days, sepsis ranks high in the list of complications and tetanus may also result. Retention of urine is another common complication due to the fact that the urethra is now covered with a flap of skin, thorns and blood clots, as well as the swelling which develops and obstructs the small opening which has been left to permit the passage of urine. Failure of the infibulation, which means that occasionally the walls of the labia majora fail to stick together. Another attempt at infibulation is usually made.

At the time of marriage, the forcible penetration of the skin barrier by the husband may cause lacerations, which may involve the perineum, the urethra, and sometimes even the rectum - particularly if a knife is used by the husband.

At childbirth, the scars of the external genitalia have very little elasticity and require being opened up in order to permit the passage of the baby through the obstructed birth outlet. Once more, infections may occur. This unnecessary suffering is imposed on the woman during every childbirth.

Other complications are rectovaginal and vesico-vaginal fistulae- the rupture of the uterus resulting in incontinence. Cystocoles, which is the prolapse of the bladder, the rectum and the uterus, are common. Pelvic inflammation also occurs due to the retention of urine and menstrual blood in the vagina and urethra. There is a constant threat of cystitis, vaginitis, cervicitis, and other infections which may develop into a chronic pelvic inflammation leading to dysmenorrhea (painful menstruation) and infertility.

Mental complications begin to affect the female child from an early age, and remain with her throughout her life. Well before the child is operated on, she hears tales of horror relating to the act of infibulation. At the same time, girls who have undergone FGM taunt those who have not with insults and call them 'unclean'.

In this frame of mind, of fear mixed with a sense of inferiority, the girl reaches her turn for the surgery. Many of the physical wounds will heal; their pain and discomfort subside. But at each stage of her later life, further mental injuries are added.

The slow trickle of urine (as opposed to the strong jet of urine coming from her bladder) reminds her constantly of the operation. The onset of menstruation, with its accompanying discomfort and odors, forces her to recall her agony. Marriage and the opening up of the infibulation to permit the consummation of the marriage is an ordeal. The birth of the first child and the knowledge that subsequent deliveries are not going to be any easier on her scar-riddled genitals, haunt every women constantly.

In spite of her own suffering due to infibulation, the knowledge that she will have to subject her daughters to the same ordeal adds further to her mental agonies." [26]

Edna Adan Ismail was the first woman and health professional to speak in public in Somalia on the health problems resulting from excision and infibulation when she addressed the Congress of the Somali Democratic Women's Organization (SWDO) in March 1977. The 500 participants attending the Congress unanimously condemned the practice and expressed their support for "abolishment of female circumcision."

This led to the formation of a National Commission to Abolish Female Circumcision under the guidance of the Somali Democratic Women's Organization and gained the support of the President of Somalia and the Ministries of Health, Education and Religious Guidance (see "Case HIstory: Somalia").

In Somalia, FGM has always been practiced in the extreme form of infibulation according to the earliest reports available (see "History"), and this continues today involving almost the entire female population - with terrible results - as Edna Adan Ismail above describes. It is, therefore, quite remarkable that in a few years after the Khartoum Seminar where a large delegation from Somalia participated including Edna Adan Ismail, the most comprehensive program to eradicate FGM was organized. It began to be implemented in 1986/87 by the government led by the Somali Women Democratic Organization with the collaboration and financial contribution of AIDoS - the Italian Association for Women in Development. [27]

This effort had the full backing of President Mohamed Siad Barree, who had been in power since 1969. All ministries and the entire school system participated in this groundbreaking national program. Besides organizing local and national meetings to mobilize leaders on every level as well as running education and training programs of all kinds, it culiminated in an international conference in June 1988, organized by the SWDO and AIDoS jointly and held in the Parliament. [28] (See "Case History : Somalia)

This unique and well-publicized international meeting - nothing like it had ever been done before or since anywhere in Africa - was extensively discussed and widely broadcast by the media all over Somalia, where until quite recently, the very mentionining of FGM was frowned on. (See "Case History: Somalia") In 1988, at the time of the conference in Mogadishu, the political upheaval that now engulfs the whole country had already started in the north of Somalia. At this writing in Autumn 1992, what started as a civil war is now threatening the very existence of the country with anarchy and the worst famine anywhere in Africa. Women and children are starving, brutalized and raped by their own Somali men, who fight each other and hijack all the food brought by international rescue groups. These are the very men who have enforced infibulation and made it into a 'cultural tradition' as price for marriage in a society where women have no alternatives.

The Somalian initiative and program to eradicate infibulation, however, can serve as a model and an inspiration. The educational materials, including videotapes and programs developed by AIDoS, are now being adapted by them for Ethiopia, Gambia, Nigeria and Sudan together with their national Committees affiliated with the Inter-African Committee (IAC). (See below and "Women and Health").

SURVEY OF POSITIVE DEVELOPMENTS

Here the positive developments are summarized following the opening of international discussion of FGM at the WHO Seminar in Khartoum in 1979. (See "WHO Seminar)

It took nearly five years for any positive actions to start in Africa. At a nongovernmental seminar in Dakar, Senegal, in 1984 on "Traditional Practices Affecting the Health of Women and Children" held as follow-up to the Khartoum Seminar with the participation of WHO and UNICEF, the Inter-African Committee (IAC) was organized for African women by Berhane Ras Work from Ethiopia.[29] The IAC developed an action plan based on the Khartoum Recommendations and since has provided the leadership and the organizational framework which is essential for such a huge effort. By now groups have been formed in more than twentytwo countries with IAC support to implement their Action Plan. Burkina Faso at present, after the collapse of Somalia, is the only country where the Government is directly involved in actions all over the country to eradicate FGM. (See "Case History: Burkina Faso")

The IAC affiliated groups in different African countries have attracted local support from women and at least verbal support from government ministries but depend almost entirely on international financing. UNICEF, which claims to support the eradication of FGM as well as WHO and UNFPA (United Nations Population Fund), generally pay lip service: Actual assistance depends on their local representatives, most of these are men who do not want to get involved and claim they have "other priorities." UNESCO still ignores FGM altogether. (See "The Politics of FGM")

"We cannot interfere in traditions and customs" continues to be a much used excuse which in part is based on the politization of the issue in Kenya. (See "Case History: Kenya") Yet the very idea of development requires change and the rejection of many customs that all confirm the past and refuse education and change. Anthropologists, who are always hired as consultants to development programs furthermore make their living from supporting traditions, which means reconfirming patriarchal power. As a result, many programs by development agencies fail, as they confirm traditions that oppose change. They also exclude women who are the most productive members of all African societies.

How very political this issue is and how deeply rooted it is in the patriarchal system was shown at the 1980 UN Mid-Decade Conference in Copenhagen, when a group of African women stormed into the room where I spoke on FGM, based on the research I had published and presented in Khartoum in 1979. Mary Angelique Savane from Dakar, who led the group, gained a lot of media attention - which was her purpose - by shouting so loud that no one could speak or be heard. Savane now has been rewarded with a high administrative post at the United Nations in Geneva by the male decision makers. She even protested UNICEF's offer to assist African Community groups to protect children from the mutilations - charging "interference" This charge is still the weapon used in Africa by those who seek power for themselves and who object to any assistance that is offered without consulting them first.

The Press at the Copenhagen women's conference in turn was delighted to blow up this issue which serves their patriarchal objectives by reporting that women from different cultures and countries would never agree or work together. In all this turmoil, the terrible suffering and devastating mutilations of thousands of helpless little girls in Africa were quite forgotten: To talk about that had been the purpose of my presentation. [30]

The IAC represents a new group of educated African women working for their own interests and health, not beholden to the patriarchal African system that has always used 'culture' and 'tradition' as code words to keep women poor, barefoot, pregnant and subservient - much like the patriarchal system everywhere.

The message of the IAC has been accepted throughout Africa and the Middle East. By now, in almost all countries where a major part of the population is affected by FGM, groups of women have organized under IAC leadership to work against damaging **"traditional practices affecting the health of women and children"** a heading that is not controversial and covers other damaging traditions besides FGM, including child marriage, all kinds of food tabus - especialy during pregnancy - and other abuses such as force feeding young girls, tribal markings and other damaging surgery.

In Nigeria, by far the most populous African country with very different ethnic groups most of whom practice FGM, many activities have been organized by women. The Nigerian National Committee, affiliated with the IAC, is engaged in all kinds of initiatives. [31] (See "Country Report: Nigeria") A campaign was organized by the professional nurses and midwives of Nigeria which took the message to stop FGM all over the country.

Sudan now has an active national committee affiliated with the IAC headed by Dr. Osman Modawi, who for years was the Chief of Obstetrics/Gynecology at the University and the Khartoum Hospital, (see "Case History: Sudan"). [32] In Sudan many programs against FGM have been organized over the years, but for the most part they have reached only the educated elite.

Practically all actions to eradicate FGM are financed from abroad and despite the direct and large costs of FGM outlined above to the African governments, especially in health expenses, governments and their health departments have done very little to educate the population to stop FGM. It would cost far less to organize really effective campaigns to stop FGM, as Dr. Koso Thomas of Sierra Leone has proposed in her thesis and book. [33] (See "Case History: Sierra Leone").

President Daniel arap Moi of Kenya in 1982 categorically prohibited FGM, but this important move by the head of the government was not followed by any education campaigns. There has been very little action in Kenya since, until quite recently, when Maendeleo Ya Wanawake, the largest national Women's Organization made a survey of the extent of FGM and polled opinions in preparation of a campaign to stop the practice, (see "Case History: Kenya).

It is striking that men, except for a few physicians, have been largely silent - especially African men whose families are directly affected . At the Second Regional IAC Conference held in Addis Ababa in November 1990, [34] there were a few male delegates who represented the affiliated national committees, most of them physicians. But in most of Africa, men are still silent. Yet the real reason why FGM continues today all over Africa is that men will not marry women who are not mutilated according to local custom.

Though prominent African men in many countries have taken the lead in publicly speaking out on the prevention of AIDS which is overwhelming Africa, few men have ever spoken out on stopping FGM. Not one of the African political leaders and diplomats who can be seen at international meetings have had the courage to publicly announce that FGM will not be practiced in his family and that his sons will not marry women who are mutilated. And this is the kind of leadership that is really needed that would make an impression and could effectively change attitudes.

One can but wonder how many of the men who claim to be leaders in Africa have their own daughters mutilated and who arrange the marriages of their sons with excised or "well-closed" brides. What is more, physicians all over Africa make money by mutilating the daughters of wealthy African men who have gone to European or American universities. How can we respect men who mutilate their own children?

Following the WHO Seminar in Khartoum and to support the implementation of the recommendations that stressed especially health education and information for the general public, I developed **The Childbirth Picture Book/Program (CBPB)** with the help of a small grant.[35] (See "Women and Health - Actions for Change"). With their additions to prevent excision and infibulation, these teaching materials in English, French and Arabic are used by the thousands all over Africa on the grass roots level. That they are effective is confirmed by hundreds of letters from community groups requesting more; they are understood regardless of language and literacy which is important, as in most rural areas, only very few women can read. The multi-ethnic pictures by Marcia Williams speak more effectively than words. Thousands of books are sent to midwifery schools, to community health centers and tto local groups who, in turn, distribute them. Enclosed in each book is a short note asking readers to renounce FGM - that is, to state that they will not submit their own children to FGM, now that they have learned about the damaging results from this book.

The distribution of the CBPBs to local groups on the grass roots level has been remarkably effective as our growing correspondence from many areas shows. The books are widely circulating among large numbers of people - men and women, see **WIN NEWS**, section on FGM where responses from users are reported, The letters show that large numbers of people reject FGM once they have learned from the pictures the real damage that results from the operations. The biological facts about reproduction are still quite unknown in Africa today among the majority of the people. In the Middle East, girls and women are still "protected" from such information or any knowledge of their own bodies, with terrible results for their health. The many damaging myths about women's health take a terrible toll.

The experience with the distribution of the CBPBs in Africa and the Middle East over the past ten years shows that a great deal could be accomplished very quickly by distributing the CBPBs on a large scale. This would be quite inexpensive, as no highly trained experts need to be involved. The books reach people from all walks of life giving them an opportunity to learn the facts and decide for themselves. Besides stopping FGM, wide distribution of the CBPBs would also substantially improve the health of women and children as the books deal with the basic facts of reproduction, with pregnancy, nutrition and family planning. They also provide essential information regarding the prevention of AIDS. (See "Women and Health - Actions for Change").

We hope that now that considerable experience with the CBPBs has been gained, some major grass roots education program will be started in several areas to conduct large scale programs to test the effectiveness of these teaching materials. Mass-distribution of the CBPBs could turn out to be the least expensive way to persuade whole populations to stop mutilating their children and could be very useful in campaigns against AIDS.

In the past, it was possible to hide FGM, and secrecy for centuries has concealed the terrible reality. This is no longer possible now. Due to greater mobility and constant civil wars in Africa, more and more African refugees are coming to Europe, North America and all parts of the world where FGM is a criminal offense quite aside from the fact that FGM is an internationally recognized human rights violation. Therefore, the issue has to be dealt with on the governmental and public level.

To those who still claim that African customs must be protected and that it is racist to interfere by protecting African children from the mutilation, let me ask: Would you have your daughter subjected to FGM? Real racism is to claim that a child because she is black or brown, should be forced to submit to this horrible torture with lifelong health damage and suffering - something you categorically reject for your own child!

All over Europe and recently in Canada health ministries have had to warn their personnel that FGM is illegal - as some African immigrants bring their children to publicly funded health services demanding to have them excised and/or infibulated. In France FGM is a criminal offense - see above - and in Britain, special legislation was passed after a drawn-out debate in Parliament when it was discovered that private surgeons were doing FGM on African women. Other countries all over Europe have warned their government funded health serices that these mutilations are illegal.

Somalian refugees are fleeing their country in large numbers. Every Somalian woman is infibulated because most Somalian men, despite education, still insist on FGM. Besides immigrating to Europe and the United States many Somalians are also coming to Canada - where considerable efforts by the medical community are being made to stop FGM and educate the immigrants. (See: "Case History: Somalia") For instance, the College of Physicians and Surgeons of Ontario banned "the performance of female circumcision, excision or infibulation" as announced in a press release in spring 1992 and instructed physicians how to take care of infibulated women in childbirth. [36] Unfortunately physicians in the United States and the American Medical Association have not been heard from despite several inquiries by **WIN NEWS**.

It is important that African women get factual information, education and support to stop the mutilations in their own families. It must be made clear to African men who still insist on the mutilation of their daughters, even if they have moved to another part of the world, that governmental social services in Europe, in North America and, indeed, all over the world where such services exist are required to protect children and to remove them from families where they are threatened with physical harm. To mutilate a child is a criminal offense, no matter what the African customs. It is only fair that each immigrant family be informed on entering a country where they want to settle, that FGM is prohibited, much like they are informed that they must observe all other laws. .

In the past, the mutilations were practiced in secrecy with the collusion of all international agencies, including UNICEF, who kept silent. This is no longer possible and with more and more refugees from Africa settling all over the world, FGM is spreading unless action is taken to stop it now. Immigrants have to observe the laws of each country where they choose to live. Culture and tradition are no excuses when the life and health of a child are at stake. FGM is not a secret or hidden practice. It goes on in African and Middle Eastern capitals and in at least twentysix countries. The mutilations are also practiced by physicians, by trained health personnel and in hospitals, including all over Egypt.

When I first started to investigte FGM, I had no idea that it was so widespread. After traveling all over Africa repeatedly and visiting maternity hospitals, I became aware that many millions of girls and women were involved. In 1979 at the Khartoum Seminar, I estimated about thirty-five million girls and women were mutilated. Since then I had to more than triple that figure to an estimate of about 110 million, and the numbers are steadily increasing as population growth is very high in Africa (2.5 to 3.5 percent per year average). So far population growth outstrips any reductions of FGM achieved through education and all other actions combined, because most African men are failing to renounce and fail to effectively oppose FGM.

Finally, we must be quite clear what FGM really means for girls and women, which is documented in this report - and we all must speak out. Family violence has also been hidden for centuries - what this really means is male violence and assault including sexual assault against women and girls. It goes on in every society and country - but women are finally speaking out all over the world and are demanding change, as reported in every issue of **WIN NEWS.** In the United States male assault and violence are the predominant causes of injuries and deaths of women - most of them by husbands or "lovers."

FGM is the systematic practice of male violence against girls and women and no matter what the myths, traditions or embellishments - it is a crime. It is practiced to keep women under the control of men - a fact that is frequently and openly stated all over Africa. FGM continues and spreads for one reason: because men support it, men demand it or men tolerate it. If they did not, it would vanish all over the world. The responsibility to act rests on men if they are ever to gain our respect.

To eradicate FGM, since male leaders are refusing to take effective action, we must strengthen African women and provide them with all the resources and the education they need to gain economic independence so they are able to reject FGM, refuse male domination and punish male violence. The future of Africa is in women's hands - women have always been the productive force of Africa. If we really care about Africa we must support African women in every way to bring peace, health and productiveness to this continent which is collapsing due to male violence.

FOOTNOTES

1. Women's International Network-**WIN NEWS**, "an open participatory quarterly journal by, for and about women" started publication in 1975 and reports on women's development from all regions of the world. Editor/publisher Fran P. Hosken, 187 Grant St., Lexington, MA 02173 USA. **WIN NEWS** has featured a section on FGM in every issue since summer 1975, (third issue).
2. Hosken, Fran P. **The Childbirth Picture Book/Program**, - "A picture story of reproduction from a woman's view.", pictures by Marcia L. Williams. Published since 1980 by Women's International Network News, address above. Books, flipcharts, color slides in English, French, Spanish, Arabic (also printed in India in six languages, in Nepal and the Marshall Islands). Additions to prevent excision and infibulation in English, French and Arabic. Nutrition supplements in English, French and Spanish. For community health workers and families worldwide.
3. **The Inter-African Committee on Traditional Practices Affecting the Health of Women and Children**. c/o Economic Commission for Africa, ATRCW, P.O. Box 3001, Addis Ababa, Ethiopia. Inter-African Committee, 147, rue de Lausanne, CH-1202 Geneva, Switzerland.
4. Widstrand, Carl Gosta. "Female Infibulation", **Studia Ethnographica Upsaliensa**, Vol. XX, 1964.
5. Thiam, Awa. *La Parole* **Aux Negresses**. Denoel/Gonthier, 19 rue de l'Universite, 75007 Paris, France, 1978.
6. "College of Physicians and Surgeons of Ontario, Canada Prohibits Female Genital Mutilation". 80 College St., Toronto M5G 2E2, Canada. See **WIN NEWS** Vol. 18-2, Spring 1992, p. 46.
7. "Female Genital Mutilation - Is It Practiced in USA?". See **WIN NEWS** Vol.16-3, Summer 1990, pp. 28-30; From **American Medical News**, 27 April 1990, published by the American Medical Association.
8. United Nations Center for Human Rights, CH-1211 Geneva, Switzerland. "United Nations Seminar on Traditional Practices Affecting the Health of Women and Children". E/CN.4/SUB.2/1991/48 12. June 1991. April 29 - May 3 1991, Ouagadougou, Burkina Faso. See **WIN NEWS** Vol.17-3, p. 31 and 17-4 p. 29-31.
9. Shandall, Ahmed Abu-El Futuh, M.D. "Circumcision and Infibulation of Females", **Sudan Medical Journal**, Vol. 5, No. 4, December 1967.
10. Cook, Robert, M.D. Regional MCH-Nut Advisor, World Health Organization, Regional Office for the Eastern Mediterranean, P.O. Box 1517, Alexandria, Egypt. "Damage to Physical Health from Pharaonic Circumcision (Infibulation) of Females: A Review of the Medical Literature", 1976.
11. Verzin, J.A., M.D. "Sequelae of Female Circumcision", **Tropical Doctor**, Oct. 1975.
12. Baasher, T.A., Dr. (Frc Psych). Regional Advisor on Mental Health, World Health Organization, EMRO, P.O. Box 1517, Alexandria, Egypt "Psychological Aspects of Female Circumcision".
13. Kenyatta, Jomo. **Facing Mount Kenya**. Vintage Books, Division of Random House, New York, October 1965.
14. Lantier, Jacques. **La Cite Magique et Magie en Afrique Noire**. Librarie Fayard, 1972.
15. Hosken, Fran P. "Female Circumcision in the World Today: A Global Review", **Traditional Practices Affecting the Health of Women and Children**, WHO/EMRO Technical Publication No. 2, Vol. 2, 1982 (Background Papers to the WHO Seminar), pp. 195-214. The same article was revised and published as "Female Genital Mutilation in the World Today: A Global Review", published in **International Journal of Health Services**, Editor-in-Chief, Vicente Navarro, Baywood Publishing Co., 120 Marine St., P.O. Box D, Farmingdale, NY 11735 (Vol. 11, #3, 1981, pp. 415-430.).
16. El Dareer, Asma Abdel Rahim, M.D., Dept. of Community Medicine, Faculty of Medicine, University of Khartoum, Sudan, "An Epidemiological Study of Female Circumcision in the Sudan", thesis submitted for the degree of M.Sc. in Community Medicine, 1980/81. See also **WIN NEWS** Vol. 7-2, Spring 1981, p. 37, and **WIN NEWS** Vol. 7-3, Summer 1981, pp. 38/9.

FOOTNOTES (Continued)

17. "Final Report on Position of Female Circumcision in Nigeria", signed by Dr. O.A. Adelaja, Sr. Consultant, Medical Statistics, Federal Ministry of Health, Fed. Secretariat, Ikoyi, Lagos, Nigeria (March 1981). See **WIN NEWS** Vol. 7-3, Sum. '81, p. 41..
18 Pratiknya, Ahmad Watik. Prof., Faculty of Medicine, Gadjah Mada University, Yogyakarta, Indonesia. "Female Circumcision in Indonesia: A Synthesis Profile of Cultural, Religious and Health Values" p. 51-56. **Female Circumcision: Strategies To Bring About Change**. Proceedings of the Seminar on Female Circumcision 13-16 June 1988, Mogadisho, Somalia. published by AIDoS - Italian Assoc. for Women in Development, Via dei Giubbonari, 30 - 00186 Rome, Italy.
19. Ghadially, Rehana, Dpt. of Humanities, Indian Institute of Technology, Bombay, 76 India "The Practice of Female Circumcision among the Bohra Muslims of India", **WIN NEWS** Vol. 18-2 Spring 1992, p.45.
20. Ploss, Heinrich, **Das Weib**. 1885 (first edition / in German) also: Ploss and Bartels **Das Weib** 1886-1908 (second - ninth editions / in German).
21. Bakr, Salah Abu, Dr. "Circumcision and Infibulation in the Sudan: Its Effect on the Innervation of the Vulva", paper presented at the Vth Obstetrical/Gynaecological Congress, Khartoum, Sudan, 1977. (Copy in author's file).
22. Shandall, op. cit.
23. Masters & Johnson, **Human Sexual Response**, Little Brown Co., 1966.
24. Hite, Shere. **The Hite Report**, Dell Publishing Co., Inc., New York, 1976.
25. Taba, A.H., M.D. "Female Circumcision", **World Health**, World Health Organization, 1211 Geneva 27, Switzerland, May 1979, p. 10.
26. Report of the World Conference of the U.N. Decade for Women: Equality, Development and Peace, Copenhagen, 14-30 July 1980, Document #A/CONF. 94/35, p. 34.
27. AIDoS - Italian Association for Women and Development. Via dei Giubbonari 30 - 00186 Rome, Italy. Daniela Colombo, Director.
28. **"Female Circumcision: Strategies to Bring About Change"** - Proceedings of International Seminar on Female Circumcision, 13-16 June, 1988. Mogadishu, Somalia. Report by AIDoS. (See above.) See **WIN NEWS** Vol. 14-3, Summer '88, pp. 28-31
29. Seminar on: **"Traditional Practices Affecting the Health of Women and Children"**, Dakar, Senegal, February 10-14, 1984. Conference report and recommendations: Inter-African Committee (IAC), c/o Economic Commission for Africa, ATRCW, P.O. Box 3001, Addis Ababa, Ethiopia; IAC, 147 Rue de Lausanne, CH-1202 Geneva, Switzerland. See **WIN NEWS**, Vol. 10-2, Spring 1984, pp. 35-36.
30. United Nation Mid-Decade Conference for Women, Copenhagen, 14-30 July, 1980. UN Press Release (Conference Round-Up) WOM/C/P-21, 30 July 1980. See **WIN NEWS** Vol. 6-3, pp. 2-22 (Forum, see p. 20)
31. Inter-African Committee (IAC), Nigeria. Director Dr. Irene M. Thomas. IAC Office, Mandilas Moters Complex, 9-13 Atitebi St., (Off Apapa Rd.), Ebute, Metta, Nigeria.
32. Sudan National Committee on Traditional Practices Affecting the Health of Women and Children. (SNCTP) President Dr. Osman Modawi. P.O. Box 10418 Khartoum, Sudan. See **WIN NEWS** Vol. 17-4, Autumn 1991, pp. 32-35.
33. Koso-Thomas, Olayinka, M.D. **"The Circumcision of Women: A Strategy for Eradication."** Zed Books, Ltd., 57 Caledonian Rd., London M1 9 BU, England. See **WIN NEWS** Book Review, Vol. 13-1, Winter '87., pp. 34-35.
34. Second Regional Conference, Inter-African Committe (IAC), Addis Ababa, Nov. 19-24, 1990. Conference Report available from IAC, address above. See **WIN NEWS**, Vol. 17-1, Winter 1991, pp.38-44.
35. **"The Childbirth Picture Book/Program"**. With additions to prevent excision/infibulation. English/French/Arabic. Also flipcharts and color slides. Published by **WIN NEWS**, see footnote 2. See **WIN NEWS** Vol. 18-3, Summer 1992, pp. 30-33 for summary of campaign to stop female genital mutilation.
36. "College of Physicians and Surgeons of Ontario, . ." Ibid. See Footnote 6.

THE WORLD HEALTH ORGANIZATION SEMINAR:

"TRADITIONAL PRACTICES AFFECTING THE HEALTH OF WOMEN AND CHILDREN"

KHARTOUM, SUDAN - FEBRUARY 10-15, 1979

Unknown to most of the world, a historical meeting for women was held in February 1979 in Khartoum. The Seminar, **Traditional Practices Affecting the Health of Women and Children,**[1] organized by the Eastern Mediterranean Regional Office of the World Health Organization (WHO/EMRO), took place in a quiet conference room of the impressive new Friendship Hall, built with Chinese assistance, on the banks of the Nile. Hosted by the Sudan, official delegations from health departments of nine African and Middle Eastern countries participated as well as observers from many more countries and representatives of United Nations agencies, invited experts and physicians.

Most international meetings hosted by the Sudan are held at that time of the year, as the heat is least oppressive and the twin desert cities of Khartoum and Omdurman, on opposite banks of the Nile, are free of sandstorms that often envelop the whole area later on. The Nile, flanked by large trees, vegetation and green fields, is the life line of this largest but scarcely populated African country. Most of the Sudan is covered by sand and seemingly endless deserts. The land provides a scant living to the many different ethnic groups or tribes who for many centuries have followed their herds of camels, sheep and goats, battling a harsh and hostile environment.

Khartoum is a city of contrasts. On the wide streets, many flanked by sand-filled ditches and sandy sidewalks, one can meet sheep and goats besides cars. Traditional life can be observed in the large market area, surrounded by government buildings and mosques. Most of the trading is done by men dressed in their flowing white robes. A long queue of men waits daily outside the largest movie theater in the center of town. A few women, almost all of them dressed in the traditional tobe - a 6 to 10 yard piece of colored cloth draped around the body and covering the head - can be spotted here and there: But both in modern Khartoum and in the traditional city of Omdurman, most of the shopkeepers, as well as the shoppers and pedestrians - indeed most of the people in the streets - are male. Practically all the people working in the air-conditioned, modern hotels (where the WHO seminar participants were housed), many of them along the Nile, are also men. Yet every day a group of women students from the nursing and midwifery schools of the Health Ministry attended the Seminar sessions, dressed in spotless white tobes. But they never spoke or participated in any way.

The topic of the Seminar, **Traditional Practices Affecting the Health of Women and Children**, which had been prepared by the Eastern Mediterranean Regional Office of WHO included a number of subjects: Nutritional practices and food tabus during pregnancy, traditional practices related to childbirth, breast-feeding, weaning and nutrition of both mother and baby were discussed, also early teenage childbirth and the health problems related to child marriage. But the main subject to which most of the time was alloted was female circumcision. This term is still used in the Sudan - though infibulation is what is practiced all over Khartoum and the Sudan (See "Health Facts and Overview"). In Africa and the Middle East a variety of genital and sexual operations to which young female children are subjected are popularly called female circumcision. This was the first time ever that this subject was discussed from the health point of view at an international gathering.

Delegations from the health departments of the participating countries and UN agency representatives as well as many Sudanese physicians and health officials attended this meeting. Egypt, Somalia, Djibouti, South Yemen, Oman, Ethiopia, Kenya and Nigeria sent health officials, and an observer from Burkina Faso (called Upper Volta in 1979) attended. Many others were invited, especially from West Africa, as the WHO African Regional Office located in Brazzaville, Congo, collaborated in this seminar. But travel difficulties in Africa due to fuel shortages prevented many from coming.

For the first two days, traditional practices relating to nutrition, pregnancy, childbirth and breast-feeding were discussed, but the main subject of the Seminar was female genital mutilation (FGM.). After five days of extensive presentations and discussion four recommendations were unanimously voted by the delegates at the end of this ground-breaking meeting:

- Adoption of clear national policies for the abolishment of female circumcision.
- Establishment of national commissions to coordinate and follow up the activities of the bodies involved including, where appropriate, the enactment of legislation prohibiting female circumcision.
- Intensification of general education of the public, including health education at all levels, with special emphasis on the dangers and the undesirability of female circumcision.
- Intensification of education programmes for traditional birth attendants, mid-wives, healers and other practioners of traditional medicine to demonstrate the harmful effects of female circumcision, with a view to enlisting their support along with general efforts to abolish this practice.

The topic was introduced by Fran P. Hosken with a global review of FGM to document where FGM is practiced today, by whom and how many people are involved as well as what operations are practiced. [2] Then, the delegations from participating countries made their national reports, outlining the situation in their countries from research and case histories, including Egypt, Sudan, Somalia, Nigeria, Djibouti, Ethiopia and Kenya. A number of obstetricians and gynecologists from the Sudan discussed the terrible health problems they encountered daily in their practices and provided some clinical surveys of the incidence of various infections and disabilities resulting from the operations.

Dr. Asma El Dareer of Sudan made a progress report of her findings as the chief investigator of the first and only nationwide study (done province by province) of the epidemiology, that is, the spread and distribution of genital operations to which girls are subjected at different ages. This provided an overview of the situation in the Sudan, showing that the vast majority of the women are infibulated. (see "Case History : Sudan"). Sudan is the only African country where extensive medical and clinical research exists.

One of the informal recommendations that was made at this technical meeting was to hold another similar seminar in Francophone West Africa, where the operations are very widespread, but little research and no clinical surveys have been made. Hardly any reports have been published in the French medical literature.

In 1984, the issue of FGM was finally taken up again, following the above recommendation, at a nongovernmental meeting in Dakar with participants from Francophone countries with the support of WHO and UNICEF and hosted by the Health Ministry of Senegal. At that conference the original Khartoum Seminar Recommendations were re-confirmed and amplified and the **Inter African Committee on Traditional Practices Affecting the Health of Women and Children** was founded, which since then has greatly expanded and is now working all over Africa (see below).

The significance of the Khartoum Seminar is evident from the recommendations which have become an effective basis for all future action. But it took the WHO more than 20 years and a worldwide press campaign by **WIN NEWS** to decide to hold such a meeting to discuss the health problems of FGM. Already in 1958, the United Nations Commission on Women had requested that WHO should investigate the health aspects of these traditional practices. Female genital operations were also discussed at the United Nations seminar on **The Participation of Women in Public Life,** which was held in 1960 in Addis Ababa for African participants. The report on this seminar includes these statements in paragraphs 60/61/62, summarized here:

> "Many participants expressed strong concern at the continuance. . . of those customs and practices which led to the mutilation and scarification of the physical person. . It often caused severe haemorrhage and septicaemia, resulting in some cases in death. By preventing generalized dilation at childbirth such operations. . . endangered the lives of both mother and child. . .

> . . . while it was the duty of all African women to further the development of African culture. . . they should join in condemning those customs which were deleterious to health and indeed dangerous. . .
>
> . . . the view was expressed that the World Health Organization could show that this mutilation has no medical justification and that rather it is harmful to health and should be abolished forever."[3]

In 1975, Women's International Network News (**WIN NEWS**) started to publish a column on FGM where all the facts including the health damage due to genital operations are documented and discussed. Since summer 1975 every issue of this quarterly journal, which is distributed worldwide, reports information about FGM. Before that, the operations were quite unknown, especially among women outside of Africa and the Middle East, and the subject was silenced among UN agencies and all organizations working in Africa (see "The Politics of Genital Mutilation").

WIN NEWS broke this silence and made great efforts to distribute information on FGM as widely as possible. At first journals and newspapers would not print my articles stating "this subject is not acceptable."

In the late 1970s, before the WHO Seminar, my articles outlining the health problems and facts of FGM based on my investigations going to hospital maternities all over East and West Africa and talking to the midwives were published in health and women's journals all over Europe. WHO was repeatedly challenged to at last take up this issue, which they had refused to do for so many years. Finally, my article on "The Epidemiology of Female Genital Mutilation" based on field work and previously published medical articles on FGM came out in July 1978 in the prestigious international medical journal **Tropical Doctor,** published in London.[4]

Shortly after its publication, I was invited by WHO to participate in a Seminar to be held in Khartoum in February 1979 on **Traditional Practices Affecting the Health of Women and Children**. It evidently was organized as the facts that I had documented in this article could no longer be denied - that FGM is a major public health problem that damages the health of millions of women and children in a large region of Africa and the Middle East. Twenty years after the UN Commission of Women first requested that WHO should address the health problems related to FGM, and under the growing pressure of women worldwide, the Seminar was scheduled with Sudan offering to host this meeting.

First, the physical problems of the operations were discussed, mainly by Sudanese gynecologists (See: "Health Facts and Overview"), citing many examples. The psychological problems and dangers were presented next in a research paper by the Secretary of the Conference, Dr. T. A. Baasher, the Mental Health Adviser of the WHO Eastern Mediterranean Regional Office in Alexandria. Dr. Baasher, a physician from Sudan, is quite familiar with all aspects of the problems resulting from the operations. He also explained the Sudanese customs and traditions related to FGM to the Seminar participants. His research paper was an analysis and survey of the opinions of educated Sudanese and Egyptian women on FGM and their personal experiences, based on a questionnaire.

Two of the country reports stand out: the one from Somalia, a ringing appeal to abolish the practice and the one from Egypt because of its comprehensiveness.

Raqiya Haji Dualeh, a delegate and a member of the Somali Women's Democratic Organization (SWDO), delivered the paper of Somalia where "all females with very few exceptions are still subjected to infibulation and frequently at a very young age. . ."

> "Female circumcision may be considered as another form of female sexual oppression, the manipulation of women's sexuality in order to ensure their control, domination and exploitation. In specific terms it serves to harness women into a secondary, submissive role by giving them a negative concept of themselves . . .
>
> The women and people of Somalia consider that as long as women are subject to measures which discrimiate against them or restrict them in the flowering of their human potential and in the exercise of their political and economic rights, their society will become weak. . ."

> Women are victims of outdated customs, attitudes of superiority which men still have. . . The roots of women's sexual oppression, then, can be said to exist in the family, the society, the state, and religion. . ."[5]

After praising the Somali Revolution, Dualeh admitted that women had a long battle ahead:

> "We still have to fight the struggle at the level of traditions, oppressions, prejudices, outmoded concepts and ideologies of contempt for women, denial of their abilities, robbing them of confidence in themselves, and other hangovers from the past. ."

And she expressed hope in the then newly organized Somali Women's Democratic Organization with the help of the Revolutionary Government. She emphasized the need to provide the basis to build a new generation free of traditional prejudices against women's rights, needs, and responsibilities.

> "Among our society female circumcision is still widely practiced. The majority of the population practice infibulation or Pharaonic Circumcision, the most drastic form. . . We believe it is the most cruel and abusive operation that could be done to a human being, the destruction of a human being's physical nature. . . Millions of young girls who cannot speak for themselves are victims of this brutal practice. . .
>
> It is a horrible ordeal and a sad experience for all those women who undergo this cruel operation. Also at marriage time it is a terrible and miserable period of suffering for women, because they have to undergo another operation in order to have intercourse. Many women have problems in childbirth as well as post-partum difficulties.
>
> We want to abolish the custom. It can only be accomplished through education and the emancipation of women. . ."[6]

Dualeh did not describe the operation - infibulation - or the health consequences, since in this technical meeting, the medical problems had already been discussed and were known to all participants.

Dr. Mohamed Warsame, the Director of the Banadir Hospital for Women and Children in Mogadishu, a member of the Somali delegation, estimated that in one year (1978) the costs of taking care of the mutilated women and children brought to the hospital amounted to many hundreds of thousands of Somali shillings - in a country that is one of the poorest in the world. Of course, only a tiny fraction of the inhabitants of Mogadishu, the capital, have access to health services and hospitals (See "Case History: Somalia").

The hopes expressed by Dualeh sound ironic now when this society is literally being torn apart by the horrendous violence of men, victimizing their own women and children most of all, who are brutalized and starving - as shown for months now on TV. Perhaps the senseless violence that has been going on in Somalia between male clans and tribal groups is another manifestiation of the long hidden brutal violence practiced against women and girls, imposed on them by men - infibulation - as Dualeh describes.

The sickening performance of every Somali man of cutting open his bride to satisfy his sexual desires by raping a screaming bleeding girl - wreathing in pain, often hardly more than a child - connotes a depravity and a corruption of values that are hard to fathom, let alone comprehend. And this is sanctioned all over Somalia as an accepted "family tradition". It took great courage for a Somalian woman to speak on the horrendous treatment of women in her country at an international meeting. The same male violence has now erupted all over Somalia with rape and murder of women and children high on the list of atrocities reported daily and shown on TV.

The Egyptian country report consists of several research studies which document that excision of the clitoris, contrary to what is generally believed, is very widespred throughout Egypt, including in Cairo and other cities, and is almost universally practiced in all rural areas. Dayas, the traditional midwives, do much of the operating; so do barbers and physicians as well as trained nurses and midwives in the cities. In addition infibulation is practiced in the upper Nile Valley bordering Sudan, where it has existed for many hundreds of years (See: "Historic Background").

The Egyptian report includes a study by Eleanor W. Smith, Professor of Maternal Child Health Nursing, on "Knowledge and Attitudes of Nurses in Alexandria Towards Female Circumcision", based on a structured interview of 135 nurses working in obstetrics. What stands out in that study is that 33 percent of the nurses asked stated that they would circumcise their daughters either for aesthetic reasons or to decrease their daughters' sexual desire and protect the girls from delinquency. The study showed positive correlation between age and education and the intention to circumcise their daughters. Younger nurses were less inclined to circumcise their daughters than the older ones. More than threequarters of the nurses in the sample were themselves circumcised.

Another study made at a family planning clinic in Cairo in January 1979 was presented by Mary B. Assad. The study shows that 90 percent of the women interviewed were circumcised and nearly half of them had already had their daughers circumcised, while a third more intended to do so. Almost all the respondents stated that their sisters were also circumcised. "Dayas", the traditional midwives performed more than half of the operations; barbers next; physicians operated on 12 percent of the girls and trained nurses did the rest. This had changed little from the mothers' to the daughters' generations, according to the questionnaire.

Most of the respondents answered they experienced fear, severe pain, bleeding, inflammation and urinary disturbances. The reasons given were in this order: attenuation of sexual desire, family custom, hygienic purposes [7]. But what is shocking is that the trained women employed by the family planning clinic had, or planned to, circumcise their own daughters. These are women who teach on reproductive health and contraception.

One must conclude that family planning organizations not only fail to inform the clients they serve about the basic facts about reproduction and how their bodies function, but worse, their own female employees are kept in ignorance about the biological facts and sexuality so they subject their own children to FGM. Family planning in Egypt, as elsewhere, is internationally subsidized using international training methods. As is once more shown here, women's health seems of little concern to the international organizaitons working on population control.

The Seminar participants and delegates developed recommendations after each topic was presented. More health education for the public as well as improvement and enlargement of health services were the principal means recommended for all the subjects discussed from nutrition to teenage childbirth. That was easy. But clearly more specific guidelines were needed for the chief topic of the Seminar - FGM - to which most of the time was allotted.

A committee of five representatives experienced in such matters was charged with preparing the recommendations. Six recommendations were presented on the last day for approval by all the delegates. The first two recommendations were accepted at once (see above). The other four concerned with education and initiatives for change, were condensed into two, after a long and difficult discussion.

Dr. Bertha Johnson, a physician and a psychiatrist from Nigeria and Vice President of the Seminar, asked the crucial question about the last recommendation, concerned with educating health personnel, including midwives, birth attendants, and traditional healers. "Education for what?" she asked. The recommendations, as developed by the committee, simply advocated "intensification of education for traditional birth attendants, midwives, healers. . ." without any mention for or against what. The recommendation, as first drawn up, had left the objectives quite ambiguous.

The question of Dr. Johnson opened a long discussion. She pointed out that, as prepared by the committee, the recommendations could be interpreted to teach health personnel to perform excisions and infibulation operations "better"; that is, more efficiently, using modern tools and antibiotics and even teach how to perform the mutilations in aseptic ways in hospitals. It soon became apparent that it had been the intention of the committee to leave this recommendation "open" for different interpretations. This might have passed except for the vigilance of Dr. Johnson.

This discussion of the last two recommendations went on for hours, and all the different motivations by the participants soon came out. It was claimed by those in favor, all of them men, that to perform the operations "under sanitary conditions" was a good "intermediary step" to save children from infections and other mishaps! Many of the male Sudanese gynecologists supported this "intermediary step".

Dr. R.H.O. Bannerman, a physician from Ghana in charge of theTraditional Medicine Program for WHO in the Geneva headquarters office, insisted that "Africans would not give up their important social traditions", and advocated the "intermediary step". One can but wonder about the claim that a sexual mutilation performed in a Western hospital with Western tools using Western antibiotics is an African social tradition. Dr. Bannerman had been a member of the committee formulating the recommendatins.

This so-called "intermediary step" quickly became the center of the debate. Under the euphemistic cover "to prevent worse harm", the recommendation as first proposed by the committee, would have smoothed the way to perform sexual castrations and infibulations on nonconsenting female children in hospitals by physicians in Africa and the Middle East, with international assistance, financing and support; and the physicians would make handsome profits from the operations.

All the women, led by Dr. Johnson, opposed all ambiguity which could permit the introduction of sexual mutilations into the modern sector with international approval. The question before the participants was not just the formulation of two paragraphs of these recommendations. The question was, Would a WHO-sponsored, international, technical meeting on women's health approve of genital mutilations performed on female children by trained health personnel and physicians in hospitals, including those supported by international assistance? It would also mean that female sexual castration could be subsidized from abroad and eventually introduced all over the world - wherever African immigrants settled. Since most African men refuse to marry women who are not mutilated according to their traditions, FGM would soon spread all over the world with the health care systems at taxpayers' expense mutilating African children at their fathers request , providing a steady income to physicians. That is the reality of the medicalization of FGM, and we should never forget it.

The economic incentives to modernize the operations are, of course, evident. In the Sudan, in Egypt and Kenya, in Nigeria and Mali, and indeed, all over Africa, where these operations are practiced traditionally, trained health personnel, aside from traditional operators, are making a handsome income from the operations. The Egyptian country report, presented earlier, showed that a sizable number of physicians and trained nurses were involved in the mutilations.

In the Sudan, at the Fifth Obstetrical and Gynaecological Congress in 1977, the Secretary of the Women's Union, Kateera Yassin, accused the physicians and midwives of making fortunes from doing the operations on the children of the rich. In the general hospitals of Mogadishu and Bamako, the operations were done routinely, as documented in the country reports. When FGM was prohibited in Kenya in 1982 by President arap Moi in a widely published statement, the chief medical officer of Kenya immediately sent a warning to all hospitals under the Kenyan Health System - including missionary hospitals - that henceforth all female circumcision must stop: This documents that Kenyan hospitals performed FGM routinely. No doubt it is also done in many other hospitals in Africa.

Dr. Bannerman of Ghana is not alone arguing for the continuation of all African traditions- even though speaker after speaker detailed the suffering and health damage. This is an amazing attitude for a physician sworn to uphold health and who works for an international agency concerned with health all over the world. There are all kinds of "enlightened" United Nations officials and others working for international development who still argue that FGM should be performed in hospitals under the pretext that "this will save lives." It will, of course, save the lives of a few children of the wealthy - mostly of politicians - who have access to good hospital services and who will be sexually castrated in a sanitary way. As a result, the plight of the many who are operated on in the rural areas in the traditional environment will continue to be ignored. It will also institutionalize sexual mutilation and provide a large source of income for physicians and health care personnel, who will, therefore, promote the operations.

The modernization and medicalization of FGM were discussed at length at this international technical seminar devoted to women's health. The same issue of performing sexual mutilations as surgical interventions sanctioned by the international health and medical systems comes up again and again. Therefore, it is necessary to be quite clear what we are really talking about.

The real question is: Do we support the introduction into the health care system of an operation on healthy girls which has no medical reason but is designed to permanently impair female sexuality? The operation surgically removes a healthy functional organ and the natural capacity of females to experience sexual pleasure and orgasm. And, do we support a surgical alteration of the normal and healthy personality development of female children to make them inferior to males and subject to control by men?

The physical and sexual effects of the operations are known and have been established. (See "Health Facts and Overview") But the personality changes that these mutilating operations provoke and entail have never been properly investigated and are rarely discussed. Because then the true purpose and nature of the operations would be revealed - which does not change whether the mutilations are performed in the hospital or in the bush. These operations violate the essence of our female sexual beings, the vitality and independence of female personhood and our power of reproduction which men seek to control at any price - even at the price of our lives - as this Report documents.

All kinds of fears are aroused when any planned manipulation of the human personality or psyche is discussed. Such fears are associated by men with political control, as for instance described by Huxley and Orwell. This fear is used to discourage discussion of the fact that these mutilations in reality are a systematic attack by men - using "culture and tradition" as pretext on the female personality by surgical means to make all females submissive to all males.

We must also recognize that these mutilations have a meaning that goes beyond the physical intervention: No matter where or how they are done, they represent a systematic attack by all males on all females, with the objective of establishing male sexual superiority. To gain control over females is, of course, a universal male objective: It is the essence and goal of all patriarchal societies, which are based on the patriarchal family structure. Male bonding - where control of women is concerned - is the real reason why nowhere men have acted forecefully to stop FGM.

In order to effectively deal with the abolishment of these mutilations, it is necessary to recognize that we are concerned here with a basic power issue: The issue is control of female reproduction and sexuality, that is, control by all males over all females - or the ordering of society along patriarchal lines.

These basic motivations were, of course, never stated at this Seminar in Khartoum, nor are they ever mentioned when the subject of "female circumcision" is discussed in the context of the health care system - or what has been cynically called the "modernization of female circumcision to save lives."

The issue of male superiority is basic in all institutional arrangements of the male-dominated health care systems all over the world, with vast political implications: Women are made into disenfranchised recipients and consumers who are being told by male physicians what is "good for them" and what is going to be done to them in the name of "health" - at a staggering price! Men decide on what is done to women's bodies; whether by "tradition" or whether by reason of "health", it makes no difference - as long as it assures male superiority. This became entirely clear in the discussions at Khartoum.

That this is also an international issue is shown by the Western hospital experience where operations, especially if performed on women, have a way of proliferating in proportion to the income they generate for the male-dominated medical profession, as for instance, the proliferation of hysterectomies in the USA shows. The number of hysterectomies increases in proportion to the insurance financing available; and the same is true of cesareans in many hospitals. It also is clear that the modernization of sexual operations of females is a potential source for huge incomes for physicians as well as a means to institutionalize male sexual control over women in modern health care systems especially in African, Arab and Middle Eastern societies.

European and US physicans also have tried repeatedly in the recent past to introduce female sexual mutilations in different forms into the health care system in Britain and the US giving various medical reasons, quite aside from performing sexual operations on their private patients as various cures or to enhance sexuality usually for exorbitant fees (see "The Western World").

There is little doubt that attempts are being made now on many levels with the collusion of male-dominated health systems to spread these operations well beyond their traditional areas in Africa and the Middle East. With increasing mobility, African and Middle Eastern immigrants are settling all over the world and are bringing these mutilations with them wherever they go. The operations have been recently documented among immigrants in France, Great Britain, Sweden, Italy and are said to be practiced in Australia and the USA as well. Helpful physicians are glad to oblige and do the operations - for a high fee, of course. Canada is making an effort to educate the many thousands of Somali refugees to stop mutilating their children with physicians leading thie effort,. while the physicians in the Netherlands are trying to legalize FGM and to introduce the mutilations at taxpayers' expense in the hospitals - under the pretext of "preserving tradition" (see "The Western World" and "Health Facts and Overview").

It is also a curious fact that men who advocate the modernization of genital mutilation as an "intermediary step" - as was done at the Khartoum Seminar - never offer a plan for what to do after the operations are introduced into hospitals and safely institutionalized. How are we ever going to get rid of them?

At the WHO Seminar in Khartoum, after hours of inconclusive discussion during which the Sudanese physicians all spoke for the "modernization" of the operations, Dr. Baasher, as Secretary of the meeting and representative of the sponsoring office of WHO, urged the delegates to consider very carefully if these traditional operations really have a place in modern health care. He asked the physicians and health professionals present to examine if sexual mutilations are an appropriate concern for professionals working to improve health. But Dr. Baasher was the only man who raised the issue of medical ethics. Since then, the issue of "modernization" of female genital mutilation has come up again and again (see chapters "The Politics of Genital Mutilation " and "The Western World").

The refusal by Dr. Bertha Johnson, who was the ranking female physician and elected Vice President of the Seminar, to accept the ambiguous recommendations that were proposed initially, started this whole discussion. It was her vigilance that uncovered the underlying issues of this debate. Dr. Baasher's admonition raising the ethical issues finally settled it: The recommendations were unanimously approved by all participants in an unequivocal form (see above).

In the May 1979 issue of **WORLD HEALTH**, the official publication of WHO, an article "Female Circumcision" was published, written by Dr. A. H. Taba who was the Director of the Regional Office of WHO which organized the Seminar. After a description of the Seminar and its recommendations, Dr. Taba states:

> "These recommendations should be helpful to all the countries concerned in dealing with this problem. Putting them into effect will call for collaborative efforts at all social and political levels, with close coordination between religious, educational health institutions and community agencies at large.
>
> These increasing efforts on the part of national authorities together with collaborative actions at the international level, will make effective inroads into this difficult field. It is to be hoped that the day when female circumcision will be completely abolished is not too far distant."[8]

Dr. Taba's call for "collaborative actions at the international level" is especially important. Until the seminar, FGM was a forbidden subject at international meetings, and all discussion was shunned. United Nations agencies including UNICEF, which is supposed to work for mothers and children, pretended that FGM did not exist and refused to acknowledge the widespread health damage and needless deaths. The Khartoum Seminar, by stating the facts openly and in an international governmental Seminar, opened international discussion, and the article in **WORLD HEALTH**, published in nine languages, put the issue in the public domain: No one can any longer pretend ignorance.

The recommendations, which express the wishes of African and Middle Eastern health departments directly concerned with FGM, open the way for international action and support, including those by governments and private organizations working internationally. These four concise recommendations effectively direct future actions and deal with the essence of what needs to be done: They have and are serving as landmarks.

What is more, these recommendations have removed all the excuses for doing nothing, professed for so long by governmental organizations - including UNICEF and all international family planning organizations led by IPPF (International Planned Parenthood Federation) hiding behind such statements as "we cannot interfere" or "these are cultural traditions" and "such practices exist only in a few remote areas" (see "The Politics of Genital Mutilation").

For instance, IPPF, which had refused to recognize the existence of FGM, printed an abbreviated version of the WHO Seminar recommendations in their magazine, **PEOPLE,** which is distributed worldwide. But what they printed was cut in such a way that it could be interpreted that FGM should be medicalized! My letters of protest were ignored for nearly a year until they finally printed a short correction. IPPF has utterly failed to provide any leadership in this area. In fact, they have ignored FGM until 1988, when they printed my article on the International Conference to Eradicate FGM held in Mogadishu (see "Case History: Somalia"). Then, in 1991, IPPF belatedly recognized the existence of FGM by printing a small leaflet on the subject. No action has followed.

As statistics unfortunately show, only too clearly, family planning all over Africa has utterly failed. The birthrates are the highest in the world and continue to increase in practically all African countries, despite famine and AIDS. But family planning gets more funding than health programs, especially women's healt; therefore family planning programs must be made to deal with FGM.

The WHO Seminar, despite its lack of advanced publicity, received worldwide attention and was reported by the international press all over the world. WHO stated that never before did they have so many requests for information and seminar reports, which were printed in several languages including Arabic. Even UNICEF, the agency designated to work with mothers and children which had failed to participate in the Seminar in Khartoum and afterwards tried to ignore the recommendations, had to finally acknowledge that FGM was a major health hazard for female children as well as a major public health problem affecting the health and lives of many millions of families as I had documented.

The statistics and the figures I initially presented at the Khartoum Seminar had to be increased many times as, at first, the extent of the problem in West Africa remained unclear for lack of documentation. French colonial authorities completely ignored the problem, and no French medical research and publications exist similar to those from Sudan and Kenya and other areas that were under British colonial rule. There are unfortunately no medical research publications by Africans on the subject. Even now, factual information on FGM in Francophone Africa is hard to find (see "Health Facts and Overview").

Population growth in Africa (average 2 1/2 to 3 percent per year) results in the number of mutilations steadily increasing, as so far actions to implement the WHO recommendations have been unable to reduce FGM sufficiently to balance the large number of births. Also, the mutilations, especially in urban areas, are now done on ever younger children where it was formerly a puberty rite. Activities to prevent FGM are based on local initiatives in countries that are suffering from severe economic restrictions. The World Bank/IMF (International Monetary Fund) imposed austerity has resulted in the slashing of all health and education programs that could have dealt with FGM.

In 1982, WHO followed up on the 1979 Khartoum Seminar with a "Statement of WHO Position and Activities." This statement, referring to the Seminar recommendations encourages governments as well as local groups and especially women's organizations, to take action against FGM. But the key statement of this position paper is:

> "WHO has consistently and unequivocally advised that female circumcision should not be practiced by any health professionals in any setting - including hospitals or other health establishments."[9]

This statement strongly reconfirms the opposition of WHO to all attempts to introduce FGM into health care systems, that is, WHO unequivocally opposes the medicalization of FGM.

One would assume that this would settle the issue and stop the debate. But unfortunately, this is not the case as has been shown again quite recently in summer of 1992. Physicians in the Netherlands confronted with a large influx of Somali refugees tried to persuade the health department to introduce FGM into the health care system, which in that country is funded by the government. Therefore, for physicians to get paid for performing the mutilations on female children of immigrants in the hospitals, the government would have to approve. That means women in the Netherlands, or, in fact, in all countries where health care is funded by the government, would be forced to subsidize with their taxes the mutilation of female children of immigrants.

All these ramifications were in the balance in the debate of 1979 in Khartoum which was of enormous importance not only to African or Middle Eastern women who are directly affected but indeed to the status of women everywhere in the world.

There have been many other attempts by physicians to 'medicalize' the mutilations. For physicians to introduce FGM as a legitimate operation is of course potentially enormously profitable, and groups of physicians have tried, quite independently from African customs, to introduce FGM as a counterpart to male circumcision, for instance in the USA. (See "The Western World").

There are, of course, physicians all over Africa as well as nurses, midwives and trained health workers who do the operations for money, using the hospitals and often donated pharmaceuticals and tools. Indeed, I was contacted by a British physician who suggested **WIN NEWS** should publicize his method of doing excisions 'safely.' He wrote as his 'contribution' to women, he was willing to teach this method to anyone concerned. He had developed this method after working in a hospital in Sierra Leone where he saw many cases of girls badly butchered by local excisors. He suggested **WIN NEWS** should announce his offer (see "The Western World").

Given the attitudes by physicians about women, it is essential to continuously emphasize opposition to the medicalization of FGM, quoting the position of WHO.

To implement the WHO recommendations requires a continuing commitment. Even though, as stated above, the Seminar and the recommendations were publicized all over the world, the impact in Africa in affected countries was minimal for some years as I saw myself on a trip through East and West Africa in 1983, where I visited many of the hospitals and maternities I had seen before and talked to WHO and UNICEF representatives, health ministries and women's organizations.

Since the 1979 Seminar was held in Khartoum with the participation of Anglophone countries, it was suggested then to hold another similar meeting for Francophone and West Africa. In October 1980, I was invited by WHO to come for a consultation to their regional office in Alexandria which had sponsored and organized the 1979 Seminar. I proposed to set up a regional educational network to develop and distribute educational materials on FGM with the support of the WHO and UNICEF network. There were no teaching materials or publications on the subject for the general public - and they were very much needed - as I pointed out.

But after the success of the 1979 Seminar, a larger conference by nongovernmental organizations was what WHO preferred to implement the recommendations. I had to point out that Women's International Network was in no financial condition to support such a major conference, nor, as a network, did we have a membership base to take on such a responsibility. Most of all, in order to have any impact and have results, any follow-up actions would have to be organized by African women and in Africa.

Women's International Network continued to publicize the WHO Seminar and its recommendations. To do so in a concrete way, we developed **the Childbirth Picture Book/ Program (CBPB).** A prototype of the book was sent in English and French to UNICEF offices, WHO representatives, family planning and other organizations working in health; it was also sent to midwives and physicians all over Africa for comments and suggestions,

The book and slide program was also shown and discussed at the United Nations Mid Decade Conference in 1980 at the FORUM in Copenhagen. UNICEF had a team of their workers, including some midwives from Africa at the FORUM and Dr. Bertha Johnson from Nigeria, who had played such a pivotal role in the 1979 Seminar, and others came to the meetings to discuss the CBPB and its usefulness.

FGM was now 'presentable' at international meetings due to the Khartoum Seminar, and obviously an issue of concern to women. UNICEF distributed a press release at the Conference offering support to all groups willing to take on this problem. [10]

A panel discussion, including speakers from Kenya, Somalia, Egypt and Sudan, was scheduled in a large conference room, but few people came as "Female Circumcision" was omitted from the announced title. [11] The presentations dealt with health education and each speaker outlined the activities in her country regarding FGM, but no one explained what FGM was all about to an audience that had never heard of it before.

At a meeting where I was scheduled to speak about the spread of FGM around the world, about the WHO Seminar and to provide some factual information based on my research, a group of women led by Marie Angelique Savane from Dakar, the president of an African women's group AAWORD, began to shout and broke up the meeting. AAWORD has a policy of excluding all white women, but it was never made clear where the line is drawn, according to Hitler's racial purity laws or the Apartheid rules of South Africa or what the racial requirements are. Savane used FGM to attract press attention to herself.

Savane also strongly objected to the UNICEF statement offering assistance to community groups in Africa interested in stopping FGM; she charged interference after claiming that African women had other problems. She also published an article in a widely read international journal on children, claiming that FGM was an "important tradition" that African girls looked forward to. [12] The international press used her statements to play up the controversy - which was publicized by the media for years after the Conference in Copenhagen to show that women cannot work together internationally. Savane's activities paid her dividends; she was appointed to a high post at the United Nations in Geneva - her devisive activities did not go unnoticed by male decision makers at the UN.

In 1983, I went on an extended trip to East and West Africa to introduce the **UNIVERSAL CHILDBIRTH PICTURE BOOK** [13] in English and the recently made translation into French, to offer free copies to midwifery schools as well as to discuss their use with health ministries, with UNICEF and WHO representatives and with internationally sponsored health programs. I found that by then the WHO Seminar was forgotten and its recommendations never implemented anywhere, including in the countries that had sent delegations.

The CBPBs were well received everywhere, and we have followed up since by sending many hundreds of books regularly to midwifery schools, to UNICEF, WHO and UNFPA offices all over Africa for distribution, and to hundreds of local groups. The demand by grass roots organizations has been steadily increasing as reported in **WIN NEWS** in the section on FGM, where excerpts are printed of some of the many letters from local health workers and midwives (see "Women and Health"). On the 1983 trip all this was started by personal contact. But it also became clear that an organized effort was needed in every country where FGM is practiced to deal with this problem in an organized way.locally.

The 1984 Conference in Dakar on **Traditional Practices Affecting the Health of Women and Children** organized by nongovernmental organizations (NGO), initiated such an organized effort. Supported by NGOs based in Geneva and with the participation by WHO and UNICEF and the Health Ministry of Senegal, representatives of women's groups from all over Francophone and West Africa came to participate in this meeting which already had been proposed in Khartoum in 1979. This Dakar Conference took up the recommendations of Khartoum and amplified them into an action plan for the IAC (Inter-African Committee) which was founded at that meeting with Berhane Ras Work of Ethiopia, who had organized the conference, as its president. [14] The IAC has its headquarters in Addis Ababa at the ECA (Economic Commission of Africa) working together with the ATRCW (African Training and Research Center for Women) and has administrative and fund-raising offices in Geneva.

At the 1985 UN Decade Conference in Nairobi, the IAC organized an impressive series of meetings with speakers from all over Africa, after silencing women like Savane who could no longer misuse the issue to attract press attention. Against great odds and financial problems, the IAC helped organize local groups in more and more African countries - the latest 1992 count is some 22 affiliated groups from Egypt to Sierra Leone and most countries in between. Many well-known African women joined and organized local groups and numerous information and education programs have been initiated locally. The African leaders of many countries not only have been persuaded to accept the IAC but also have supported the eradication of FGM by their statements. In two countries, major national initiatives were organized independently.*

The IAC organized two regional conferences in Addis Ababa: The most recent one in November 1990 [15] was held in Africa Hall, the headquarters of the ECA. The conference was opened with speeches by the ECA Executive Secretary, by the OAU (Organization of African Unity) representative and the Health Minister of Ethiopia. This official support is remarkable in view of the fact that until the 1979 WHO Seminar, no one in any official position in Africa would acknowledge that FGM existed, let alone speak about it publicly.

The problems of building an organization that spans from East to West Africa including such a diversity of countries are daunting especially on "Traditional Practices" long regarded as an absolute tabu subject. This quite aside from anthropologists who as a profession support all traditions - no matter how damaging for women - as this is how they make their living. Besides FGM, the IAC has taken on other traditional practices that affect women's health, such as nutritional tabus especially for pregnant women, child marriage and other locally practiced damaging traditions, many related to childbirth. All these practices were already discussed in 1979 in Khartoum (see footnote 1).

The IAC has succeeded against enormous odds, not only to gain the support of the African leadership but also to mobilize African women around this issue. They have initiated actions including conferences, meetings, education and training programs of all kinds to raise consciousness and bring the issue out in the open. The 1991 IAC Activity Report, for instance, outlines a variety of actions in some 15 African countries, including Egypt, where the Cairo Family Planning Association started to work against FGM several years before the IAC was organized (see "Country Report : Egypt"). [16]

The IAC has gained support from many organizations as their biannual newsletter reports. They also are now collaborating with AIDoS [17] - the Italian Association for Women and Development - who are adapting the training materials and programs they developed for Somalia for other countries. Teams from several African countries are now beginning to use them in their countries.

All these activities to stop FGM were started by the Khartoum Seminar of 1979 - which not only broke the ice by bringing the issue finally into the international action domain but also provided the guidelines by formulating recommendations which stand out for their comprehensiveness and brevity. To be sure, such action was long overdue. Even now some thirteen years after the Seminar it is still not possible to record any measurable positive results in terms of numbers, and there are still too many people who are not only uninformed on FGM but also unwilling to acknowledge the facts. Typically the international press reporting on African living conditions never mentions FGM.

The immeasurable damage these traditions cause to African families and African economic development is never discussed. In the chapter on Health Facts, a cost accounting method is outlined. But the huge emotional costs and psychological impediments created by these mutilations cannot be measured, quite aside from the appalling, unnecessary human suffering and the loss of productive energy. With AIDS spreading all over Africa more rapidly than on any other continent to which these and other African sexual practices greatly contribute, it seems imperative for African men to finally face the facts and most of all face themselves and their responsibilities.

---

* Somalia under the now evicted President Siad Barre and Burkina Faso are the two countries where major national campaigns were organized with full governmental support. See also **WIN NEWS** section on FGM.

SubSaharan Africa today is the region with more civil wars, more famine, more poverty, more violence than any other region of the world. It has the largest infant and maternal mortality, the highest illiteracy, the worst health conditions and a steadily declining per capita food production. It is also the region where absolute patriarchy is the rule, where women are deprived of property and land rights, where polygamy and wife abuse are the rule and where male domination is absolute both in the village as well in national governments. It is, therefore, clear that men are responsible for the worsening conditions of Africa: women and children are the abused and voiceless victims

The time to blame colonial powers is long since over - but the time for African men to take a look at themselves as persons and human beings in our modern world is long overdue - given the accelerating downtrend of subSaharan Africa according to all worldwide recognized measuring methods. If the quality of life in Africa is to change, African men must change and face their responsibilities. Most of all they must face their responsibilities vis a vis their women, children and families: Because men are responsible for the mutilation of their daughters and their abuse of women, for polygamy and for the killing spread of AIDS as this Report documents. The behaviour of men must change, if African life is to improve. But first of all each man must face himself and change.

FOOTNOTES

1. **Traditional Practices Affecting the Health of Women and Children: Report of a Seminar** (Khartoum, 10-15 February 1979). World Health Organization/Eastern Mediterranean Regional Office Technical Publication No. 2 (1979). WHO/EMRO, P.O. Box 1517, Alexandria, Egypt. (Report available in six languages). Vol. 2, No. 2, Background Papers (1982).
   WHO SECRETARIAT:
   Secretary of Seminar: Dr. T.A. Baasher, Reg. Advisor on Mental Health
   Programme Coordinator, Sudan: Dr. R. Khan.
   Programme Manager, Traditional Medicine, Geneva: Dr. R.H.O. Bannerman.
   Temporary Advisor: Edna Adan Ismail, Training Depart., Health Ministry, Somalia.
   Temporary Advisor: Fran P. Hosken, WIN NEWS, USA.
   Conference Officer: C. Cartoudis Demetrio.
   National Preparatory Committee: Chair: Dr. Hamid Rushwan, Sudan.

   PROGRAM: (Friendship Hall)
   Sat. Feb 10. Opening. Nutritional Tabus and Traditional Practices in Pregnancy and Lactation including Breastfeeding.
   Sun. Feb. 11. Traditional Practices in Relation to Childbirth.
   Mon. Feb 12. Female Circumcision: A Global View/Country Reports.
   Tues Feb. 13. Female Circumcision: Psycho-Social Aspects.
   Wed. Feb. 14. Child Marriage and Early Teenage Childbirth. Summary Report and Recommendations. Closing.
2. Hosken, Fran P. "Female Circumcision in the World Today: A Global Review", **Traditional Practices Affecting the Health of Women and Children: Background Papers to the WHO Seminar**. World Health Organization/Eastern Mediterranean Regional Office Technical Publication No. 2, Volume 2, (1982), pp. 195-214. WHO/ EMRO, P.O. Box 1517, Alexandria, Egypt.

   Hosken, Fran P. "Female Genital Mutilation in the World Today: A Global Review", **International Journal of Health Services**. Baywood Publishing Co.,, 120 Marine St., P.O. Box D, Farmingdale, NY 11735, Vol. 11, No. 3, 1981, pp. 14-430 (An updated version of the above).
3. Document ST/TAO/HR//9 from United Nations Seminar "On the Participation of Women in Public Life". Addis Ababa, 1960, Paragraphs 60, 61 and 62.

FOOTNOTES (Continued)

4. Hosken, Fran P. "Female Circumcision and Fertility in Africa", **Women and Health**, Issues in Women Health Care, Vol. 1, No. 6, Nov/Dec, 1976, pp. 3-11. State University of New York, College at Old Westbury, Old Westbury, NY 11568.
   German Translation:
   "Klitorisbescheidung: Genitale Verstummelung von Frauen in Afrika", **Courage**, Bleibtreustrasse 48, 1000-Berlin 12, W. Germany (Sept. 1978).
   Italian Translation:
   "Mutilazioni Sessuali Delle Donne Africane", **Effe**, Piazza Campo Marzio 7, Rome, Italy (Oct/Nov 1978, Issue IV, #10/11, pp. 3-8).
   French Translation:
   "Les Mutilations Sexuelles en Afrique", **Questions Feministes**, Editions, TIERCE, 1 rue des Fosses-Saint Jacques, 75005 Paris, France. (Vol. #8, May 1980).
5. Dualeh, Raqiya Haji. "Female Circumcision in Somalia", **Traditional Practices Affecting the Health of Women and Children: Background Papers to the WHO Seminar**. Op. cit., pp. 261-264.
6. Ibid. (See also unabbreviated edition cited in the chapter on "The WHO Seminar", **Hosken Report: Genital and Sexual Mutilation of Females** (Second Ed.), published by WIN NEWS, 187 Grant St., Lexington, MA 02173 USA (1979).
7. Assad, Mary B. "Female Circumcision in Egypt: Current Research and Social Implications". **Traditional Practices Affecting the Health of Women and Children: Background Papers to the WHO Seminar**. Op. cit., pp. 229-250. All papers presented at the Seminar are included in this publication.
8. Taba, Dr. A.H. "Female Circumcision". **World Health**, May 1979, p. 12. (Official magazine of the World Health Organization, Avenue Appia, 1211 Geneva 27, Switzerland).
9. World Health Organization, "Female Circumcision Statement of WHO Position and Activities" June 1982. Submitted to the UN Sub-Commission on Prevention of Discrimination and Protection of Minorities. Working Group on Slavery. June 1982, WHO, 1211 Geneva 27, Switzerland. (Copies available from **WIN NEWS**).
10. **UNICEF Information:**"Female Excision: UNICEF's Position", 7 July 1980 (IN80/8) UNICEF Information Division, United Nations, New York, NY 10017.
11. **WIN NEWS** Vol. 6-4, Autumn 1980, p. 42/43 Report from the Mid-Decade Forum/ Copenhagen Forum Panel Discussion / "Sex Education / Female Circumcision".
12. Savane, Marie-Angelique, Sociologist, President of AAWORD, "Matters of Concern: Genital Mutilation", **International Child Welfare Review**, #40, March 1979 (p. 37).
13. Hosken, Fran P. **The Childbirth Picture Book (CBPB) Program - A Picture Story of Reproduction from a Woman's View**, drawings by Marcia L. Williams, **WIN NEWS**, 187 Grant Street, Lexington, MA 02l73 USA. Additions on Excision and Infibulation in English, French and Arabic. (The book is also available in many other languages.)
14. Inter-African Committee on "Traditional Practices Affecting the Health of Women and Children", Berhane Ras Work, President; **Inter-African Committee Activity Report 1991**, and **Bi-Annual Newsletter**; Headquarters: c/o ECA/ATRCW, P.O. Box 3001, Addis Ababa, Ethiopia and 147, rue de Lausanne, CH-1202 Geneva, Switzerland.
15. Second Regional Conference on Traditional Practices Affecting the Health of Women and Children, November 19-24, 1990, Addis Ababa, Ethiopia; Inter-African Committee on "Traditional Practices Affecting the Health of Women and Children" - Berhane Ras Work, President (address above), Conference Report available; See also **WIN NEWS** 17-1, Winter 1991, "IAC Second Regional Conference", pp. 38-42.
16. Cairo Family Planning Association, Aziza Kaamel Mahmoud, Coordinator, 50 Goumhouria Street, Cairo, Egypt "Project on the Physical Violation of Young Females"; See **WIN NEWS** 18-4, Autumn 1992, p. 36. **WIN NEWS** 18-1, Winter 1992, pp. 36-37. **WIN NEWS** 16-4, Autumn 1990, pp. 32-33 and other issues.
17. AIDoS (The Italian Association for Women and Development), via dei Giubbonari, 30 int. 6, 00186 Rome, Italy.

HISTORIC BACKGROUND

To document the history of a traditional practice such as female genital mutilation (FGM), which has existed for more than two thousand years steeped in myths and shrouded by secrecy, is quite beyond the scope of this Report. Therefore, the term "history" needs to be qualified. It is used here to indicate that this chapter deals with the past, as opposed to the present: The objective is to provide the background and access to historic sources that describe these traditional practices that still go on today, much as they did in the past.

To write a true history of FGM would require tracing the many migrations of African peoples from West to East Africa and back, across the huge, inhospitable African deserts and the enormous, almost empty savannahs. It would require investigating the wanderings of migrant ethnic groups and tribes, to examine their feuds, conquests and local wars. It would be necessary to follow the voyages of Arab traders by land and sea and to investigate their far-flung commercial activities and their extensive slave trade: especially their trade in women, in West and East Africa and the Middle East. Written accounts by the many indigenous populations involved in these traditional practices are not available as many of them have no written language and these activities are secret, protected from all outsiders and often steeped in magic and irrational beliefs. In many areas of Africa, FGM is an inherited trade and therefore those who practice it are careful to keep it secret and protect their income and the prestige they derive from this practice.

The origin of female genital operations is unknown. There is no consensus if the operations originated in one area and spread or if they were "invented" by different ethnic groups in different areas at different times. Some claim that they started in the Middle East on the Arab Peninsula and were spread from there by Arab traders. Others claim that this is quite unlikely. Asim Zaki Mustafa, [1] a research assistant in the Department of Obstetrics and Gynecology at the University of Khartoum, states that these operations are so widespread that it is unlikely they had a common origin. Other sources, however, claim that these practices orginated in the Middle East, most likely Egypt.

One thing seems certain: that male circumcision preceeded the female operation, which however, has a different purpose and quite different physical results, even where both operations are undertaken as puberty or coming-of-age rites. It also is a fact that both operations existed long before Moslemization in East and West Africa as well as what today is called the Middle East; but they were accepted and propagated by Islam.

Male circumcision operations are represented in a relief of the Egyptian tomb of Ankh-Ma Hor of the Sixth Dynasty (2340-2180 B.C.). Other Egyptian representations of pharaonic times show the circumcised penis: Male circumcision evidently has been practiced in Egypt for many thousands of years.

No similar records exist for female genital mutilation, though many speculate that it started in the same area as a parallel to the male operation or at puberty. Since the Egyptian records are unique and no similar ones are available from anywhere else, it is impossible to make any conclusive statements either about the origins of the male or female operations or about their spread.

In the absence of any historic, medically-confirmed documentation, the origins of these practices have provided much room for speculation but very few facts. It is, however, certain that in all societies where female excision is practiced, male circumcision is also performed. But the male operation exists in many more societies, both in the past as well as now, than operations on females.

The purpose here is to provide a basic historic record of female genital mutilations by coordinating information from many sources and field work. It is hoped that the many gaps will be filled in by researchers. Much work is needed to gain an understanding of the historic origins of these operations, which are shrouded in magic beliefs and myths, and are distorted by hypocrisy, discrimination, secrecy and sexual tabus.

Unfortunately, Africanists and historians concerned with Africa have not investigated the background of genital operations performed on females. Yet, it appears that on no other continent are these practices so widespread or have found such ready acceptance among so many very different ethnic groups, and they continue to spread today. Genital operations on females, as is recorded in this report, at present also are practiced on the southern part of the Arab Peninsula and along the Persian Gulf as well as by some Moslems in Indonesia and Malaysia. It is claimed that the operations practiced in Asia are of a less-damaging kind than those in Africa (see "Health Facts and Overview").

The absence of historic or social research and documentation on FGM is especially remarkable, since these mutilations have such an important influence on social behavior and on family life as well as on economic and national development. It is also astounding, if one looks at the prolific publications of African researchers, especially anthropologists, to find only silence on this subject. Countless other African customs, including remote practices of specific population groups, have been documented, illustrated, recorded and discussed at academic meetings. However, female genital mutilation has been almost entirely ignored and until recently deliberately excluded as a subject from all academic meetings concerned with Africa and the Middle East.

It was necessary to turn to medical publications to get any facts. The ethnographic and anthropological literature, written mostly by men, ignores the mutilations and conceals their true results and effects on African life. Most of the publications cited here are from British sources covering East Africa - unfortunately there are almost no French medical or factual articles according to a computer search.

Women's lives in Africa have recently been extensively investigated from the viewpoint of development. Numerous publications describe the contributions of African women, many written by Africans. But the customs of excision and infibulation, so widespread all over Africa, which have a dramatic influence on the mental, physical and social well-being of millions of women and children and their health, remain entirely hidden.

It is interesting to note that Alex Haley, who describes himself as a historian, in his well-known book **Roots**[2] never says one word about FGM. Yet he describes life in the Gambia, where his ancestors came from. Even today, most girls in the Gambia and all over West Africa are subjected to these mutilations - with terrible results for their health.

The only book, written by an African woman, that provides substantive research and information on female genital mutilation as well as personal accounts of the operations by the victims, is that of Awa Thiam, **La Parole aux Negresses,** [3] published in spring 1978. The other publication by an African that contains a description of the rituals of excision is the book by Jomo Kenyatta [4] while he was a student of anthropology in London in the 1920s. It is limited to a description of excision performed by the Kikuyu of Kenya, though as a man, he was not allowed to be present at the operation.

The cause of the practice of excision and infibulation is lost in the distant past; typically, no one in Africa today can give a plausible explanation for genital mutilation of girls that is not tied to myths, magic, misconceptions and ignorance of the biological facts. One can only guess how long it has taken to bring about the unquestioned acceptance "as our custom and tradition" of these terrifyingly sadistic and permanently damaging mutilations, that are even now considered an essential requirement for marriage in many African countries. Women still today feel compelled by tradition to mutilate their own children, much as they have done for many centuries - or their daughters would be unacceptable for marriage - the only career and option even today for almost all women in Africa and the Middle East.

The control of women by men, especially of women's bodies and sexuality, goes on in every society - only the means of control are different. Genital mutilations are one way to control the female behavior of a society. Mutilating the genitalia of female children, and thus altering their normal and natural personality development, renders women subservient to men. The final achievement of exerting control over women is to make them internalize the need for their own mutilation and carry out the operations on their own daughters. This can be observed all over Africa today with women stating that "it is required by our traditions"

Everywhere, secrecy is paramount. The operations have been traditionally surrounded by tabus, and this continues at present. In some areas, especially in West Africa, for instance in Sierra Leone, there are threats and penalties for revealing what takes place at the initiations of the secret societies of women - called "Bundu". These initiations include excision and surround the actual operation with magic of all kinds. The prohibition against revealing the secret proceedings is said to be so potent that no one dares to describe them, even now. How old these rites and beliefs really are, no one knows; they are handed down from generation to generation, nothing is written down. For an eyewitness account of a traditional initiation. (See: "Case History: Sierra Leone")

Nevertheless, it appears that both in the past as well as now, the immediate physical danger of the operations was and is known. The extirpation of sexual satisfaction of women - indeed, the sexual castration of women - is the purpose of the operations, as stated throughout the historic literature. However, the dangers of the operation for childbirth were and are not understood. Deaths in childbirth of both mother and child are never related to the operations, and this continues to be hushed up and ignored today. The highest maternal and infant mortality rates in the world are documented in the regions of Africa where female genital mutilations are widely practiced, a fact that has never been acknowledged by any internationally sponsored health or family planning programs.

The continuing silence about genital mutilation has no excuse. The ignorance about their own bodies and health - which is the lot of women everywhere, especially where women are illiterate and segregated - is the cause of endless and needless suffering.

There is one basic difference between past and present that must be made clear from the start: The practices described here were performed traditionally in the absence of any knowledge of the medical fact or biology. The basic health and sexual facts are now available to everyone who can read; they could also be made available to everyone who can listen to a radio or look at pictures but they are not. Such knowledge is available in every country where these operations exist; however, this information is retained by a political professional elite who are not making it available to the majority of the population who practice these mutilations.

Information and education about women's health and especially about reproduction and sexuality continue to be concealed, distorted, exploited and misused everywhere in the world for the purpose of controlling women. There is no valid reason today for concealing from women the knowledge and health facts about sexuality and reproduction that girls and women most urgently need. What is different today from all the past and the history given here is that we have mass communication tools. Why, then, don't male African leaders free their populations of such damaging practices and myths that are contrary to their national as well as personal goals of modernization and development?

There is no excuse for the continuing silence about genital mutilation!

Ploss and Bartels **Das Weib** [5] **(Woman)*** is the most frequently used historic source. Ploss and Bartels are quoted and requoted throughout the medical and anthropological literature up to the present time. None of the writers who quote this work have checked to see if the practices described still exist today. Medical writers especially often use Ploss as reference for the spread and incidence of the operations, though the descriptions are nearly 100 years old and unconfirmed.

---

*The original edition of **Das Weib - in der Natur und Volkerkunde (Woman - An Ethnographic Study)**, by Dr. Heinrich Ploss, goes back to 1885. Dr. Ploss was a famous German physician who published many articles on medical anthropology. His other well-known historic work is **Das Kind (The Child)**. Dr. Ploss died at the end of 1885 and the first edition of his book was exhausted within one year. The Anthropological Society of Germany then asked Dr. Bartels to develop another edition, using the extensive research that Dr. Ploss left behind. From then on, numerous steadily enlarged editions were published, edited by Dr. Bartels. In 1935, the work was finally translated into English, edited by Eric John Dingwall (William Heinemann Medical Books Ltd., London, 1935). A contemporary version called "Femina Libido Sexualis" is the same book by Dingwall, arranged by J. R. Brosslowksy, published by the Medical Press, New York, 1965.

Reliable primary sources of historic facts about genital mutilations of females are very scarce. What is more, one soon discovers that researchers use the same original records that are reworded according to the interpretations of the male writer.

In the absence of publications by Africans, written historic information for the most part consists of observations by travelers in East Africa, Egypt and the Sudan and information by ethnographers and physicians. Almost all are men. Sources about female genital mutilation from West Africa are even more limited. Indigenous reports, if they exist, have not been published. It is hoped that this account will be instrumental in bringing to light new information by African historians.

Two types of operations are described in the literature: excision/clitoridectomy and infibulation. The term "infibulation" as explained by Widstrand [6] and others is derived from the Latin "fibula", which means a clasp. A fibula was used by the ancient Romans to hold together the folds of their toga, a loose garment worn by both men and women. A fibula or clasp in the form of a ring was put through the prepuce or foreskin of gladiators or slaves in Rome to prevent them from tiring themselves with women. There are also other reasons given; but the objective was to prevent sexual intercourse. In the case of women, one or more rings were inserted through the labia to enforce chastity. Sometimes, additional devices were used, such as tying together the rings or closing them with a padlock. Slave girls in ancient Rome were infibulated in this way to prevent conception, as childbearing would hinder their work, a practice evidently learned from the Middle East.

This mechanical method of infibulation, which is also described by Remondino [7], besides being practiced on slaves in ancient Rome, was also documented in a few isolated cases in Europe much later (see "The Western World"). The practice is well-known to the veterinary profession. For instance, the infibulation of mares is done when the horses are sent out to pasture to prevent them from conceiving.

The Oriental method of infibulation, which is discussed here, is accompanied by excision/clitoridectomy and means the closing of the vulva by scarification and practiced still today. The two raw sides of the partially sliced off labia majora are held together with various devices until a scar is formed, which closes the entrance to the vagina except for a tiny opening for elimination of urine and menstrual blood.

When excavating Egyptian graves, archaeologists found mummies that were excised - so state several medical publications from Egypt and the Sudan. Some archaeologists claim that the mummies were so well preserved that not only clitoridectomy could be established but infibulation as well. Others deny the mummies were infibulated, but it is generally agreed that excision was practiced already in ancient Egypt by the ruling class.

For instance, in a general discussion of female circumcision, Dr. A. Huber [8], who worked for many years in Ethiopia, states that in a female Egyptian mummy of the 16th century B.C., signs of excision were detected. Dr. Shandall [9], in his study of female circumcision and infibulation in the Sudan, states that "A large number of circumcised females were found among the mummies of ancient Egyptians, but only a few infibulations were encountered."

"Infibulation was practiced by ancient Arabs long before Islam" [10], relates Dr. Shandall; and he adds that this was done to protect shepherd girls against likely male attacks, while they were out alone minding the sheep.* Protection against rape is frequently cited as a reason for infibulation in Sudan and Somalia, even at the present time.

Herodotus (484-424 B.C.) found the ancient Egyptians practicing excision when he visited their country around the middle of the 5th century B.C., and he reports on it.

---

*This reasoning must be questioned. What is to prevent a rapist from doing what every bridegroom does: accomplish penetration by force and/or by using a knife? Infibulation does not protect against rape. This implies that every man in societies where women are mutilated or segregated is out to rape every female he meets. It also establishes that men are unable to control their sexuality and not women, as claimed in Sudan and other Moslem societies.

A Greek papyrus in the British Museum dated 163 B.C. refers to operations performed on girls in Memphis at the age when they received their dowries. The Egyptian physicians Drs. Karim and Ammar added that there is an Egyptian plaque from about the same time (160 B.C.) "recording the details of a legal suit to recover the costs of clitoridectomy." [11]

In the 14th edition of **Das Weib**, by Ploss and Bartels, the same story about the girls of Memphis is related. Many medical writers repeat this story from Ploss/Bartels, often without specific reference. From this report, it was concluded that all girls in Egypt were subjected to circumcision at the time they were given their dowries, that is, just before marriage. Widstrand also refers to the same papyrus in the British Museum which describes the legal proceedings to recover the money given to the mother of a girl "for excision and dowry".* Some sources related that clitoridectomy was a sign of distinction and was practiced first on the females of the royal families of Egypt. It was also reported that women in ancient Egypt could not inherit unless they were circumcised.

Strabo, the Greek geographer, reported at about 25 B.C., that this operation on girls was a custom in Egypt when he visited this country. Strabo also described the people he found living along the East Coast of the Red Sea and calls them "mutilated"; he states that they excise their women like the Egyptians.

In a research study of a Nubian village in upper Egypt, John G. Kennedy [12] states that female circumcision was a custom of ancient Egyptians. The operations continue today much as in the past. Kennedy describes that the mutilations are performed on girls in Nubia long before puberty, accompanied by the chants of Koranic incantations and by shouting by the assembled women to drown out the screams of pain by the victim. The operation he describes actually is infibulation and the rituals quite resemble what is practiced in Khartoum and all over the Sudan at the present time: All kinds of precautions are taken against the threats by evil spirits or "jinns" who are believed to be dangerous and are said to be attracted by genital blood.

In Egypt and Sudan, traditionally and up to the present time, it is claimed that the only way to blunt the sexual wildness of girls and preserve their chastity is through excision and infibulation because women have an inherently wanton character which is physiologically centered in the clitoris. Since the family honor, according to Arab tradition depends on the virginity of the daughters, their purity has to be protected by excision and infibulation, as females are unable to control their sexuality.

Many texts try to relate FGM, historically, to the male operation. The male operation was widely practiced in the Middle East in ancient times, including in Egypt. It is reported by all sources that the male operation was practiced much earlier than operations on females.

The Mufti of the Sudan, Sheikh Ahmed-el-Taher, stated:

> "Circumcision was a practice followed by the Prophets and the first of them to be circumcised was the Prophet Abraham. The Koran says: 'When his Lord made trial of Abraham by commands which he fulfilled' Sura II, Verse 110." [13]

Some anthropologists also speculate how or if the tradition of male circumcision, the removal of the prepuce, is related to cutting off the entire penis which was offered as a sacrifice to the gods. This is said to have been practiced in Ancient Egypt. The custom to use the male genitals as war trophies was also widespread, as reported in Middle Eastern history, and has also been recorded by the ancient Egyptians.

The Gallas, Somalis and the Abyssinians, it is related, cut the complete genital apparatus off their enemies. Some warriors offered the genitalia of their enemies as trophies to the girls they chose to marry. To use the male genitalia as war trophies continues to the present in some parts of Africa; for instance, it was reported in the two recent upheavals in Zaire- in Biafra and Shaba Province. It was also reported in the Vietnam war.

---

* The document in question is in the British Museum, ed. F. G. Kenon, London, 1892, N. 24, p. 32, according to Widstrand.

Circumcision of both boys and girls came into fashion long before Islam and was practiced in many different areas in Africa. The practice was unknown to the Romans until they conquered Egypt and the Middle East. The Copts in Egypt and the Abyssinians (Ethiopians) have practiced circumcision of boys and girls (at a much younger age than the typical puberty rites of sub-Saharan Africans) from prehistoric times.

It is stated that both the Jews and the Arabs learned circumcision in Egypt, rather than vice versa. The rule in the Middle East, as well as in sub-Saharan Africa, is that a boy cannot get married unless he is circumcised. The same rule applies to excision, which has acquired much the same rhetoric and similar, though less important, rituals as the male operation. All rituals connected with men are more important than those with women in the Middle East as well as in most of Africa because of the dominant position of men. But the real purpose and the result of excision and infibulation are quite the opposite of the male operation, though they are often correlated, a fact which was and is not at all unknown to the practitioners.

The origins of excision and infibulation are also discussed by Awa Thiam [14] and others stating that excision goes back to the prophet Abraham - whose first wife, out of jealousy, had one of her co-wives excised. Assitan Diallo from Mali, in her thesis on "Excision Among the Bambara" [15], writes that excision has existed in West Africa long before Islam was adopted by the Bambara (see "Case History : Mali"). It is practiced to affirm the sex of the individual because it is believed that the clitoris represents a male element in a female and that the prepuce of the penis represents femininity in a boy. Hence, the girls are excised and the boys circumcised in order to establish their sex in society.

In all the literature, it is stressed time and again that genital mutilation is not a religious rite but rather that it is a custom of the people or certain ethnic groups. It was and is practiced by members of all religious denominations in Africa, including Christians; that is, Copts, Ethiopian Christians, Catholics and Protestants as well as Animists and Moslems, none of whom oppose it on religious grounds. Neither does the leadership of any of the Christian or Moslem denominations publicly speak against the mutilation of female children. However, some Moslem leaders propagate the operations on girls in the name of religion, especially in West Africa, and have done so throughout the past. Animists often state that the operations are done because it is "the wish of the ancestors."

In classic Arabic, female circumcision or clitoridectomy is called "Khafd", but the term "Taharo" is more frequently used - both mean purification. It is widely believed for instance in the Sudan that a female is polluted and must be "cleaned" by excision before she can become a woman and is fit for marriage (= child bearing).

Mohammed, the Prophet of Islam (580 A.D.) advised his followers against practicing a drastic type of operation. Shandall quotes the exact statement of Mohammed (in two versions) who is alleged to have said to a woman who was performing circumcision in the Medina "do not go deep; this is enjoyable to the woman and preferable to the man" (Omatiya); the other version frequently quoted is "do not go deep. It is more illuminating to the face and more enjoyable to the husband" (Razeen). (See "Case History : Sudan").

In Moslem literature, this statement is attributed to Mohammed: "Circumcision is an ordinance in men and an embellishment in women."

One must ask: Why did Mohammed the Prophet not speak against the mutilations of females? His advice, "Do not go deep", has furthermore been quite ignored by the Moslem religious leaders. Infibulation (Pharaonic Circumcision) - that is closing the entrance to the vagina by various devices or by scarification after excising the clitoris - today is performed only by Moslems, according to all available records. But no religious justification can be found anywhere to support infibulation. On the contrary, it is said to be against the Moslem prescription to hurt or injure anyone. It appears that the Moslem religious leadership has entirely failed to communicate the true creed to their followers, many of whom mutilate their daughters claiming "it is demanded by their religion." This is said, for instance, in the Sudan.

Contempt for uncircumcised women by Moslems is mentioned frequently in the literature. Indeed, one of the worst insults in Moslem Africa and especially in the Sudan is to be called "son of an uncircumcised mother."

Moslemization is rapidly progressing in Africa. Local Marabouts (Moslem holy men) in West Africa are reported to advocate genital operations by stating that the operations have religious importance and that they are "demanded" by the Koran. In a study made in 1991 in rural Senegal by ENDA (Environmental Development Action in theThird World) the local Moslem religious leaders insisted that FGM must be continued on religious grounds and rejected all change .

Moslem women are often led to believe that FGM is a Moslem religious command. Since there is no central authority in Islam (such as the Pope with the Catholic Church), a large number of "interpretations" of the Koran exist in different countries. The different interpretations of the Koran depend on local customs and are used by the local religious leaders to support patriarchal power and male privilege by curtailing women's freedom and access to education using religion. But the concept of the inferiority of the female is firmly anchored in the basic Islamic philosophy of the segregation of the sexes.

H. H. Hansen reports about his interview in 1965 with the Grand Mufti Sheikh Hasan Mahmoon, who was at the time the supreme religious authority in Egypt and the Chancellor of the influential Moslem Al-Azhar University.[16] The Grand Mufti stated that the operation consisted in the removal of the external genitalia of girls of eight to ten and that the term "taharo" which means purification, is frequently used for the procedure. The Grand Mufti was well informed on genital mutilation and so is the highest Moslem leadership in all countries where the operations are practiced, as FGM is done on their own children. Marriage is compulsory according to the Moslem religion and its wealthy leaders all practice polygamy; thus their experience with genital mutilation is firsthand.

No Moslem leader today or in the past has publicly opposed FGM, according to the literature. Only one published statement on the subject is available from the Moslem religious authorities in the Sudan, made in 1945 before the legislation prohibiting the operations was passed upon urging by the British Administration, and that statement falls far short of a prohibition on religious grounds. (See "Case History : Sudan".)

Since historically Egypt and the Nile Valley and the Red Sea coast were centers for female genital operations, one cannot help but wonder if these practices were adopted by the Jews during their stay in Egypt. Elizabeth Gould Davis writes: "The Jews. . . denied that they practiced it upon their daughters, but there is evidence to the contrary."[17] She quotes Sir Richard Francis Burton as saying that the rite was practiced by the Jews until the days of Rabbi Gershom (1000 A.D.), who denounced it as a scandal. The only Jewish population group in Ethiopia, the Fellashas, who lived near Gondar, practiced the operation on their girls to the present time. The Fellashas as Jews were recently brought to Israel by air as a result of the Ethiopian famines and political upheavals.

The earliest description of infibulation in the historic literature is that of a Venetian historian called Pietro Bembo, in a posthumous history published in the middle of the 16th century. He transmits reports of travelers to the Red Sea: "These areas are inhabited by black, exellent men, brave in war." Bembo then describes that in this part of Africa, virginity is held in such high esteem that "the private parts of girls are sewn together immediately after birth. . . when adult, the girls are given away in marriage. . . The husband's first measure is to cut open with a knife the solidly consolidated private parts of the virgin." [18]

In the medical literature, the astonishing notion that the clitoris has to be amputated on medical grounds begins to appear early: Soramus, a Greek physician who practiced about 138 A.D. in Alexandria and Rome, supplied a detailed description of the operation of excision, including what instruments were used. He also claimed that "In some cases the clitoris is so large that it presents a shameful deformity," which brings about over-excitement and excessive sexual intercourse (venery). Soramus treated such cases by cutting away with a scalpel "what seems to be too much." [19]

Aetius, another physician (502-575 A.D.) as quoted by Karim and Ammar, describes the operation in similar ways. He approved of the Egyptian custom of amputating the clitoris of a girl "before it grows too large." The girl is placed on a chair and her legs are held open by a person sitting behind her. "The surgeon standing in front seizes the clitoris with a large pair of forceps and pulls it out with his left hand; with the right hand, he resects the body close to the teeth of the forceps." [20]

Paul (or Paulus) of Aegina, a Greek physician in the 7th century A.D., described the same operation, stating that an enlarged clitoris is a shameful thing that could "erect like a penis and could be used for lesbian coitus,"[21] so Karim and Ammar report.

Asim Zaki Mustafa (see above), in his research article about female circumcision and infibulation, states that Jesuit missionaries came to Abysinnia (Ethiopia) by the late 16th century and converted the people to Roman Catholicism. They met great resistance when they tried to prohibit the excision operations on girls as "pagan." Mustafa quotes almost verbatim from Dr. Sequeira, who wrote several years earlier about the same event in an article in the **Lancet**[22], a British medical publication. Sequeira states he learned what he described from Ploss.* In the fourth edition of Ploss, it is related that when Roman Catholic missionaries first came to Ethiopia, they prohibited excision because they thought it was a Jewish rite; but when the girls were grown up and ready to get married, "those parts" were sometimes so large and protruding that they were offensive to the eye and to the touch.

When the men were ready to choose wives, they rejected the Catholic converts and instead married girls who had undertaken excision. "Thus the Catholic community diminished and the people returned to their heathen misconceptions", Ploss reports.

The missionaries appealed for help to Rome, to the Collegium of Cardinals "de propaganda fide" (for the propagation of the faith), who sent a mission of skilled and experienced physicians to make a clear report about the facts of this situation.

These physicians declared, when they returned, that either through the heat of the climate, or some other natural condition, such a change in the development "of these parts" resulted, that they were very different from the women in other countries. This situation created disgust in the men; consequently, it was an impediment to marriage. As a result, the Catholic clergy agreed to the operations, but they asked the people of Ethiopia to declare that this operation "in no way had any Jewish religious intentions. . ." It was then determined "that all impediments for marriage should be eliminated." Thus, excision was, and is still today, sanctioned by the Pope and the leadership of the Catholic Church.

In the 18th century, James Bruce, the famous Scottish explorer, who rediscovered the source of the Blue Nile, travelled south along the Red Sea (1768). He went inland to Gondar, which was then the capital of Ethiopia. Ploss reports that Bruce was told when he visited Ethiopia (then called Abyssinia) that the abnormal size of the clitoris of Ethiopian women was a hindrance to reproduction. Therefore, to remedy this evil, the parts that protruded were cut off. "All the Egyptians, Arabs and the nations in the southern area of Africa, including the Agows, the Gafats, and Gonges, undertake these operations on their children," Bruce relates. "No specific time is set; however, it is always done before they get married."[23]

Dr. Sequeira, in his article in the **Lancet**, notes that "a congenital hypertrophy of the pudenda is common in Abyssinian women."[24] But he presents no medical evidence or case histories, nor does he define what is meant by "hypertrophy." Similar statements about hypertrophy of the clitoris can be found in all subsequent medical publications on the subject of clitoridectomy that give Sequeira in their bibliography. But no medical writer presents a shred of evidence or a single, firsthand observation as to what this alleged hypertrophy is all about.

Dr. Alfons Huber[25], an Austrian gynecologist who worked for many years in Ethiopia in the 1960s, states that he himself has examined many thousands of Ethiopian women of all ages. He never found any "hypertrophy" or unusual enlargement of the female genital organs or clitoris to be any more frequent in Ethiopia than elsewhere.

In 1977, I inquired in Addis Ababa at the largest family planning organization of Ethiopia if they had observed any hypertrophy of the genitalia of Ethiopian women. They had not observed any abnormalities. And family planning clinics are in a good position to know, since they insert IUDs.

---

*This shows again that most of the information on the subject is copied by different researchers from Ploss without any verification.

During the circumcision controversy in Kenya in the 1920s and 1930s and beyond, when Protestant missionaries, led by the Church of Scotland Missionary Society, prohibited the operations to their converts, the Catholic leaderhsip did not object to the mutilation of the daughters of their converts. The Catholic Church never did anything to discourage the mutilations of female children. The results are reflected today in the much greater number of excised girls in Catholic parishes in Kenya as compared to Protestant girls, as Jocelyn Murray established in her study of the controversy surrounding the prohibitions of female circumcision in Kenya. [26] (See "Case History : Kenya").

It should be added here that Catholic missionaries have officially condoned the operations everywhere in Africa, with the blessing of the Pope, ever since the envoys from Rome established the "necessity" for the operations at the end of the 16th century in Ethiopia, no matter how many girls and women died as a result.

Nor did the Christian Ethiopian Orthodox Church ever oppose genital mutilation, though it was all-powerful until recently. Practically all Ethiopian girls are excised, usually before 40 days old. In Ethiopia, this custom is strictly guarded and surrounded by secrecy, and it is especially concealed from foreigners. For instance, Dr. Huber reports that a Swiss man named Ilg, who was the personal advisor of Emperor Menelik (who ruled in the latter part of the 19th century), had lived for many years in Ethiopia and knew the country very well. Yet, Ilg had no idea that female circumcision even existed!

Dr. Huber also states that according to the oldest records of Ethiopian legislation, female circumcision is considered to be a "religious custom" but not a law. In the articles of faith of the Emperor Claudius, who ruled in the 16th century in Ethioipia, female circumcision is mentioned and defended in the meetings with the emissary sent by the Pope. Evidently, this representative of the Roman Catholic Church thought that female circumcision was a religious command, much like male circumcision of the Jews; and therefore, he objected to the practice. The Emperor claimed that it was a custom of the people, much like tatoos or facial scarring, and had no religious significance.

M. Niebuhr, the German traveler and sole survivor of the first European scientific expedition to Arabia, Egypt and Syria, reported on the practice of excision in 176, and stated that "In Oman, on the shores of the Persian Gulf among the Christians of Abyssinia, and in Egypt among the Arabs and Copts, this latter custom was prevalent. Much has been said concerning the origin of the custom. . . which seems, at first view, so absurd." And he states that "Out of cleanliness, and to render ablution easier, that the practice of circumcising women has been first adopted. No law has appointed it. . . it is usage, not a religious duty." [27]

Nearly 100 years later, Sir Richard Francis Burton (1821-1890), the indefatigable voyager and linguist who traveled all over the world, described his experiences in his books about Asia, Africa and the Americas. He mastered dozens of languages including Arabic, and made the pilgrimage, forbidden to nonbelievers, to Mecca and Medina in 1853, disguised as an Arab notable. He reported this feat in a book published in 1855/ 56 . [28] While exploring Africa, he visited Ethiopia, found Lake Tanganyika and searched for the source of the Nile.

Of course, Burton knew African and Middle-Eastern society and customs intimately. He reports in a footnote* written in Latin in the book on his pilgrimage to Mecca and Medina that circumcision among the Arabs is the practice for both sexes, relating the story of Abraham. He states that excision, the amputation of the clitoris - the seat of pleasure, according to Aristotle - is performed because otherwise the women would be insatiable and indulge in excessive sexual intercourse.

---

* Burton's footnote on female circumcision is written in Latin, evidently so that the average Victorian reader of his famous travel books would not be shocked. Nevertheless, it was taken out by the publisher from the later editions. However, after his death, his wife Isabel Burton edited his works and put it back in. In the edition of 1898, on pages 19 - 20, the entire footnote in Latin is printed.

Burton also talks about the immoderate growth of "these parts", therefore, amputation is necessary. He also describes the effect this allegedly has on coitus for men. He relates that the Somalis, besides the clitoris, cut off the labia and all external genitalia as well, and adds that female circumcision is practiced universally throughout the Egyptian area (Egypt at that time controlled a very large part of the Middle East).

Burton spent most of his life traveling and had a unique ability to adapt himself to local customs; he lived undetected for long periods of time among the Arabs and the people of Ethiopia and Somalia. He also went on many voyages including one to Harar (inhabited by Somalis). In his book **First Footsteps in East Africa** [29], the marriage customs are explained:

> "The Somali, when they can afford it, marry between 15-20; the marriage portion (bride-price) may be as high as fifty sheep. Dowries are unknown. The arrangements are made by the parents. The bride, as usual in the East, is rarely consulted. Sons of chiefs, arrived at manhood, immediately marry four wives. They divorce the old and unfruitful ones. . . allow themselves an unlimited number. . . Daughters, as usual in Oriental countries, do not 'count' as part of the family. They are, however, utilized by the father, who disposes them to those who can increase his wealth and importance. Divorce is exceedingly common." [30]

The marriage, he stated, is celebrated in the towns with feasting and music. "On first entering the nuptial hut, the bridegroom draws forth his horsewhip and inflicts memorable chastisement upon the fair person of his bride."

Burton also reports that right after the wedding, "during the space of a week, the spouse remains with his espoused, scarcely ever venturing out of the hut." [31] Burton did not explain the reason why the bride could not leave the house: after her infibulation had been cut open, she had to remain secluded with her legs spread apart, until the wound was healed. She was subjected to frequent sexual intercourse, as custom required, until the newly cut opening to her vagina assumed the size needed by her husband for penetration for his pleasure.

Burton's observations coincide with those made recently, especially by Annie de Villeneuve [32], as well as by Dr. Guy Pieters [33] (See "Case History : Somalia"). At my visit to Somalia in 1979, the same custom of locking a bride and bridegroom into a room for about a week still goes on according to discussions with midwives in Mogadishu. The bridegroom is honor bound to penetrate the wife he has acquired for a steep price - after opening her with a knife or other sharp instrument, as his natural weapon is usually unable to overcome the artifically created obstruction. Intercourse then is frequently repeated through the open wound to keep it from closing again - without any regard for the terrible pain inflicted. The helpless bride, who often has barely reached her teens, must remain on her back with her legs wide open for days to keep the wound and vagina from closing. Women remember with horror their weddings for the rest of their lives.

In a letter in the Munger Africana Library of the California Institute of Technology in Pasadena written by Sir Samuel Baker White, he discusses infibulation of young girls which he observed in East Africa. Sir Samuel explored the sources of the Nile in 1861, discovering Lake Albert in 1864. He describes infibulation as an operation to insure chastity and a practical preventive measure which makes connection with the male organ impossible. A sketch shows how the labia are cut and sewn together, with a reed inserted to keep a tiny aperture and he describes the wedding night:

> "On the night of marriage, the cicatrice is reopened by a pointed instrument and one rip does it. The girl is then led immediately to the hut of her husband and thrust in while the bridesmaids wait outside the door until the husband appears and gives them a bloody cloth as proof of his wife's virginity." [34]

A drawing of the curved, pointed knife used to rip open the scarred genitalia accompanies this letter.

Widstrand also quotes from a great many accounts of travelers to Egypt and the upper Nile Valley - the present-day Sudan - who describe genital operations on women and remark on these terrible customs. Several state that despite or because of infibulation, virulent syphilis is frequent.

Ruppel, one of these travelers, describes the situation from his voyage in 1829:

> "The removal of the occlosure or opening of the vulva does not take place before the brideprice is paid, and the opening is made to suit the husband - larger or smaller. When the time of birth approaches, the vulva is opened more by a few new incisions and after the partus the hole is closed again. This closure remains intact as long as the child is nursed, and then a new operation is prepared. This procedure is repeated, three, four times. . . the husband decides the matter." [35]

To what length the obsession with virginity and the manipulation of women's genitalia can be carried is detailed by another traveler, Pallme, who went to Kordofan (Sudan) in 1843. He writes that at the time of marriage, "the bridegroom presents a model in clay or wood of his erected membrum, which is used as a measure when the bride is opened." [36]

A similar story is related by Ashley Montague, where he quotes from a description of Werne from 1853.

> "When a girl whose virginity has been preserved in such a revolting manner becomes a bride, further cruelties are practiced. One of the women who perform infibulation visits the bridegroom immediately before marriage in order to obtain exact measurements of his member. She then makes to measurement a sort of phallus of clay or wood and by its aid incises the scar for a certain distance and leaves the instrument wrapped round with a rag - in the wound in order to keep the edges from adhering again. The wedding feast is celebrated with hideous din. The man leads his bride home - every step she takes means pain - and without giving the fresh wound time to heal or scar, he exercises his marital privileges. Before a child can be born, the vulva has to be opened again throughout its length, but after delivery, infibulation is again inflicted according to the husband's orders, either to the original or other measurements and so the process continues." [37]

Dr. Peney, surgeon-in-chief to the French forces in the Sudan, wrote in 1859 about the practices he observed among the Sudanese population, including infibulation. He describes the infibulation operation performed on children, as quoted by Ashley Montagu:

> "Between the age of 7 and 8 the girl is handed over to the matron whose office it is to perform the operation. Some days beforehand the mother of the family invites all her female relations and acquaintances to assemble in her abode, and the ceremony is preceded with food and merriment. When the hour comes the child is laid on a bed and held down in position by the assembled women, while the matron, kneeling between the patient's thighs, begins by slicing off the tip of the clitoris and the edges of the inner lips. Then the razor shears along the rim of the outer lips, removing a ribbon of flesh about 2 cm. wide. It lasts between four and five minutes. In order to drown the shrieks of the girl, the assembled guests and kin raise the loudest and shrillest din conceivable until the process is over. Then, when the flowing blood has been staunched the girls is laid flat on her back, her legs extended and tied firmly together so that she cannot walk, otherwise the desired effect would not be produced. Before leaving the girl to the healing process of nature, the matron introduces a hollow cylinder of wood, about as thick as a goose feather, into the lower portion of the vagina, between the bleeding edges of the wound and this is kept in place until the scar is completely formed. For purposes of micturition and menstruation this tiny orifice is all that remains of the vaginal outlet." [38]

In the early 19th century, travelers from Egypt related that excision was practiced on all girls in Egypt (Cairo) but infibulation was not. However, infibulation "was quite general in the case of female slaves to prevent them from becoming pregnant." [39] Infibulated slave girls were brought to Egypt mostly from the south, from Nubia and the Sudan; "the slave dealers. . . took care to acquire infibulated girls, who naturally fetched a higher price on the Egyptian markets." [40]

Other sources related that the notorious slave markets in East Africa were mainly for female slaves, especially young girls bought by Arabs, as the mortality rate of women was very high.

During Napoleon's Egyptian campaign, the Surgeon General of the French Army noted in 1803 that excision was performed on young girls, "but that this is not the only cruelty that the jealousy of the Turks - who ruled in Egypt at that time - had invented", by which he refers to infibulation.[41] In all 19th century accounts from Egypt and East Africa on this subject, the importance of virginity is stressed: hence infibulation.

The Anthropological Society of Bombay in 1890 published a paper "On the Practice of Female Circumcision and Infibulation Among the Somal and Other Nations of North East Africa"[42], written by one Major J. S. King, who evidently had spent some time in East Africa. His historic information confirms what has been discussed above. He adds that throughout the Somali and Dankali countries, also in Shoa and the city of Harar, "female circumcision is invariably combined with infibulation."[43]

The description of the operation itself is quite the same as the ones given before. After the wedding ceremony (the bride being about 15), "some young men take a pride in piercing what may be called the velum virginale with no other instrument than that furnished by nature; but in general a knife is used."[44] The operation usually is performed by an experienced woman of an outcast tribe (midg'an):

> ". . . the husband holds the wife to prevent her struggling. Dancing and singing, accompanied by hand clapping, in lieu of musical instruments, are vigorously maintained outside, to drown the cries of the bride. Among the Somal in the interior of the country, the husband generally severs the velum virginale himself, while two of his male relatives hold the bride."[45]

During the preliminaries of the match, the man meets the girl to be his bride in a hut. "He then bids her to strip and proceeds to critically examine the whole of her nude form." Subsequently, the bride-price is negotiated and during that time, the husband-to-be is allowed private meetings with his fiancee, for each of which he has to pay a fixed price. And King concludes:

> "Somalis themselves admit that infibulation is a relic of paganism, but they are so thoroughly conservative, in the worst sense of the word, that they dare not relinquish the custom."[46]

Many of the sources quoted state that infibulation is a custom of the people, especially the poor, as girls often have to work together with men, while in wealthier families the women live segregated. Clearly, the economic value of a girl depends on the bride-price, which in turn, depends on her virginity; and this has not changed up to the present time, as reported in the case histories. (See "Case History : Somalia")

The economics involved is confirmed by a recent publication by Rose Oldfield Hayes[47], who taught in the early 1970s at the University of Khartoum. Her analysis alleges that there is positive support for infibulation from an economic point of view. She also shows that the concept of family honor, which depends on the virginity and chastity of the females, further reinforces the operations as well as the traditional role of the male as head of the family. A woman in this patriarchal society is defined in terms of her relationship to men: her father, her husband, and finally her sons.

The "History of Circumcision from the Earliest Time to the Present" by P. C. Remondino, M.D., published in 1891 in Philadelphia, is a collection of facts and stories from many parts of the world. Most of the book is concerned with male circumcision but in one chapter, Remondino talks about infibulation of women:

> "Infibulation was known. . . for centuries and in those rude times it seemed as the most natural and effective mode of accomplishing the object (to insure chastity). It was not as barbarous an operation as emasculation of the male, as it only temporarily interfered with his functions."[48] *

---

* Typically, Remondino regards the practice of infibulation exclusively from the male view; that is, the male is prevented from having sexual intercourse ("his function") only temporarily by infibulation. Once he has paid the bride-price, he can cut open the obstruction and take his pleasure. The mutilation and pain of the women involved are of no concern to Remondino.

And Remondino relates:

> "In Ethiopia, when a female child is born the vulva is stitched together, allowing only the necessary passage for the needs of nature. These parts adhere together and the father is then possessed of a virgin which he can sell to the highest bidder, the union being severed with a sharp knife just before marriage. In some parts of Africa and Asia a ring transfixed the labia, which to be removed, required either a file or a chisel; this is worn only by virgins. Married women wear a sort of muzzle fastened around the body; locked by means of a key and padlock, the key being only in the possession of the husband. The wealthy have their seraglios and eunuchs that take the place of the belt and lock. Another method is a belt worn about the hips, made of brass wire, with a secret combination of fastenings, known only to the husband. In the museum of Naples are to be seen some of the belts, studded with sharp pointed spikes over the abdominal part of the instrument, which was calculated to prevent even innocent familiarity. . . to say nothing of greater evils." [49]

Harems were kept throughout the Middle-East and East Africa until quite recently by the privileged, the rich and the Moslem ruler. Segregation of females to the back of the house was the next best thing for those who could not afford a harem. For the poor, according to the prevalent social values, there seemed to be no alternative but infibulation. One must therefore conclude that rape of any female that came along was the accepted practice by men in these societies; otherwise, infibulation would not be needed.

Remondino reports that rape in the historic past was punished by loss of the virile organ; for instance, it was part of the penal code of the ancient Egyptians. The same punishment was also used by the Spaniards and Britons, he writes. But "the difficulty of proving the crime as well as the ease with which the crime could be charged through motives of revenge, spite or cupidity. . . resulted. . . in the punishment going out of use." [50]

Instead, women were made to pay the price for rape by being mutilated, infibulated, and segregated while males in Middle-Eastern and African societies and elsewhere as well are encouraged to "prove" their manhood - thus encouraging rape.

To operate a harem successfully, eunuchs were needed. Thus, eunuch factories were established in Egypt where African boys were gathered from the Sudan, Ethiopia and other neighboring countries - the children being either kidnapped or bought. Remondino describes a large eunuch factory on Mount Ghebel-Eter, operated by Coptic monks "who do a thriving business with Arabia, Constantinople and Asia Minor." A complete eunuch (ablation of all genital organs) fetched about four times more than a castrated one. And Remondino states it is estimated that 35,000 little boys from the Sudan and other areas of Africa were sacrificed annually to produce an average of 3,800 eunuchs.

Remondino remarks "on the useless barbarity and the really unnecessary need of such mutilations of humanity" and suggests that such practices should be abolished. But he says nothing about abolishing harems or the mutilation of females. Harems and eunuchs are gone by now. However, the senseless and brutal mutilation and infibulation of little girls and women continue to this day.

Remondino also cites a publication of one Colonel DuBisson, "Les Femmes, Les Eunuches et les Guerrieres du Soudan" ("The Women, the Eunuchs and the Warriors of the Sudan"). DuBisson, who traveled in Abyssinia, Egypt and the Sudan, wrote about what he saw and learned. He noticed that, contrary to Oriental custom, many harem women were allowed to go about "unattended by the usual guard of eunuchs" and he observed that they walked in a painful, hesitating and impeded manner.

> "On inquiry, DuBisson learned that this was due to the fact that each woman carried a bamboo stick, about eight inches in length, three inches or more being inserted in the vagina so as to effectively fill the opening, the balance projecting beyond, between the thighs of the person; this bamboo stick, or guardian of female virtue, was held in place by a strap with a shield that covered the vulva, the whole apparatus being strapped about the hips and waist, and the whole being held in an undisplaceable position by a padlock. This was affixed to the woman whenever she was allowed outside the harem grounds, put in position by the eunuch, who carried the key at his girdle. In such a harness virtue can be considered perfectly safe." [51]

At the end of DuBisson's tale, Remondino, a true representative of the male species, states:

> "In the Sudan there are no divorce courts, hence the probable necessity of the apparatus. . . the woman is not obligated to wear it unless she chooses to go out unattended. . . In the United States such a practice might do away with considerble divorce proceedings." [52]

What is most striking, perhaps, about these accounts is how little has changed. The descriptions given, the male attitudes revealed here from the past are much the same today. The patriarchal attitudes about virginity, chastity and seclusion and the tacit approval of excision and infibulation continue to this day and in all parts of the world. As this report shows, such attitudes are not at all limited to the countries where female genital mutilation is actively practiced. Rape and sexual assault, often given as reasons by men why the mutilation of women is "necessary," are nowhere stopped or prevented by punishing men. At present, sexual assault and rape are the most underreported international crimes everywhere in the world. What is more, wherever such statistics are kept, rape is the fastest growing crime.

One question that was raised in **WIN NEWS** must finally also be asked here: It must be raised with all men, in all families and societies and in all parts of the world:

> "Where are the men speaking and organizing against sexual assault by men? Where are the men opposing male violence against women and most of all rape who are willing to punish and stop it? Where are the male peer groups who make it known that violent behavior against women is unacceptable among men?" [53]

The ideology of rape as a crime of power is documented by Susan Brownmiller in her book **Against Our Will: Men, Women and Rape.** [53] The same ideology that rape cannot be controlled - that is, patriarchal societies do not wish to control it - to keep women in fear and dependent on "male protection" supplies the rationale for genital mutilation and especially infibulation. Fear of rape makes infibulation inevitable is the logic provided by men. As Brownmiller says: "Fighting back on a multiplicity of levels, that is the activity we must engage in, together, if we - women - are to redress the imbalance and rid ourselves and men of the ideology of rape" [54] - which is so closely related to the ideology of genital mutilation.

At present - in autumn 1992 - we have seen for many months on TV the terrible, senseless violence of the civil war in Somalia: dying shrunken children held by desperate women in rags - often too famished to eat when they are finally reached by international rescue teams. These pictures of utter human degradation are followed by pictures of young Somali men and boys, well fed and laughing, brandishing their automatic weapons and visibly enjoying the violence.

Somalia is now reaping the results of customs of extreme violence against women under the label of "tradition" - a total breakdown of society into anarchy. The last Somali Government tried to eradicate infibulation with a national initiative that was internationally supported. (See "Case History : Somalia") But the majority of the male population refused change, and revolting against the Government, they are now indulging in unlimited violence. Women and children always are the victims of men out of control. Societies based on this most brutal male violence against helpless women and girls have no viability in today's world. And that is what is happening now in Somalia and in other African countries beset by constant civil wars and local tribal assaults.

The customs and traditions described in this history still go on all over Africa and the mentality of the men who continue them has hardly changed - though many of them now wear suits, drive cars and watch TV. They can also be found at the United Nations in New York. They must be held responsible. But the countries where men practice these brutal customs against women are also the poorest in the world. Women everywhere must join together to stop male violence, which goes on all over the world - we have no other choice. When I first began to speak about FGM, no one wanted to believe me and too many women still do not want to see the truth under the cover of "custom and tradition." This report, I hope, shows the reality which we must change here and now.

FOOTNOTES

1. Mustafa, Asim Zaki. "Female Circumcision and Infibulation". **Journal of Obstetrics and Gynaecology**. British Commonwealth, April 1966, p. 302.
2. Haley, Alex. **Roots**. Doubleday, New York, 1976.
3. Thiam, Awa. **La Parole aux Negresses**. Denoel/Gonthier, Paris, 1978 (in French).
4. Kenyatta, Jomo. **Facing Mount Kenya**. Vintage Books, Division of Random House, New York, October 1965, (originally published in the 1930s).
5. Ploss, H. and Bartels, M., editors. **Das Weib in der Natur und Volkerkunde,** Leipzig, Th. Griebens Verlag, Fourth Edition, October 1895, p.173 (in German). Similar accounts on female circumcision appear in all previous and also later editions with very little new information added. First edition 1885.
6. Widstrand, Carol Gosta. "Female Infibulation", **Studia Ethnographica Upsaliensa,** Vol. XX, 1964, pp. 95-6.
7. Remondino, P.C. **History of Circumcision from the Earliest Times to the Present**. F.A. Davis Co., Philadelphia, 1891.
8. Huber, Alfons. "Die Weibliche Beschneidung", **Tropenmedizin und Parasitologie**. Stuttgart, Vol. 20, No. 1, March 1969, p. 3. (in German)
9. Shandall, Abu El Futuh. "Circumcision and Infibulation of Females: A General Consideration of the Problem and a Clinical Study of the Complications in Sudanese Women", **Sudan Medical Journal,** 5, 1967, p. 178.
10. Ibid.
11. Karim, Dr. Mahmoud, and Ammar, Dr. Roshdi. "Female Circumcision and Sexual Desire". Ain Shams University, Faculty of Medicine, Cairo, Egypt, 1965, pp. 3-4.
12. Kennedy, John G. "Circumcision and Excision in Egyptian Nubia", **Man**. London, Vol. 5, No. 2, 1970, pp. 175-91.
13. Pridie, E.D.; Lorenzen, A.E.; Cruckshank, Dr. A.; Hovell, J.S.; and MacDonald, D.R. **Female Circumcision in the Anglo-Egyptian Sudan,** 1945, from the Foreword by Sheikh Ahmed-El-Taher.
14. Thiam, Awa, op. cit.
15. Diallo, Assitan. **L'excision en Milieu Bambare**. Thesis of the Ecole Normale Superieure de Bamako, Mali. 1977-78. (in French) See also **WIN NEWS**, Vol. IV, No. 3, Summer 1978, translated and summarized from French.
16. Hansen, H.H. "Clitoridectomy: Female Circumcision in Egypt". **Folk**. Vol. 14-15, 1972-73, p. 18.
17. Davis, Elizabeth Gould. **The First Sex**. Penguin Books, 1972, p. 15.
18. Widstrand, op. cit., p. 102.
19. Karim and Ammar, op. cit.
20. Ibid.
21. Ibid.
22. Sequeira, J.H. **Lancet**. Vol. 2, November 7, 1931, p. 1054.
23. Bruce, James. (Ploss, op. cit., p. 178, Fifth Edition, 1897).
24. Sequeira, op. cit.
25. Huber, Alfons. "Die Rituelle Beschneidung der Frau, Sinn und Verbreitung." **Mitteilungen Anthropologische Gesellschaft,** Wien, 101, 1972, p. 81 (in German).
26. Murray, Jocelyn Margaret. **The Kikuyu Female Circumcision Controversy, with Special Reference to the Church Missionary Society's "Sphere of Influence"**. University of California, Los Angeles, Ph.D., 1974, pp. 334-60.
27. Niebuhr, M. **Travels Through Arabia**. Vol. II, Edinburgh, 1972.
28. Burton, Richard Francis. **Personal Narrative of a Pilgrimage to Al-Medinah and Meccah**. Vol. II, George Bell and Sons, London 1898, pp. 19-20.

FOOTNOTES (continued)

29. Burton, Richard Francis. **First Footsteps in East Africa, or an Exploration of Harar.** Memorial Edition, Vol. I., Tylston & Edwards, London 1894, p. 85.
30. Ibid.
31. Ibid.
32. DeVilleneuve, Annie. "Etude sur une Coutume Somalie: Les Femmes Cousus". **Journal de la Societe des Africanistes.** Tome VI, Paris, 1937, pp. 15-32. (in French)
33. Pieters, Dr. Guy. "Gynaecology at the Country of the Sewn Women", **Acta Chirurgica Belgica,** No. 3, May 1972 (in French).
34. Hosken, Fran P., "Genital Mutilation of Women in Africa", **Munger Africana Library Notes,** California Institute of Technology, Pasadena, October 1976.
35. Widstrand, op. cit., p. 103.
36. Ibid.
37. Montagu, Ashley. "Infibulation and Defibulation in the Old and New Worlds", **The American Anthropologist.** Brief Communications N.S. 47, 1945, p. 465.
38. Peney. "Etudes sur. . .Soudan". **Bull. de la Societe de Geographie.** Paris, 4 Ser, T. 17, 1959, p. 399 (quoted in Ploss and Bartels, ed. Dingwall, London 1935, Vol. 1, p. 357) and in Montagu, Ibid., p. 465.
39. Widstrand, op. cit., p. 102.
40. Ibid.
41. Ibid.
42. King, Major J.S., Bombay Staff Corps. "On the Practice of Female Circumcision and Infibulation Among the Somal and Other Nations of North East Africa", **Anthropological Society of Bombay,** 1890, ii, pp. 2-6.
43. Ibid.
44. Ibid., p. 3.
45. Ibid., p. 5.
46. Ibid., p. 6.
47. Hayes, Rose Oldfield. "Female Genital Mutilation, Fertility Control, Women's Roles and the Patrilineage in Modern Sudan: A Functional Analysis". **American Ethnologist.** Vol. 2, No. 4, November 1975.
48. Remondino, op. cit., p. 48.
49. Ibid., p. 51.
50 Ibid., p. 97.
51. Ibid., p. 51.
52. Ibid., p. 52.
53. **WIN NEWS,** Vol. 8-2, Spring 1982, "Editorial", p. 1.
54. Brownmiller, Susan. **Against Our Will: Men, Women and Rape.** Simon and Schuster, New York, 1975, p. 404.

CASE HISTORY : SUDAN

The Fifth Congress of the Obstetrical and Gynaecological Society of the Sudan was held in February 1977, in the Medical School of the University of Khartoum. [1] The key panel of this professional meeting was concerned with "female circumcision" as female genital mutilation (FGM) is called popularly as well as by professionals in the Sudan. The most drastic operation - infibulation, or Pharaonic Circumcision - continues to be widely practiced in the most populous areas of the Moslem region of Sudan, including the twin cities of Khartoum and Omdurman.

The Congress, which I attended as a guest, was jointly sponsored by the Sudanese Obstetrical and Gynaecological Society and the Ministries of Health and Social Affairs. The government had asked the Congress to make recommendations concerning the ongoing genital operations to which female children continue to be subjected in most of the Sudan, except those living in the southern provinces who are different ethnic groups from the rest of the country and where a civil war has raged for many years.

The Sudan is the largest country of Africa but has a population estimated at only about twenty-five million. Its history goes back thousands of years. Along the Nile Valley, the monuments of ancient kingdoms can be found. Different rulers from the north or south conquered and reconquered parts of the Fertile Nile Valley, which is still the most densely inhabited area in this sparsely settled country, where deserts cover huge areas. Many local rulers, kings, sheiks and sultans fought local wars for centuries to control this area.

The present territory of the Sudan had been part of the Roman and later British empires. Arab, Turkish, Ethiopian and Egyptian conquerors invaded and ruled the land along the Nile during past centuries. Sudan finally became its own master only quite recently, with the first Sudanese Parliament inaugurated in January 1954. A drawn out civil war in the south, which started shortly after independene, was settled in 1972 but flared up again and continues today.

Besides conquerors and invaders, many thousands of pilgrims going to Mecca from Moslem West Africa have crossed and recrossed the savannah belt of the Sudan, which is called "the Broadway of Africa." [2] Many of these pilgrims, traveling in groups on the way to Port Sudan to cross the Red Sea to Saudi Arabia, stopped on the way to rest from their long and arduous journey. Quite a few of these West African pilgrims never went home but settled in the Sudan, which has plenty of land and few people.

It is impossible to determine where and how genital operations on girls started and spread all over the Sudan, among the many different ethnic groups, each with strong tribal loyalties. FGM is recorded in the Nile Valley already in ancient Egypt (see "History") . But it is not known who might have introduced such customs, which are now anchored in most Moslem population groups all over the Sudan, except for the non-Moslems living in the southern area. At present, due to the civil war in the south which spreads Moslemization, FGM is also being spread through southern Sudan.

Some knowledgeable Sudanese claim that these operations originated along the Red Sea coast, especially Pharaonic Circumcision (infibulation), which continues to be practiced today in the most radical form by the majority of Sudanese ethnic groups.[3] The medical facts and descriptions of the operations are given under "Health Facts and Overview"; they will not be repeated here but should be read first as they serve as reference.

Dr. Fatma Abdel Mahmoud, who was Minister of Social Affairs in 1977, a gynecologist by profession and also a member of the Sudanese Society of Obstetrics and Gynaecology, made the opening speech of the Ob/Gyn Congress, delivered in Arabic. Here are some of the high points:

> "I am addressing. . . my colleagues and greeting this Conference, and asking for your help and direction. We must explore ways and means to create a new society.
>
> This new society must be concerned with the child and care for it, even before it is born. Maternal care must change.
>
> With the cooperation of the Ministry of Social Affairs and the Ministry of Health, we shall solve our. . . development problems and social ills. . .
>
> Pharaonic Circumcision is one of those ills. We want to try to liberate men and women from such impediments and to protect mothers and children.
>
> Our new legislation is concerned with the family and the protection of mothers and children. Special studies are being undertaken to research circumcision and solve this problem. . .
>
> The liquidation of this practice can only be accomplished through education and thus by raising the consciousness of women. Ninety percent of the women are illiterate, compared to seventy-five percent of the men. . .
>
> The gathering here of physicians and colleagues provides a unique opportunity: We wish you every success."[4]

The special panel discussion on FGM was scheduled for an evening meeting in order to enable more of the busy professionals and members of the University to participate. The Director of the Sudanese Family Planning Organization, Dr. Ali Bedri, who had worked all his life for the abolishment of the operations, chaired the meeting, which lasted well into the night.

After many presentations by panelists discussing the damaging health results of FGM, the formulation of the recommendation requested by the Ministries of Health and Social Affairs was debated. This debate focused on whether to recommend outright prohibition of all forms of circumcision, or whether to recommend that Sunna Circumcision (the removal of the prepuce and tip of the clitoris - the "mildest" form of the operations) should be permitted.

A very similar debate took place two years later (1979), also in Khartoum, at the World Health Organization (WHO) Seminar; at that time the question was whether or not to sanction the "mildest" form of the operations internationally, and to enable health personnel to perform it under sanitary conditions, again under the pretext to prevent "worse harm." And this debate continues to this day with advocates for FGM always male.

In 1977, the gynecologists could not agree on how to medically define the operations and draw a clear distinction on medical grounds as to what could be cut and what not. Everyone in the room, of course, knew that the traditional midwives - operators who do most of the surgery - understand nothing about anatomy and would not be deterred by any medical definitions.

Then, Kateera Yassin, the Secretary of the Sudanese Women's Union, asked to speak. She boldly challenged the gynecologists. First, she described the terror of the operation and the ordeal that children are made to suffer. She accused the physicians of having debated the issue for thirty years, yet nothing has been accomplished. "Children continue to be mutilated, and the medical profession does not speak up," she said . "Many doctors make money from doing the operation on children brought by their parents, instead of opposing it. Some of them become rich." And she also accused midwives of profiting from these practices.

The doctors, embarrased by her public accusations, especially after they themselves had discussed at length the terrible results of the mutilations, had to act. As no agreement could be reached on what should be allowed to cut or how much and after a very long evening - it was getting very late, this statement was finally unanimously passed and sent to the Ministries: **"All forms of circumcision should be abolished."**

Unfortunately no one made any suggestions as to how this might be accomplished.

The presentations by panelists and contributions from many Congress participants gave an overview of the health problems of women in the Sudan concerning Pharaonic Circumcision (infibulation). Some of the presentations were especially noteworthy.

Dr. Suliman Modawi, the president of the Ob/Gyn Society, and his brother, Dr. Osman Modawi, a senior member and chief of the Department of Gynecology of the University and the Khartoum Hospital, summarized the problems physicians encounter with their patients, for the benefit of the visitors from several countries who attended the Congress.

> "Pregnancy can take place in the absence of full penetration, and there have been cases of labour with a pin hole introitus. If early abortion occurs, the foetus remains in the vagina, and severe infection follows. In antenatal clinics, it has been noticed that there is a high percentage of cystitis and vaginitis. . .
>
> Infertility is sometimes due to difficulty in penetration, sometimes due to infection of the infibulation wound. . .
>
> The fear with which a woman approaches her labour, a reflection of her early experience of circumcision, causes inertia and delay in the first stage of labour. Retention of urine during labour is fairly common and the passage of a catheter difficult.
>
> Obstruction of labour is sometimes due to stenosis of the vagina and scarring following circumcision. This causes atrophy and fistula formation in the rectum and vagina. Perineal tears are common and often extensive. . .
>
> Incision of the scar has to be done for the birth of the head, and often lateral and posterolateral incisions have to be made as well, to give sufficient room. Untrained midwives leave these wounds open, or approximate the gaping edges. The wound takes a long time to heal by granulation. In some cases, a secondary circumcision (infibulation) is performed to close the wide opening." [5]

The recent history of female circumsion in the Sudan was presented by Dr. Asim Zaki Mustafa, Research Assistant at the Department of Obstetrics and Gynaecology, University of Khartoum.

Dr. Mustafa related that already in 1943 a Medical Committee had been set up by Sir Hubert Huddleston, who then was the Governor General, to study the problem of female circumcision. This Committee decided that Pharaonic Circumcision was cruel and harmful, and that it should be abolished. The heads of the main Moslem religious groups in the Sudan supported this Committee. A booklet explaining these views was written both in Arabic and English and widely distributed with support from the press and radio.

But all this had no positive results; therefore, in 1946, the government resorted to legislation. People raced to have their children operated before the law came into effect. Girls as young as two years were infibulated with a terribly high incidence of fatalities.

According to the new law, midwives performing Pharaonic Circumcision could be imprisoned for up to seven years and fined up to fifty Sudanese pounds. People reacted violently to the first arrest made of a midwife, and there was a riot. The operations continued in secrecy, well protected by families who were in favor of it. The legislation forced the midwives and relatives of the girls to hide the complications. As a result, even more damage was done. After that no more arrests were made. [6]

Then, Dr. Abu el Futuh Shandall spoke and updated his reserach study of 1967, **Circumcision and Infibulation of Females: A General Consideration of the Problem and a Clinical Study of the Complications in Sudanese Women,** [7] where he tabulated the case histories of 4,024 women, all his patients at the Khartoum Hospital: More than 3,000 of the women were infibulated, and the rest, except for about 200 - mostly non-Sudanese - were excised.

The study tabulates all complications encountered as a result of these operations and is the most thorough and complete clinical study ever made on infibulation. The new data presented at the Congress were from Dr. Shandall's private practice; that is, from a higher income group. The number of Pharaonic Circumcisions, especially of schoolgirls, had been somewhat reduced in Khartoum, compared to the earlier clinical study at the public hospital. His figures, nevertheless, showed that at the present rate of decrease, it may take several generations before this practice is abandoned, unless some effective actions and prevention campaigns are undertaken.

Dr. Shandall's study established clinically the morbidity (disease) resulting from the operations. However, the mortality rate remains unknown in the Sudan, as well as in the rest of Africa. Not only are primary fatalities concealed everywhere, but death in childbirth, which is said to be frequent especially where infibulation is practiced is not attributed to the operations. Death from infections or tetanus in the absence of any knowledge by the people of the causes of infections is never related at all.

Accurate clinical statistics especially concerning women, are very difficult to get in most of Africa. Where they exist, they are from a tiny fraction of women and girls who have access to modern medical help, mostly from the higher socioeconomic groups living in urban areas.

Next, Dr. Salah Abu Bakr discussed his research, a study of the histology, that is, the microscopic examination of tissue of the genital area of women before and after excision. This study established that excision physically eliminates a woman's capacity to experience sexual stimulation and thus orgasm, due to the removal of the nerve endings and especially the clitoris, the most sensitive organ of a woman. (See "Health Facts and Overview").

Dr. Bakr also presented the results of questionnaires which he had given to secondary school students, young married women and older women to describe their personal experiences with the operation.

The questionnaire established first that with very few exceptions, all the women (selected at random) were Pharaonically Circumcised. The schoolgirls, though most of them had undergone the operation about eight to ten years ago (about the age of five), all remembered it as a horrible ordeal and a traumatic experience. The older women (all of whom were married) regardless of age vividly remembered not only the torture of the operation but also their marriage and first intercourse as a terrible ordeal. Several of the women had to be operated on (cut open by midwives) in order to have intercourse. Many had problems in childbirth, as well as post partum difficulties.

The psychological aspects of female circumcision were discussed by Dr. T. A. Baasher, a Sudanese mental health specialist who worked in the regional office of the World Health Organization in Alexandria. In 1979, Dr. Baasher came back to Khartoum to take charge of the WHO Seminar on "Traditional Practices Affecting the Health of Women and Children", where a great deal of time was devoted to the topic of the social and psychological aspects of the operations.

Dr. Baasher explained that FGM is deeply anchored in Sudanese life and traditions:

> "It is mainly a women's affair and the pattern of behaviour, cognitively and emotionally, follows century-old cultural practices. The family usually celebrates the occasion, and relatives and friends actively participate in the ceremony. On the day of the operation, a Sudanese girl puts on her best clothes, wears a golden ring and bracelets, smells profusely of Oriental perfumes and her palms and soles are carefully painted red with henna. More significantly, she may be referred to as the 'bride'. This is a clear indication of her coming of age and future connection with marriage and expected sexual role.
>
> Long before the operation, she is apt to hear about it, but seldom allowed to attend or observe its side effects. As she grows within cultural norms, she may become familiar with the common social assumptions that the 'girl who is not circumcised is unacceptable': **el beydourha meno!** (who wants her?) **el beyaresha meno!** (who marries her?) and so forth."[8]

The celebration and the gifts which are bestowed on her, especially in more well-to-do families, as well as the language used conceal the real nature of the operation.

> "To make it socially and psychologically acceptable, all of the side effects of circumcision may be semantically covered under such usage that the girl has been embellished 'sammahpah'. . . In the same vein an uncircumcised girl may be considered as 'nigsa' (unclean). . . this too may explain the use of the generic term of "Tahara" for circumcision which implies purification. . ."[9]

Dr. Baasher's presentation reported on the results of a questionnaire of seventy women living in Alexandria, most of them Sudanese and Pharaonically Circumcised. Most of the respondents rejected the practice; several stated that female circumcision "infringes on women's basic human rights." One stated that "circumcision is not the best method of controlling female sexual desire. Indeed, education, guidance and faith are the correct way of doing so. . ." Another one said "it is not right to deprive one from a natural feeling created by God."

Some respondents were more outspoken and called the operation "cruel" and "criminal," as well as "primitive, barbaric," and "it should be done away with". Yet twenty-seven percent supported it; typically allegiance to family custom and religion and tradition were cited as reasons; and also attenuation of sexual desire, hygienic purposes, and aesthetics.[10]

To get conclusive findings on the psychological effects of the operations on personality formation and mental health, it would be necessary to compare over a period of years the development and lives of a group of operated girls and women with a similar group of girls and women allowed to grow up normally and without any mutilations.

But, no one has even suggested such research in the Sudan no doubt because it would reveal some very unpleasant realities and would quite demolish the claims made by male anthropologists about the importance of traditions. The question must be raised: important for whom? For men, of course - to preserve male authority, male privilege and control of women. Why are anthropologists never heard discussing any of the terrible physical damage done to women and children which results from many customs and traditions - for instance, those documented in this report.

A real examination of the psychological and social effects of genital mutilation would also show that the mutilation of women is entirely incompatible with the national goals of economic development set by every African and Middle Eastern government, including the Sudan. Almost all the African and Middle Eastern countries where genital mutilation is practiced are desperately poor by all standards, and some are on the verge of economic collapse, quite aside from social upheavals caused by the frequent civil and tribal wars and male violence against women and children.

Genital mutilation is a traditional practice that reflects a social organization that is entirely incompatible with present-day economic goals. These mutilations are an obstacle to the political, social and economic development of each country and society, both on physical and health grounds, but especially for psychological reasons.

Poverty is not the cause of traditional practices like genital mutilation as some claim, but the opposite is true. Many traditional, social practices, and especially those that psychologically oppress women or otherwise limit their activities and development, are the cause of poverty of a nation. How could it be otherwise, since women are half the population and are in charge of rearing each new generation, transmitting to the young the same damaging and oppressive psychology during the most formative years?

In the Sudan, much more is known than elsewhere about genital mutilation and its effects on the social structure and vice versa. The Sudan is a striking example of a society unable and/or unwilling to free itself from these traditions, which are recognized by the educated Sudanese for their damaging health results on the lives of individual women and families: but nowhere is the enormous social and psychological burden understood that not only stifles the lives of individuals but also negates the very development objectives of the whole society and nation, as the failure of Sudan to reach any of its economic goals demonstrates. This failure imposes terrible hardships on the population and continuous insecurity on all citizens.

The constant civil wars that Sudan has engaged in as well as flights into religious fundamentalism cannot conceal the failure of this society to develop and govern itself. These are based on customs and traditions that are incompatible with contemporary life and destroy much of the productiveness of half the population - women.. Decisions in the government as well as in each family are made by men: As long as these men put traditional male power, male privilege and absolute male control of women first and ahead of change, the country will remain in absolute poverty with a large segment of the population malnourished, illiterate and in poor health.

The necessary change requires a fundamental alteration of the social structure and the status of women to enable them to effectively participate in development. According to recent statistics, Sudan, ruled by a succession of dictatorships, is one of the world's poorest countries with a deteriorating economy despite vast agricultural and mineral potential. [11] Millions of people are refugees, displaced by continuing warfare and unable to sustain themselves, let alone lead productive lives. In addition there is a large nomadic population who, much like in other countries, rejects education and change. Widespread belief in evil spirits, all kinds of supernational powers, witchcraft and jinns governs the lives of many people all over Sudan and especially women, most of whom are still illiterate and have no contact with contemporary life.

Genital mutilation is still the requirement for marriage by the vast majority of men, and marriage is obligatory for all women and men in this Moslem country. As long as men refuse to change and instead resort to violence, nothing else will change.

As one of the physicians and gynecologists remarked at the 1977 Congress, where it was shown that the operations do not even accomplish the stated objective of preventing sexual intercourse, as a woman can have herself re-infibulated anytime: "Why do men insist on these operations. . . Why?. . . It is all in their heads," he said. And this is the key to the situation in the Sudan and all over the world: it is all in the heads of men - it is men who must change or be made to change by women. But as the recent history in Sudan and much of sub-Saharan Africa shows, the male answer is war and violence.

The recent history of genital mutilation in the Sudan was briefly summarized at the Congress, especially the legislation of 1946. This legislation prohibiting Pharaonic but permitting Sunna Circumcision is still on the books but has never been implemented after its first and only enforcement raised local protests.

Though British colonial administrators made it a rule not to interfere with local customs or religious practices anywhere, there were exceptions in cases of severe ill treatment or torture. For instance, widow burning in India was prohibited, excision in Kenya was taken up when medical missionaries pressed the case.(See "Case History Kenya"). But Pharaonic Circumcision in the Sudan remained unknown or was ignored for a long time. Women had no contact with the male physicians of the medical system that was part of the British administration of Sudan. Sudanese women were secluded. Male doctors could not attend Sudanese women least of all in childbirth. In some Moslem areas, male doctors are still prohibited from taking care of women even if it means a woman's death.

In the early 1920s, a British army nurse, Ms. Mabel Wolff, came to the Sudan and started the first midwifery service. Her sister, also a nurse, joined her a few years later. Besides attending women, they began to teach and set up a midwifery school, the first ever in the Sudan. Mabel Wolff, who saw the terrible health problems and suffering of women as a result of Pharaonic Circumcision in her work every day, made these problems known to the medical service. She worked and taught all her life against the mutilations, which were accepted as "natural" by all women at the time: they had never known anything else.

Even now, both in the Sudan and in many other areas in Africa, women are not aware that FGM is not "necessary" and not practiced in most of the world. In 1979, while in the Sudan, several women journalists including myself visited a maternity clinic some distance from Khartoum. The women there with whom we talked could not believe that none of us were infibulated - they just laughed. There was no way to convince them. No woman would ever admit she is not "closed" because it means she is a prostitute.

At the time the Wolff sisters started their pioneer work in the 1920s, only a few women from the leading families could even read and had any contact with the world outside their own families. Both men and women accepted infibulation as perfectly natural. Health problems or mishaps resulting from the operations were ascribed to evil spirits and jinns of all kinds who lurk everywhere and were feared as the cause of most troubles: And they still are at the present time

The advocacy of Mabel Wolff convinced the medical service to investigate the situation. As a result the Midwifery School was set up in Omdurman: It educated a growing number of women to become midwives who, in turn, trained others - all of them taught against infibulation and tried to make women aware of the dangers of these operations.

In the 1930s, the issue began to be discussed in England including in Parliament. It also reached the consciousness of more and more Sudanese especially those who were educated abroad, and who began to speak against the practice. [12]

As a result of these various actions, the Sudanese government finally decided that something had to be done.

Dr. Suliman Modawi, in a study, describes the background:

> "For ages the Sudanese performed the operation on their boys and girls who were equally proud of the occasion which they celebrated as an initiation ceremony of significance. The attention of our generation was first focused on female circumcision as a social problem and stigma in the late 1930s. A member of the British Parliament attacked the custom and urged the Sudan British administration to take steps to prohibit it by law and warned against its spread to the Southern Sudan.
>
> The subject was then widely discussed by the British press and medical journals. In the Sudan, the majority of the British administrators and enlightened Sudanese discussed the problem with extreme caution. Very few Sudanese nationals and religious leaders at the time suspected the government, rightly or wrongly, of unnecessary interference in Sudanese intimate affairs. . ." [13]

"Interference" has now become the watchword by which proposals to better the lives of those most disadvantaged - too often women - are frequently turned away. "Interference" has been charged by governments of developing countries in the United Nations and other public occasions so often that international development organizations wait paralyzed and do nothing, even while people are dying before their eyes. "Interference" is also the motto of Africans who want, for whatever misguided reasons, to ignore the mutilation of their own children, and "we cannot interfere" is used by international agencies, for instance UNICEF, as an excuse to do nothing for the children whom they are supposed to protect. (See "The Politics of Genital Mutilation") .

In the 1940s, there were fewer qualms about helping those most exploited and abused, especially women and children. The British colonial administration has a long record of trying to assist the victims in societies under their protection or rule: besides widow burning in India and circumcision in Kenya - both mentioned above - foot binding in China, slavery in Arabia and the Middle East, and infibulation in the Sudan were some of the issues taken up. Though it is claimed that the initiatives in Sudan and Kenya only resulted in stiffening resistence to change, the facts documented in this report do not bear that out. Other colonial administrations, for instance, the French in West Africa who faced the same problems of FGM did nothing and ignored the mutilation of girls and women in the large regions of Africa under their administration. As a result, Francophone Africa has the highest maternal and infant mortality,

Though the British administration failed to accomplish any immediate results in the Sudan, the way to change was opened for the first time in a society that had been immovable and closed for centuries as far as the position of women was concerned. As Dr. Modawi describes, FGM was not even recognized as a problem before the British health service came to the Sudan, and before the Wolff sisters began to teach women about basic hygiene and midwifery. The British took up the issue by first publishing a report in 1945, written by the Sudan Medical Service and signed by nine physicians, "the writers being either Sudanese or Friends of the Sudanese." [14]

The first signature of the report is that of Dr. Ali Bedri, who chaired the panel on female circumcision at the1977 Ob/Gyn Congress, (see above) and who had worked against the mutilations all his life. The Foreword, written by the Governor General, Sir Hubert Huddleston, is an amazingly frank statement on behalf of women:

> "During my long association with the Sudanese, I have noticed that while educational and technical progress have taken place on a large scale, the social and domestic advances which should accompany it have been mostly absent, and this lag in the emergence of a healthy and well-balanced community is without any doubt due in general to the inferior position of women and in particular to their forcible subjection to the harmful practice of Pharaonic Circumcision. . ." [15]

Huddleston urges the Sudanse to give up "such a cruel custom. . . an offense against humanity. . . unworthy of an enlightened people." And he adds, "a carriage cannot be drawn. . . at a smooth and rapid speed if one horse is lame and lags behind. . ." He concludes:

> "I am not asking for the rapid political emancipation of women. . . But I do wish to ask for a reasonable status for Sudanese girls and women within your households, based on humanity of treatment and an opportunity for sound domestic progress. Neither of these can be attained so long as the evil of Pharaonic Circumcision is allowed to rot the fabric of your home life." [16]

This Foreword is followed by one of the Mufti of the Sudan, Sheikh Ahmed El Taher, the highest Moslem authority, giving the Sharia opinion. Two versions of the Prophet's words on the subject are given:

> "Abu Daud. . . related a saying of Om Attiya that the Prophet said to a woman who used to undertake this operation in Medina: 'Do not go deep. That is enjoyable to the woman and is preferable to the husband'. . . Bureain related another version of this statement of the prophet. 'Do not go deep. It is more illuminating to the face and more enjoyable to the husband.'" [17]

The Mufti then explains that the Prophet meant "slight excision would serve to ... improve the complexion in addition to being more conducive to pleasure . . . " [18]

A number of other opinions of Imams and Sheiks and various Moslem religious authorities quoted from books of religion and tradition are related, including the following one said to be conveyed by the Prophet:

> "Purity is accomplished by five things: circumcision, removal of hair from the pubis, trimming of the moustaches, paring of the nails, and plucking of hair from under the arm pit." [19]

Circumcision for the male is a command, but as the Mufti reiterates by quoting numerous religious authorities, for females it is "preferable," an "embellishment," and "commendable". Though some contrary opinions are also given.

Some of the religious authorities quoted are quite explicit, stating that the "removal of the lower part of the protruding skin at the top of the vagina" is the kind of circumcision recommended (but not obligatory). "However, this is not what is practiced in the Sudan," the Mufti states. "The operation practiced in the Sudan is excessive excision (infibulation) and is against religious commands," he claims.

In the rest of the Mufti's statement, a long list of quotations and opinions is given from Moslem theologians, discussing whether circumcision is "obligatory" or "simply preferable" for women. They add up to a majority claiming that female circumcision is an "embellishment." And the Mufti states that the upper classes in Egypt have abandoned female circumcision ,and so have the people of Hedjaz, the Prophet's land (the area in Arabia where Mecca and Medina are located).

The Mufti concludes: "It is therefore the duty of the Moslems to follow the tenets of their religion and give up repulsive customs which have no origin in the Book of the Tradition, and are not substantiated by the opinions of learned Moslems." [20]

To the above introductions, statements by important Sudanese officials are added. A Foreword by El Sayed Sir Ali El Mirghani Pasha simply states that all customs take a long time to disappear. In yet another introductory statement, El Sayed Sir Abdel Rahman El Mahdi Pasha thanks the Governor General and the medical men for their statements, which "have come up at the right moment" He adds that he has published in the **El Nil** newspaper a statement "advocating care for the education and uplift of Sudanese women in combating Pharaonic Circumcision with a view to its replacement by the Sunna. . ." He concludes: "I am full of hope that this movement will spread. . ." [21]

The main part of the report written by the nine physicians of the Sudan Medical Service gives a detailed description of the Pharaonic Circumcision operation, including a brief description of the anatomy and functions of the female organs involved in the operation.

After the operation is described and the physical dangers outlined - both immediate and in childbirth - the effects of the operation on the personality and the psychological development of women are also discussed. This was the first time any medical report had paid attention to that.

> "These. . . psychological results. . . may be particularly serious. Certain psychological traits common among Sudanese women may possibly be attributable to circumcision. A feeling of guilt induced by the implied presence of immoral organs which have to be removed before a woman is accepted as morally clean and safe.
>
> The removal of certain external sexual organs, as a result of this operation, lessens the sense of sexual gratification and consequent relaxation and so may result in increased desire on account of the imperfect satisfaction. This may eventually lead to various types of minor psychosexual aberrations. .
>
> Circumcision precludes the full and proper social development of the Sudanese woman in that it contributes to her submissive attitude and inferiority complex and the corresponding cruelly masterful tendency on the part of the man.
>
> Female circumcision is an ancient primitive practice which should not be tolerated by an enlightened people. The resulting widespread pain, suffering and mutilation cannot be justified on any count. . ."[22]

The reasons most frequently given for the practice are outlined next and summarized here:

- Religious grounds - this has been denied by Moslem authorities;
- To promote chastity - experience shows that the operations are useless for that purpose. . . chastity is the result of individual responsibility and education;
- To prevent pregnancy out of wedlock;
- To increase pleasure of the male - pleasure is not increased by a passive partner;
- To prevent disease - this has been refuted.

At the end, the report summarizes:

> "A nation can only progress when all its members advance. Mutilation of women by circumcision debases them. They are responsible for the care and upbringing of the children. . .Circumcision tends to retard the mental development of girls and to make more difficult their adjustment to a life which is rapidly becomig more complex. . .
>
> It is a question of vital importance to the Sudanese people. . . The future progress and status of the Sudanese must be seriously jeopardized unless they put their house in order. . . It is appalling to think that little girls in the Sudan should be subjected to such brutality for no justifiable reason. . .
>
> Circumcision is one of the major social problems of the Sudan. It is a legacy of dark ages. . . it is the duty of the present generation to do away with it. . .We feel that the time is overdue for a concerted drive in the interests of the international reputation, well-being and future progress of the Sudanese people."[23]

This report, signed by nine members of the Sudan Medical Service - all men - including the above mentioned introductions was widely distributed in Arabic and English. Unfortunately, only a tiny fraction of women in Khartoum could read at that time; and it is doubtful that more than a few of those even learned about the existence of this report. Despite its support by the Sudanese leadership, this report probably did not reach many outside of Khartoum/Omdurman and other large towns, least of all women the vast majority of whom are illiterate even today. At that time, radios were not generally available or affordable in the Sudan, tape recorders did not exist. A large part of the rural population are nomads following their herds: all of them practice FGM.

In 1946, a year after the report was published, legislation prohibiting the operations followed. This legislation, which is still on the books, has been ignored ever since its first implementation raised protest and a demonstration. No attempt was ever made to implement this law after Sudan became independent nor has the government even tried to organize the kind of educational effort that is essential to make it effective.

A letter from a Sudanese Judge who played an active role in the legislation, provides the background, as he was directly involved:

> "It is not at all difficult to trace the history of Pharaonic Circumcision in the Sudan. The Kushite or Nubian Empire which embraced the whole of the Northern Sudan up to Khartoum, existed side by side with its adjacent Egyptian Empire of the Pharaos since the third millenium before Christ. They had the same civilization, and perhaps common religious customs, since they frequently invaded each other and mixed freely. By the middle of the 7th century after Christ, when both civilizations were in a state of rapid decline, Islam conquered and occupied Egypt and, though not totally subjecting Nubia, the Arabs started to infiltrate into it. They came gradually across Egypt, the Red Sea, and the Western desert. They brought with them their religion, language and customs. They mixed with the Nubians, intermarried and finally outnumbered them.
>
> Among the customs this mixture of races developed and maintained, was the custom of female circumcision. The Muslim Arabs, though insisting on their traditional way of removing the projecting part of the clitoris, adopted the way of their hosts by effecting an addition to it, the sewing up of the labia of the girl, not heeding the great pain this combined operation was causing to the non-consenting child.
>
> However, this custom of Pharaonic Circumcision, with all that can be said against it, continued to be rigidly followed in the Sudan for the last ten centuries or more. No cry of any sort had ever been raised against it from within, until perhaps sometime in the 1940s. Then, some of the wives of the high-ranking British rulers of the Sudan, who had the chance of mixing with the Sudanese society and studying their customs, raised a terrible hue and cry against female circumcision in the Sudan.
>
> Those gentle ladies with the cooperation of some of the educated Sudanese men (female education was then in its infancy) campaigned vigorously for the abolition of Pharaonic Circumcision. The atmosphere was so tense that in the end, it aroused the government to find a solution for the problem. With all the enthusiasm of a reformer they issued the following amendment to the Sudan Penal Code of 1925:
>
> **"UNLAWFUL CIRCUMCISION:**
>
> **'Section 284-A(1)** Whoever voluntarily causes hurt to the external genital organs of a women is said, save as hereinafter excepted, to commit unlawful circumcision.
>
> **Exception:** It is not an offence against this section merely to remove the free and projecting part of the clitoris.
>
> **(2)** Whoever commits unlawful circumcision shall be punished with imprisonment for a term which may extend to five years or with fine, or with both.
>
> **Explanation:** A woman can, by causing hurt to herself, permit an offence under this section.' " [24]

This legislation is frequently cited by both those who advocate traditions ("the legislation failed"), as well as those working for abolition ("it is the first step in the right direction, but it was misapplied"). It must be noted, however, that the legislation permits clitoridectomy - but forbids infibulation: This makes it useless in practice. Obviously, every operator will claim that the "legally permitted" operation was performed. To establish otherwise requires a gynecological examination to which no girl or woman will submit. But this was never considered at the time, nor the fact that excision is also a very damaging mutilation especially when extensive cutting is involved as the scars narrow or even close the entrance to the vagina. Excision exposes a child to the same infections as well as castrating the girl sexually.

The judge then describes from personal experience what happened when the new law was implemented for the first time:

> "The first offence of unlawful circumcision under the new law was detected by the police in Rufaa town of the Blue Nile Province, which is about hundred-twenty kilometers south of Khartoum on the eastern side of the Nile. The population of the town is fairly sophisticated, with many educated people among them. . .

> The Police lodged a complaint under the new Section 284-A(1) against the midwife who performed the unlawful circumcision, and against the mother of the child as abettor of that offence, and obtained a warrant for their arrest from the local Magistrate. The arrest took the people by surprise and there was resistance to it. As the townspeople heard of it, they joined the resistance and demonstrations of a serious nature followed." [25]

The judge goes on to describe that as a result of this riot, the new legislation was modified and he adds:"As far as I know, very few prosecutions under the new law for unlawful circumcision had further been made. . ." [26]

Yet Dr. Shandall reports in his clinical study [27] that the Minister of Health claimed that in the Khartoum area, the incidence of Pharaonic Circumcision had been reduced by seventy-five percent in the next year. Dr. Shandall's clinical study made in the 1960s or twenty years after the legislation shows that nothing of the kind is true. Nor do the surveys cited at the 1977 Ob/Gyn Congress or those at the 1979 Khartoum WHO Seminar allow much room for optimism. At the present time infibulation continues to be widely practiced under a government whose priorities are Islamic Fundamentalism and the war in the south.

It is true that there are now women at the university and some women in all the professions. The development of women's organizations was promoted and supported by previous governments on political grounds. However, the vast majority of women outside Khartoum are still illiterate and follow traditions as in the past.

The judge then describes in glowing terms the great progress of women. Like many others also in other areas of Africa and the Middle East, he is misled by appearances. That girls go to school and some also participate in higher education does not mean they are not mutilated: As long as men make infibulation a marriage requirement FGM, will continue.

But even the enlightened judge's convictions seem to collapse when confronted with the reality of the lives of the majority of the Sudanese, who live dispersed all over the countryside, many of them as nomads following their herds:

> "I have every doubt, however, that Pharaonic Circumcision can effectively be combatted among the nomadic and pastoral tribes of the Western Sudan, as long as they maintain the way of life they are now leading. Adult lads and full grown girls - meet freely in the grazing fields or watering places unobserved. They naturally flirt. The very rigid and tight Pharaonic Circumcision practiced by these tribes is perhaps intended to guard against human weaknesses which these meetings stir up. I wonder if the continuity of practicing that type of circumcision is not counter-balanced by the risk involved in its abolition among these tribes. ."[28]

This shows that it is widely believed in the Sudan, and elsewhere in Africa - for instance in Somalia - that the operations are "necessary for the protection of girls." The statement implies that evidently any man may sexually assault any woman he meets anywhere and that by working outside the segregated family compound makes every female available for rape. That a man is responsible for controlling himself apparently does not occur to the judge nor that infibulation does not protect a woman against rape as any man can use a knife on her much as a bridegroom does.

Despite the many positive statements about the "great progress of women in Khartoum," the judge seemingly cannot understand that young people of both sexes, who are brought up without suspicion and fear of each other, can meet and work together without becoming sexually involved. Perhaps the judge - himself a victim of the sexual tabus and myths of his society about the need for segregation of the sexes and exaggerated fear of sex - cannot conceive of another way of life. Or perhaps the judge knows something he does not tell us about his society: that sexual assault by men is the order of the day and that no woman is safe from male assault if she leaves her house. Yet even if that is so, infibulation, as has been shown, is not a protection against rape.

Dr. Shandall makes some important recommendations in this regard in his study of 1967 that are entirely valid today. He proposes that all children, boys and girls alike, should receive sex education at school and the young should be taught something about the social and physical implications of circumcision of girls.

Dr. Shandall also recommends that midwives and health personnel should be increased and trained to teach the people about the grave health risks of the operations and the consequences of depriving their children of sexual pleasure. Most important, Dr. Shandall suggests that the religious leaders should set an example with their own families, renouncing female circumcision and urging that their followers do the same.

About three years after enactment of the legislation prohibiting Pharaonic Circumcision, an eyewitness account of the operation written by E. Hills Young, the principal of the Midwives Training School of the Sudan Medical Service, was published in **The Nursing Mirror**, a British professional publication. Hills Young states that this was the first time she had witnessed an operation carried out by one of her own school staff midwives, "under more hygienic conditions than were customary."

Two little girls, aged six and nine, dressed in new clothes, were operated on early in the morning in a courtyard in Omdurman, which was filled with women and children who had come to watch. As is traditional a piece of round matting, with a hole in the center, had been placed in the middle of the sandy yard on the ground.

Hills Young describes what she witnessed:

> "The trained midwife prepared a bowl of swabs, a sterile cut-throat razor, and a bottle of iodine, and brought them on a tray. . . the old grandmother then squatted on the edge of the matting and an old brown blanket was placed in front of her crossed legs. All this time, the courtyard was getting more and more congested, while there was an endless babble of voices and the beating of tom toms. . .
>
> The midwife washed her hands and the smaller girl was brought to the mat. She was then made to walk three times around the hole before seating herself on the blanket, leaning against the grandmother with her legs wide apart each side of the hole. The grandmother held her arms whilst two or three other women held her legs. The midwife swabbed the external genitalia with iodine, then gripped the labia majora in her first finger and thumb, took up the razor and quickly incised off these parts, including the clitoris, in two movements. After this she swabbed the wound with a solution of lysol and warm water.
>
> There was surprisingly little bleeding. The wound was then nipped together by the midwife's fingers for a few seconds, after which the women tied the little girl's legs firmly together, with strips of rags and carried her to the bed.
>
> The other little girl was then brought to the mat. . . The babble of talking and the noise of the tom toms drowned the feeble cries of the little sister. In spite of this, the elder child seemed much more frightened. . .
>
> On sitting down, the little girl covered her face with her hands, but this was not permitted and the grandmother firmly held her arms while the other women held her legs. The child struggled violently but the midwife quickly performed the operation and swabbed the wound. The grandmother protested that the excision had not been sufficient but the midwife firmly repudiated this fact and refused to do anything further.
>
> . . . It is the custom before the little girls are permitted to rest and have some food that they are taken to the Nile or nearest running water to have their faces and hands ceremoniously bathed. This practice is thought to ensure easier menses and early marriage. In districts where only well water is available this is brought to the courtyard for the ceremonial bathing.
>
> The ablutions having been completed, the little girls have their legs tightly tied together and remain like this for at least fifteen to twenty days, or until the wound is completely healed.
>
> Should any sepsis occur the mother and grandmother are not unduly perturbed because they think that the scar tissue will become more firm and thus the 'seal of chastity' made more secure." [29]

After she witnessed the above operations, Hills Young, as head of the Midwives Training School, took steps to prevent future operations from being conducted by staff midwives.

Government trained midwives had been taught to perform less extensive operations using more hygienic methods, but this was stopped. And Hills Young explains:

> "It was, of course, essential that midwives should be taught how to open up the scar during labour and the best method of dealing with the gaping wound after delivery was completed. . . The trained midwives are also taught how to treat brides when they or their husbands desire remedial repair of the impossibly small vaginal orifice.
>
> . . . Young mothers who have some education and admit that this is a harmful, cruel practice, have no assurance that their daughters will find a husband unless they are circumcised. To refer to a man as the son of an uncircumcised woman or to a girl as 'uncircumcised' is still the greatest insult in the Sudan." [30]

Midwifery is an all important profession in the Sudan. Traditional midwives or birth attendents in most countries where genital mutilation is practiced did (and many still do) not only the excision and infibulation operations but also all the surgery during and after each birth that is necessary as a result of the genital operations - all of it without anesthesia. In the Sudan the opening of brides - which often is done secretly and for a high fee to assure silence, - is another most lucrative operation. The manliness of the bridegroom is measured by his ability to penetrate the artificial closure with nothing but his natural weapon, a feat that is often impossible to accomplish. Hence, the assistance of the traditional midwives' knife is secretly enlisted - for a price. However, one can also find in the hospitals many young brides whose impatient husbands used their own knives or other sharp instruments to open the way for their pleasure - often with terrible results. But only a few, lucky young women get cared for in a hospital.

That this continues to this day was confirmed by a special BBC documentary program on FGM in Sudan which was shown in London on TV in early 1983. It also included some scenes from one of the hospitals in Khartoum. [31] A seventeen - year - old bride was brought in for surgery because her genital area including the rectum was slit open and one huge gaping bleeding wound: This was the result of the loving attention of her husband who had paid a hefty price for her. He could not wait to take his pleasure and to satisfy himself so he used his knife. The surgeon explained they get quite a few cases like that, while getting ready to try to repair the damage. He also added that the slashes were so extensive that it would be difficult for the young woman to ever deliver a child normally quite aside from the terrible psychological trauma that would follow her throughout her life. But of course the Sudanese husband was quite within his rights - no one would fault him. If his wife can't have children he can - according to African custom and tradition - return her to her parents and get back the bride-price.

Since men and women live segregated, everything concerning childbearing is a women-only affair. Midwifery education introduced first by Mabel Wolff and her sister in the 1920s began by training the illiterate village women and establishing simple hygiene which was quite unknown. It took enormous perseverance and persuasion by the Wolff sisters to convince the local birth attendants to accept their new methods through personal demonstrations. Their selfless work over many years bore fruit with the establishment of the first midwifery school in Omdurman - which still exists today. All participants in the WHO Seminar in 1979 were invited to visit the school which now trains midwives not only from the Sudan but from neighboring countries as well.

"Besides improving midwifery services, illiterate village women have played an important part in reducing the incidence and severity of Pharaonic Circumcision in the Sudan," writes Dr. Ahmed Bayoumi in an article on the "Training and Activities of Village Midwives in the Sudan." [32] The article describes the remarkable success of the Wolff sisters' work in reducing maternal and infant mortality under very difficult conditions. Practically all women were infibulated when the Wolff sisters started the school, and Pharaonic Circumcision requires that the midwives learn to perform a midline anterior episiotomy in order to enable the women to deliver at all.

The traditional method of delivery was for the women to hold on to a rope hung between the rafters of the hut or house or be suspended from it with ropes while the traditional birth attendant is sitting under her on the ground. The midwife waits until the occlusion bursts open, literally tearing the woman apart. Armed with a knife, the birth attendant tries to assist in this process by making incisions at random to help the baby come out.

Predictably, the maternal and infant mortality rate was staggering. Indeed, the population in the Sudan had greatly declined at the beginning of this century, as the demographic records show, due, it is said, to constant internal warfare. However, there is no doubt that customs such as genital mutilation killed a very large number of women of reproductive age which decimated the population.

The important work of Mabel Wolff, who is still remembered and highly respected in the Sudan, was continued by Miss Hills Young, who came from England in 1941 and enlarged the training program of the Midwifery School in Omdurman; it continues its important work to this day.

The candidates for training at first were local women already working as birth attendants; but gradually, other younger women were recruited, mostly relatives of the "hereditary" village midwives. Most of the candidates were married women between twenty and thirty-five. The consent of the husband had to be obtained first in each case.

A document by Hills-Young, the principal of the Midwives Training School (see above) "The Training of Midwives in the Sudan" [33] describes the teaching methods and syllabus exactly. Teaching was almost entirely oral, since hardly any of the trainees could read or write. This syllabus still provides an excellent model for what needs to be done not only all over the Sudan but also in most of the vast rural areas of Africa if the health of women is really to be made a priority. More women die of childbirth than of any disease in most African and some Middle Eastern countries - so the World Health Organization statistics confirm - and quite needlessly. Health ministries, all run by men, ignore the situation and spend their scarce resources on importing sophisticated, expensive medical technology, installed in the university hospitals to serve the politicans and their families.

But the urgent health needs of women, especially in connection with childbirth, are entirely ignored, and they are similarly ignored by international programs, including those supported by the World Health Organization. [34] Recently a "Safe Motherhood" initiative has been started by WHO together with the World Bank and other international agencies. Though several conferences have been held in Africa, this international program has ignored FGM, despite the fact that it is the cause of most deaths in childbirth. Though the World Bank claims to sponsor "Safe Motherhood", the bank's economic "austerity programs" forced on African governments have resulted in dramatically cutting all health programs and especially maternity services. Even the large hospitals in the African capitals, including Sudan, have no drugs, no sheets, not even cotton or soap, let alone any surgical tools, and electricity is often cut off. The maternities of the many hospitals in Africa that I have regulalry visited are always the most neglected areas.

Yet most African men are literally obsessed with having more children, using women as reproduction machines to bolster their egos and legitimize themselves.

A new midwifery school was built in the1940s to house the growing number of trainees coming from all over the country; updating and retraining courses for practicing midwives were also organized, as well as regular inspection and recruitment tours.

The teaching at the school was consistently directed against all genital operations teaching the midwives the dangers involved. Though the school was and is unalterably opposed to these traditional practices, it is a fact that even today, midwives do the operations - as Kateera Yassin, the Secretary of the Women's Union, pointed out at the Fifth Ob/Gyn Congress in 1977. This was again discussed at the World Health Organization Seminar in Khartoum in February 1979, where it was shown that trained midwives who then got only the paltry sum of two pounds a month from the government for their work, try to augment their income by doing circumcision operations, mainly infibulation.

Time and again, women in the Sudan took up the issue of circumcision, trying chiefly by education to change these damaging customs. In 1945, a declaration against circumcision was signed by women school teachers all over the country:

> "We, the citizens, hereby undertake to serve our beloved country to our utmost and work for the welfare of the women with loyalty and sacrifice. We undertake to follow our leaders and the modern methods encouraged by our young people, and should refrain from the habit of circumcision which denotes barbarity.

> This habit brings evil both to the girl and woman and we shall support those who stand against it especially H. E. the Governor General, Sir Sayed Ali and Sir Abdel Rahman, the Mufti and native doctors."[35]

This pledge by the women teachers is often cited. In addition, so Ina Beasley, who in the 1940s was Controller of Girls' Education in the Sudan, states that "definite teaching against the operation was undertaken, as well as extending girls' education in general." Specific lessons were drawn up at the Training College to discourage the practice of Pharaonic Circumcision and sent to all headmistresses. There were posters made and tours arranged for senior Sudanese schoolmistresses to visit remote school districts. Similar tours were arranged for Sudanese midwives from midwifery schools to speak against the operations. Unfortunately, all these efforts reached only women, while men continued to demand infibulated brides - and they do to this day.

Beasley discusses some of the problems these actions for change encountered not the least of which was that "no one could advance a convincing and adequate reason for the operations except custom, and its acceptance as a part of life. . ."

> "It may have been easy verbally to demolish arguments about cleanliness, virginity, chastity and equality to demonstrate that any connection with the Muslim religion was erroneous, but reasoning seldom shakes the sort of unassailable conviction that prevailed. . .
>
> And for the women in general, it was even harder to receive such a novel idea. Strict seclusion had been the rule until about the period of the 1940s when schooling for girls was beginning to impinge on this, but the number of literate women was still very small. . . thus with no outside contacts, it was hardly to be expected that the old beliefs would be readily discarded. . .
>
> In addition, over the centuries, the way in which religion had become bound up with the idea was important to a religious-minded community. . ."[36]

"Religion requires it" is even now one of the most frequently cited reasons in the Sudan for subjecting girls to the operation. But, as all Moslem religious scholars insist, there is no religious requirement for the operation on women, indeed Pharaonic Circumcision is considered to be against Moslem teaching, which is opposed to all physical harm. However, one does not hear Moslem leaders preaching against the operations in the mosques in the Sudan or elsewhere, though the mosques are used frequently for political and social purposes, much like churches elsewhere.

Beasley points out that the belief that an uncircumcised girl will not find a husband is widely held by women, especially mothers, and "without marriage it is impossible to envisage a future for any women." This belief to this day is responsible for the ongoing mutilation of countless children: Men are doing nothing to dispel this belief.

Where are the Sudanese men who discourage such ideas, from the president and his entourage to the religous leadership? Why does no man in the Sudan speak publicly to other men on this issue even now? Why is there only silence on the part of the male leadership who know very well that their failure to speak is responsible for the continuation of these mutilations of their own daughters?

When independence from British rule became the overriding issue, Beasley shows that women's needs once more were pushed aside: "What is of paramount importance in all this is to lessen the sufferings and handicaps which the operation brings. . . But when politics enters this sphere, what happens to the women in pain and hardship appears to be of scant concern. . . In the heady atmosphere of politics. . . matters of compassion are lost. . ."[37]

Independence in the Sudan, as elsewhere in Africa, has brought too few changes for women's lives. There were no campaigns for women's freedom from the impediments of the past, such as genital mutilation. Men achieved their ambitions, but that women might have equal aspirations was neither discussed nor anyone's concern, least of all that of the male decision makers. Yet the Sudan is the only country where not only extensive medical research studies have been made but there is also official recognition among the educated elite, that genital mutilation **is** a problem.

At the 1977 Ob/Gyn Congress, it was announced that a countrywide study to document the incidence and spread of genital mutilation would be undertaken by the Medical Faculty of the Department of Community Medicine of the University of Khartoum, with the assistance of the World Health Organization. A number of other donors later also contributed, including the Government of the Netherlands and IPPF (International Planned Parenthood Federation). Dr. Asma El Dareer, who had done previous surveys on FGM, was appointed to direct the study. She named its objectives:

"(1) to determine the prevalence of the practice and types of female circumcision in the Sudan;

(2) to identify the health problems encountered as a result of this practice;

(3) to outline the social, religious, and traditional attitudes towards the practice of female circumcision and hence to discuss possible ways which can lead to abolishing female circumcison." [38]

Separate questionnaires for women and men were developed and first tried on a limited, sample population. A Preliminary Report was made by Dr. Dareer at the WHO Seminar in 1979. [39]

In spring of 1981, Dr. Dareer published a study on the provinces of Khartoum, Blue Nile, Kassala, Kordofan and Darfur of 3,210 female and 1,545 male respondents. The tabulations show that more than 82 percent of the women were Pharaonically Circumcised, 12 percent were partially infibulated, and only 1.2 percent were not circumcised at all. Nearly half of the women were re-infibulated after delivery, despite the complications in childbirth; the reasons given were to please their husbands and tradition; 80 percent of the husbands who were asked, wanted their wives to be re-infibulated.

Traditional untrained midwives do nearly 60 percent of the operations and 34 percent are done by government-trained midwives, 1.6 percent by physicians, the rest by other operators or nurses. The most frequently used instruments are special knives, razors, and scissors, in that order.

The opinions of the respondents are revealing. Dr. Dareer writes:

> "More than 80 percent of the female respondents said they approved of the continuation of circumcision, regardless of type; however, the younger and more educated women preferred Sunna or were against it.
>
> More than 87 percent of the male respondents approved of the operations but only 16.1 percent preferred Pharaonic (infibulation).
>
> Fathers said that they did not interfere; by adopting this passive attitude, which amounts to approval, I believe that they actually participate in subjecting their daughters and sisters to this ordeal." [40]

Questions on sexual response were included, though often not answered, as sex is a tabu subject for women; sexual pleasure is only for men. Fear of sexual intercourse is widespread among women, which affects sexual life and, as reported also in other studies, often leads to divorce.

The findings of Dr. Dareer's study show that "the main reasons for approving of circumcision in general are related to tradition and religion. . ."

> "The findings also support the previous conclusion that the type of circumcision depends on the education of the parents. . .
>
> The main reasons why women said they oppose circumcision were firstly the complications encountered during marriage and labor, and secondly, the troubles experienced from the time of circumcision for the rest of their lives. . ." [41]

A long list of recommendations summarized here includes first of all more education for women and men; it is important that fathers are persuaded to face their responsibilities toward their daughters: It is not a "woman's affair"; but men have a critical role. The opinion of Islam should be clarified: Most people give religion as the reason for the operation, though it is stated repeatedly by scholars that Islam does not approve of the operation.

Since the mutilations provide income for midwives, a substitute income must be found for them; Dr. Dareer recommends more midwives should be trained and paid better salaries by the government. The mass media should be enlisted, especially radio, which now can reach most areas all over the country, making known the truth about the suffering of women and the health complications. The broadest support of leaders and health personnel should be enlisted.

Finally, a standing committee should be organized to coordinate and direct all efforts to work against the operations.

The study covers a larger geographic area than any previous one made and for the first time includes a large number of male respondents. It is revealing that more men than women approved of the operations and an even larger number of husbands wanted their wives re-infibulated after delivery. Yet the educational level of men is considerably higher than that of women, and men have far more opportunities to learn about the rest of the world than women, whose contacts often are still limited to their families.

Though men continue to claim "circumcision is a women's affair," it is a fact that men pay for the operations and for the often expensive celebrations that accompany the painful mutilations of their daughters. Men control the expenditures of every family, as very few women work outside the home, and those who do are mainly in the urban areas, and work only if men approve. Men pay the considerable costs involved with the mutilations; if they did not the operations would cease to exist. As Kateera Yassin of the Sudan Women's Union and others have frequently stated: Fortunes are being made by the operations. But no one asks who makes it all possible and who therefore must be held responsible: the fathers who pay for the mutilations of their own children and the men who refuse to marry women who are not mutilated.

Re-infibulation, which immeasurably adds to the pain and complications of childbirth, had "greatly diminished," according to the study of Dr. Shandall in the 1960s. But, the latest figures show that even in Khartoum, it is now widely practiced again. Some physicians claim that since more women deliver in the hospital, traditional operators, who thus lose the fee for the delivery, persuade the older women of the family that the new mother must be re-infibulated.

Pressure of the older women in each family is very great - almost all of them are illiterate. They firmly believe that a girl who is not infibulated is unmarriageable and a prostitute, a disgrace for the whole family. The young wife of each son is required to move into the home of her husband's family. The husband's mother often is in charge of her children. Frequently, these grandmothers insist on having their young granddaughters operated on - sometimes against the wishes of the child's mother. A typical story illustrates the generation gap in Khartoum:

> "The grandmother, now aged fifty-eight, the mother of three - bears testimony to the horrors of the operation. A member of the Hadenowa tribe, she was circumcised Pharaonically at the age of seven. The shock and pain of this ritual. . . was repeated each time she gave birth, hanging traditional style, hands tied to the ceiling.
>
> Each time she suffered the torture of rupturing the tightly sewn area, re-sewn after each birth according to practice.
>
> Her eldest daughter is now thirty years old. Unlike her mother, she was fortunate enough to have been circumcised Sunna style with only the clitoris removed. Nor does her face bear the same deep knife cuts as her mother - once considered a sign of beauty. . .
>
> Mother and daughter are engaged in a bitter conflict over the seven-year- old child of the daughter. The grandmother thinks it is time for her to be circumcised like all good Sudanese girls. Her daughter is vehemently opposed to the practice. She is a university graduate who has travelled extensively. She and her friends have begun to rebel against the sufferings caused by these practices. . ." [42]

Since men and women still live quite separate lives, the older women control the younger ones - while the necessity to please men, who control the purse strings of every household, is, of course, the paramount need: A man, after all, can divorce a wife anytime, for any reason or any whim.

Young women in contemporary Western societes are often told about the warmth and advantages of the large "traditional family" where three generations and all unmarried family members lived together. What is never mentioned is that these families are based on the unpaid hard labor of the young girls and women who have no rights, have no freedom and are mercilessly exploited - often they even lack sufficient food and are never allowed to rest while education or any innovations are only for boys and men.

An examination of family law in Sudan shows that despite the fact that women have equal rights according to law, a man can still divorce a woman in the traditional manner, simply by declaring his intention before witnesses. A man can absent himself from his home without any explanation to the wife. The wife does not take part in family meals (men and women eat separately in all Moslem societies, with the men always eating first and the best food). Nor does a woman take part in any male socializing; thus, a wife finds herself often alone for considerable periods of time. [43] All houses have separate quarters for men and women.

According to Mrs. Nagwa Kamal Farid, the first female judge working in Khartoum, when women initiate divorce, "the main reason is cruelty by the man. Another frequent cause for divorce, according to psychologists and doctors, is the sexual and psychological problems arising from female circumcision." [44] Many women seem to resign themselves to sometimes impossible situations because they cannot tolerate the idea of losing their children; that is, children of each marriage are the property of the husband. An analysis of the social and economic situation and status of women in the patriarchal system of the Sudan in relation to FGM is given by Rose Oldfield Hayes, who in the early 1970s worked and taught for several years in Khartoum at the university. She claims that as a social scientist, she observed few signs that would lead to the conclusion that any changes are imminent as far as most of the women are concerned.

> "The majority of women in Arab Moslem Sudanese society are village peasant women, whose lifeways have been altered only slightly by modernization attempts on the part of the government. . . The most often enforced ideal. . . is that of a woman who remains behind the mud walls of the family compound, tending to the domestic chores, the children and any domestic livestock. . . Men occupy all positions of institutionalized authority in traditional Sudanese society, the role of the grandmother is perhaps the single exception." [45]

The traditions, which go back for centuries, essentially remain the same today, with the exception of a few women of prominent families who have gained access to education. And, as Oldfield Hayes relates, formal education has made some changes in the lives of elite women, enabling them to function in modern economic life.

> "These new roles require behaviour quite different in several respects from that expected of traditional Arab Moslem Sudanese women. . . However, the activities permitted to elite women have been expanded only enough to allow them to make their professional contribution to the modernizing state and little more." [46]

She states that many women teach in schools for girls, some work as interpreters, newspaper correspondents, radio broadcasters, librarians, and the like. Public appearances of young women are restricted to a few cultural events and the movies, either in a group or escorted by a male relative. Local travel is by closed taxi; marriages are arranged by parents; and the traditional dress, the tobe, is worn.

> "Marriage restricts an elite woman's freedom even further, as it does for traditional women. . . It is her male relatives who remain responsible for her comportment and for administering punishments for what they consider to be transgressions." [47]

While women's lives have begun to change somewhat in response to economic needs of the modern sector, where women's labor is required, the lives of rural and nomadic Moslem women continue much as in the past.

> "In the traditional nomadic and semi-nomadic societies of the Northern region, the men are responsible for the main herds - whether cattle, camels or sheep and goats - while the women take care of cultivation or food gathering, the animals kept in or near the settlement, setting up and dismantling camp, and making and repairing household goods. . ." [48]

Women in these rural communities have some economic independence, as they can sell their products in the towns, such as baskets, leatherwork, and dairy products, and they are not restricted to their houses.

A considerable segment of the population still follows their herds. A report from the camel-herding nomadic tribes of North Kordofan Province describes the life of Moslem nomad women, who without exception, are infibulated. A primary health care program in the region also found a high incidence of venereal disease (syphilis and gonorrhea), which flourishes despite, or rather because of, infibulation. While men seek treatment, women, because of the dual standard of morality, are inhibited from getting such health care. Men have many sexual partners due to polygamy and promiscuity, and they are the ones who spread venereal disease.

The report by a member of the health team sent out to investigate the health conditions/ needs of nomads, states:

> "Nomadic girls are, virtually without exception, Pharaonically Circumcized ('tahoor el arab') at the early age of five or six years old. . .The procedure is usually carried out with a razor blade and the cost varies, although the most common price seems to be around three Sudanese pounds in cash or kind. The procedure therefore provides quite a lucrative income for midwives (although not all midwives carry out the practice) in the winter months - the traditional time of circumcision.
>
> The difference between the government and traditional midwife in the performance of circumcision is one of finesse. The former has some concept of hygiene (which often means merely using a clean razor blade) and may be able, at least for the wealthier clients, to provide local anesthetic and even on occasions, needle and thread. It was interesting to note that the Harvard International Institute's health project in Abyel, South Kordofan, working through the University of Khartoum, and coordinated by U.S. Agency for International Development (AID), considers that giving clean razor blades to traditional midwives will be a contribution to community and nomadic health in that area. . . ."[49]

The reasons given for the mutilations are much the same as in Sudanese towns, with "religion" ("prescribed by the Prophet Mohammed") and "insurance of virginity and faithfulness" the most often cited ones, though both are false. The marriage customs, which are similar in many nomadic societies, are by arrangement at a very young age, sometimes girls as young as six are married off, though consummation takes place later: twelve or thirteen is a common age for marriage with fifteen in wealthier families, though the couple often do not set up their own tent until later.

The men leave with their herds for extensive periods of time (often for months) in summer; the women and children stay in the camp sometimes quite alone - - which would be unthinkable in Moslem urban areas.

The situation of women in the modern and urban sector in Sudan was analyzed in a feature story in **Sudanow** [50], a magazine that was published by the Ministry of Culture and Information of Sudan. Only ten percent of the women work in the modern sector; the rest are occupied with traditional chores. For women who live in towns, there are more choices than in the past; but it is a great problem to combine working (whether by choice or necessity) with taking care of a family.

> "There are actually very few jobs available to women without qualifications or training. Doors are often closed to women as a result of social pressure. For instance, the service sector jobs taken mainly by women in industrialized countries, in shops, restaurants and so on -- are considered unsuitable for women in the Sudan because of their public and unsegregated nature.Though education can open doors to a career, it is frequently seen as a bonus in the home rather than a key to the outside world.
>
> In view of the complex of attitudes and logistical problems that confront the urban working woman, it is perhaps not surprising that so few actually follow a career. In the country as a whole, the ratio of boys' schools to girls' is two to one at primary level, three to one at general secondary level. . .

> "In the field of clerical and general office work, another well-accepted sphere of female employment, women are outnumbered three to one by their male colleagues." [51]

Though more young women now get a professional education, once they are married and have children, they often have no time to combine home and career.

> "There is clearly an ideal in Islam that women should not have to work. . . Motherhood is always women's chief profession. . . Islam provides for a woman as mother, wife or sister . . . Women leaders have resorted too much to recommendations on paper for increasing women's participation, rather than concrete plans of action. . . the same gap between theory and practice applies to political representation. . ." [52]

And the article concludes that both in the rural sector and in town, there is a crying need for attitudes to change.

In March of 1979, a few weeks after the WHO Seminar, Ahfad University College held a symposium to celebrate its seventy-fifth anniversary as the country's first secular school for girls. The topics discussed ranged from famous women of the Sudan and the social, economic and political status of women, to family planning and female circumcision.

> "Female circumcision was the best-attended session, with speaker after speaker condemning the practice. The abolition of all forms of circumcision was unanimously agreed to be the goal; how to accomplish this was also discussed. More education was the recommendation demanded by all the women at this first-ever, open women's meeting in Sudan, where women from all over the country came to speak their minds. . ."

A leadership training workshop didn't mince words about the needs and problems of women in the provinces:

> "Lack of education; malnutrition among children; complications from female circumcision and traditional methods of childbirth; excessive bride-price; lack of water supply; women aren't taught new techniques in agriculture. . . The consensus was that in spite of real progress in certain areas, Sudanese women still lagged very much behind men in education, legal and political rights, health and nutrition and social matters. . ." [53]

Another workshop was held in Ahfad College two years later in March 1981. This time, the main topic was "Eradicting Female Circumcision in the Sudan." [54] The meeting was sponsored by the Babiker Badri Scientific Society for Women's Studies. Health Minister Khalid Hassan Abbas addressed the opening session. He said that the program of the workshop to eradicate female circumcisions would find its point of departure from the religious heritage and would make use of scientific progress. He pledged the ministry would give full consideration to the workshop's resolutions and recommendations.

A number of gynecologists and obstetricians, midwives, National Council for Social Welfare representatives and some Arab and African delegates attended and spoke. Many of the physicians who had spoken at the 1977 Ob/Gyn Congress, at the WHO Seminar, and on many other occasions discussed again the health problems before this audience. A representative from the religious leadership, Sheikh Siddig Abdal Hai, again assured the audience that the operations had no religious basis. Yet in all recent questionnaires in Sudan, "religion" is given as the main reason why children are subjected to the mutilations and the religious leaders do nothing to dispell these beliefs.

Dr. Asma El Dareer, who chaired the Babiker Badri Scientific Society for Women's Studies, addressed the meeting on the opening day and said that the problem has captured for a long time the concern of those interested in the welfare of the Sudanese family. On the second day, three groups worked on formulating recommendations to assist in eradicating female circumcision. The participants called for holding an annual enlightenment week to campaign against circumcision. They urged the Imams to preach in all mosques each Friday on the bad effects of circumcision They further appealed to the Ministries of Education and Health and all guidance associations to launch information campaigns. Finally participants adopted an **Anti-Circumcision Declaration** which was signed by all who attended the meeting.

This Declaration includes these statements:

> "We, as members of the workshops for the campaign to eradicate Female 'Circumcision' in the Sudan, taking our initiative from the Babiker Badri Scientific Society for Women's Studies. . . having learnt of the medical and social ill-effects caused by it (circumcision), having heard the views of our religious, medical and social scientist leaders, we hereby declare with complete conviction, that we shall fight this harmful custom which damages the bodies that God has given us, and harms women physically and psychologically, endangers their health and even life itself. . .
>
> We shall start with our own families, and then work with our friends, our neighbors, our colleagues at work, those we meet by chance and those in the Organizations to which we belong, and through all other possible means, in the service of the country at large. . ." [55]

The Babiker Badri Scientific Society for Women's Studies did assume the responsibility for implementing the recommendations of the workshop. They formulated an action program over three years, which includes the making of a film.

Unfortunately, this remarkable statement created by local initiative and backed by the prestige of the educational elite and leadership of women, was no more successful than the other efforts described above, which have had few or no positive results or are still limited to paper recommendations with no plans to implement them.

Except for some small private grants and contributions, international assistance has not been forthcoming, though by now, the facts of the mutilations are quite well known through a number of international publications. A continuing section on Female Genital and Sexual Mutilation is published in **WIN NEWS** [56] in every issue (quarterly) always providing new information. International agencies of the United Nations have been aware of these initiatives by women and their health needs but have never ever tried to help with the development of any viable health programs that include and deal with FGM. USAID (US Agency for International Development) supported a primary health program in Sudan in the early 1980s. But FGM was ignored. No other country - not even Britain where FGM is well-known and extensively documented - tried to seriously support any of the local initiatives such as the ones described above.

It should be added here that the issue of sexuality was never discussed at the WHO Seminar or at other meetings: though the research shows that the effect of the operations on women is to destroy their capacity for sexual pleasure and orgasm. The objective of the operations "to keep women faithful" is openly stated by traditionalists all over Africa, which means that women must be deprived of sexual pleasure and satisfaction. In the Sudan, the myth that women are unable to control their sexuality is especially prevalent. Segregation of the sexes makes open communication between women and men about sexuality impossible. The operations not only create fear of sex but also often make sexual intercourse a painful ordeal that women must suffer - indeed, they have no choice.

For instance, the extensive research study by Dr. Shandall, who also questioned husbands of infibulated women, shows that many men took second wives because their first wives could no longer conceal the terrible pain of sexual intercourse. Sexuality is a tabu subject among most people in the Sudan, and sexual problems are never discussed; the many men and women who experience such problems are concerned only with hiding the facts for fear that it might reflect on their status in the community. Thus, the sexual problems resulting from genital mutilation both for men and women remain hidden, unfortunately, though they affect the lives of most families, destroy countless marriages and cast a shadow over the whole society.

Family planning education was recently introduced in Khartoum; a seminar on "Family Education" met in 1978 "to discuss the most delicate subject ever treated in a Sudanese conference: sex education". [57] The topics of the papers given at the strictly academic gathering covered many subjects. Only one person, Ms. Awatif Bashir, a nursing sister spoke up for sex education in the discussion that followed. She talked about the increasing number of cases of nervous breakdowns of women that are coming to light -- all due to sexual causes

The research study that Dr. Asma Dareer first proposed and for which she received support by the Obstetrical - Gynaecologivcal Society of Sudan in 1977 (see above) which was also discussed at the WHO Seminar in Khartoum in 1979, attracted international attention and support. As a result, a male physician of the university faculty took over its direction and finally Dr. Dareer was dismissed from her own study, due to professional jealousy, before the work was completed. However, Dr. Dareer had spent years gathering information in a large part of the country. Her results and analysis were sufficiently comprehensive to be published in book form. **Woman, Why Do You Weep - Circumcision and its Consequences** came out in London in winter 1982 /'83. [58]

This book is the most comprehensive work ever published to establish the facts regarding infibulation in Sudan. The results are very discouraging as overall some 82 percent of the more than 3,200 women interviewed were in favor of continuing the practice, but the number of men was even greater - more than 87 percent. What is more, Dr. Dareer found that re-infibulation after the birth of a child was again being practiced and increasing. While the gynecologists had claimed at the 1977 conference (see above) that this practice was disappearing, Dr. Dareer's research shows that nearly half of the more than 2,200 married women she asked had been re-infibulated.

The reason why the women subjected themselves to such repeated ordeals was to please their husbands or at the request of the husbands. Women are totally dependent on men. Any husband can instantly divorce his wife - if she no longer pleases him sexually, and a tight vagina is more exciting it is believed - hence re-infibulation is practiced.

Dr. Dareer worked relentlessly for many years organizing initiatives and actions to convince her society to give up this terrible practice of FGM, the results of which she knew only too well as a physician.

How great a price is paid by women in the Sudan is illustrated by this typical case history, which is just one of too many similar tragedies that can be found in the files of gynecologists:

> "I was infibulated when I was five years old. I remember every bit of it still - the terrible pain and lying tied up for several weeks. It hurt so much that I cried and cried. I could not understand why this was done to me.
>
> When I was nearly twelve, my aunts one day examined me. They declared that I was not closed enough. They took me to the midwife who lives a few streets away. When I noticed where they were taking me, I tried to run away, but they held me tight and dragged me into the midwife's house. I screamed for help and tried to free myself, but I was not strong.
>
> They held me down and put a cover over my mouth so I could not scream. Then they cut me again; and this time, the woman who operated on me made sure that I was closed.
>
> They carried me home. The pain was terrible. I was tied up and could not move. I could not urinate, and my stomach became all swolen. I was terribly hot one moment, then shaking with cold. This was during the dry season of the sandstorms, when it is hard to breathe. I don't know how many days I was lying there. Then the midwife came again. I screamed as hard as I could, as I thought she was going to cut me again. Then I lost consciousness.
>
> I woke up in a hospital ward. There were moaning women all around me. I was terrified; I did not know where I was. I was in terrible pain; my legs were propped up and my genital area was all swollen and hurt all the time.
>
> Later I was told that the infibulation had been cut open to let the urine and the puss out. I was terribly weak, and I did not care anymore. I wanted to die. Why would my mother permit this? What had I done to be so terribly hurt?
>
> It is years later now. The doctors told me that I could never have children because of the infection. Therefore, no one will marry me; no one wants a wife who cannot have a child. I sit at home alone and I cry a lot. I look at my mother and my aunts, and I ask them: 'Why did you do this terrible thing to me?'"

Unfortunately most girls don't get taken to a hospital; they are just left to die.

The economic conditions of the Sudan have been getting steadily worse. The country, much like the rest of Africa, first was hard hit by the increase of oil prices. Then, a well-publicized investment plan by Saudi Arabia in the 1980s to make Sudan into the bread basket of the Middle East was first scaled down and then abandoned. Most other development plans based on foreign investments failed, and the World Bank/International Monetary Fund (WB/IMF) imposed drastic economic measures to curtail government expenditures in return for urgently needed loans. The per capita income of the Sudan remains one of the lowest in the world. The country is in dire economic straits.

After more than a generation of self-rule, formal independence began on January 1 , 1956, with a parliamentary system which is now suspended. Sudan now is worse off than ever, according to all economic measurements. Sudan has accumulated one of the largest debts to the IMF, and there are severe shortages of foreign exchange with imports greatly exceeding exports. The terribly violent civil war in the south which started up again with a vengeance is further depleting all resources. Perhaps because of all these failures, an upsurge of traditional Islamic beliefs, which started as a result of events in Iran, has swept the country. Recently after repeated political upheavals, another military dictatorship has taken over following a military coup in 1989, which is implementing strictest Sharia (Islamic) law. The civil war in the southern part of the country is pursued by the present regime to Moslemize this region which is inhabited by very different ethnic groups from the largely Arab population in the northern regions and Khartoum. In the process FGM is spreading through the south.

How does all this affect women? Men who are failing at everything are taking out their frustrations on women. Women are no longer permitted to wear the traditional dress the "Tobe", which covers the head, but now they must be completely veiled as in Saudi Arabia, with no hair showing. Women need permission to travel from the men of their family and are subject to increasing restrictions of all kinds. They are the ready-made victims as they are unable to defend themselves.

As the study of Dr. Dareer documents, men have no intention of giving up infibulation, which is their means of control of women, but by doing this they also rob the country of a large part of its productive force and of effective participation in the modern economy. There is no doubt that if men rejected FGM as a marriage requirement, the mutilations would stop. Until men reject FGM and the male leadership declares publicly that their own daughters will no longer be mutilated nor will any of their sons marry a mutilated woman, nothing will change. One can but speculate what effect liberation from FGM would have on this unfortunate society and the development of the country.

Despite the economic hardships and the political upheavals, there have always been small groups of educated people who have continued to work against the mutilations and have tried to convince others to join them.

Recently, under the guidance of Dr. Osman Modawi, who as head of the Obstetrical Gynaecological Society and Chief of the Ob/Gyn Department at the Khartoum Hospital has been the recognized leader of his field for many years, the **Sudan National Committee on Traditional Practices Affecting the Health of Women and Children** was organized. [59]

Previously a National Committee for the Eradication of Female Circumcision had been initiated by a ministerial decree in 1981 within the Ministry of Social Welfare. But after the Inter-African Committee (IAC) on Traditional Practices Affecting the Health of Women and Children was organized in Dakar in 1984 (see "The Health Facts and Overview" and "The Khartoum Seminar"), it was proposed at their regional conference in 1987 in Addis Ababa that non-governmental groups in different African countries should be formed in order to affiliate with the IAC. In 1988, the present Sudan National Committee was set up with Dr. Osman Modawi as president. [60]

The Committee has developed a large number of programs for which it is seeking support and funds. A survey made first showed that among younger people 74 percent still support continuing FGM while among older groups it is 80 percent. But 48 percent opted for a less drastic form of FGM. The survey also found that the reason most often cited for continuing the practice is "tradition" and concluded that there is a great need for extensive information/education campaigns and most importantly it was proposed "men should be involved".

A comprehensive work plan has been developed and large numbers of posters and leaflets with graphic messages and warnings are printed and distributed.

Given the present desperate economic situation as well as the ongoing civil war, it is clear that all such campaigns depend on international support. Sudan has never lacked leadership among its still very small educated elite. According to official figures, literacy is only 20 percent, and for women it is undoubtedly much less. The war is creating large numbers of refugees as well as enormous hardship of every kind. It would be quite unrealistic to predict much positive change.

Large parts of the northern region of Sudan where FGM is practiced including the area around Khartoum are a sandy desert or stony wasteland with a very harsh climate and frequent sand storms that make everyday life often very difficult. Why would any people continue to create for themselves additional misery, incredible pain and suffering that make much of their personal lives a continuous ordeal? Yet information is readily available to everyone. Indeed, the facts are by now known especially to urban residents that any claims that FGM is "necessary" are a lie.

It is not true that these mutilations of helpless children cannot be stopped. It is not true that people cannot change and that these practices based on ignorance, misconceived fears and desire for power as well as false pride will not yield to reason. Do we have so little faith in human nature that we give up and give in to irrational practices that deliberately torture thousands of helpless children systematically year after year, for no other reason than that they are female?

If Sudanese men, who are responsible for these continuous revolting tortures, refuse to change, do the rest of us just watch and do nothing using "tradition" as an excuse? We can no longer plead ignorance or innocence - FGM has officially been recognized by governments as a human rights violation. The charge of "racism" and "interference" no longer holds - the real racism is practiced by those who claim that a little girl because she is black or brown needs to be mutilated, while it is categorically rejected for those who are white.

By doing nothing, we are condoning the wholesale torture of female children as well as the perpetuation and spread of FGM, which is now being exported all over the world with the influx of African refugees.

In the Sudan, all the necessary information is available and known to all government officials and the men in control. How many of them have their own children infibulated? It is not true that FGM is a "women's affair" as men claim, because men pay for the mutilations and because they refuse to marry anyone who is not mutilated. Communication can and does reach the farthest corners of this earth - often instantly. We can reach and teach people to free themselves and we have the means to stop those who are unwilling to give up such torture and brutalities. All of us have an obligation to protect children, nomatter where they live.

First of all the heads of the governments must be held responsible and challenged before the whole world. The international campaign against apartheid in South Africa has been successful in showing that the leadership of a country can be held responsible. Starting with the Sudan where an educated leadership that opposes FGM can set an example, all African leaders must be challenged to organize national campaigns against FGM and held accountable for the continuing torture of their girls and women.

Female genital mutilation is intolerable in our world today and that must be made clear to all the men who refuse to work for change - they will be made to answer publicly, before the whole world, for the systematic mutilation, torture and death of countless women and girls before an international human rights tribunal - just like the leadership of Nazi Germany was.

FOOTNOTES

1. **WIN NEWS**. "Vth Sudanese Congress of the Obstetrical and Gynaecological Society of the Sudan, Khartoum, Feb. 14-18, 1977", Vol. 3, No. 2, Spring 1977, pp. 29-30.
2. Balamoan, G. Ayoub. **Migration Policies in the Anglo-Egyptian Sudan, 1184-1956**, Harvard University Center for Population Studies, 1976, Cambridge, MA 02138 USA.
3. Modawi, Dr. Suliman. **The Impact of Social and Economic Changes in Female Circumcision**. Sudan Medical Association, Khartoum University Press, 1974.
4. **WIN NEWS**, op. cit., p. 29. Speech by Dr. Fatima Abdul Mahmoud, Minister for Social Welfare.
5. Clark, Isobel, and Diaz, Christina. "A Slow Change in Attitudes", **Sudanow**. Ministry of Culture and Information, Khartoum, Sudan, March 1977, p. 44. (This article is a summary of the statements made by the Doctors Modawi.)
6. Shandall, Dr. Ahmed Abu El Futuh. "Circumcision and Infibulation of Females: A General Consideration of the Problems and a Clinical Study of the Complications in Sudanese Women", **Sudan Medical Journal**, Vol. 5, No. 4, 1967. (This study includes a summary of the historical background of the prohibition of female circumcision.)
7. Ibid.
8. Baasher, Dr. T.A. "Psychological Aspects of Female Circumcision". (Regional Advisor on Mental Health, World Health Organization Eastern Mediterranean regional office, P.O. Box 1517, Alexandria, Egypt). Paper presented at the Vth Obstetrical/ Gynaecological Congress, Khartoum, Sudan, February, 1977, p. 4.
9. Ibid., p. 11.
10. Ibid.
11. Gupte, Pranay. "Sudan Is Facing Hard Economic Choices", **New York Times**, November 16, 1981.
12. Passmore Sanderson, Lilian. **Against the Mutilation of Women: The Struggle to End Unnecessary Suffering**, Ithaca Press, London, 1981, pp. 71-77.
13. Modawi, op. cit.
14. Pridie, E.D.; Lorenzen, A.E.; Cruickshank, Dr. A.; Hovel, J.O.; and MacDonald, D.R. "Female Circumcision in the Anglo-Egyptian Sudan". Sudan Medical Service, Khartoum, January 3, 1945. The nine men who signed this report are: Ali Bedri, Abdel Halim Mohd, Abdulla Omer Abu Shamma, El Tigani Homd, El Maki, E.D. Pridia, J. S. Hovell, A.E. Lorenzen, D.R. MacDonald and A. Cruickshank. Included also are a foreword by His Excellency the Governor General, Major General Sir Hubert Huddleston, KCMG, CB, DSOMC.
15. Ibid.
16. Ibid.
17. Pridie, et al (Ibid.) "Foreword" by Sheik Ahmed El Taher.
18. Ibid.
19. Ibid.
20. Ibid.
21. Pridie, et al. (Ibid.) "Foreward" by El Sayed Sir Abdel Rahman El Mahdi Pasha, p. 6.
22. Pridie, et al. (Ibid.), p. 7.
23. Ibid.
24. Letter from a practicing judge in Khartoum, dated September 5, 1976, copy in the author's files. The name of the judge is confidential.
25. Ibid.
26. Ibid.
27. Shandall, op. cit.
28. Letter from practicing judge in Khartoum, op. cit.

FOOTNOTES (Continued)

29. Hills-Young, E., MBE, DN. "Female Circumcision in the Sudan". **Nursing Mirror**. March 12, 1949, pp. 377-78.
30. Ibid.
31. **WIN NEWS** Vol. 9, No. 2, Spring 1983, p. 66.
32. Bayoumi, Ahmed. "The Training and Activity of Village Midwives in the Sudan". **Tropical Doctor**. Vol. 6, No. 3, July 1976, pp. 118-25.
33. Hills-Young, E., MBE, DN. "The Training of Midwives in the Sudan", London University. The complete document is available from London University. Ms. E. Hills-Young has kindly made a copy available from her files. A training outline is provided. Also, see Hosken, Fran P. "Case Histories: Sudan", **Hosken Report: Genital/Sexual Mutilation of Females** (Second Revised Edition), **WIN NEWS**, Lexington, MA., USA, 1979, pp. 12-13.
34. Hosken, Fran P. Ms. Hosken testified as Editor of **WIN NEWS** in the U.S. Congress on women's health as a prerequisite for development: March, 1981: Foreign Affairs Committee, House of Representatives, Clement J. Zablocki, Chair; April, 1981: Foreign Relations Committee, Senate, Senator Charles Percy, Chair; May, 1981: Appropriations Committee, Subcommittee on Foreign Operations, Senator Robert W. Kasten, Jr., Chair.
    These testimonies describe three multi-million dollar health programs in Africa (Sudan, Mali, Somalia) funded by the U.S. Agency for International Development (USAID), and the Program for Strengthening Health Delivery Systems (SHDS) in 20 countries in Central and West Africa, with the collaboration of the World Health Organization. Only a small part of these programs is concerned with mother and child health (MCH), and even less with childbirth. Yet all health statistics show that MCH and childbirth-related problems are the greatest unmet need. In the countries where the above cited programs operate, death in childbirth and infant mortality (much of it at birth) are the highest in the world: This was ignored in these programs. (See "Women and Health: Actions for Change").Testimonies available from author.
35. Beasley, Ina M. "Female Circumcision", **Women Speaking**, July-Sept 1976, pp. 21-23.
36. Ibid.
37. Ibid.
38. El Dareer, Asma Abdel Rahim, MD, "An Epidemiological Study of Female Circumcision in the Sudan". Thesis submitted for the degree of M.Sc. in Community Medicine, Department of Community Medicine, Faculty of Medicine, University of Khartoum, Sudan (1980/81). See also **WIN NEWS** Vol. 7, No. 3, Summer 1981, pp. 38-39.
39. Preliminary Report on the above study presented at the World Health Organization Seminar on "Traditional Practices Affecting the Health of Women & Children", Khartoum, Sudan, February 10-15, 1979. Published March 1979. Available from WHO/EMRO, P.O. Box 1517, Alexandria, Egypt.
40. El Dareer, op. cit.
41. Ibid.
42. **Middle East Magazine**, March 1978, p. 49.
43. "Divorce in the Moslem World", **Middle East Magazine**, Cover Story, March 1978. See also **WIN NEWS**, Vol 4, No. 2, Spring 1978, pp. 64-66.
44. Ibid., p. 68.
45. Oldfield-Hayes, Rose. "Female Genital Mutilation, Fertility Control, Women's Roles and the Patrilineage in Modern Sudan: A Functional Analysis", **American Ethnologist**. Vol 2, No. 4, November 1975, p. 632.
46. Ibid.
47. Ibid.
48. "A Woman's Place", **Sudanow**. Ministry of Culture and Information, Khartoum, Sudan, November 1977.

FOOTNOTES (Continued)

49. Chell, Angela. "Nomadic Sexual Practices: Case Study-Sudan". Acord/Cuso Office, P.O. Box 44997, Nairobi, Kenya. See also **WIN NEWS**, Vol. 6, No. 1, Winter 1981, p. 41.
50. "A Woman's Place", **Sudanow**, op. cit.
51. Ibid.
52. "Awakening In Sudan", **Front Lines**, April 26, 1979, p. 5.
53. Summarized from Workshop Program of the Babiker Badri Scientific Society for Women's Studies on "Eradicating Female Circumcision in the Sudan". Ahfad College for Women, P.O. Box 167, Omdurman, Sudan. Chair: Asma El Dareer, MD. See also **WIN NEWS**, Vol. 7, No. 4, Autumn 1981, p. 34.
54. Ibid.
55. Ibid.
56. **WIN NEWS** has had an ongoing column on "Female Circumcision: Genital and Sexual Mutilation" in every issue since Summer 1975 (Vol. 1, No. 3). All issues available: for more information write to **WIN NEWS**, 187 Grant Street, Lexington, MA 02420 USA.
57. "Too Delicate to Discuss", **Sudanow**. Ministry of Culture and Information, Khartoum, Sudan, April 1978, pp. 40-41.
58. El Dareer, Asma Abdel Rahim, MD. **Woman Why Do You Weep - Circumcision and Its Consequencies**. Zed Press, London. See **WIN NEWS** Vol. 9, No. 2, Spring 1983, pp. 60-61. Book Review by Fran P. Hosken.
59. Sudan National Committee on Traditional Practices Affecting the Health of Women and Children, Amna Abdel Rahman Hassan, P.O. Box 10418, Khartoum, Sudan. See **WIN NEWS**, Vol. 16, No. 1, Winter 1990
60. Ibid., affiliated with Inter African Committee (IAC) on Traditional Practices Affecting the Health of Women and Children, 147 rue de Lausanne, CH-1202, Geneva, Switzerland. See **WIN NEWS**, Vol. 17, No. 4, Autumn 1991.

SUDAN: ECONOMIC/SOCIAL FACTS & SUMMARY

Sudan:	Largest country of Africa, divided into 5 northern and 3 southern regions with two or more provinces each.
Climate:	Desert in North to tropical in South.
Population:	25 million estimate. Khartoum (capital), 3-4 million. **Annual Growth Rate**: 3% (estimate 1987)
Life Expectancy:	49 years // **Infant Mortality**: 112/1000.
Government:	Military Dictatorship. Constitution suspended. Independence: January 1, 1956.
Ethnic Groups:	Arab African // Black African.
Languages:	Arabic (official) // English // Tribal languages.
Religions:	Islam (about 70%) // Animist // Christian (about 5%).
Literacy:	20% (women much less).
Education:	Compulsory 9 years attendance 50%.
Annual/Capita Income:	$300, (1990 estimate). Inflation, 75% (1989).
Economy:	Growth Rate: 0.0%. Cotton, peanuts, gum arabic, sorghum, sesame seeds, livestock, other agricultural products. Imbalance of trade: imports nearly double of exports. Large foreign debt. Major markets Egypt, Gulf states, Saudi Arabia.

CASE HISTORY : SOMALIA

In Somalia, infibulation is practiced by the entire population - indeed by all ethnic Somalis wherever they live. This practice has existed for as long as anyone can remember and is recorded in the earliest historical accounts (see "History"). Though it is traditionally called "circumcision", the extreme form of the mutilations to which little girls are subjected is not accompanied by any rituals, festivities, or celebrations such as is done traditionally in Sudan or other African countries designed to disguise the harshness and brutality of the violence.

Here below is an eyewitness account of what is done to all Somali girls because men still today refuse marriage with an uninfibulated, or what is called "open", bride. And without marriage there is no future for a girl:

> "With the Somalis, the circumcision of girls takes place in the home among women relatives and neighbors. The grandmother or an older woman officiates. At each occasion, usually only one little girl or at times two sisters are infibulated; but all girls, without exception, must undergo this mutilation as it is a required for marriage.
>
> The operation itself is not accompanied by any ceremony or ritual.
>
> The child, completely naked, is made to sit on a low stool. Several women take hold of her and open her legs wide. After separating her outer and inner lips, the operator, usually a woman experienced in this procedure, sits down facing the child. With her kitchen knife the operator first pierces and slices open the hood of the clitoris. Then she begins to cut it out. While another woman wipes off the blood with a rag, the operator digs with her sharp fingernail a hole the length of the clitoris to detach and pull out the organ. The little girl, held down by the women helpers, screams in extreme pain; but no one pays the slightest attention.
>
> The operator finishes this job by entirely pulling out the clitoris, cutting it to the bone with her knife. Her helpers again wipe off the spurting blood with a rag. The operator then removes the remaining flesh, digging with her finger to remove any remnant of the clitoris among the flowing blood. The neighbor women are then invited to plunge their fingers into the bloody hole to verify that every piece of the clitoris is removed.
>
> This operation is not always well-managed, as the little girl struggles. It often happens that by clumsy use of the knife or a poorly-executed cut the urethra is pierced or the rectum is cut open. If the little girl faints, the women blow pili-pili (spice powder) into her nostrils. But this is not the end. The most important part of the operation begins only now. After a short moment, the woman takes the knife again and cuts off the inner lips (labia minora) of the victim. The helpers again wipe the blood with their rags. Then the operator, with a swift motion of her knife, begins to scrape the skin from the inside of the large lips.
>
> The operator conscientiously scrapes the flesh of the screaming child without the slightest concern for the extreme pain she inflicts. When the wound is large enough, she adds some lengthwise cuts and several more incisions. The neighbor women carefully watch her 'work' and encourage her.
>
> The child now howls even more. Sometimes in a spasm, children bite off their tongues. The women carefully watch to prevent such an accident. When her tongue flops out, they throw spice powder on it, which provokes an instant pulling back. With the abrasion of the skin completed according to the rules, the operator closes the bleeding large lips and fixes them one against the other with long acacia thorns.
>
> At this stage of the operation the child is so exhausted that she stops crying but often has convulsions. The women then force down her throat a concoction of plants.

> The operator's chief concern is to leave an opening no larger than a kernel of corn or just big enough to allow urine, and later the menstrual flow, to pass.The family honor depends on making the opening as small as possible because with the Somalis, the smaller the artificial passage is, the greater the value of the girl and the higher the bride-price.
>
> When the operation is finished, the woman pours water over the genital area of the girl and wipes her with a rag. Then the child, who was held down all this time, is made to stand up. The women then immobilize her thighs by tying them together with ropes of goat skin. This bandage is applied from the knees to the waist of the girl and is left in place for about two weeks. The girl must remain lying on a mat for the entire time while all the excrement evidently remains with her in the bandage.
>
> After that time, the girl is released and the bandage is cleaned. Her vagina is now closed - except for a tiny opening created by insertion of a straw or reed and remains closed until her marriage. Contrary to what one would assume, not many girls die from this torture. There are, of course, various complications which frequently leave the girl crippled and disabled for the rest of her life." [1]

This description by Jacques Lantier matches a very similar report published by Annie de Villeneuve [2], who watched the operation performed on two sisters one morning at dawn in Djibouti, where the same Somali ethnic groups live and practice the same mutilations. Infibulation continues to be done today on almost all female children throughout Somalia and wherever ethnic Somalis live as Edna Adan Ismail, who headed the Midwifery Training Department of the Ministry of Health in Somalia, confirms. (See "Health Facts".)

Dr. Guy Pieters, who worked in Somalia from 1966 to 1968 as a gynecologist and surgeon in the Hospital of the European Common Market, reports that the Somali nurses whom he questioned described to him the procedure much as above; it continues today in all rural areas where Somali families live because Somali men insist on it and will not accept for marriage a girl who is not infibulated.

However, in Mogadishu, the capital, and in other Somali towns, the operation recently was "modernized". It was performed in some government hospitals by specially trained Somali male nurses: boys were circumcized and girls were infibulated in sanitary ways. This modernization of infibulation affected only a small part of the most modernized sector of the Somalis living in urban areas. The vast majority of Somalis traditionally are nomads following their herds; they have no contact with the modern world or urban life. Dr. Pieters writes about his experiences practicing medicine in Mogadishu:

> "Each Sunday (Sunday is not a holiday in Moslem countries), the General Hospital in Mogadishu does about fifteen circumcision operations on little boys, and an equal number of infibulation operations on little girls. One team of male nurses works on a table on the boys and another team on the girls in the main operating theater of the hospital. The little girls, aged 4-8, are brought by their parents to the door of the surgical unit of the hospital; the parents wait outside.
>
> Each little girl is brought into the large operating room and strapped onto one of three tables in the gynaecological position with her legs held apart by two male nurses dressed in surgical gowns with masks and gloves. The operation starts by disinfecting the child with Mercurochrome. Local anesthetic is given by four injections into the small lips and under the clitoris, but it is not sufficient to control pain.The small lips are then clamped and cut off with surgical scissors; next the entire clitoris from top to bottom is excised. 'This is the nerve that must be taken out', the officiating male nurse explained to the doctor.
>
> The bleeding usually is not very profuse and wiped off with tampons. The two sides where the cuts were made are then brought together along the entire length of 2-3 centimeters, sutured with catgut and sewn together with silk, about 5-8 stitches. It is important, the operator explained, that only a tiny opening as small as a pencil point remains. . . After more disinfectant is applied locally, the little girl, who frequently screams, is taken off the table and returned to the parents at the door. They pay about a dollar for the operation and take her home. At certain times, when infections seem more frequent, each child is given an injection of penicillin on two consecutive days. But there are rarely any immediate complications. . . " [3]

Dr. Pieters adds that in the cities, some well-to-do families go to private physicians (there are not many) to have the operations done on their children under general anesthesia. Others who have relatives in villages have the operations done on their children in the traditional way. But either way, Dr. Pieters states, there are no religious implications or traditional rituals involved.

When questioned about his experiences in Somalia, Dr. Pieters states:

> "I saw myself all that I described in my article. What I could add is this: In Somalia all little girls are infibulated between 4-8 years old. In all cities, the operation is performed in the hospitals. Although the psychological effects are very bad, the custom which has continued for many hundreds of years is universal. . . " [4]

At the United Nations Conference on Human Settlements in Vancouver, B.C., in July 1976, Mr. A. J. Abdille, the managing director of the Somali Settlement Development Agency, headed the Somali delegation. He gave a rousing speech about the accomplishments of modernization by his government under President Mohammed Siad Barre. He spoke about "the abolition of harmful traditional beliefs such as tribalism which acted as great obstacles to accomplish unity." And he added: "One of the main decreed proposals of our October 1969 Revolution was to build a new socialist society based on social justice, self-reliance, hard work, and above all, freedom from exploitation . . ." [5]

Abdille then named some of the steps taken, including introduction of popular participation, self-help programs, the role of women and youth, the abolition of illiteracy and of harmful traditional beliefs. A national literacy campaign was also conducted all over Somalia.

In a private interview after his speech, I asked Mr. Adbille about women in Somalia - there were none in his delegation. He said the literacy campaign was a great success, and his own wife, the mother of six living children including two girls, had recently learned to read. I also inquired about other traditions, such as he had mentioned in his speech. "Yes, the government is putting great emphasis on modernization and change", he said. As head of the Settlement Development Agency, it was his responsibility to help the nomadic population groups toward a sedentary way of life and self-support.

Then I asked Mr. Abdille about women's health and about infibulation. First, I established the fact that I knew all about the mutilations and that it was useless to try to tell me that these operations did not exist, as so many Africans try to do. But Mr. Abdille did not mind talking about this at all. "Yes, of course, all women in Somalia are infibulated", he said. I asked about his wife. "Naturally, she had been infibulated long before they were married, but that was long ago", he said. "What about your two daughters?" I asked him. Yes, of course, he had them infibulated, he replied. I asked him why. He was startled at the question. "But everybody does this. There is no question about it; of course it is done." "Everybody?" I asked again. "Do all the men in the government have their daughters infibulated?" "Yes, it is the custom", he replied. "But you just talked about changing customs in your speech and you said your government was abolishing harmful traditions!" He was amazed at my question. "But not that; it is a very old custom, and you know people don't like to give up their traditions. . . "

Finally, I asked Mr. Abdille about doing the operations in the government hospitals: "Is that true", I asked. "It is, after all, not the customary way." "No," he said; "but it is much better to do it in the hospitals." "Why not give up such a tradition instead of using the hospitals" I asked. Clearly such a possibility had not occurred to him. "Perhaps the World Health Organization or UNICEF might help," I suggested, since this was at a United Nations conference. "But we don't want any help!", he asserted; "and nobody wants to change that custom."

At the United Nations International Women's Year Conference, held in Mexico in 1975, changes in the lives of Somali women, initiated by the government, were described in glowing terms. The leader of the Somali delegation, Ms. Marian Haji Elmi, explained some of the new measures:

> "From the very beginning, the Somali Revolution in 1969 understood the role and contribution of women and began to implement the principles of equality. . .

> Here are some comparative data: In 1969, about 4,106 girls were enrolled in primary schools; this figure rose to 20,837 in 1974. At the secondary level, from 134 in 1967, the figures have risen to 1,773 in 1974. There were only 11 girls enrolled in the so-called University Institute before October 1969, while the Expanded National University of Somalia enrolled about 200 women in 1974. In 1971, the Somali Women's Organization was established by a presidential decree as one of the major branches of the Political Office. A 15-women Central Committee has been established in each district.
>
> . . . a comprehensive family law was passed ensuring equality in matters of marriage, divorce, family support and inheritance. There are specific limitations to marriage involving an additional wife; the marrying age is set at 18, though girls may marry at 16 with the consent of a guardian. Both husband and wife have the right to initiate divorce proceedings. . . Somali women were granted equal property rights in January 1975. Between 1974 and 1975 the Somali Revolutionary Government launched a major rural development campaign. . . As a result of this campaign, 426,192 women became literate." [6]

These truly revolutionary changes in a very conservative country were inspired by the USSR, which was a major influence in the political development and modernization of the country. But as is true with all legislative initiatives where women are concerned and especially in countries where most women cannot read, the vast majority of the women, unfortunately, does not even know that such legislation exists. Somalia never had a written language in the past; the present written language was developed in the late 1960s with the help of UNESCO, the United Nations Educational, Scientific and Cultural Organization. But since there is no written literature, Somalis have to learn another language to get a higher or technical education.

After the government initiated the literacy campaign and encouraged the education of women in the late 1960s - there were no schools for girls, as in other traditional Moslem countries - some Moslem religious leaders began to preach against education for women in the mosques, in opposition to the government decree. After many warnings, the government finally ordered the public execution of five sheiks (some sources report ten) for preaching disobedience to the government. That was in 1975; since then, opposition to education for women has stopped.

The government needs women to fill clerical and other service jobs in its offices; hence, the education campaign. Young women were also encouraged to join the military service of the revolutionary government as part of the modernization program. But, of course, all girls continue to be infibulated at an early age as tradition demands. The operations in the hospitals continued, as was confirmed by Mr. Abdille in 1976 and again in 1978, when I asked the ambassador of the Somali Democratic Republic to the UN Mr. Abdiraza Haji Hussein, this question; yes, the hospitals, where available, are used for that purpose. And he added proudly - as this was an intervew for WIN NEWS: "You know, of course, women in Somalia have equal rights." [7]

The mutilations continued to be done in the hospitals - except for the Benadir Hospital in Mogadishu whose director, Dr. Warsame Ali Mohammed, was one of the strongest opponents to FGM and also had been a delegate to the Khartoum Seminar in 1979. Finally at the International Conference in Mogadishu in 1988 on "Strategies to Eradicate Female Circumcision" (see below), the Health Ministry announced that henceforth no trained health worker or midwife would be permitted to do infibulations.

A view of the reality of life of the women in Somalia is given by Dr. Pieters, though it must be said first that only very few women have access to a physician or a hospital, as the majority of the rural people are nomads following their herds. Dr. Pieter's description is summarized here:

> "The usual age of marriage is between 12 and 15. The mother carefully watches for the start of menstruation. But it is the father who disposes of the girl and sells her for a payment, arranged between the families, in money, in camels, goats, or sheep. . . After the sale is arranged, the mother or sister of the husband-to-be comes to inspect the girl to be sure that she is a virgin, that is, 'closed'.

> If all is in order, the husband can take possession of the girl; but no matter how virile he is, the obstacle is insurmountable. The girl has to be opened first. This task is usually delegated to one of the aunts. The operation is generally made with 'a little knife'. The opening is just big enough to allow penetration, which has to take place frequently during the early days and weeks of the marriage to prevent the open wound from closing again. After a while, a new scar forms around the opening. Men who do not wish to have their wives opened in this brutal way with a knife may take weeks until they are able to consummate the marriage. . . in cases when the girl does not agree to the marriage, she is cut open by force." [8]

And Dr. Pieters goes on to relate from his experience as a gynecologist some of the case histories that provide an insight into the way of life of women in Somalia who came to the hospitals in the towns. The majority of the people rarely seek medical help in the modern sector. The very few Somali women who are highly educated and sent to international meetings, some of them stunningly beautiful, lead quite a different life; but they are also infibulated as practically all Somali women are, though some of their daughters may now be spared.

Dr. Pieters, who lived in Somalia for several years, states that most of the men have several wives as permitted by Moslem law; it seems that divorce for both men and women is very frequent, though apparently re-infibulation is required each time a woman is divorced to guarantee paternity to the new husband. Each woman must wait a few months before she can be married again to make sure she is not pregnant from her previous husband.

A woman who is divorced returns to her father's family, and the father negotiates another union involving another payment of the bride-price. Sometimes when men marry very young girls, the marriage is not consummated immediately, as the men have several other wives. Dr. Pieters reports that not only men but also women can get divorced quite easily; however, in that case, a part of the bride-price must be returned.

Similar family arrangements involving payment of a brideprice prevail in much of Moslem Africa, though it is generally very difficult for women to get a divorce, and it means abandoning her children, as by tradition the children belong to the husband. (See "Case History : Egypt"). One of Dr. Pieters' patients had been divorced five times. The fifth divorce was initiated by the wife because she could not get along with the first wife of her husband. She was married to a sixth man whom she liked but had no children with him. Her husband, however, had five children already with his two earlier wives; three of the children had died. During her thirteen years of what she said was a happy marriage, her husband entered five other marriages with different women.

Another woman who consulted the doctor because of pregnancy problems was married for the fourth time, though only twenty-five, and was expecting her fourth child. Dr. Pieters recorded and tabulated the histories of some of his women patients. In each case, the time the woman remained divorced was also recorded, which means she had to go back to live with her parents. Often it is only a few months before her father closes another deal.

For example, the price for a wife is from 3,000 Somali shillings (first marriage at fourteen) to 300 shillings plus "goods" (lowest). By comparison, a Somali camel at that time was 500-600 shillings, a donkey 60-90 shillings and a cow 200-300 shillings. The duration of the six marriages of one woman was from five days to thirteen years. Half of the marriages were with cousins, which is a typical Moslm arrangement in order to keep the bride-price in the family. The examples, recorded by Dr. Pieters, are quite usual for women in Mogadishu.

After each divorce, a woman is immediately re-infibulated to restore her to the "original condition of virginity", at least in appearance and thus enabling her father to collect another bride-price. The infibulation, according to a local informant, is needed as protection against rape, as rape is a constant threat. Sexual intercourse implies great pain for women: But their only purpose in life is to have children and thus, they must suffer it. A woman is inspected each time she is traded to a man to be sure that she is closed before the bride-price is paid in order to guarantee that any child of hers is her husband's. That is a man pays the bride-price for the use of a woman's genitals for his pleasure and to produce offspring that he owns - including daughters whom he can trade.

It is clear from this description that women in societies which require payment of a bride-price, are nothing more than merchandise traded between men to obtain what men want - offspring as well as sexual and personal services - for which they pay other men. The women get nothing at all and have no say in the transactions. In many societies, women have no right to their children nor to own property; rather, they are property. In fact, they are slaves of men.

Before a Somali woman can give birth, she has to be cut open some more with the 'little knife', as the cut for intercourse is not large enough for the baby to come out. After the birth, the vulva are sewn up again as in the original infibulation. She is again tied up until the wound is closed - to be cut open again with the 'little knife' for intercourse after the baby is weaned. And so it goes on.

The 'little knife' is the governing instrument in the life of each Somali woman, so Dr. Pieters states. (See also the description by Edna Adan Ismail in "Health Facts and Overview").

Many different pathological problems arise as a result of all these operations, including cysts of all kinds, as well as complete occlusions, menstrual problems and more. Dr. Pieters enumerates a list of case histories of severe health problems which required surgery, due to infibulation. His observations were made on women who came to the hospital where he worked; but, of course, only a tiny number of women have access to a hospital, and even fewer seek help from male doctors.

Most women suffer all their lives; no one knows how many die. Mortality statistics are not available for women separately in most societies that practice genital mutilation. No doubt they are staggering.

The psychological traumas of these horrible mutilations are not investigated. The unusual sadness of Somali women, who always seem depressed, can be obseved and is frequently described in literary works. "Young Somali women, who are among the most beautiful in Africa, never smile, and they are of an astonishing coldness," Dr. Pieters states.

For a Somali woman, what we call 'to make love' means excruciating pain; yet her desire for a child can be satisfied only by undergoing a harrowing ordeal of sexual intercourse. As a village woman remarked, women of Somalia always suffer. As a child she must suffer the infibulation. She suffers when she is opened and when she has intercourse; then she must go through torture to give birth. Each child reminds her of her own terrible pain; and she knows that each one of her daughters will have to go through a lifetime of the same misery.

The women are the martyrs of this custom, of which they are unable to rid themselves. The 'little knife' is always there, accompanying every stage of their lives with more pain.

This question must be raised with Somali men who are responsible for this torture: Why? Can any man really enjoy imposing such senseless violence on his wives and children? What do men gain from this? Do they enjoy buying their "male superiority" at such a price? Are they totally insensitive to the torture they inflict on their own wives and children? Yet as long as infibulation is a requirement for marriage, it will continue - as women have no other way of life. And why do so few men in Western countries speak to this issue? Even physicians have been mute! Dr. Pieters is the exception.

Somalia changed its foreign policy due to the war with Ethiopia in 1977. The Somalian military government, under the leadership of President Mohammed Siad Barre, sought to annex the Ogaden area, inside the borders of Ethiopia, where ethnic Somalis live. This invasion took place in the second half of 1977 and was finally rebuffed in 1978.

Ethiopia turned back the Somali invasion with USSR help. For many years the USSR had given technical assistance and help to Somalia since the 1969 Revolution, when the Marxist military government took power. It was expelled from Somalia in 1977. Relations with the USA and the West, which had been only minimal since 1969, were strengthened as US military assistance was sought by the Somalian government for the 1977/78 war.

As part of the new politics, development assistance was provided by the USA. One program was the development of a major rural health delivery system, with assistance of the US Agency for International Development (US/AID), which included the training of health personnel. The project paper stated:

> "The purpose of this project is to assist the Ministry of Health of the Government of Somalia Democratic Republic in developing an institutional capability to provide comprehensive Primary Health Care Services to the rural poor and nomadic population of Somalia. . . By the end of the five-year project period some 800,000 rural poor and nomadic population in four regions of Somalia will receive Primary Health Care Services." [9]

This program - one of the most ambitious of the health programs developed by US/ AID in cooperation with different African countries - was not only comprehensive but could have made a major impact on the health and well-being of a very large part of the Somalian population including women. It was addresed to an up-to-then completely neglected population and was designed to lay the groundwork for providing health services for the majority of the population by developing training programs to reach rural and nomadic people. It had been planned to replicate this initial program throughout the country to bring health care to areas never reached before.

A health expert team was sent by US/AID to Somalia in March/April 1979. The team report [10] is a comprehensive document that lists all the health problems and needs of Somalia.

Women are mentioned as suffering from nutritional deficiencies. High infant mortality is also reported, and there is a short section on mother and child health in the recommendations. But in the entire report there is not one word about infibulation, though this is the major cause for maternal and child morbidity and mortality.

The failure to recognize genital mutilation as a health problem in Africa by internationally assisted health and family planning initiatives is responsible for the continuation and spreading of these mutilations into the modern sector and health services, as is shown in this report. The failure of US/AID to even mention the operations as cause for severe damage to women's and children's health in Somalia was interpreted by the Somalian government as approval of the mutilations, especially since all other adverse health conditions were specifically cited in the US project papers except genital mutilations.

Therefore I contacted the US/AID Office responsible for the guidance of this program and sent the staff health and medical information on infibulation and statistics showing that these practices persisted throughout Somalia as well as the health damage due to these mutilations. The second follow-up team sent by US/AID to Somalia to finalize the program with the Somalian Health Ministry was given printouts of the information on FGM I had provided and given specific instructions on the subject.

> "Attached you will find a packet of materials developed by the Women's International Network (WIN) / Fran P. Hosken, Publisher/Editor.
>
> The materials point out the extent and consequences of female circumcision in Somalia (and neighboring countries). . .
>
> We request that the team include as part of the documents it produces a commentary . . . and plans, if any, for GSDR (Government of Somalia Democratic Republic) official action which may be taken to discourage its continuation. The team's recommendation on what would be an appropriate, realistic attitude for AID and the US Government to take concerning female circumcision will be of assistance."

The report of the second US / AID health team made upon their return in January 1979 includes discussions with the Health Ministry of Somalia about infibulation, which is always called female circumcision in Somalia:

> "With regard to the prevalence and health implications of female circumcision, a custom that has been universally practiced, and that has health implications, official governmental opinion is strongly opposed to FC. A commission composed of the Ministers of Health, Education and Religion and the Somali Women Democratic Organization (SWDO) is studying the issue. The positionof the SWDO is that passing a law against the custom is premature at the moment. They feel that a massive educational campaign against the practice is required before a law will be accepted and confirm already changed attitudes. . .

> The official position of the government and the typical opinion of educated men and women in urban areas are opposed to circumcision. It is in rural areas that ideas about the rights of women are slow to penetrate. The AID supported outreach of health services and health education will be the first step forward changing traditional attitudes towards customs such as circumcision that are harmful to the well-being of women and children." [11]

The US/AID Health Program with a budget of $14.5 million was at that time one of the largest of several health programs in sub-Saharan Africa in areas where FGM is practiced: Others were in Sudan and Mali. Most of them failed and since then US/AID has curtailed all health activities in Africa. But the design of the Somalian program still can serve as a model - except that the MCH (mother and child health) area would have to be greatly strengthened. The implementation of the program plan, undertaken by a contractor chosen from several bids for this government contract as the law requires, failed completely due to a series of mistakes and unexpected problems.

The program was to be implemented from two different health centers located in the north and south of the country. But they never got started. This, however, was the first time that any internationally supported health program even looked at FGM and was prepared to deal with it in cooperation with the government, which at that stage had not taken any official position publicly opposing FGM - as they strongly did a few years later.

Until US/AID brought up the issue of FGM as a health problem in the framework of the first major internationally supported health program, no one had ever discussed the issue officially with the health ministry. For instance, none of the many private international organizations working in Somalia during the drought in the 1970s in the refugee camps ever dealt with it - and they still do not today.

Dr. Kevin Cahill, an expert in tropical medicine who had worked for years in Somalia, was called back to Somalia during the drought of the 1970s. Upon his return he published an article in the **New York Times** about the famine stating that women and children were the chief victims and the majority in the refugee camps. [12]

When I asked Dr. Cahill as a health expert on Somalia about his experience and his advice regarding infibulation, he told me: "FGM is of no interest to me. My research is concerned with the major illnesses of Somalia. Infibulation is not one of them." But that infibulation is the cause of a whole series of major health problems including many unnecessary deaths was evidently of no concern to this physician, and his attitude is unfortunately quite typical for medical professionals.

Health problems resulting from FGM, quite aside from the terrible suffering and disruptions of daily life, also cost African governments - which must pay for hospitals and health care - a great deal of unnecessary expenses and professional time, which they can ill afford. In turn international health assistance is also sharing in these costs.

In 1979, Dr. Warsame, the Director of the Benadir Hospital for Women and Children in Mogadishu and a delegate to the Khartoum Seminar, stated that his hospital alone spends several hundred thousand Somali shillings each year on emergencies and injuries from the infibulations, both as an immediate result of the operations as well as in childbirth. Edna Adan Ismail, who headed the Midwifery Training School of the Somali Ministry of Health, spoke to this issue as a member of the WHO Secretariat of the Seminar in Khartoum. She described her own long experiences and the terrible injuries that frequently result from the operations that the midwives and the hospitals have to deal with on a daily basis and that occupy much of their professional work and time.

That FGM is practiced in refugee camps which are under international sponsorship by the United Nations High Commission of Refugees and assisted by large numbers of non governmental organizations who run the camps and its various programs was documented in detail at the National Council for International Health Conference in June 1983. [13] Dr. Sandra Gove (MD, MPH) presented a paper on her experience working with a health team of Medical Volunteers International in a refugee camp in Bo', Somalia. Apparently the camp authorities were doing nothing to stop the mutilations to which children were subjected right in the camps with the knowledge of the international agencies including those running the essential health services of the camps.

In her research paper, Dr. Sandra Gove describes the situation she found in the camps at Bo', Somalia:

> "Of the expatriate doctors and nurses, less than half knew of the existence of the procedure (FGM) before working in Somalia. . .
>
> As medical workers and educators in the camp, expatriate contact with the results or complications of the procedure was common. It is a radical procedure with many medical complications. Hemorrhage can be severe from the dorsal artery of the clitoris or the labial branches of the pudendal artery. . .
>
> Called to where eight girls had been circumcised two days before, four had high fevers and pus coming from the sutures and thorns. Most had lost their voice from prolonged crying. Wound infection can result in sepsis and occasionally tetanus. Infection often involves the urine and can cause ascending pelvic infection. Urinary retention can result from urethral damage or too tight infibulation requiring re-operation. The knife can slip on a struggling girl, resulting in rectal and other lacerations. Some girls faint from the intense pain and blood loss. . ." [14]

The paper then goes on to discuss in detail all the medical complications in childbirth including that as a result of FGM, "infertility can be as prevalent as 30%". But what is astonishing and quite unacceptable is that according to Dr. Gove, her medical team as well as the many other doctors and nurses working in the Somalian camp at Bo' decided not to interfere!

> "There was general agreement among volunteers interviewed that a refugee camp such as Bo', where the peoples' society and culture are already under major assault, is an inappropriate setting for a campaign to eliminate the practice. There was also general agreement that Westerners are not the ones to initiate change, that change must come from within the culture - from women and perhaps the religious leaders. . ."

Though the paper also stated that FGM raised personal and ethical conflicts the physicians and health workers did nothing to protect the little girls. This was several years after the Government of Somalia had sent a delegation to the WHO Seminar in Khartoum committed to work against tinfibulation and the Health Ministry as well as the government supported SWDO (Somali Women's Democratic Organization) were actively working for the eradication of the practice. But the international health personnel in the camps evidently never asked the Health Ministry or of anyone about FGM.

It is outrageous that internationally supported health personnel supposedly committed to minister to refugees failed to carry out their mandate as physicians and health workers by failing to protect girls and women from life-threatening permanent mutilations. But they also failed to inform themselves regarding the official policies of the Somalian Health Ministry which, as shown above, already had begun work to stop FGM.

The cultural excuse, considering that FGM is internationally recognized as human rights violation simply is a sham and for physicians and the international health personnel to fail to prevent the mutilations of children implicates them in the crime - which is doubly offensive in the case of refugees. By definition refugees must learn to adapt to other cultures, countries and societies if they are to survive. To keep refugees in ignorance that FGM is unacceptable in most of the world and to fail to teach them about the biological facts of reproduction makes the international refugee camp personnel and especially those concerned with health responsible for this violence against women and girls.

The excuses made by the physicians, including the writer of this paper, a woman physician, are simply unacceptable. Why as a physician did she not provide much needed leadership in teaching the people under her care and organizing preventive education?

But the final responsibility for mutilating children under their care and in their camps - for whom they are responsible - rests with the United Nations because the camps are set up under their jurisdiction and international initiative. Unfortunately, what is described above goes on in all UN refugee camps in areas where FGM is practiced; for instance, in Sudan, Ethiopia and once more now in Somalia as well as in all other amps that take care of Somalian refugees.

Already in 1979 at the Khartoum Seminar on "Traditional Practices Affecting the Health of Women and Children", where Somalia participated with a large delegation, Raqiya Haji Dualeh spoke for the SWDO (Somali Women's Democratic Organization) stating that they had already formed a national commission "composed of representatives of the various Ministries: Education, Health, Justice and Religious Affairs, Social Welfare, Information, in addition to workers' unions, youth organizations, doctors, psychologists and other members of the general public." [15]

The SWDO, as a political organization, supported by the Siad Barre government functioned throughout the country to reach all women with their message for change, with the objective of mobilizing the entire female population.

The SWDO had their own headquarters in Mogadishu, where national actions were planned. When I first went to Somalia after the Khartoum Seminar, I was warmly received. The SWDO jointly with Dr. Warsame of the Benadir Hospital for women and children arranged a public meeting on female circumcision at the Medical School. I was invited to speak as member of a panel to summarize the information on FGM I had presented at the Seminar in Khartoum.

The meeting was announced in the papers and on the radio in Mogadishu; on the designated evening, the auditorium was packed. Besides the vice presidents of the SWDO and Dr. Warsame, a representative of the Ministry of Justice and Religious Affairs as well as several physicians spoke and there were many members of the Medical School and community leaders as well as representatives of different embassies in the audience.

A question period followed in which the audience eagerly participated and that continued for hours until late that night. People from the audience including midwives and physicians described the problems they encountered when they tried to spare their own children from undergoing the operations.

The girls who are not operated on are ostracized by their classmates in school and teased by their friends. They are unmercifully taunted and ridiculed as unclean until many girls asked their parents to be circumcized, though they are never told what the operations are all about. But all girls believe that it is necessary to become "grown-up".

One midwife described the dilemma: Whether a girl is operated on or not, she is a victim. "I cannot sacrifice my child. Either way, she suffers. What am I to do", she asked. "As a midwife, I know the terrible health results. As a mother, I know how the child suffers from being teased, insulted and excluded by her friends. She will face even worse problems later when the family of the man to whom she will be given in marriage may turn her down as 'unfit'. How can we stop these operations as long as we know that if our girls are not circumcized, they will not find husbands and they will blame their mothers: their lives will be ruined either way!" [16]

Dr. Warsame then described how a group of people, including his own family, met this problem, which had been worsened in Mogadishu since all girls went to school. There is no way to keep any secrets among children. The majority of the girls were brought up in the belief that the operations are essential for their status and acceptance in society.

To prevent the victimization of their children, Dr. Warsame said that a group of parents who refused to have their children operated on formed a mutual support organization. The girls are brought in contact with other girls who are not circumcized - for mutual support. When they are teased that they are dirty and bad because they are not operated, they can find support from their friends who also are not mutilated and they are taught to say: "We are better than you because we are whole and you are cut. We are the way Allah made us and Allah knows best".

The meeting at the Mogadishu Medical School provided an important guide post for consciousness raising for the SWDO campaign to rid their society of these terrible mutilations by galvanizing the leadership and making them listen. The SWDO as a national and political organization supported by the government reached women all over the country with their activities and had developed an extensive program for educating for change which included these important points:

> "To combat the negative aspects of traditional culture that are standing in the way of progress. . .
>
> To participate fully in the political, economic, social and cultural aspects of the Somali society. . .
>
> To combat ignorance, hunger and disease; and to raise the educational standard of women and their political consciousness. . .
>
> To create women centres. . . and cooperatives of various types. . . to facilitate women's participation in the economic development of the nation. . .
>
> To cooperate with other organizations of the society. . . to strengthen. . . friendship . . . throughout the world." [17]

It was clear, however, that despite the plans to work against FGM the many efforts by the SWDO to raise the consciousness of the leadership in their country and the awareness by the health ministry of the terrible harm done by the mutilations, no one in Somalia could finance what amounted to a prolonged educational effort and national campaign which was essential if any real change was to be made.

The attitude of the international nongovernmental organizations especially those concerned with health was to ignore the issue even in the refugee camps as shown above. And there were many different international organizations including church groups working with the extensive refugee population with large camps outside of Mogadishu and other towns, as refugees are attracted to urban areas in their search for food, water and subsistence.

Since Somalia, specifically the southern part of the country including Mogadishu had been an Italian Colony, Italy had many ties in Somalia as well as extensive development programs. The SWDO made contact with the then recently organized AIDoS group - the Italian Association for Women in Development - who agreed to collaborate with them on the campaign to eradicate FGM. Based on the success of a previous effort in 1984/85 supported by Sweden in organizing a series of seminars in Mogadishu, the SWDO and AIDoS launched a major "Information Campaign to Eradicate Infibulation" in Somalia in 1987/88. [18] The program paper states:

> "The Italian Association for Women in Development (AIDoS) is currently implementing a project which is designed to give technical, organizational and material support to the SWDO to carry on and expand its information campaign on the health consequences of infibulation. The project consists of the development of several 'information packets' to be used as a teaching aid by instructors who will conduct informative seminars for various target groups. . .
>
> The focus of the approach is to present the subject of infibulation primarily as a health issue in an effort to remove the discussion from its religious and cultural connotations. . .
>
> The project will work among the following social groups:
>
> - women and mothers who are accepted and/or influential within their community;
> - secondary school pupils;
> - religious leaders; and
> - medical and paramedical personnel."

Information packages were developed for specific target groups and eventually all government ministries were involved in the delivery of the information in written and visual form. AIDoS sent some women experts to Mogadishu - two of whom stayed to work with the SWDO women for several years - setting up a communication center at their headquarters including computers and printing equipment to enable them to produce their own teaching materials. The ILO (International Labor Office) Training Center in Turin, Italy, assisted in the development of teaching programs for different target groups and sent an advisor to Mogadishu to help with the production and the field testing of the teaching materials.

To focus attention on these efforts, a "National Seminar on the Health Hazards of Female Circumcision and Its Eradication in Somalia" was held March 14-16, 1988, in Mogadishu with the objective to "Formulate a Definite National Policy for the Eradication of Female Circumcision". [19] A list of recommendations was developed with specific requests addressed to different ministries including Ministry of Health, Ministry of Justice and Religious Affairs and Ministry of Interior. These Mistries were asked to play a major role in implementing the SWDO/AIDoS program.

Under the leadership of Murayo Garad Ahmed, the president of the SWDO, other important government leaders participated in the conference as well as representatives of international agencies such as UNICEF. Much of the SWDO/AIDoS program was being integrated into various existing programs by different ministries and especially by all schools and information programs.

This national seminar served to alert the people to the upcoming much larger international meeting on **Strategies to Bring About Change,** which took place June 13-16, 1988, in the Parliament of Mogadishu with opening and closing ceremonies attended by representatives of Somali ministries, United Nations agencies, the ambassador of Italy and representatives of other embassies. [20] The Big Hall of the Somali Parliament was a unique setting for this extraordinary conference, as the central figure of the huge fresco that covers the entire wall behind the speakers is a Somali woman in traditional dress with raised arms floating in a column of light above a backdrop of hundreds of Somali people.

The working part of the seminar was divided up into four different subjects: health, law, religion, training and information. First the presentations from invited speakers were made with an introduction by Daniela Colombo, the director of AIDoS. I presented "World Review of Actions to Abolish Female Circumcision/Genital Mutilation." Berhane Ras Work, the director of the IAC (Inter African Committee on Traditional Practices Affecting the Health of Women and Children) spoke about the IAC activities and programs all over Africa. Stella Efua Graham Dorkenoo gave an overview of her work in London to protect children of immigrants.

Then representatives from other countries with groups working to stop FGM outlined their activities and programs including Egypt, Nigeria, Sudan and the Gambia. A physician from Indonesia spoke who explained how the physical operations had been reduced in his country to a ceremony that no longer included any cutting but was purely symbolic to satisfy the traditional aspects. Both the legal and religious implications were extensively debated as well as the health and cultural aspects by Somalian leaders in their fields. The health problems and experience were presented by Somali physicians including Dr.Warsame.

Finally, the SWDO/AIDoS program was discussed and some of the videotapes of specific training modules developed in Somalia were shown by the representative of AIDoS and the ILO training center who had worked in Mogadishu together with the SWDO women to develop these teaching materials and were continuously trying them out in the field.

In her opening speech Muraio Garad Ahmed, the SWDO president, provided the context to the campaign:

> "In Somalia, infibulation is a deeply rooted cultural practice that concerns all Somali families: men and women, mothers and fathers, male and female children. . . The magnitude of the problem calls for urgent search of solutions. . . all the resources must be utilized. . . The SWDO plans and hopes to completely eradicate infibulation in Somalia before the year 2000 and has sought assistance and collaboration from international agencies both governmental and nongovernmental." [21]

This conference represented the largest international effort the SWDO had ever organized with the assistance of AIDoS to make it clear to all those concerned with development that women had a voice and women were committed to the eradication of all damaging traditions and especially FGM. Representatives of embassies, of United Nations agencies and many other international organizations working in Somalia came to the meetings, which were continuously covered by the local press and media. especially the formal opening and closing ceremonies of the conference in the Parliament.

After this, international organizations working in developing countries and especially in Africa can no longer claim that women wish to continue all traditions: Just the opposite is true. The recommendations of the WHO seminar, furthermore, deal with the eradication of "Traditional Practices" from an international and health view . What is more, FGM is a human rights violation internationally recognized by the Human Rights Office of the United Nations in Geneva. Men who run the health sector all over the world and who make the political decisions, including at the United Nations, must be made to listen to women. speaking for and demanding change. But never before was the case for change so strongly made as at the conference by the SWDO in 1988 in Mogadishu.

At the closing session of the conference, a poem by Dahabo Elmi Muse that won first prize in a national poetry compeition was read in the Parliament:

> "Pharaoh, who was cursed by God/ Who did not hear the preaching of Moses/ Who was led astray from the good word of Torah/ Hell was his reward! Drowing was his fate! The style of their circumcision/ butchering, bleeding, veins dripping with blood! Cutting, sewing and tailoring the flesh! This loathsome act never been cited by Prophet nor acknowledged by the Hadith! Non-existing in Abu Hureyra/ No Muslim ever preached it! Past or present the Koran never preached it (Pharaonic Circumcision) / And if I may think of my wedding night, awaiting me was caresses, sweet kisses, hugging and love/ No never!
>
> Awaiting me was pain, suffering and sadness/ In my wedding bed there I lie groaning, curling like a wounded animal, victim of feminine pain.
>
> At dawn awaits me ridicule/ My mother announces, yes she is a virgin. When fear gets hold of me/ When anger seizes my body/ When hate becomes my company or companion/ I get feminine advice, it is only feminine pain they say, and feminine pain perishes like all feminine things!
>
> The journey continues, or the struggle continues as modern historians say! As the good tie of marriage matures/ As I submit and sorrow subsides/ My belly becomes like a balloon/ A glimpse of happiness appears/ A hope, a new baby, a new life! Ah, a new life endangers my life/ A baby's birth is death and destruction for me! It is what my grandmother called the three feminine sorrows and if I may recall my grandmother said, the day of circumcision, the wedding night and the birth of a baby are the three feminine sorrows.
>
> As the birth burst: And I cry for help the battered flesh tears. No mercy, push they say! It is only feminine pain and feminine pain perishes.
>
> When the spouse decides to break the good tie, when he concludes divorce and desertion, I retire with my wounds. And now hear my appeal! Appeal for dreams broken/ Appeal for my right to live as a whole/ Appeal to you and all the peace-loving people. Protect, support and give a hand to innocent little girls who do no harm, trusting and obedient to their parents, elders and all they know are only smiles. Initiate them to the world of love, not to the world of feminine sorrow!" [22]

In 1988 while the SWDO/AIDoS conference took place in Mogadishu, the civil war had already started in the north of Somalia. Less than a year later it spread all over the country. Another drought even worse than the previous one resulted in hundreds of thousands of starving refugees, mostly women and children. The civil war not only escalated but the whole country has broken down into warring clans with warlords hijacking food shipments and threatening international efforts to feed starving women and children. All law and order has collapsed with male violence totally out of control. Men armed for years by the two competing international powers - the USSR and then the USA - are now power crazed using these weapons against the helpless and their own women and children to capture all food supplies brought to sustain the starving people. A society where men traditionally use their power to mutilate their own female children is not viable in our world. Men accustomed to practice such brutality on their families know no restraint: Somalia is reaping the results of its own traditions. The victims once again are girls and women and their young children. But no one speaks for them!

SOMALIA: ECONOMIC/SOCIAL FACTS & SUMMARY

Somalia:	15 regions
Climate:	Hot and dry with seasonal monsoons.
Population:	5.4 million (1985 estimate). Mogadishu (capital), 700,000 (estimate). **Annual Growth Rate:** 3%
Life Expectancy:	47 years // **Infant Mortality:** 145/1000.
Government:	Republic. Independence: July 1, 1960. Somalia Revolutionary Socialist party until 1990. Civil War started 1989.
Ethnic Groups:	98.8% Somali // 1.2% Arab and Asian.
Languages:	Somali. Written language developed end of 1960's with UNESCO assistance.
Religions:	Islam (99%).
Literacy:	40% (women much less).
Education:	Compulsory 12years. Attendance 50% primary, 7% secondary.
Annual/Capita Income:	$300 (estimate). Inflation 30% (1985).
Economy:	Growth Rate: 3.1%. Imports exceed exports by factor of three. Agricultural products: livestock, bananas, hides and skins.

FOOTNOTES

1. Lantier, Jacques. **La Cite Magigue et Magie en Afrique Noire**. Libraries Fayard, Paris, 1972, pp. 277-9 (in French).
2. Villeneuve, Annie de. "Etude sur une Coutume Somalie: Les Femmes Cousus", **Journal de la Societe des Africanisters**, Tome VI, Paris, 1937, pp. 15-32 (in French).
3. Pieters, Dr. Guy. "Gynaecology in the Country of Sewn Women", **Acta Chirurgica Belgica**, No. 3, pp. 178-79. An abbreviated summary of the article, "Infibulation in the Horn of Africa" appeared in the **New York State Journal of Medicine**, April 1977, pp. 729-31, co-authored by Albert Lowenfels.
4. From personal correspondence with Dr. Guy Pieters (1977-78) in author's files.
5. Abdille, A.J., Managing Director, the Settlement Development Agency. Statement as head of the Somali delegation at HABITAT - The United Nations Conference on Human Settlements, June 7, 1976.
6. Excerpts from the "Statement of the Leader of the Somali Delegation in Mexico, Ms. Marian Haji Elmi, President of the Supreme Revolutionary Council, Mogadishu, Somalia Democratic Republic." See also **WIN NEWS**, Vol. 1, No. 4, Autumn 1975, p. 64.
7. **WIN NEWS**, Vol. 4, No. 2, Spring 1978, pp. 6-7.
8. Pieters, op. cit., pp. 182-3.
9. "Rural Health Delivery Project Paper", US/AID/SOMALIA, January 1979, Annex L. Section 611 (3) Certification. Project No. 649-0102. Agency for International Development, Department of State, Washington, DC 20523 .USA
10. **US/AID Field Trip Report to Somalia**, March/April 1978. Summary, Conclusions and Recommendations. (Available from AID Agency for International Development, Department of Information or Bureau for East Africa - AID, Department of State, Washington, DC 20523 USA).
11. "Rural Health Delivery Project Paper," op. cit., Part 4. Results of specific project analyses, p. 25. (Available from AID/address above.)

FOOTNOTES (Continued)

12. Cahill, Kevin, MD. **New York Times,** Sunday, July 13, 1975.
13. National Council for International Health, 1701 K St., NW, Suite 600, Washington, DC 20006 USA. See **WIN NEWS** Vol. 9, No. 3, Summer 1983, p. 29.
14. **Medical Team Interaction with Female Circumcision in a Refugee Camp, Bo', Somalia.** By Gove, Sandra MD, MPH, and Diamondstone, Laura RN, PH.N, volunteers with Medical Volunteers International, 2546 Great Highway, San Francisco, CA 94116. See **WIN NEWS,** Vol. 10, No. 3, Summer 1984, pp. 38-40.
15. Dualeh, Raqiya Haji. Somalia Country Report. Somali Women's Democratic Organization. Paper delivered at World Health Organization Seminar, Khartoum, Sudan, February 10-15, 1979. See also **WIN NEWS,** Vol. 5, No. 2, Spring 1979, p. 18.
16. Meeting on female circumcision at University of Mogadishu, February 1979, Mogadishu, Somalia. See also **WIN NEWS,** ibid., p. 24.
17. **WIN NEWS,** Vol. 5, No. 2, Spring 1979, p. 23. (Includes a summary of the Statutes of the SWDO - Somali Democratic Women's Organization.
18. AIDoS Information Campaign to Eradicate Infibulation in Somalia - 1987/88.Via dei Giubbonari, 30 00186 Roma, Italy. Contact: Daniela Colombo, Director. See **WIN NEWS,** Vol.13, No. 4, Autumn 1987, pp. 19-21.
19. Report on National Seminar on Health Hazards of Female Circumcision and Its Eradication in Somalia. See **WIN NEWS,** Vol.14, No. 3, Summer, 1988. pp. 32-33.
20. **Female Circumcision Strategies to Bring About Change.** Proceedings of the International Seminar on Female Circumcision. June 13 -16, 1988. Published by AIDoS, address above. See **WIN NEWS,** ibid., pp. 24-31.
21. Opening address by SWDO President, Muraio Garad Ahmed at International Seminar on Female Circumcision. See Footnote 20.
22. Poem by Dahabo Elmi Muse. Proceedings of the International Seminar on Female Circumcision, op. cit., pp. 135-136.

CASE HISTORY : EGYPT

To a first time visitor, Cairo seems nothing so much as a huge, traffic congested, busy metropolis, replete with new, luxurious high-rise buildings along the banks of the wide, majestic Nile. The idea that half the female children and most of the older women are sexually mutilated may seem quite incredible. Yet, this is a fact.

In the villages around Cairo, literally all girls continue to be mutilated - so Dr. El Sayyad, the Director of the Mother and Child Health Division of the MInistry of Health - candidly confirmed in October 1980 when I went to see him. And despite many efforts, described below, families in rural areas cling to the traditions they have practiced for centuries. Cairo and all other Egyptian cities are crowded with immigrants from the rural areas: They continue their traditional family practices, and excision of all girls is one of them.

The Egyptian country report at the Seminar of the World Health Organization in Khartoum in 1979 on "Traditional Practices Affecting the Health of Women and Children" included a survey made earlier that year at a Cairo family planning clinic in a low-income neighborhood: 90 percent of the women coming to the clinic during one typical week were excised and most of them had or were planning to have their daughters operated on. (See: "The World Health Organization").

H. H. Hansen relates in his study published in 1972 on clitoridectomy in Egypt that he was personally informed by a woman doctor that practically all women of her generation (born about 1920) were subjected to "circumcision" [1], as female genital mutilation (FGM) is called all over Egypt; this term is used for all different types of mutilations including infibulation, which is practiced in southern Egypt near the border with Sudan.

Though all kinds of studies and books and publications exist on women in Egypt, genital operations are almost never even mentioned, nor the damaging influence that they have on women's well-being, health, personality and family life. Family planning clinics and maternity hospitals in greater Cairo see large numbers of mutilated women. Hansen, in his study, states that 100 percent of the women coming to family planning clinics in the 1970s were found to be circumcised. [2]

Nawal El Saadawi also describes in her book that practically all girls of her generation (born in the 1920s) were excised, and she was from a well-educated Egyptian family. [3]

In Egypt traditionally all forms of female genital operations have been practiced for thousands of years: The earliest records of FGM available anywhere are from Egypt. It has been claimed that the operations can be detected on some Egyptian mummies. (See: "Historic Background"). In southern Egypt, infibulation was practiced traditionally, and this continues up to the present time as documented in a study of Egyptian Nubia published in 1970, [4] which describes infibulation much as it is performed in the Sudan. Egypt administered the Sudan in the 19th century and even today, many Sudanese live in Egypt and continue to subject their female children to infibulation. This also was shown in a study made in 1977 [5] of Sudanese women living in Alexandria, who were infibulated, or Pharaonically circumcised.

A survey made in 1980-1981 in Alexandria (a city of about four million people) by the Family Planning Association estimates that 80 percent of the people of Alexandria practice excision. [6] Some two-thousand cases a year are brought to the hospitals in Alexandria with the girls in shock, according to this study. But, for the most part, people refrain from seeking help except in dire emergencies, as there is legislation prohibiting these operations. However, it is rarely enforced (see below).

It is claimed that traditionally genital mutilation was not practiced along the Mediterranean coast or in Alexandria. Yet it appears that now due to greater mobility of the people, these customs are spreading to ever larger areas.

The survey from Alexandria found also that the reasons given as to why the operations are done are quite similar to those claimed in Sudan and also in sub-Saharan Africa: tradition, religion, control of female sexuality; cleanliness is also cited as a reason for the operation as well as beauty.

The claim that the operations are done to make a women more beautiful is made in various Egyptian surveys as well as in the Sudan. Since sexual ideas about women originate with men, one can but wonder about the attractiveness of mutilated female genitalia for Egyptian and Sudanese men!

For instance, a young woman doctor who was expecting a baby informed Hansen (so he reports in his study on clitoridectomy in Egypt) that "if the baby should be a girl, she would do the operation herself, as physicians in Cairo were reluctant to perform the operation". But why should a mother, and an MD, maim her own daughter? First, she gave religious reasons - the young woman was a Moslem. But Hansen adds that most of the Christian Copts in Egypt also practice clitoridectomy. The second reason was aesthetic and cosmetic - she wished to remove something disfiguring, repulsive and ugly. The third reason was that the little girl should be protected from sexual stimulation; as a fourth reason, tradition was given and that the majority of husbands preferred their wives to be circumcised. [7]

The young Egyptian woman physician's view on the aesthetic appearance of the female genitalia as reason for excision is shared with other Moslems, for instance, in the Sudan. A Moslem bride is "prepared" for her husband by completely removing all body hair, especially in the pubic area, which is considered ugly as are her external genitalia. There is something "unfinished" about them, and thus, they are cut off. The idea is that excision makes the female body more beautiful and "clean". The clitoris and the female genitalia are ugly, dirty and shameful. In Arabic, the word for excision is "tahara" which means cleansing or purification.

The survey in Alexandria shows that the operations are mostly done at home, usually one girl is operated on or, at times, sisters or cousins together. The operators are mostly "dayas", the traditional midwives. Sometimes a trained midwife does the operation, or a barber officiates. Barbers traditionally are associated with performing minor surgery. In some parts of Nigeria also, excision is done by barbers, who are always men, while in most of the Moslem societies, excision is a strictly female affair.

In Egypt the operations are also done at clinics in the modern sector and in towns or at the private offices of physicians. Though it is claimed that by now most physicians refrain from doing the operations, the Egyptian country report contributed to the WHO Seminar in Khartoum states that both physicians and trained health personnel are involved, serving the middle class, as the operations are a lucrative source of income.

In a study on sexual mutilation in Cairo by Dr. Mohamed Badawi, MD, MPH, in 1985 of women in Cairo most of them in their twenties and Moslem (except for 6%) he found that the mutilations were done mostly at home by dayas (over 60%), next by physicians (22%) and the rest by barbers. Most of the women questioned had gone to high school, a quarter of them to college and only 2% were illiterate. That is among the middle class in Cairo, FGM continues to be widely practiced on girls aged 6-11 who are subjected to the mutilations by force so Dr. Badawi states:

> "Most of the women reported that they were deceived, assaulted, chased and violently immobilized to be forced to have their genitals mutilated. The remaining percentage of women reported that they were misinformed and misled as to the imminent danger of physical violence and genital mutilation. Their 'consent' was not 'informed' in any legal sense of the word." [8]

Here are some of the personal comments made by women which Dr. Badawi recorded:

> "I was terrified to say No // I dare not say No // I wasn't fully comprehending what was happening to me. I wanted someone very much to explain what was being done to me - in vain. // I was shocked and never was I able to comprehend until it was over // Please don't make me remember what happened, I am trying to forget // I cried and screamed for help and no one helped // I cried like mad, shouting you all cheated me // They told me: You must be purified like the rest of your sisters, you are no exception // They attacked me by surprise // I saw the Daya holding a razor, then she hurt me // I couldn't believe my mother was with them; they all attacked me one early morning while I was still sleeping."

Dr. Badawi concludes that mothers are the ones primarily responsible for making the arrangements for their daughters' mutilations. However, where there is no male head of family, for instance, due to divorce, separation or death or where the mother is financially independent, few subject their daughters to this ordeal that has lifelong effects. Religious affiliations, that is, those affiliated with Islam, are primarily responsible for this practice, despite the fact that "there is no clear and definite statement in the Koran, the principal authority of Islam, that supports the practice of female genital mutilation," so Dr. Badawi concludes.

Educated Moslems make time and again the very same statement in other countries all over Africa where FGM is practiced. But they and the religious Islamic leaders have done nothing to effectively share their knowledge. Hansen reports that he spoke on this subject to the Grand Mufti Sheikh Hasan Mahmoon, who was at that time the supreme religious authority in Egypt and the Chancellor of the Moslem al-Azhar University, which has great influence on religious decisions throughout the Moslem world including Egypt. This important religious leader was well informed on FGM, which is called **Khafd** in classic Arabic. (See "Historic Background") But that FGM is not an Islamic requirement has not been widely communicated by him or any other Islamic authority through religious or other channels to the community not even in Egypt where TV, radio and all kinds of media are readily available and widely used. Dr. Badawi states:

> "Female genital mutilation is a common and popular practice throughout Egypt where every day thousands of young girls are subjected to this torture and mutilation. Religious institutions and ancient social customs are primarily responsible for the genital mutilation of female children. The full social and psychological consequences of mutilating the genitals of female children have yet to be evaluated. Preliminary evidence, however, suggest that the psychological consequences of female genital mutilation are very similar to that of rape victims. . ." [9]

Egypt has a statute which goes back to 1959 prohibiting the operations; and it was further reinforced in 1978. In 1959, on the basis of a resolution by the Minister of Public Health, a committee was formed to investigate the question of female circumcision. Besides the Undersecretary of the Ministry of Health, who served as chairman, the Grand Mufti, the Governor of Cairo, and five directors from the ministry made up the all-male committee.

The following resolution was formulated, signed by the Minister and the Undersecretary of the Ministry of Public Health:

> "Circumcision as performed at present is physiologically harmful for girls whether before or after marriage. Although Islamic Jurists basing their arguments on verified shadith (sayings of the Prophet) have differed on whether Khafd (reduction, meaning female circumcision) is a duty, a sunna, or makrama (ennobling) yet they have all agreed that it is an Islamic ritual and Sharia law forbids the total clitoridectomy. Therefore, the committee sees the necessity to proceed with the Khafd operation in the following order:
>
> 1. It is absolutely forbidden for others than doctors to perform the operation.
>
> 2. For those who desire circumcision, the operation should be partial and not total clitoridectomy, in accordance with the by-laws to be formulated at a later stage." [10]

In June 1978, another document, "Facts on Female Circumcision", was issued which referred to the above-cited document of 1959. In addition, it states that: "Female circumcision is forbidden in the public health units for scientific and health reasons. It is not permitted for certified dayas to perform any surgical operation including female circumcision." [11]

In the country report contributed by the Egyptian delegation from the Ministry of Health to the 1979 World Health Organization Seminar in Khartoum, this legislation is cited. An investigation of the implementation of this resolution shows that doctors do not report - nor do the hospitals - the many cases of mutilated children brought to the hospitals usually due to hemorrhage, that is, uncontrolled bleeding. And the Egyptian report continues:

> "In the 30 percent of the cases that are reported because of obvious mutilations and severe hemorrhage, usually no serious action is taken against the parents. The case is closed once the parents are reprimanded by the police officer." [12]

This Egyptian legislation is frequently cited for its "effectiveness" in the Sudan, as private physicians who serve wealthy Egyptians see fewer excised women and, therefore, claim at medical meetings that the practice is decreasing. Egyptian women in the modern sector who go to international meetings frequently also claim that these operations no longer exist in Egypt because they are no longer practiced among the highly educated upper class or among their own friends. Such women have never visited public clinics or investigated what goes on in the squatter settlements among urban immigrants to Cairo or in the villages and are not aware of the sexual practices of the vast majority of the population.

The Egyptian country report is discussed in more detail in the chapter on the World Health Organization Seminar: it does show, however, an astonishing ignorance of the basic biological and sexual facts, even on the part of the trained health personnel including nurses working in obstetrics. For instance, in a survey made by professor Eleanor W. Smith, who taught maternal and child health Nursing in Alexandria, fully 83 percent of the obstetrical nurses working in hospitals in Alexandria, believed there were "no disadvantages" connected with the mutilations. A third of the 135 nurses questioned said they would have their own children operated for "aesthetic reasons" or "to protect their daughters from delinquency"! [13]

Many trained workers in family planning clincis (such training programs are often planned and organized with US and other international assistance) similarly are recorded to opt for excision of their daughters for instance in the Egyptian survey made and presented at the WHO Seminar. One can but wonder about the training in family planning that these women receive: It is largely up to these family planning workers who are in constant contact with the people that come to the clinics, whether or not family planning is positively accepted and practiced. Yet, the family planning workers clearly do not know the basic biological facts about female anatomy or they would not have their own daughters excised.

Family planning programs in Egypt as well as in much of Africa, are often the only organized way by which women and also men can get factual biological information on reproduction and personal health. Such information is quite incompatible with traditional myths and the customary beliefs about their own bodies, sexuality and reproduction that girls are traditionally taught and that have terrible results for their health. The myths about the necessity of genital mutilation are one obvious example. They would not be believed, except for the lack of factual information and total ignorance about the functions of the human body that prevails. But nowhere have family planning organizations addressed this issue. The international family planning organizations and programs - both governmental and non governmental - have altogether failed to teach reproductive health as part of family planning activities.

Family planning in Egypt is supported by the government and all major international family planning organizations, but so far it has failed to effectively reduce population growth. The answer may be that women who are kept in total ignorance about their bodies and health have little motivation to practice birth control. Not even trained nurses and family planning workers know the facts about genital mutilation - as shown above.

The myths and misinformation or, alternatively, the lack of knowledge on reproduction and on the biological facts of the female body is both cause and reason why these mutilations continue today and why family planning programs are ineffective as population statistics show, even though family planning has been official government policy in Egypt for more than 20 years or longer than anywhere else in Africa or in the Middle East.

The population of Egypt continues to grow, though by now basic foodstuffs have to be imported at an ever-larger rate. Productive acreage per person in Egypt is the lowest in the world in a country where most of the land is desert. In Egypt, as elsewhere, family planning programs concentrate on acceptors, that is, they try to persuade as many women as possible to accept contraceptives; but little or no time is "wasted" to teach women about reproduction and sexuality; the harmful effects of genital operations are never mentioned at all.

In a society where the status of most women depends on the number of her sons and where Islam prevails, which makes marriage compulsory, family planning cannot possibly succeed. There also is a direct relationship between the education of a woman and the number of children she has, as all population statistics show. The vast majority of Egyptian women continues to be illiterate, and nothing effective is done to remedy that situation.

A young woman reporter of **El Ahram**, the leading paper of Egypt, put it quite succinctly: when she told me that in Egypt family planning is a prime political problem as everything is related to the population explosion, which is rapidly engulfing the country.

Egypt is the first country in Africa where family planning was made official government policy. As elsewhere, it was first introduced by private initiatives. Aziza Hussein of Cairo, long active in international affairs, is credited with starting the first family planning activities in Egypt by organizing the Cairo Family Planning Association, which she still leads. Later she also served as president of International Planned Parenthood Federation (IPPF) the largest worldwide association of national groups. Recently she talked to me about the beginning of family planning in Egypt, which required a new way of thinking quite different from traditional Egyptian and Middle Eastern concepts and attitudes:

> "At first, no one wanted to talk about family planning; but we finally succeeded in getting the subject out in the open for public discussion. We introduced IUDs to physicians in Egypt and called in international family planning organizations for assistance. Twenty-five family planning clinics were organized and functioning before the government program was started in 1966." [14]

The really revolutionary ideas represented by family planning as a woman's right need to be put into the context of the status of women in the Middle East. In her book, **Veil of Shame**, [15] Evelyne Accad provides the background of the status of North African and Arab women including Egyptians. The status of women in these Moslem societies, seen through contemporary fiction, provides a far more penetrating background than any academic, sociological study could. "Spoliated in spite of the laws, sometimes sold, often beaten, bound to forced labor and assassinated almost with impunity," this description characterizes the lot of the Arab woman in North Africa and the Middle East; Accad adds: She is "one of the serfs of our age." [16]

In an introductory chapter on "The Social Position of Women in North Africa and the Arab World", the background is provided, urging the reader to discard all preconceived notions which are, for the most part, derived from European cultural history.

The life cycle of a woman is typically defined by customs which operate today in Egypt as well as in most of Northern and Moslem Africa and much of the Middle East. Here are some highlights:

> "In North Africa and the Arab world the birth of a child is a time for rejoicing - provided that child is a male. . . If, on the other hand, the child is a girl, her birth will be treated differently: the mother is likely to be sad at the prospect of her daughter repeating her own fate; the father is annoyed because he must bear the burden of guarding the girl's (and the family's) honor and must find her a husband. . ."

> From early childhood, a girl is brought up in constant fear of losing her virginity. There are several psychosocial explanations for this virginity mania. . . It (is) evidence of exclusive possession, proof that the merchandise is brand new. . .
>
> . . . It represents the 'honor' of the girl and, more importantly, of her family. In the event that a girl brings dishonor to her family by losing her virginity, it is considered normal for her brother to murder her in order to avenge the family's honor. . . Public opinion permits such ritual murder. . . So far, no court has ever handed down a sentence of capital punishment for a man judged guilty of having murdered a woman for 'misconduct'. . .
>
> . . . Marriage is of paramount importance. But marriage is unlikely to be a joyous affair for the bride, first because she will have no part in choosing her future husband, and second because marriage becomes, for most women, a state of oppression and imprisonment. . .
>
> . . . when the day of the leilat-al-dokhla (literally 'night of penetration') arrives, a ritual of preparation takes place. . . Every trace of hair (is removed) from the bride's body. . . the removal of the pubic hair removes the bestial stigma from the female genitalia.
>
> On the marriage night the relatives generally gather outside the nuptial chamber and, after the consummation, the mother-in-law (and sometimes others as well) troop in to view the sheet or handkerchief stained with the hymenal blood.
>
> Procreation of numerous children is a religious virtue. . . So while women are treated as factories for producing the yearly offspring, their partial redemption lies in fulfilling this role successfully. At the same time, women unable to assume this function are regarded with disdain and contempt. . .
>
> The woman's position in marriage is rendered even more precarious and unsatisfying by the institutions of polygamy, concubinage and divorce by repudiation. Since in most countries in North Africa and the Middle East there is no distinction between secular and religious law, it is legal for a Moslem male to have as many as four wives and an unlimited number of concubines. . .
>
> A wife must practice ta'a, the submission of the woman to her husband's will and desires. . . She does not have the right to leave his house (or the conjugal bed). He on the other hand has the legal right to keep her under his roof and make her submit to his will. He can appeal to the police and have them bring his wife back by force if she has left his house without permission. . . In the quest for obedience, ta'a permits the Arab male to beat his wife with a stick. . ."[17]

Family planning is of enormous importance for the status of women as it carries the seeds of revolution by providing the opportunity for women to control their reproduction. Traditionally such control is vested in the male, especially in Moslem societies and in Africa. For the first time, women at least are addressed and encouraged to participate in the decision of whether or not to have a child. The very possibility for such a choice is something entirely revolutionary for a woman whose every decision about her own body has always been made for her, without the slightest consideration for what she wanted herself or her health.

Family planning, though it is generally accepted by Moslem societies and is not in conflict with the teachings of Islam, nevertheless has aroused opposition among orthodox Moslem groups also in Egypt, who oppose all change, especially where women are concerned, and who regard women as chattel and tools to be used by men.

The Cairo Family Planning Assocation, which was instrumental in introducing family planning in Egypt more than 25 years ago under the leadership of Aziza Hussein, a revolutionary step at that time, also took the initiative in championing divorce legislation, that is, reform of family law. In a Seminar held in 1978 on "Law, Women and Family Size", the connection between population growth and the status of women in the family was established:

> "Studies and research indicate that the status of women in family law, currently carried out in Egypt, does not offer women a proper position in the family, a fact which leads to insecurity not only to women but also to their families. To be constantly threatened by unrestricted divorce and polygamy causes women to lose psychological, social and economic security. . . As a result of which they resort to more childbearing in the hope of attaining this security of which they are deprived." [18]

The seminar makes a number of recommendations. Among them are to draft a comprehensive family code similar to the existing civil or penal codes. This code would enable each member of the family to know his or her rights and obligations which could not be interpreted by local authorities in different ways.

The minimum age of marriage should be raised and the right of a woman to work cannot be restricted because of marrriage.

A married man would have to get the permission of a judge to marry another wife, such permission would have to be justified financially and both wives would have to consent.

Similarly, divorce could only be transacted by a judge and not unilaterally. All parties would be punished should the divorce take place outside the court. A daughter would remain in her mother's custody until marriage; a son would remain with her only until the age of fourteen, at which time he could choose the parent with whom he wished to live.

The legislative response at first was positive and a new code was drafted and enacted. However, most recently with the gain in power of Islamic fundamentalism, judges have been unwilling to implement the legislation.

Another ground breaking initiative organized by the Cairo Family Planning Association and a first in Egypt, indeed in Africa, was the "Seminar on Bodily Mutilation of Young Females" held in October 1979, half a year after the WHO (World Health Organization) Seminar in Khartoum on "Traditional Practices Affecting the Health of Women and Children", where the issue of female genital mutilation was discussed for the first time by delegations of African and Middle Eastern health ministries including Egypt. (See above.)

The objectives of the seminar in Cairo were outlined as follows:

> "to point out the historical, social, health and psychological aspects. . . to ascertain the prevalence of this custom, the factors contributing to it and the effects resulting from it in order to formulate a clear policy. . . aimed at correcting some of the misconceptions surrounding it, as well as arousing awareness regarding its harmful effects on women's health and psychology. . ." [19]

A large number of both national and international organizations were represented at this meeting including the World Health Organization, UNICEF, the Arab League, the medical departments of leading Egyptian universities and many media organization representatives. The seminar attracted a great deal of media attention as it was the first time this issue of FGM was publicly presented.

The meeting was opened by Dr. Amal Osman, Minister of Social Affairs. The speakers, especially those from the medical schools, established unequivocally the adverse effects of the operations on the health of women and on the Egyptian family. A long list of well thought out recommendations were developed. This list can serve Egypt as well as other affected countries as an example of what needs to be done and provides a remarkably detailed outline for useful actions. Among these recommendations the following ones stand out and are applicable in most areas where genital mutilation is practiced:

> "To organize a national campaign. . . through mass media for both rural and urban areas, with the objective of arousing consciousness about the health, psychological and social damage resulting from female circumcision. . .
>
> To inform and educate the parents. . . through different agencies, especially . . . Family Information and Education Programs. . . Maternal and Child Care Centers, Parents Councils in schools, etc. . .
>
> To provide simplified booklets including instructive materials relating to female circumcision practice and the bad effects resulting from it. . .

To give attention to the role of women's organizations and. . . women's committees in political parties. . .

To convince midwives to work in eliminating this custom. . . providing them with suitable work that may prevent them from continuing to gain out of practicing such operations.

To include in the Medical Faculties and the Nurses' Schools, appropriate courses and programs. . .

To include in the Ministry of Education schools curricula, the necessary instructive material showing the damages caused by female circumcision. . .

To carry out further scientific research. . .

To formulate the legislation necessary to forbid female circumcision."

El Ahram, the most influential paper of Cairo, published extensive articles on the seminar which established the fact that there is no Islamic tenet that female circumcision is a religious prescription - on the contrary. Well-known Egyptian physicians who spoke at the seminar were also cited in the press coverage on the detrimental psychological and physical results of the operations. One of the key medical speakers at the meeting was Dr. Roshdi Ammar from the Obstetrical/Gynecological Department of the Medical School of Ain Shams University.

Dr. Ammar, together with Dr. Karim, had published already in 1965 a clinical research study of 331 women on the effects of excision on orgasm. Based on their research, the two doctors summarized their findings: "circumcision is a harmful practice, it is a cause of sex trauma, and has a definite effect on orgasm and to a lesser degree on sex desire." They added that "Orgasm has a definite effect on the general nervous system. . . over forty percent of the women who were unable to obtain orgasm had been diagnosed as seriously psychoneurotic. Of the women who did obtain normal orgasm less than two percent were regarded psychoneurotic." [20]

The seminar by the Cairo Family Planning Association in the autumn of 1979 became the beginning of a continuing initiative and once more stressed that FGM is not required by the teachings of Islam - though male circumcision is. This issue was and is stressed every time FGM is discussed in a Moslem country. It is of course a fact that genital operations on females are practiced by all religious groups, including by all Christian denominations both Catholic and Protestant as well as by members of the African and Middle Eastern Christian churches such as the Ethiopian Church and the Coptic Church, quite aside from most African traditional religious beliefs called animist.

However, as experience shows, some religions more than others encourage the practice or fail to oppose it or simply ignore it. Though FGM is not required by the Koran, large numbers of Moslems practice it because they believe that it enhances their religious standing. Much of the Moslem religious leadership does not discourage such beliefs. There are areas in Africa where local Moslem leaders support such ideas. It is said frequently by Moslem scholars that according to various interpretations the Prophet said "Circumcision for men is an order, for women a noble act." [21]

Protestant Christan denominations at times oppose the practice strongly (see "Case History: Kenya"), but the Roman Catholic Church never has and is doing nothing even now to discourage the mutilation of the female children of their converts. (See "Case History: Ethiopia"). The members of the Ethiopian Christian and Coptic Christian churches have practiced FGM traditionally for centuries with the full knowledge of the religious authorities. And African indigenous or animist religions are deeply involved in the traditional cultural beliefs which embrace and support FGM.

In Egypt, about ten percent of the population belong to the Coptic Christian Church (about six million people), most of whom traditionally excise their female children. The WHO Seminar and the resulting discussion of the health issues, which in the past were never mentioned publicly let alone in Egypt, prompted the Coptic Church authorities to investigate the practice and its effects on the health of their female followers.

In the summer of 1980, the Coptic Church authorities, specifically the Department of Education and Women's Programs, developed a program, "The Project on Combatting Female Circumcision"[22], and asked the UNICEF office in Cairo, then headed by Mr. Ulf Kreuger, for assistance. This proposal, which included an extensive plan of action, a three-year training and education program, the development of educational materials and training sessions for religious and community leaders throughout the Coptic community of Egypt, represented one of the most thorough and practical plans developed on the community level. The project involved the entire Coptic Church membership and community leadership in an outreach program designed to address every section of the Coptic community.

But Dr. Maurice Assad, the Assistant General Secretary of the Coptic Church, who is an educator by profession, and helped in the development of the plan, was refused all UNICEF help by the Cairo office. This despite the fact that the International Office of UNICEF, following the WHO Seminar in Khartoum in 1979, had announced worldwide that UNICEF was ready to assist all national and local efforts to abolish the practice of female circumcision". This policy was officially announced at the end of 1979 [23] and confirmed in a press release which was widely circulated at the United Nations Mid-Decade Conference in Copenhagen in May 1980.

UNICEF in this four page press release states that in order to eradicate female circumcision the agency will make "strong advocacy efforts towards national policy and decision-makers - all health personnel - and the general public; and UNICEF will provide "support to individuals and organizations. . . foster action oriented research and disseminate. . . results of successful action".[24]

Yet the first UNICEF representative who was asked to support a well-planned community program - Mr. Ulf Kreuger of Egypt - refused. When his refusal was brought to the attention of the UNICEF headquarters in New York and Executive Director James Grant, UNICEF ignored the whole matter. Yet it was UNICEF headquarters in New York that had announced and distributed the new poilicy regarding FGM, after years of deliberately looking the other way by the international agency specifically set up to concern itself with women and children. But as in all other UN Agencies the leadership is by men - including many from Africa and the Middle East. No one knows if they do not have their own daughters mutilated - and no one asks!

Women worldwide wrote letters of protest about this refusal of assistance by a UNICEF representative. More than any other international agency UNICEF depends on private donations and especially on the good will of women volunteers. Despite an open letter to Mr. James Grant in January 1981 published in **WIN NEWS**[25] asking UNICEF to comply with its own internationally stated policies concerning genital mutilation, UNICEF has not provided assistance to the Coptic Church program.

UNICEF's assistance to any programs to stop FGM has been at best reluctant and very limited. While UNICEF headquarters in New York make paper statements and claim to make policies, what goes on in the field is quite different. Action is left to the local representatives, mostly men, who do whatever they wish or what pleases the local decision makers almost always men who have other "priorities" and are certainly not concerned with working against FGM.

There is no leadership on the part of Mr. Grant in New York, though he travels around and is frequently quoted in the press. But he has always avoided doing or saying anything effective regarding FGM - indeed UNICEF has and is the international agency most reluctant to deal with the issue despite its mandate to work for children and their mothers - though some individual officers within this huge bureaucracy at times have been most helpful. (See "The Politics of FGM").

The Cairo Family Planning Association after the great success of its initial seminar in autumn 1979 developed a program which was the first organized action anywhere to prevent FGM. By 1981, a special office of Coordinator of Female Circumcision was set up and took over the many activities of implementing all the recommendations made at the seminar held in October 1979, which had created a great deal of attention.

Ms. Aziza Kameel Mahmoud took over as coordinator of the female circumcision project and has guided the many activities ever since as part of the ongoing programs of the Cairo Family Planning Association. These represent a large variety of meetings, personal interventions, publicity campaigns, consciousness raising activities, education programs and teaching assignments addressing many different audiences of Egyptian society.

The "Project of the Physical Violation of Young Females" now publishes an annual report which lists the many activities carried out during the previous year and provides a remarkable list of initiatives for anyone interested in effectively working on stopping these mutilations.[26] Over the years the Cairo Family Planning Association and Ms. Kameel have gathered more experience than anyone else as to what is effective and what needs to be done. The activities organized are mainly addressed to the health and social service sector in Egypt and to the extensive educational institutions in Cairo especially in the field of nursing and medicine that train professionals who work all over the Middle East.

In addition, in 1991 a television and broadcasting project was organized, and special TV messages were developed as well as programs for training broadcasters. Messages on FGM were integrated into selected TV programs. Another recent project is concerned with a survey of all educational materials on FGM including booklets, prints, posters, leaflets, videos, models, and more.[27]

The Egyptian program is now affiliated and works together with the Inter African Committee on Traditional Practices Affecting the Health of Women and Children-(IAC), which has affiliates in more than twenty-two countries in Africa.[28] The Egyptian program was organized some years before the IAC was organized in 1984. Egypt is by far the most urbanized member country of the IAC with very different living conditions from most of sub-Saharan Africa. Certainly the programs developed and implemented in Egypt provide a useful learning experience about activities to stop FGM in many other African countries. But the Egyptian government refused to give permission to the Cairo Family Planning Association to host the IAC Regional Conference of 1990 in Egypt stating that a private group in Cairo could not host an international seminar.

An overview of the activities of the Female Circumcision Project was effectively presented at the 1988 seminar held in Mogadishu, Somalia, on "Strategies to Bring About Change" The report by Aziza Kamel stated that their program was based on an extensive survey which documented that 80% of the 500 women aged 20-30 questioned had been circumcised, with custom and tradition given as the main reasons. Some of the programs and actions listed below can serve as examples:

> "Producing educational and scientific messages // Booklets and printed materials in English and Arabic // Producing video cassettes in form of messages // Gaining the attention of journalists, radio and TV broadcasters and informing them about FGM // Holding seminars in higher nursing institutes and university hospitals and Ministry of Health hospitals // Training leaders among nurses, social workers in the villages of greater Cairo // Educating students of secondary schools // Educating young men at community centers // Educating women factory workers // Organising face to face campaigns at different meeting places using audio-visual methods // Using mobile units headed by social workers to pass out information to reach different countries as well as families."[29]

The annual reports of the project detail many more activities to reach the growing and very diverse population of Egypt, a country that has been the seat of many different societies, empires and civilizations going back as far as recorded history.

Egypt's unique monuments that are still being explored by archaeologists go back to prehistoric times. But what is disconcerting to learn is that the archaeologists who investigated the lives, accomplishments, artifacts and customs of these remarkable and productive ancient societies also found when excavating burial sites and evaluating the human conditions of the mummies that the females found in these magnificent tombs bore evidence and unrefutable signs of genital mutilation! (See "Historic Background").

SOME PERSONAL HISTORIES:

These personal stories of women are from the Egyptian country report presented at the Seminar in Khartoum and other sources.

Mona is a 23-year-old graduate of a commercial school and a Copt. She is single and works as a secretary in a college in Cairo. She was operated on at the age of nine:

> "My mother had nothing at all to do with the whole process. . . It was a decision between my father and his sister. My aunt told me that she was taking me on an outing when I realized that we were going to the doctor's clinic. . ."
>
> My aunt and the young Muslim doctor and his male assistant caught hold of me. The doctor explained that this was necessary for my future, to guarantee my marriage. They held me tight and I couldn't run away. The male assistant stretched my legs apart, and the doctor cut off the tip of my 'clitoris' with his scissors. . .
>
> My aunt followed the same procedure with my cousins, as well as my three sisters . . . The people around me still explain that circumcision is as important as keeping clean and is a prerequisite for mariage. . .
>
> The dayas (traditional midwives) emphasize the importance of the operation, and claim that what is cut off is ugly and the husband would not experience any pleasure if it is not cut off. All girls I know in my neighborhood are circumcised. . ."

Enayat is 22 years old, a Muslim and a graduate of the Faculty of Commerce, who was born and raised in Cairo. She married an army officer who is also a university graduate. Her father is a lawyer. Enayat and her two sisters were circumcised when they were less than nine years old.

> "My grandmother and my father decided that I should be circumcised according to custom and tradition. A daya came and performed the operation at home. I didn't know about it except on the day itself when my grandmother told me it was necessary. I was very afraid, especially when the woman came, opened her bag, and produced the razor and the disinfectant. I screamed from pain, and my grandmother and my aunt were greatly concerned. It took me one week to resume my usual activities. . .
>
> I don't intend to circumcise my daughter because this is an old custom that does not fit with our modern way of thinking. . . People circumcise their daughters to avoid nervous tensions from which uncircumcised girls suffer. An uncircumcised girl is considered to cause trouble in marital life. The dayas support female circumcision because it is a source of income."

Here are more statements by Egyptian women from different backgrounds who were asked their opinions about the operations. Many women are led to believe that the mutilations are essential for marriage and for acceptance by their society. But it is clear that all of them lack essential information on their own bodies and how they function.

> "A daya performed the operation on me while her assistant twisted my arms under my legs and held me down. I screamed from fear and pain. Later I learned they had cut off all the clitoris and the two leaves (labia minora). I stayed in bed five days and for seven days I was given chicken for lunch. . .
>
> During the earlier years of my married life, my husband had intercourse with me almost evey night. I felt it was wrong, but had to submit out of duty. I came from a strict house; sex was never mentioned. I don't know if my cold feeling was due to circumcision. When I was about to circumcise my eldest daughter at the age of eight, an enlightened lady whom I met explained all the fallacies regarding the practice and advised me against it. I persuaded my husband and my girls were spared. My neighbors followed my example. . .
>
> I am convinced it is wrong, and I know of many cases of hemorrhage after the operation. One girl bled to death, though she was taken to the hospital. The parents were taken to court and penalized. Unfortunately, the operation is now done in secret, and serious cases are not taken to the hospital for fear of punishment.

> The daya did the operation with a razor, after putting some alcohol on the place first. Of course, I felt great pain and screamed, but I was given a glass of lemonade and carried to bed. They took the pieces of flesh, rolled them in salt, and wrapped them in a rag which was tied around my arm for a week."

Another woman relates she could not move for three days and could not urinate for eight hours. Then her mother made her sit in warm water with disinfectant, which helped; but it still burned. The doctor checked the wound twice and she was fed chicken and liver to make up for lost blood. The doctor cut off the clitoris and the labia minora: "Whenever I wash myself, I feel there is nothing there." Nevertheless, she is in favor of the operation.

Another believer in circumcision is having all four of her daughters mutilated: "The daya cut off a part of the clitoris and the two leaves (labia minors) of each child with her razor, one right after the other, while I held them down" she relates. She believes that cirucmcision helps children to grow and develop. "It fattens them up.," she says. "All must be circumcised - my husband is a believer in circumcision. He reminded me of the necessity to circumcise our daughters. It is shameful not to be circumcised. . . no man likes to have an over-sexed woman. . . her organ would prick the man, an uncircumcised woman is like a man - only foreigners do not circumcise their daughters."

The "deflowering" of the bride is another Middle Eastern custom also practiced in Egypt. This is considered all-important as it visibly confirms virginity and absolute male control over the female reproductive organs. It is ironic that Middle Eastern men and male heads of families believe their "honor" is hinged to the status of the genitalia of their daughters. Female genital mutilation is practiced because, according to male perceptions, this is the most efficient way for men to control female sexuality and virginity.

The "deflowering" of the bride demonstrates visibly that she is a virgin by producing a bloody cloth upon first penetration, and is the high point of each Middle Eastern marriage ceremony. The formal "deflowering", which is done by the husband or by a daya, requires that a bloodied piece of cloth or handkerchief be shown as proof of the bride's virginity to the families, who are assembled outside the bride's bedroom. This is to confirm the family's honor - that is, the honor of the father of the bride - showing that the merchandise is new, for which he gets a considerable bride-price. This practice, accompanied by drums and celebration, still prevails not only in Egypt but also all over North Africa, the Middle East and other Moslem societies.

It is astonishing that virtually nothing has been said by the World Health Organization about the obvious danger of AIDS infection by this medieval custom, though the link between FGM and AIDS has been cited frequently. But obviously their honor is more important to these Moslem men than the lives of their daughters, and now they are risking the very future of their own families and societies in order to keep their honor - read supremacy - in place rather than protecting them from infection with AIDS..

Infection with AIDS, which is a death sentence that no one can escape to date, is the silent ever-menacing background and inevitable result of the sexual customs and traditions of Africa and the Middle East. Sexual mutilations, polygamy, rape, child marriage and prostitution are imposed by men on the most defenseless members of their societies and families. Women and girls are the victims. To defend these traditions is no longer just a human rights violation but a death sentence as well: And this should be remembered by the men in Western societies and international agencies who so glibly speak about "the importance of preserving traditions". How dare men uphold these sexual customs for their own aggrandizement and satisfaction - customs that kill those on whom they are imposed by force with no choice of their own: girls and women?

Egypt has all the educational and intellectual resources, the communication facilities and health networks as well as infrastructure to effectively deal with the problem: Sexual mutilations and male imposed sexual customs are a growing death threat due to AIDS, which is spread by men. Where is the leadership of Egypt, where are the men to finally say **STOP - we must change our customs**, we must change **ourselves**! And in the end each man must face **himself** and change! .

EGYPT: ECONOMIC/SOCIAL FACTS & SUMMARY

Egypt:	26 Governorates. President (elected). Most urbanized country of continental Africa.
Climate:	Hot and dry summer. Most of the country is desert except for Nile Valley and Delta. Arable land: 3%.
Population:	54.8 million (1989 estimate). Cairo (capital), 12 million. Alexandria, 4 million. Nile Valley and Delta are most densely populated regions in the world. **Annual Growth Rate:** 2.6%.
Life Expectancy:	59.3 years // **Infant Mortality:** 93/1000 (1989).
Government:	Republic. Independence: 1922. Constitution 1971. Universal suffrage over 18 years old. President/Prime Minister/Cabinet. People's Assembly (legislative).
Ethnic Groups:	Egyptian, Bedouin Arab, Nubian.
Languages:	Arabic (official). English, French.
Religions:	Sunni Muslim (90%). Coptic Christian.
Literacy:	45% (women much less).
Education:	Age 6 to 12 compulsory, free. Twelve major universities.
Annual/Capita Income:	$680 (1987 estimate).
Economy:	Growth Rate: 2% (1987-88). Exports: 2.5 billion. Imports: 10.1 billion. (Foodstuffs, machinery, equipment.) Basic foods are subsidized and rationed. Oil export. Film industry.

FOOTNOTES

1. Hansen, Henny Harald. "Clitoridectomy: Female Circumcision in Egypt" **Folk**. Vols. 14-15, 1972/73, pp. 15-26.
2. Ibid., p. 18.
3. El Saadawi, Nawal. **The Hidden Face of Eve: Women in the Arab World**. Zed Press, London, 1980, p. 8.
4. Kennedy, John G. "Circumcision and Excision in the Egyptian Nubia", **Man**. London, Vol. 5, No. 2, 1970, pp. 175-191.
5. Baasher, T.A., M.D. (Regional Advisor on Mental Health, World Health Organization, Eastern Mediterranean Region, P.O. Box 1517, Alexandria, Egypt) "Psychological Aspects of Female Circumcision", paper presented at the 5th Obstetrical/ Gynaecological Congress, Khartoum, Sudan, 1977.
6. Summary of Survey on Female Circumcision in Alexandria, Egypt. conducted by the Family Planning Association of Alexandria, 17 Sidi El Metwally St., Alexandria, Egypt. See **WIN NEWS**, Vol. 7, No. 1, Spring 1981, p. 34.
7. Hansen, H. H. Op. cit., p. 18.
8. Badavi, Mohamed, M.D./ M.P.H. "Epidemiology of Female Sexual Castration in Cairo, Egypt". **The Truth Seeker**, July/August, 1989, pp. 31-34.
9. Ibid., p. 33.
10. Assaad, Marie Bassili. "Female Circumcision in Egypt: Current Research and Social Implications". Country Report on Egypt. World Health Organization Seminar, **Traditional Practices Affecting the Health of Women and Children**, Khartoum, Sudan, 1979, p. 18.
11. Ibid.
12. Ibid., p. 19.
13. Ibid.

FOOTNOTES (continued)

14. Aziza, Hussein, President, Cairo Family Planning Association. See **WIN NEWS**, Vol. 3, No. 2, Spring 1977, p. 44.
15. Accad, Evelyne. **Veil of Shame. The Role of Women in Contemporary Fiction of North Africa and the Arab World**. Editions Naaman, C.P. 697, Sherbrooke, Quebec, Canada, 1978. See **WIN NEWS**, Vol. 3, No. 3, Summer 1977, pp. 52-54.
16. Ibid., p. 19.
17. Ibid., Chapter 2, pp. 19-31.
18. Law, Women, Family Size Project, February 14-16, 1978. Cairo Family Planning Association, 50 Goumhouria Street, Cairo, Egypt. **The Legal Status of Women in the Family and Its Effect on Their Attitude Towards Childbearing**. See **WIN NEWS**, Vol. 4, No. 3, Summer 1978, p. 40.
19. Report on "Seminar on Bodily Mutilation of Young Females", October 14-15, 1979, published by Cairo Family Planning Association. See **WIN NEWS**, Vol. 6, No. 2, Spring 1980, p. 38.
20. Karim, Dr. Mahmoud, and Ammar, Dr. Roshdi. **Female Circumcision and Sexual Desire.** Published by Ain Shams University Press, Cairo, Egypt, 1965.
21. Ibid.
22. Summary of "Project on Combating Female Circumcision", Middle East Council of Churches (Coptic Church of Egypt), Dept. of Education, Women's Programs, 1127 Corniche El Nil Street, Cairo, Egypt. Dr. Maurice Assad, Asst. General Secretary. See **WIN NEWS**, Vol. 7, No. 1, Winter 1981, p. 38.
23. "UNICEF's Position on Female Circumcision", UNICEF Information Bulletin, No. 21. UNICEF, 3 UN Plaza, New York, New York 10017, USA. See **WIN NEWS**, Vol. 6, No. 3, Summer 1980, p. 36.
24. "UNICEF Conference Statement on Female Excision", #IN/80/8, UNICEF, Information Division. See **WIN NEWS**, Vol. 6, No. 3, Summer 1980, p. 36.
25. Open letter to Mr. James Grant, Exec. Director, UNICEF, January 1991. See **WIN NEWS**, Vol. 7, No. 2, Spring 1981, p. 38.
26. "Project of the Physical Violation of Young Females". An on-going program by Cairo Family Planning Association (summarized in annual reports). See **WIN NEWS**, Vol. 15, No. 4, Autumn 1989, pp. 28-29; **WIN NEWS**, Vol. 16, No. 4, Autumn, 1990, pp. 32-33; **WIN NEWS**, Vol.18, No. 1, Winter 1992, pp. 36-37; **WIN NEWS**, Vol.18, No. 4, Autumn 1992, p. 36.
27. Activity Report 1991 **Project on the Physical Violation of Young Females**. Cairo Family Planning Association. (See **WIN NEWS**, Vol. 18, No. 4, Autumn 1992, p. 36.)
28. **Inter-African Committee on Traditional Practices Affecting the Health of Women and Children**, 145 rue de Lausanne, CH-1202, Geneva, Switzerland, and P.O. Box 3001, Addis Ababa, Ethiopia.
29. **Female Circumcision, Strategies to Bring About Change**. Proceedings of the International Seminar on Female Circumcision, 13-16 June 1988, Mogadisho, Somalia, pp. 70-71. Published by AIDoS - The Italian Association for Women in Development, via dei Giubbonari 30, 00186 Rome, Italy.

For further information see **Enaba, Aziza Wa Abeer** - a film on women's lives and circumcision in Egypt by Dr. Laila Abou-Saif, 19 Gamal Al-Din Abou Al-Mahassen, Garden City, Cairo, Egypt.

CASE HISTORY : ETHIOPIA

Ethiopia, which was known as the Christian Kingdom of Abyssinia in the past, has a long and fascinating history and is the oldest independent country of Africa. Herodotus, the Greek historian of the 5th century B.C. described the country in his writings. According to legend, the rulers of Abyssinia were said to be descendants of King Soloman and the Queen of Sheba. Their son, Menelik I, is credited with the establishment of the Ethiopian empire. Missionaries from Egypt and Syria introduced Christianity in the 4th century, which developed a church cut off from European Christians due to the rise of Islam in the Middle East.

The Portuguese established contact with Ethiopia in 1493 and tried to convert the country to Roman Catholicism. The ruins of medieval castles, churches and splendid stone buildings are among the attractions from a glorious past shown to tourists today in Gondar and other parts of the country. After a century of conflicts between pro- and anti-Catholic factions, all foreign missionaries were expelled in the 1630s, which resulted in hostility toward foreigners and Europeans and in isolating the country until the mid 19th century.

Only then did the kingdom begin to emerge from its medieval isolation. In 1930, the regent and cousin of the empress took over and was crowned as Emperor Haile Selassie. In 1936, the Italians under Mussolini invaded and occupied the country and the emperor was forced into exile. Repeated pleas by Haile Selassi to the League of Nations to free his country from Italian occupation were ignored. The emperor finally returned to his throne only after the Italians were defeated in World War II.

After the United Nations was organized, Haile Selassie spared no efforts to make Addis Ababa an international center. The Ethiopian capital became the seat of the Organization of African States and the Economic Commission of Africa of the United Nations, the two most important regional institutions of Africa. Haile Selassie was one of the few absolute monarchs left in the postwar world. But the people became dissatisfied with his rule and in 1974, after a period of unrest and demonstrations, the aging Haile Selassi was deposed. The military took over the rule of the country. At the end of 1976 Mengistu Haile Merriam, one of the military rulers, took over as chief of state and went to Moscow to sign a military assistance agreement with the USSR.

The socialist regime was concerned with organizing the people and modernizing the country - including carrying out a program of land reform and redistribution of property. Modernization faced enormous problems, especially in the mountainous regions due to lack of roads, transportation and communication. The majority of the people are desperately poor peasants and live a medieval, isolated life in the inaccessible highlands. Women are mercilessly exploited by an oppressive patriarchy and used solely for sexual purposes - as a physician who spent many years in Ethiopia observed. Women, besides growing and preparing the daily food, produce all the household utensils, weave and make the clothes, bear and take care of the children besides carrying water and firewood. The poverty and exploitation of women in rural areas have changed very little over time, no matter who ruled in Addis Ababa .

In 1990, the socialist dictatorship collapsed due to the continuing war with Eritrea, which was fighting for independence for more than two decades, the rebellion in the Northern part of the country and the breakdown of the USSR, which had supported the regime.

To this brief outline must be added that almost the entire female population of Ethiopia is genitally mutilated: Excison is practiced throughout the highlands by the Christian Amharas, who ruled the country until Haile Selassie was deposed. Most of the Moslem population (about 40-45%) infibulate their daughters. All along the Red Sea coast, in Eritrea and in the areas adjoining Somalia, as well as in the large region of Ogaden - mostly inhabited by ethnic Somalis - almost all girls and women are infibulated.

The war for independence of Eritrea - the "longest civil war of Africa" - took place in a region where infibulation is practiced by all ethnic groups. Some women are said to have joined the war as soldiers in order to free women from these terrible mutilations still advocated by local Moslem sheiks. The government in Addis Ababa finally collapsed, exhausted by this war, and Eritrea proclaimed independence; a provisional government took over. The form of independence of Eritrea and the future of Ethiopia will be decided in elections scheduled for 1993. It remains to be seen what the competing groups will do for the freedom of women of Ethiopia, all of whom are mutilated- excized or infibulated according to what men locally require. Except for the few highly educated of the leading families, most women of Ethiopia are among the most oppressed and abused human beings anywhere in Africa.

In Ethiopia, FGM is traditionally even more carefully concealed than elsewhere in Africa. Most international visitors, including many European admirers and supporters of Haile Selassie in the recent past, knew nothing about these damaging sexual mutilations. Even Europeans who lived in Ethiopia for many years were quite unaware that also the aristocracy and ruling families of the country (mostly Amharas) routinely had their daughters mutilated. Their baby girls are excised usually before they are 40 days old.

For instance, a Swiss man named Ilg who lived in Ethiopia for many years and was the very well-informed personal advisor of Emperor Menelik - who ruled at the turn of this century - was completely ignorant of these operations, so Dr. Alfons Huber reports. [1]

Dr. Huber, an Austrian gynecologist, states that the operations in Ethiopia have no religious implications but are a custom of the people, much like facial scarring or tatoos. Roman Catholic emissaries sent by the Pope from Rome to the court of Emperor Claudius in the 16th century objected to the practice because they thought it was of religious origin, much like the Jewish practice of male circumcision, which Catholics vehemently oppose. The Emperor assured them that female circumcision had no religious meaning; thus the practice was approved by the Catholic Church and has been approved by Catholic missionaries all over Africa ever since. (See "Historic Background").

In early 1977, while in Addis Ababa, I was invited to join a private gathering of several young wives of high placed government officials - all mothers of young children - to discuss the status of women in Ethiopia. The women described the extended family system of Ethiopia and the custom that most girls marry very young, often at barely fourteen. Since they have children immediately, many are prevented from getting the education they would have liked, including going to the university. This was one of the women's chief complaints. Clearly they belonged to the elite: The vast majority of the women live in rural areas where up to 95 percent are illiterate and have to do heavy household chores from an early age.

Family planning had been recently introduced as part of an integrated "Family Life Education Program", the women stated at our meeting: There is an absolute prohibition of sex before marriage, and it is a social disaster for a woman to have a child out of wedlock. However, if a woman names the father of the child, he usually accepts it and is required to marry her. Every family wants male heirs: To have sons is most important, the women stressed. In some areas, the bride-price is required; in others, a dowry system prevails. Some young people of educated families - for whom these women spoke - are trying to avoid this now, so they said.

After some frank discussions about the family system, I steered the conversation toward female circumcision. "Everyone circumcises their daughers; of course, it must be done", all the women explained. "It is our tradition; women who are not circumcised are considered to be promiscuous. It is done", the women informed me, "on baby girls before they are 40 days old". The women were speaking about the customs of the Amharas, who live in the area of Addis Ababa. To excise children so young is the tradition of the Ethiopian Christians of the highlands.

"What about health problems" I asked. "But it is a perfectly safe pratice", one of the women quickly said. "All women in my family are circumcised. I never heard of any problems and I have a very large family. We do not live isolated from our relatives, as you do in Europe and America. I would know about any problems in my family", she assured me.

Another woman related that the Department of Health is now sending information to all parents of school children in Addis Ababa about vaccinations and preventive shots. And they also send warnings that people should not cut out the uvulas* because this operation may be dangerous. But the Department of Health has sent no warnings about circumcision of girls; therefore it must be perfectly safe, one of the women said.

"I have a young daughter", another woman added "but my husband told me she must not be circumcised. He absolutely opposes it. My mother is very upset. She says we are taking a terrible chance, and I shall be very sorry later when she grows up. But my husband has forbidden it; I really don't know why."[2]

The Black Lion Hospital is one of the largest hospitals of Addis Ababa. When I visited it, one of the resident pediatricians whom I asked about circumcision told me, "We often get baby girls with all kinds of problems as a result of the operation. Some children are brought in because they are bleeding and it does not stop".

He continued: "When a blood vessel is cut by the operator, such children die without medical help. In other cases, obstructions of the urinary meatus occur from the scars and there are many infections. The girls here in Addis Ababa are operated on very young; it is the same all over the Ethiopian highlands. Often the operations are done on newborns up to 10 days old. In other areas it is a little later up to a few years old. But the operations are done all over Ethiopia with the exception of the Gojam area, where female circumcision is not performed." [3]

And the doctor added: "Here in the hospital, we teach against it. It is decreasing with literacy and in the modern sector". The literacy rate in Ethiopia outside of Addis Ababa is one of the lowest in the world. But as the conversation (above) with women from prominent families shows, most of them are indoctrinated to support the continuation of the mutilations, convinced about the importance of "their traditions". Though, as the women, who were attractive and well dressed in the latest fashions, admitted, they regretted getting a very limited education due to early marriage - another "tradition".

I also talked to two women of the Municipal Women's Organization of Addis Ababa, which was newly formed in 1977 as part of an effort to organize the people both in rural and in urban areas. They told me about the "Kebeles", the neighborhood organizations throughout Addis and all other cities. These are the urban counterparts to the many peasant associations - more than 21,000 all over the country, one of the women said. Each such peasant group has a women's group.

The women's group of the municipality, with an office in City Hall, was formed after International Women's Year in 1975, when a small nucleus of educated women in Addis Ababa organized. I asked them about traditional practices and also circumcision. "Circumcision is a bad social habit; we are just becoming aware of this. There is no movement against it at present", they added, "but women are beginning to examine all traditions, and we will decide what to do about the bad ones." [4] A nationwide women's organization, the Revolutionary Ethiopian Women's Association - REWA - was formed by the Mengistu government, which organized literacy and other kinds of training programs.

Many Ethiopian women are not aware that circumcision does not exist in other parts of the world. For many hundreds of years, it has been part of life in Ethiopia. A young woman student who had recently arrived from Ethiopia at a college in the Boston area discussed her customs with her classmates. The topic turned toward marriage customs. The young woman mentioned circumcision. The American students did not understand what the Ethiopian woman was talking about, and in turn, she could not believe that her new American friends were not circumcised. But everyone does it; it is unthinkable not to. Educated people have doctors to operate on their baby girls, the Ethiopian student said. If a girl is not operated on she becomes wild when she grows up and no one can control her. Circumcision makes her quiet and easy to manage. Everyone knows that!.

---

* It is the custom among many Ethiopians to cut out the uvulas, the little fleshy protruberance inside the mouth at the opening to the throat. This little piece of flesh is, by custom, amputated on newborn infants by cutting it, usually with a piece of horsehair. Many babies die as a result of the operation or from infections.

Many changes were carried out in Ethiopia under the socialist government including land reform; but as the women of the municipality of Addis Ababa had said to me:already in 1977 "The men just laughed at us when we talked about women's rights. These were the men who worked for the revolution. Polygamy, the women claimed, is not legal in Ethiopia; but though it is not practiced by the followers of the Ethiopian Church, it certainly exists in the rural areas and is practiced by the Moslems, who are more than forty percent of the inhabitants of the country.

An East African physician who works for an international family planning organization and who travels all over Ethiopia, sent this information in response to an inquiry about female genital operations:

> "Almost all cultural groups in Ethiopia practice female circumcision. As far as I know, it is only in some districts of the Administrative Region of Gojam. . . among followers of the 'Kebat' Christian sect, where female circumcision is not practiced.
>
> Female circumcision is done. . . by local practitioners. There have not been any reports about female circumcision being performed in hospitals. The process of female circumcision involves. . . cutting a small portion of the clitoris. . .
>
> According to the positivists of female circumcision in Ethiopia, the operation is meant to reduce the sexual sensitivity of the women so that they do not dominate male sexual performance. It also has psychological implications of complete acceptance of male dominance not only in sex but also in other activities as well.
>
> Infibulation. . . means the stitching of the labia majora of the female sex organ . . . Some ethnic groups like the Essas of the Harrar area and Somalis in the Eastern Region of the country do practice it. This is done to keep the virginity of the girl until marriage. The operation is done by elderly women of the community in early childhood. They leave a small opening in the lower part of the vulva so the girl has the chance of passing urine, and the menstrual flow is not obstructed.
>
> Just before marriage the vulva is cut open with a clean or new blade and the girl is allowed to have her first intercourse with her husband. . . If the girl gets pregnant, the vulva is opened by surgery to prevent difficult labor and partial obstruction. Such cases have been often met within modern medical practice. Some women get the vulva stitched back after birth to narrow and tighten the entrance of the penis and thus increase male sexual enjoyment. . ." [5]

Unfortunately, the doctor does not report what happens to the vast majority of girls and women who have no access to physicians to open the infibulation by surgery. The operation, with the exception of the wealthy in the cities, is done by local women who, in many cases, derive their living from this "trade". They have neither the tools nor the anatomical know-how to perform a delicate operation, such as cutting a part of the clitoris of a small baby girl. For the most part, they cut whatever they can get a hold of. For a description of an infibulation operation, see the beginning of the chapter entitled "Case History : Somalia".

Addis Ababa has the only fistula* hospital in East Africa, a 40-bed unit started, organized and run by a husband and wife team of physicians from Australia and New Zealand, respectively. The Doctors Hamlin, with funds they raise themselves, built on the outskirts of Addis Ababa a 40-bed pavilion with an attached operating room and a nurses' station whereby one nurse can supervise the whole room.[6] Every bed is always filled. Women who come from all over Ethiopia are waiting to be operated at a small, temporary hostel - waiting to have their lives restored. Because of incontinence - continuously dripping of urine and/or feces - due to the fistula or tears they suffered in childbirth, the women are outcasts of their families and communities; no one wants to be near them. Some of them walk for miles, all alone, to the hospital: Its fame has spread by word of mouth all over the Ethiopian highlands.

---

* A fistula is a rupture of the internal wall or division between the vagina and the rectum, or between the vagina and the bladder; it occurs due to obstructed labor and results in incontinence.

Many of the injured women lose their babies in childbirth, as well as their health and families. Child marriage is widely practiced in Ethiopia and is one reason for the fistulae: The girls have children before their own bodies are fully grown. Another reason is obstructed labor due to scars from genital operations. When I visited the hospital, every bed was occupied. Specialized care and bed rest are required for three weeks after the operation so the wound can heal, or the scar may break open again. Most of the women in the rows of narrow beds seemed much too young for motherhood. But it is the custom to marry girls off early. All marriages are arranged by the fathers: The bride-price the father gets is the incentive to marry the daughters off early - even if they die as a result.

The subject of female circumcision was discussed for the first time in Addis Ababa at an inter governmental meeting of Africa, sponsored by the United Nations, the "Seminar for Women in Public Life", held in Addis Ababa in 1960.[7] The participants of that meeting requested the World Health Organization to make a study of the health effects of female circumcision, but this request, though made officially, was ignored by WHO until 1979. (See "World Health Organization Seminar").

A Women's Program was started in the early 1970s by the Economic Commission of Africa of the United Nations, located in Addis Ababa. The African Training and Research Centre for Women began its activities after International Women's Year in 1975.[8] Though genital mutilation is practiced in the majority of their member countries, the ECA Women's Program did not acknowledge the damage done to women by these mutilations, which affect the health of more than 100 million women and girls in Africa, until 1984, when the Inter African Committee on Traditional Practices Affecting the Health of Women and Children (IAC) was formed.[9]

In 1977, I met with three African women sociologists of the ECA in Addis Ababa. I asked them about female circumcision. They were reluctant to admit it existed at all. When I inquired about the health of the women involved, they insisted that female circumcision was the least of the concerns of African women. "It is an African custom", they said, "it certainly is not a health problem and African women have more important problems". And they told me that this was none of my business, that these are "important cultural practices" that no outsider can understand.

This view, unfortunately, is widespread in Africa, especially among Western-educated sociologists, such as the women above, who have no training in reproductive health and are entirely ignorant of the gynecological problems and life-threatening health damage resulting from FGM. For the most narrow, chauvinistic and racial reasons, the mutilations of little children are defended by those who are neither qualified nor have any right to speak for them. It is one thing for traditional people to continue customs which they do not dare to relinquish for fear and for lack of education, but it is another thing for educated women to defend and thus perpetuate the mutilation of children on whom these practices are inflicted often by force and always without their consent.

While in Addis, I also went to the Family Guidance Association ,which then ran more than 170 family planning clinics all over the country. I asked the director about female circumcision. "People say that if a girl is not circumcised she will be promiscuous. It is done to subdue girls; it makes women calm and gentle. If a family doesn't have their girls circumcised, they are considered queer; so everybody does it, even highly educated Ethiopians".

In Ethiopia, there is no ritual or religious belief connected with the operations, a fact that is already reported in historical documents. For instance, the Fellasha, the only Jewish ethnic group - who have lived in the highlands for hundreds of years - practice female circumcision in ways similar to their non-Jewish neighbors. Recently, after a severe draught devastated that region, they were evacuated to Israel due to their faith. In an article published as long ago as 1896, Zaborowski[10] reported that the Jewish Fellasha operate on their girls when eight days old - similar to other population groups of the highlands. No matter what religion, Christian, Moslem, Jewish, or Animist, almost all Ethiopians have mutilated their daughters in the past and do so today.

Zaborowski also relates that excision as well as infibulation is practiced by the Galla - where they are in contact with their neighbors, the Somalis - who practice infibulation wherever they live.

> "The Danakil in the North along the Red Sea coast all practice infibulation, also the Massauah and the Bedja. Nowhere. . . is the importance of circumcision of boys and infibulation of girls so greatly emphasized, and nowhere is there a similar preoccupation with sex." [11]

Zaborowski also states that the Scottish explorer, James Bruce, learned about the operations when he first traveled in Ethiopia in the late 1760s and reported about them with horror. Bruce also visited Gondar, which was the capital of the Kingdom of Abyssinia at that time and which he describes in his book, **Travels to Discover the Source of the Nile, 1768-1773**.

Bruce explained that he was told the reason for the operation is hypertrophy or an abnormal enlargement of the clitoris, which was supposed to be indigenous with Ethiopian women. Bruce's report was quoted by Dr. Ploss in every edition of his famous work, **Woman**, first published in1885. (See "Historic Background"). The astonishing fact is that Bruce's tale of hypertrophy of the clitoris as reason for excision has been quoted ever since throughout the medical literature as a fact, explaining why excision is necessary in Ethiopia. Yet not one shred of medical evidence has ever been cited to confirm this alleged enlargement of the genitalia in Ethiopian women, and to this day there is not a single factual report or observation to confirm this hypertrophy anywhere in the medical literature nor from physicians in Ethiopia.

Dr. Alfons Huber, a gynecologist and an obstetrician who spent many years in Ethiopia in the 1960s as a physician for the Austrian Development Assistance, has reported in many articles about his experiences and the research he undertook concerning the mutilations of women, which he saw regularly in his medical practice.

In his activities as gynecologist in Ethiopia, Dr. Huber states he never saw any unusual enlargement or hypertrophy of the female genitalia in all the years he worked there.

The alleged hypertrophy of the clitoris and genitalia of Ethiopian women also provided the Roman Catholic missionaries with an excuse to condone genital mutilation of the daughters of their converts, as Huber [13] and others report. Catholic missionaries and Jesuits came to Ethiopia in the 17th century and for a time were very influential at the court in Gondar, the capital at that time. They prohibited the operation to their converts.

However, soon problems arose as young men refused to marry uncircumcised girls and the people objected against the prohibition. Thus, a papal mission was dispatched from Rome, including a medical man who determined that all Ethiopian women suffered from hypertrophy of "those parts" - that is an enlargement of the clitoris that represented a hindrance to intercourse. The operation, it was claimed, consisted in removing the "natural barriers to consummating marriage", and therefore, it was necessary and the prohibition against female circumcision was quickly lifted.

Roman Catholic missionaries ever since and all over Africa have used this 17th century pronouncement from Rome to condone genital mutilation of female children. Indeed, they permit the operations as "Christian" as long as the children do not participate in the accompanying "heathen rites". Thus, genital mutilation is performed on female Catholic children with the blessing of the Catholic Church all over Africa today. Even in Kenya, where the Protestant missionaries campaigned against the mutilations of the daughters of their converts and prohibited them, the Catholic parishes refused to join them.(See "Case History : Kenya".) Indeed, today all over Africa data are available that the daughters of Roman Catholics are mutilated in much larger numbers than any other group of Christians - and with no interference from the Roman Catholic Church.

Dr. Huber practiced in all areas of Ethiopia and reported that infibulation is done in the areas under the influence of Arabs and Islam, for instance throughout Eritrea and also among the Moslem inhabitants of Massaua.

> "The Danakil perform the operations already on girls three years old and the Somalis operate seven year-old female children. . . The Galla, who live in the area of Harrar evidently learned this practice only lately, that is, during the Egyptian occupation of the province in 1875. They operate on eight-year-old girls. . ." [14]

Besides the operation of infibulation, defibulation creates more problems. The bride is cut open just before she is handed to the bridegroom, who immediately makes use of his "right" to have intercourse. Not only great pain but also frequently profuse bleeding are the result. The screams of the bride are masked by the noise of the wedding feast, the singing, the dancing, and the rhythmic clapping of the guests outside the house or hut where the consummation of the marriage takes place, Dr. Huber reports.

He also states that young brides - girls in their early teens - are often severely injured. The vagina and even the rectum are torn as a result of forcible penetration by the man who acquires a young girl for an often hefty bride-price and is eager to get an immediate reward. When a child is born, more cuts have to be made; "the scars have to be cut from back to front with scissors", Dr. Huber states, and he concludes:

> "Female circumcision and especially infibulation are interventions into the personality of a woman, which are only possible where women are held in great contempt, used solely for sexual purposes. . . neither ritual nor hygienic reasons can be given for the continuation of this senseless atrophied tradition." [15]

Dr. Huber reports that many complications result from excision and from the much worse operation of infibulation. Shock sets in due to the overwhelming pain, as for the most part no anesthetic of any kind is given. Uncontrollable bleeding may immediately follow if a branch artery is cut; such hemorrhage can be fatal. The organs surrounding the area of the operation are often damaged due to the lack of understanding of anatomy on the part of the operator. The urethra, the bladder, the vagina, and even the rectum are injured. Incontinence may result due to injury of the urethra or the sphincter muscles. Since asepsis is unknown, infections of every kind occur, including tetanus, which is fatal. The closure from infibulation may make passing of urine difficult, and irritations and eczema are frequent. The infections may spread into the genital organs creating infertility. [16]

Perceptive observers visiting Ethiopia will notice few spontaneous expressions of warmth or affection between women and men and the same is true elsewhere in Africa, except among those in large cities who have copied Western life-styles. There often seems to be an invisible barrier of fear, suspicion and hostility between women and men. The sexual violence that is traditionally practiced by many African men as their "right" and carefully hidden from Western eyes undermines all human relationships, respect or mutual support between women and men.

Separation and segregation instead of cooperation between men and women are characteristic of most activities of traditional life. Men and women lead quite separate lives - and in most African societies, they neither eat together nor share their food: Men eat first and the best, even if nothing is left for women and children. Men hardly know their children - especially when they have several wives. Each wife is responsible for feeding her children and the husband as well, when it is her "turn" for him to sleep with her, much like in all Moslem societies in Africa.

Segregation of the sexes, the ideal of Islam, is spreading with Moslemization, which is progressing all over Africa and also in Ethiopia. Segregation breeds suspicion, fear and contempt and fosters a completely distorted emphasis on sexuality. Violence dehumanizes all sexual intercourse. Yet sexual intercourse is the only activity married men and women share in Moslem Africa of their otherwise segregated lives.

Female children are mutilated to make them easy to control, that is, control by men. The sexual act, considering that a child bride is sold to a man without her consent, is mostly brutal rape: it is another assertion of the power of males which all females are forced to suffer, at great pain, sometimes at the cost of their lives. Male violence rules family life, which is based on the ruthless exploitation of all women, who are kept in subservience by continuous assertion of male power through beatings to inspire fear. The violent sexual customs and traditions of African men are responsible for the spread of AIDS - with more people infected than anywhere else in the world. Yet the propaganda by anthropologists still demands the support of "culture and tradition" at any price. It finally must be clear that traditions condemn too many in Africa to torturous deaths by AIDS: Women and children again are the innocent victims of this propaganda against change.

The facts about FGM in Ethiopia were officially established by a comprehensive research study published in 1985 with the support of UNICEF and sponsored by the Ministry of Public Health. This survey covered most areas of the country including Addis Ababa and Eritrea and provides a detailed list of important recommendations based on thorough, local invesgitations questioning people directly to ascertain their opinions and find out how deeply entrenched the practice is. An advisory committee was formed consisting of the Ministry of Health, the Revolutionary Ethiopian Women's Association (REWA), the National Committee for Central Planning, the African Training and Research Centre for Women of the Economic Commission for Africa and UNICEF. The investigation had local and national governmental participation as well as international and regional support:

> "The survey highlights the harmful effects of traditional practices. . . in the hope that this sensitive issue will be discussed in relation to the general well-being of women and their daughters. There is much evidence that a sizable number of circumcised females suffer from uterine infections throughtout their lives, and that some deaths result from the complications due to circumcision. . ." [17]

It is interesting to compare these findings with the statements of the women from leading families in Addis Ababa (see above) who convincingly asserted that they had never heard of any problems resulting from excision and argued that the practice did no harm to women's health. These are the women who are sent to international meetings to represent their country where they claim that concerns voiced internationally about the damage done by FGM are quite exaggerated, often implying racism and resisting all international assistance as "interference". This has been the situation for many years preventing all international initiatives. But by now enough research studies like the one here have been made that irrefutably document the damaging facts.

The study found that over 85 percent of all women involved had undergone one of the three types of female circumcision: sunna, excision, infibulation.

> "Medical complications observed among the circumcised include clitorial cyst, urethral infections, extensive scarring, keloid formations and an increased incidence of tearing during delivery, causing fistula and excessive blood loss.More than 20 percent of those studied admitted knowing of complications due to female circumcision and half of these revealed that the complications had been fatal, or had led to irreparable damage."

The main purpose of the study - to learn what people believed to initiate change - produced some disturbing results, which may be due to the isolation of most people who have little contact with the rest of the world. Yet even those who do see no reason to relinquish their traditions.

> "The original reasons underlying the practice of female circumcision concern the basis of society. Among settled peoples, land inheritance was through the male line only, and the same was true for the cattle and camel herds of the nomadic groups. It was in the family interest, therefore, to preserve the true blood line. Hence, a premium came to be placed on the virginity of the bride and faithfulness of the wife.
>
> Influences such as formal education, adult education or urbanization do not seem to have much impact at present. This generalization stems from the evidence that over 70 percent of the literate indicated that they would have their future daughters circumcised. Over half of the total male respondents, the Elders and Youths in higher education, saw very little reason to worry about girls being circumcised."

The study concludes that literacy campaigns and specific initiatives to encourage participation by women to raise their status would help in discouraging FGM as well as decrease the high infant and maternal death rates - the latter estimated at 20 per 1000 pregnant women, according to the Ministry of Health.

The research documents that "the practice had a very strong hold on the population - extreme forms are common and indeed are dominant in Eritrea". It was also found that 20 percent of the respondents had suffered all kinds of severe health problems from fistulae to prolapse of the uterus quite aside from birth complications. The vast majority of women have no access to any kind of modern health or hospital care; therefore, the real damage may be much higher. As a result, comparative research was proposed.

The reasons for continuing FGM, the study concludes, are linked to economic gain, to control of women by men, and to protect the traditional male-only land holding patterns. Besides the bride-price paid to the father of the bride, which is an incentive for early marriage that is widely practiced in Ethiopia, there also are dowries given by some ethnic groups. For instance, the Tigrina-speaking people and others as well give dowries which represent the bride's share in her family's estate.

Land is inherited only by male heirs, hence the dowry. But if the bride is not a virgin, the dowry must be returned and so is the bride. The dowry, which is not customary in other African societies, serves the purpose of keeping the all-important land rights reserved for males and FGM serves to assure the male bloodline. That is, a bride must be a virgin and a wife must not have male children except those of her husband to protect male land ownership by the family. And land ownership is all important in agricultural societies everywhere; hence women are exluded from owning land in most of Africa.

Aside from these quite specific beliefs, many others were cited by respondents including female behavior: "Girls who are not excised run wild, it makes childbirth easier, uncircumcised women are forgetful and break things, they have an offensive odor, they seek divorces and end up as loose women." Aesthetic reasons were also cited. Some even cited sanity as a benefit of FGM and enhancement of good behavior or fidelity as well as honor to the male members of the family. The study concludes:

> "These beliefs cannot be divorced from the question of the status of women and societies' move to control females. The emotional and physical turmoil for the child undergoing circumcision between the age of seven and 12 cannot be overestimated. Such an experience may engender long lasting fear and disgust. . ."

Women are regarded as chattel to bring benefits and honor to the male member of the family. As long as the economic incentives to continue the practice by this patriarchal society are still in place, it will be difficult to persuade the male decision makers.

> "The struggle to eradicate FGM will be formidable. The campaign to suppress it will have to mobilize all possible means to change the knowledge, attitudes and practices of those who continue the operations and also of its influential advocates."

But while this study - one of the most detailed and comprehensive ones ever made in Africa - provides some reasons for the practices, it is difficult to apply this rationale to those who do not own land and the urban elite. There always has been a very large gap between the highly educated, sophisticated ruling families in Addis Ababa belonging to the once powerful Ethiopian Christian Church and the rural subsistence farmers of the highlands.

In turn, the Moslem inhabitants of the lowlands lead a very different life quite aside from Eritrea which has been fighting for independence ever since Mussolini's rule. Yet despite all these differences and despite the fact that the educated ruling families of Addis Ababa used to behave much like the European aristocracy of the past, they all mutilate their female children. Indeed, many men still require their daughters to be infibulated. To any outside observer, the question is why? How can a contemporary government and country tolerate the mutilations of nearly half its citizens because it is "the tradition"? This is not only irrational but a violation of internationally supported human rights agreements.

The Inter African Committee (IAC) on Traditional Practices Affecting the Health of Women and Children held its regional conferences in Addis Ababa, where also their African office, designated as their headquarters, is located at the ECA - the Economic Commission of Africa. The most recent conference in 1990, attended by affiliates from more than 20 African countries, was held at the impressive Africa Hall, which has extensive conference facilities built by Haile Selassie more than two decades ago. [18]

At the IAC conference in November 1990, before the fall of the socialist government, in addition to the delegations from all over Africa, numerous institutions of Ethiopia participated, and one of the opening speeches was given by the Minister of Health of Ethiopia. REWA, the government supported national women's organization, invited all participants to a social gathering and also organized a craft fair and an exhibition of the products made by women who until recently had made their living as excisors.

To do FGM operations - whatever the type practiced locally - is a lucrative occupation all over Africa. The women, mostly traditional birth attendants, who do these mutilations are usually highly respected members of their communities. Therefore, to effectively stop FGM, it is essential to find another source of income for the operators. The excisors in Addis Ababa all were trained in various traditional crafts to enable them to make a living and therefore could be persuaded to stop practicing their trade. Alternative methods of employment will have to be found and organized everywhere FGM is practiced in Africa. Otherwise prohibiting the practice simply means that it goes underground and that girls who are bleeding or badly damaged are not taken to a hospital but left to die - for fear of prosecution. This happens when prohibitions by a government or a president - such as in Kenya recently under President Moi - are decreed and no information or education campaigns are organized. Excisors who have no other way to earn their living simply continue, protected by silence from the community.

In Addis Ababa, retraining of excisors was supported by REWA (Revolutionary Ethiopian Women's Association) with the leadership of the IAC. Due to the change in government in 1991, REWA, which had developed many different training and literacy programs for women all over the country with governmental support was abolished. At this time (beginning 1993) a new national women's organization is being formed; and according to official sources many local women's groups are already active.

The Italian Association for Women in Development - AIDoS [19], who developed an extensive information and education program to eradicate FGM in Somalia (see "Case History: Somalia") including training materials and video tapes, have begun to adapt these programs for use in other African countries with the collabortion of the IAC. Ethiopia is participating in this effort; the National Committee on Traditional Practices [20] will carry out the project which, according to AIDoS, includes two main components: the training of four target groups (women leaders, youth, community leaders and medical/paramedical staff) and a number of teaching aids including seveal videotapes and slides.

A mass information campaign using both modern media (radio, TV, press) and traditional channels of communication (poetry, song and theatrical productions) will be organized. The information program is based on the training of leaders from four countries, besides Ethiopia, Nigeria, Gambia and Sudan are participating. The leaders are trained at the ILO (International Labor Office) Training Center in Turin, Italy [20], in how to organize such campaigns and how to adapt the training material packages developed by the IAC and AIDoS to local needs.

The implementation of this program in Ethiopia will also be supported by UNFPA - the United Nations Population Fund - as well as the regional IAC. The success of the project will depend in part on support by the government, which at present is being organized with a constitution being drafted. Elections are scheduled for 1993/94.

In the final analysis, in Ethiopia as everywhere else in Africa, all the decisions are made by men. Starting with each family, the condition of women - whether or not they are mutilated according to local traditions - depends on the wishes of men. As Dr. Huber also states, whose experience in this is perhaps more extensive than that of anyone else as he spent years in different areas of Ethiopia as a gynecologist: "There is no doubt that excision serves to manipulate female sexuality for the purpose of controlling it."

At the market in Gondar, one can observe the extreme poverty of the people who come there from the countryside - the emaciated, barefoot women and children in rags, always following a few steps behind men and often carrying heavy loads. The men carry what they bring to market on donkeys; the women carry it on their backs and often they carry children as well.

The natural conditions of the often very harsh African environment and life are difficult to endure: Disease, drought, crop failures and great hardship make life very problematic. But instead of joining their talents and hands in mutual support and cooperation for the sake of their children, too many men and women are separated by destructive traditions. Male violence, sexual assault and ruthless wife abuse are exercized by men under the cloak of "African tradition and culture". To exploit, oppress and dominate women is used to prove manhood and gain respect from other men.

Why do African men, so proud of their strength, find it necessary to vent their desires for power on young females, often hardly teenagers, who certainly are no match for their violence? What do men want? Why do African men fear female sexuality so greatly that they insist on destroying it?

In 1977, I flew in a small plane during the rainy season, when the highlands are green, from Addis Ababa to Gondar, the historical capital. The plane flew only a few hundred feet above the grassy slopes with cliffs and canyons and steep ravines. Everywhere small huts, the typical round, thatched peasant houses, were scattered in small clusters of five to ten, all over this bucolic looking landscape. There were no villages, no roads, no towns and certainly no electric wires nor any major rivers. Each group of huts seemed to exist in complete isolation.

No sign of activity or connection with the rest of the world could be discerned. There was nothing at all that connected these huts, scattered all over the green slopes, many hundreds of them, with the rest of the world. There were not even any paths that might indicate that those who lived there regularly walked to another one of the isolated compounds. The small plane took more than an hour to cross this astonishing highland, full of signs of human habitation, but without any signs of a cooperative way of life.

Many thousands of people starved in the droughts of Ethiopia. They were unable to seek help and to escape from their isolation. It often takes many months before news of a famine reaches the outside world. And in Ethiopia, droughts are reported every few years. When the most recent one was shown on TV - which resulted in many offers of assistance from the West - the government of Addis Ababa was only interested in continuing to fight the civil war in Eritrea and not in helping their starving people. The victims of this and other famines as one could see on TV are once again mostly women and children. The isolation of the subsistence farmers, the inhabitants of the highlands, where so many people die unknown to the rest of the world, has hardly changed up to the present time

Ethiopia, despite the efforts of the now ousted socialist regime, is one of the most traditional countries of Africa, with a long, recorded history. But the reality of this past is not the romantic image drawn in history books or by anthropologists. The reality for most rural Ethiopians, who still live in the past, means a life of misery, deprivation and sickness, hunger, superstition and fear. When the rains do not come or are late, all is lost. Predictably women, who face additional hardships such as childbearing, are the ones who suffer most. Physical strength under the conditions of subsistence farming or herding is an asset from which power is derived. Men, since they have first claim to food, are much stronger and bigger than the women of the highlands - after centuries of nutritional deprivation due to patriarchal customs and rules.

In addition or because of the greater power of men, all females are mutilated to keep them under male control. Due to continuous childbearing, though many children perish, women are quite unable to defend themselves against the violence by men. The realization that another kind of life is in their reach, or even exists, has not occurred to the women of the vast rural areas of Ethiopia - and the same is true for much of rural Africa. Most rural and peasant women still live in the past, isolated and illiterate, bound by tradition and without any hope for change or even the consciousness that change is possible. And change for these women can only mean an improvement of their painful lives of hard work and deprivation under the ruthless yoke of patriarchy and poverty.

FOOTNOTES

1. Huber, Alfons. "Die rituelle Beschneidung der Frau - Sinn und Verbreitung" (The Ritual Circumcision of Women - Its Meaning and Distribution), **Mitteilungen Anthropologische Gesellschaft Wien** (Communications of the Anthropoligical Society of Vienna), 101, 76082, 1976.
2. **WIN NEWS,** Vol. 3, No. 2, Spring 1977, p. 48.
3. Ibid, p. 33.
4. Ibid, p. 48.
5. Letter in the author's file from an African doctor dated October 22, 1975.
6. **WIN NEWS,** op. cit., p. 47. Addis Ababa Fistula Hospital, P.O. Box 3609, Addis Ababa, Ethiopia.
7. United Nations seminar held in Addis Ababa in 1960, "The Participation of Women in Public LIfe", United Nations Document st/TAO/HR/9, Paragraphs 60, 61, 62. See "World Health Organization Seminar".
8. African Training and Research Center for Women (ATRCW), P.O. Box 3001, Addis Ababa, Ethiopia. See **WIN NEWS**, Vol. 3, No. 1, Winter 1977, pp. 67-70. See also **WIN NEWS,** Vol. 3, No. 3, Summer 1977, p. 55; **WIN NEWS**, Vol. 4, No. 1, Winter 1978, pp. 65-69, Vol. 7, No. 2, p. 48; Vol. 8, No. 2, p. 51. and continuing.
9. Inter-African Committee on Traditional Practices Affecting the Heatlh of Women and Children, c/o Economic Commission for Africa, ATRCW, P.O. Box 3001, Addis Ababa, Ethiopia.; and: 147, rue de Lausanne, CH-1202 Geneva, Switzerland.
10. Zaborowski, M. **La Circonsion ses Origines et sa Reparation en Afrique et a Madagascar** (The Circumcision: Its Origin and Spread in Africa and Madagascar). Anthropologie Par. 1896, 7, pp. 653-75.
11. Ibid, p. 89.
12. Ploss, Heinrich. **Das Weib** (1885) in German. In English by Erick John Dignwall - **Woman: A Historical, Gynecological and Anthropoligical Compendium,** 1935, published by William Heinemann Medical Books Ltd., London.
13. Huber, Alfons. "Die Weibliche Beschneidung" (Female Circumcision), **Journal der Tropen Medizin & Parasitologie,** Vol. 20, No. 1, pp. 1-10.
14. Huber, Alfons. "Weibliche Zirkumzision und Infibulation in Athiopien" (Female Circumcision and Infibulation in Ethiopia), **Acta Tropica** (Basel), 23, 1, 1966, p. 89.
15. Ibid., p. 90.
16. Huber, Alfons. "Genitalverletzungen Afrikanisher Madchen durch rituelle Eingriffe", (Infliction of Genital Wounds on African Girls due to Ritual Operations), published in 1971 in Kommission Helmut Bake Verlag Hamburg. Edited by Arbeitsgemeinschaft Ethnomedizin, Hamburg, Vol. 1, No. 1, 1971, p. 79.
17. Selassie, Alasebu Gebere (Principal Researcher and Coordinator), "Harmful Traditional Practices Affecting the Health of Women and Children in Ethiopia". UNICEF/AAO, Ethiopia, P. O. Box 1169, Addis Ababa, Ethiopia. .See also **WIN NEWS** Vol. 11. No. 4, Autumn 1985, pp. 32 - 35.
18. **Inter African Committee on Traditional Practices Affecting the Health of Women and Children, Conference Report,** c/o Economic Commission for Africa, ATRCW, P.O. Box 3001, Addis Ababa, Ethiopia. Or: 147, rue de Lausanne, CH-1202 Geneva, Switzerland. See also **WIN NEWS**, Vol. 17, No.1, Winter 1991, pp. 38-44.
19. AIDoS - Italian Association for Women in Development, Via dei Giubbonari, 30, 00186 Rome, Italy. Daniela Colombo, director.
20. National Committee on Traditional Practices Affecting the Health of Women and Children, c/o Ministry of Health, P.O. Box 1234, Addis Ababa, Ethiopia.

ETHIOPIA: ECONOMIC/SOCIAL FACTS & SUMMARY

ETHIOPIA:	14 administrative Regions
Climate:	Temperate in highlands; hot in lowlands.
Population:	46 million (1986 estimate). Addis Ababa (capital), 1.5 million (1988 estimate). **Annual Growth Rate:** 2.9%.
Life Expectancy:	44.5 years // **Infant Mortality:** 145/1000.
Government:	Provisional government. Constitution being drafted. Elections to be held 1993-94; form of government and independence of Eritrea to be decided.
Ethnic Groups:	Oromo, 40%; Amhara, 25%; Tigre, 12%; Sidama, 9%.
Languages:	Amharic (official) // Tigrinya // Orominga // Arabic // English.
Religions:	Muslim (40-45%); Ethiopian Orthodox Christian (35-40%). Indigenous beliefs, (Animist) 15-25%.
Literacy:	60% (women much less).
Education:	Not compulsory. Attendance (elementary), 46%.
Annual/Capita Income:	$121 (estimate). 79.8% of work force in agriculture.
Economy:	Growth Rate: 2.5%. 39.7% GDP agriculture; 13.7% industry (1985). Coffee, cereals, pulses, oilseed, meat, hides, skins.

Note: Since this was published Eritrea became independent.

CASE HISTORY : KENYA

Kenya is always cited first when Female Genital Mutilation (FGM) is discussed, which continues to be called "Female Circumcision" in East Africa.

Kenya is always associated with FGM, though most Kenyans refuse to talk about it because of the "Female Circumcision Controversy" - the failed attempt by the British when the country was under their administration to free girls and women from these inhuman needless tortures in the name of "African Tradition."

In summer 1982 the issue once more gained world attention when President Daniel arap Moi, who had only recently succeeded 'President-for-Life' Kenyatta, prohibited all forms of the mutilations in a presidential decree. He personally denounced the mutilations after he was informed that seven girls had died the day before in a group circumcision ceremony performed in a rural area he was visiting.

The President said that "whoever will be found committing the act or encouraging it will be prosecuted" - so the Nairobi Times of July 27, 1982 - reports. The article continues to report on President Moi's speech at Baringo District: "The President advised Kenyans to maintain cultural values that were beneficial to the nation and discard those which were useless."[1]

The next day in an editorial, "Female Circumcision: Educate the Ignorant", the **Nation,** Kenya's most widely read newspaper, called for active support for the President's banning of circumcision: "We have in mind the churches", the **Nation** writes. "We also have in mind women's organizations. . . they have not taken the issue to the rural areas where the practice is still found."[2]

President Moi added that under his administration he would not allow children to be abused in this way. He also criticized the circumcisers, who, he said, were doing the operations to make money, and he called on local leaders to ensure that female circumcision was stopped.

This announcement by the President representing a total break with the past was broadcast all over the world by wire services and the press: It was an all-important, new departure for President Moi, the follower of President Kenyatta, who had used the issue of "Female Circumcision" as a centerpiece of his politics for independence.

President Moi's prohibition, only a few years since he had taken over the leadership of the country after the death of the revered President Kenyatta was especially astonishing as he is not a Kikuyu but from a small tribe with little political power - therefore following Kenyatta's leadership. Yet Kenyatta's personal politics had been to charge that Britain was out to destroy African traditions - using FGM as an example.

President Moi's prohibition was taken up by the then director of Medical Services of Kenya, Dr. Karuga Koinange, who "instructed Government and missionary hospitals to stop conducting female circumcision." [3] And the same article in the Daily Nation of September 1, 1982, reports that these instructions to hospitals were also sent to the Kenya Catholic Secretariat and the Protestant Churches Medical Association. This confirms that hospitals all over Kenya performed FGM on a regular basis - including those financed from abroad - which not only is against all medical ethics but also makes a mockery of African Traditions.

It also makes quite clear that FGM done in the Kenyan hospitals at Government expense was nothing more than a deliberate attempt by the male dominated power structure to permanently mutilate all females in order to reinforce patriarchal supremacy and control by all males over all females in Kenya and the same applies wherever FGM is medicalized.

The situation in Kenya makes this entirely clear. The politization by Kenyatta of FGM, which he made one of the keystones of his political struggle for independence, was organized after he was educated by the British in London and had lived there for years - observing British customs and the behaviour and freedom of British women. The institutionalizing of FGM, which was one of Kenyatta's mandates for an independent Kenya, was designed to keep women under absolute control of men. The very limited participation of women in decision-making positions in Kenyan politics today is one direct result. The sexual politics - using "African Tradition" - continue to this day.

Perhaps because of the fact that women are the real productive force in that country, which was recognized by Kenyatta, he insisted on FGM as a means of keeping women under the control of men. It also assured the leadership of the Kikuyu - Kenyatta's tribe - as men from all other tribes were persuaded by the sexual politics and followed Kenyatta's lead. He succeeded to get FGM on the political agenda as a positive issue for Independence and Kikuyu leadership, when any person really concerned with the welfare of his people would obviously reject the mutilation of half of the population he set out to lead.

What is worse is that Kenyatta convinced not only all the men - who of course realized that control over their own families and polygamy was at stake- but Kenyatta also succeeded to persuade women with political ambitions to follow him. Many influential Kikuyu women to this day refuse to speak on this issue let alone work effectively to free women from these terrible tortures - which still continue throughout most of the country. Though President Moi prohibited the mutilations including in the hospitals, he never asked that information and health education campaigns should be started which are essential if his decree was to have any real effect. Even now Kenya is the country where very little is said and less has been done in terms of effective education against FGM.

This situation can only be understood by an analysis of what has been called the "Female Circumcision Controversy": the mishandled attempt by the Britich in the 1920s and 1930s, and up to Independence, to persuade the Kenyans to give up these damaging mutilations of their female children. The British failed, and to the present time, a large majority of Kenyan girls are mutilated - though since Independence the subject has been shunned by all public officials in Kenya. Until President Moi's prohibition, the Kenyan press, however, regularly reported on the death of girls as a result of "village circumcisions," but no one in Kenya was or is willing to discuss the problem. Women in high government posts in Nairobi will even deny to outsiders that FGM exists. Yet all available facts and surveys point to the conclusion that at least two-thirds of the female children of Kenya continue to be excised. And Kenyan families of Somali ethnic origin living near the borders with Somalia infibulate their daughters, as all ethnic Somalis do.

The Female Circumcision Controversy in Kenya, which reached its height about 1930, attracted world attention at the time and is often cited as an example of "interference" or what not to do in dealing with cultural matters. It has also served as standard excuse by international organizations concerned with development and health to ignore the fact that many thousands of girls are mutilated every year in Kenya and in more than twenty-six other countries in Africa. The claim that nothing can be done to stop the mutilation of children all over Africa, citing the very limited Kenyan experience with the Kikuyu, is especially damaging when it becomes clear that the whole issue of FGM was and still is unscrupulously exploited by ambitious young African politicians to attract attention. .

Because the issue of FGM reached the British Parliament and was extensively discussed in the international press, it made a great impression both in Africa and abroad, quite out of proportion to the number of people involved in Kenya.

FGM was used by a group of Kenyan men, led by Jomo Kenyatta, as a means to reach their own political objectives at the time when Kenya tried to gain Independence, and thus the issue of FGM gained even more notoriety. Women continue to be the victims of and the pawns in the political battles fought by men - used and abused by all sides.

The time is long overdue to examine the record of this infamous affair from a woman's view and to analyze the events and their significance for the present. Perhaps this will persuade those in Kenya who are still unwilling to face these realities that it is time to work for change.

In his book **Facing Mount Kenya,** [4] Jomo Kenyatta gives his view of the history and background of his society, the "Gikuyu."* The book, first published in the 1930s, is derived from Kenyatta's thesis and papers for his degree in Anthroplogy, which he took under the direction of Bronislav Malinowski at the London School of Economics. It represents the classic view of anthropologists even now that somehow traditional and cultural practices are always good and must be preserved - no matter how damaging to some members of the society. Indeed according to this view still propagated today by anthropologists, foot binding in China, widow burning in India, harems and slavery all are "traditional cultural practices" of great value that should be preserved.

> "Malinowski supported much of Kenyatta's belief of the importance of all cultural practices to the integrity of the tribe. . . there can be no doubt that his book, in which anthropology is skillfully used as a weapon against colonialism, was a milestone in the modern history of Africa. . ."[5]

In the Introduction of his book, Kenyatta states that he is the grandson of a Kikuyu medicine man. This book, replete with attacks against the British and especially missionaries who educated him, is an account of Kikuyu customs before the arrival of the British in Kenya, when all the feudal and patriarchal traditions were still intact.

Most of the traditions have been abandoned now by the Kikuyu, who are in the forefront of modernization in Kenya after seizing most of the political power, which even today is still held by the Kikuyu minority. Kenyatta, their leader, was declared "President for Life" after Independence and ruled the country until his death in the summer of 1978.

Kenyatta's book gives his own often idealized view and analysis of his tribal society, but it was also written as a political statement in the struggle for Independence of Kenya and East Africa from British rule. This book provides a social analysis, especially of the status of women, which is the background to the "Female Circumcision Controversy."

Kenyatta strongly advocated the continuation of tribal customs and especially those defining women's lives. He built his political power and the Independence movement on the claim that the social integrity of African Traditions must be preserved and defended against the British - who, he claimed, were destroying African traditional life. Initiation, the coming of age rituals, including male and female circumcision, he insisted were critical to the viability of his society.

Kenyatta advocates that customs must be preserved at any price; that is the view of anthropologists which he no doubt learned in London from his teacher Malinowski, a staunch defender of tradition. Kenyatta's book describes the very intricate tribal rules and traditions of the Kikuyu, including the closely guarded rituals relating to initiation, reproduction and sex. Attacks against the British and against missionaries who tried to abolish the mutilation of female children permeate this whole work, which is obviously written for a British audience. It is ironic that the Kikuyu, who are only one fifth of the population of Kenya, have established their political supremacy and rule over the other ethnic groups precisely because they most eagerly accepted Western education, modernization and change. Kenyatta's book ignores altogether the other ethnic groups of Kenya over which he ruthlessly ruled all his political life. Indeed in his book he claims to speak for all of Africa.

He charges that the British administration was trying to destroy the social fabric of all Africans - citing only the Kikuyu - because the British opposed the subjection of female children to genital mutilation. To this must be added that the Luo (who are 14 percent of the Kenyan population) never practiced genital mutilation in any form - neither female nor male. Yet their social structure has always been as viable as that of the Kikuyu. As the political rivals of the Kikuyu with strong ambitions, Kenyatta evidently decided to ignore the very existence of the Luo in his book quite aside from working against them in his political plans.

---

* Kenyatta uses this spelling throughout his book, though "Kikuyu" is used in all the rest of the literature; hence the latter spelling is used here.

Dr. Leonard Bruce-Chwatt, who worked in Kenya for many years, described the situation in a recently published article:

> "The circumcision of boys and girls is of particular significance among the Kikuyu, because it marks the entry of young people into full membership of the tribal community and their sexual maturity. As would be expected, medical opinion was completely opposed to female circumcision. The Christian missions abhorred and condemned it. . . The government of that time regretted its continuance but took the long and rather detached view that only time and better education would put an end to it. . ."[6]

It was stated, of course, repeatedly by those who opposed FGM that they did not oppose the custom of initiation but only the physical mutilation of the girls; indeed, the custom of initiation is practiced in many parts of Africa and also the rest of the world quite successfully without subjecting girls to genital mutilation - but Kenyatta did not accept that. Obviously his purpose was to keep women under male control using "culture and tradition" for his purpose.

He states in his book:

> "For the present, it is impossible for a member of the tribe to imagine an initiation without clitoridectomy. Therefore, the abolition of the surgical element in this custom means to the Gikuyu the abolition of the whole institution.
>
> The Irua (the Kikuyu term for initiation) marks the commencement of preparation in various governing groups in the tribal administration because the real age groups begin from the day of the physical operation. The history and legends of the people are explained and remembered according to the names given to various age groups at the time of the initiation ceremony."[7]

Dr. Bruce-Chwatt provides some of the background of the controversy:

> "In 1929, the Tumutumu conference of all Protestant churches in Kikuyu-land resolved to take strong action against female circumcision and to suspend or exclude from the church all those who practiced or condoned the custom.
>
> Four medical men, all of them working in Kenya - Dr. John Arthur, Dr. J. Irvin, Dr. M. W. Brown and Dr. E. L. Davis - signed a Church of Scotland Memorandum, couched in non-medical language to give it the widest possible impact."[8]

The description of female circumcision by the physicians from the above-cited Memorandum prepared by the the Mission Council of the Church of Scotland leaves no doubt about the physical damage and pain these practices represent for girls and women:

> "This operation comprises cutting away the inner and outer soft parts lying round the birth canal. In its severest form, the cutting extends in front up on to the pubis and into the birth canal itself. The result is the replacement of much of the normal elastic tissues of these parts, with an unyielding ring of hard fibrous tissue.
>
> These parts are highly sensitive and the cutting causes great agony. The following results of this operation have been seen by one or other of the undersigned during medical practice in the Kikuyu Province. . .
>
> Infection of the bladder with danger of spread up to the kidney, sterility owing to impossibility of sexual intercourse. . . during childbirth. . . the hard fibrous ring resulting from circumcision hinders. . . stretching so that the delay, especially in first births, leads in some cases to the death of the child.
>
> Such delay. . . is treated in certain districts by incisions by the women attending. These are sometimes made so that the bowel passage is cut into. . . The wounds become septic and increase the danger to infection inside, which may be fatal or lead to prolonged suffering and sterility. We have treated many first births where owning to female circumcision the child could not have been born without either tearing or incisions. . ."[9]

This report by four physicians, all of whom had many times treated girls and women suffering from the results of FGM, must be compared with Kenyatta's romantic description of "Irua," prepared for consumption by the British. He calls the old women who do the operations specialists, with the skills of "Harley Street surgeons."

Of course, as a man, Kenyatta was not allowed to attend the operations of girls. But he nevertheless claims to be an authority on the subject. A whole chapter of his book is devoted to the initiation rites, with every detail given, stressing the singing, the feasting, the dancing and the many ceremonies. Never once are the pain and the damaging results of the operations even mentioned by Kenyatta, though the newspapers in Kenya, despite the fact that this is a tabu subject, repeatedly report the deaths of girls from circumcision. Here is the description by Kenyatta:

> "A clean cowhide. . . is spread on the ground. . . The girls sit down on the hide, while their female relatives and friends form a sort of circle. . . No male is allowed. . . Any man caught would be severely punished.
>
> Each of the girls sits down with her legs wide open on the hide. Her sponsor sits behind her with her legs interwoven with those of the girl, so as to keep the girl's legs in a steady, open position. . . She is not supposed to show any fear or make any audible sign of emotion or even to blink. To do so would be considered cowardice and make her the butt of ridicule among her companions. . .
>
> A woman. . . known as moruithia. . . her face painted with white and black ochre . . . to make her look rather terrifying. . . takes out from her pocket the operating Gikuyu razor. . . and in quick movements. . . proceeds to operate upon the girls. . ." [10]

Kenyatta claims - though he never was present at an operation - that only the "tip of the clitoris - no other part of the girl's sexual organ" is cut. But, of course, the reports of physicians who witnessed the results of the operations are quite different.

After the cutting, some herbs are applied to the wound and each girl is put in a hut where she remains until the wound is healed or she is dead. Kenyatta even claims that "at the time of the surgical operation, the girl hardly feels any pain." [11]

Kenyatta then severely criticizes the European doctors for their "irresponsible statements" about the difficulties resulting from the operations, especially in childbirth. But as a man, he was not allowed to be present at any birth.

To this must be added that all the elaborate ceremonies and rituals surrounding "Irua" have been drastically reduced and recently entirely abandoned among the Kikuyu in Kenyatta's own lifetime. However, the physical mutilations continue to the present time. Thousands of girls are still operated on every year among the Kikuyu, besides many other ethnic groups in Kenya.

Bruce-Chwatt summarizes the political events in London and Kenya at the time when the issue of female circumcision was publicly raised long before Independence:

> "A parliamentary group, led by the Duchess of Atholl, pressed the government for firmer action to abolish the custom. In Kenya, an attempt to regulate it, so that it should be performed only by skilled women and limited to the removal of the clitoris, was an utter failure." [12]

Jomo Kenyatta had become the Secretary of the Kikuyu Central Association, which had been formed in 1920. He was increasingly involved in politics and spent much time in London in the 1920s and 1930s. His book, based on his anthropological studies in London, was published after the initial prohibition against circumcision, as a defense and explanation of the Kikuyu society and their traditions. One cannot help but wonder what would have happened if Kenyatta, instead of studying anthropology, would have studied medicine, especially since he states that he was the grandson of a Kikuyu medicine man!

The Luo, who have been traditionally opposed to FGM, also were and still are the arch-rivals of the Kikuyu, as far as political power is concerned. Predictably, they are never mentioned in Kenyatta's book. The Luo could have provided positive political leadership and a positive alternative in the abrasive arguments concerning FGM, which Kenyatta so cleverly used - but they were ignored by the British..

The circumcision controversy by attracting world attention consolidated the power and leadership of the Kikuyu within the divided multi tribal society of Kenya, a fact that surely was not lost on Kenyatta, a most astute politician. Kenyatta no doubt had also learned in England the importance of gaining the attention of the international press to establish his power within Kenya and his society.

It seems strange that the missionaries and those of the British administration who worked against FGM never cited or worked with the Luo, who traditionally oppose female circumcision. Yet, the Luo's social cohesion and identity are just as strong as those of the Kikuyu - despite Kenyatta's constant claims that the mutilation of female children is essential for African society. It would have been easy to make the Luo a positive example; but they were never mentioned throughout this controversy, least of all in London.

This is only one of the many contradictions in this historic controversy which influences life in Kenya to this day. The unrelenting stand of Kenyatta as African leader and champion for genital mutilation, it must be finally said, is responsible for the deaths of thousands of female children annually all over Africa and that many thousands continue to be subjected to these damaging operations. One can but wonder why a man like Kenyatta, who spent many years in London and studied at the best universities, showed so little concern for the health and well-being of the female children of his own ethnic group and society, unless he was afraid of women and convinced that this was the only way to preserve male supremacy.

Contradictions beset not only the policies and politics between the different opposing factions, but internal contradictions beset each group.

The position of the Kikuyu Central Association (KCA), which Kenyatta led and through which he consolidated his power, was ambiguous at best.

> "The Kikuyu Central Association combined two seemingly contradictory elements. It was progressive and aimed at the spread of education for Africans, and it was in favor of training Africans. . . But while the KCA stressed African rights to live in a modern society, they also wished to retain the African past, which in its tribal institutions represented something valuable that must not be sacrificed to progress. Therefore, KCA leaders supported the peculiar value of African customs even when they clashed with modern standards of health and modern conditions of society which they, themselves, approved of. . ." [13]

The KCA, under the leadership of Kenyatta, strongly supported FGM and opposed all change where women were concerned.

The stand of the medical missionaries was also full of inconsistencies. They objected to clitoridectomy, yet tolerated other traditional practices damaging to health.

> " Why was the practice of clitoridectomy so unacceptable to medical missionaries? They might object to witchcraft, quack medicine, the mutilation of teeth, faulty diets based on superstition, but they would not crusade against them. . . But circumcision was singled out for fanatic rejection, perhaps because the ritual which accompanied it represented a non-Christian attitude towards sex which some of the missions felt therefore, obliged to combat." [14]

The KCA's political posture, which Kenyatta supported, was "that the abolition of (female circumcision) would destroy the essence of Kikuyu life. They made it known that they would not yield to pressure from Dr. John Arthur who had signed the Memorandum of the Mission Council of the Church of Scotland (see above) - who as physician and medical missionary took the lead against the operations - or any of the (Protestant) missions." [15]

As the politics of resistance developed, the KCA sided with all groups who favored the operation:

> "The KCA had definitely taken the side of. . . reactionary forces. . . and. . . made their support part of its anti-European, anti-government, anti-mission propaganda . . ." [16]

The younger progressive men of the Kikuyu community were in the forefront of opposing the abolition of the circumcision operation, led by Kenyatta. As a result, the government policies opposing the operations waivered:

> "J. Pease, senior commissioner of Kikuyu Province, wrote to the secretary in Nairobi: 'I consider the general policy of government towards female circumcision should be one of masterly inactivity'. . ." [17]

It is interesting to note that throughout, women were never asked by either side, and one searches documents in vain for any statement by a woman or from a female view. Women were and still are the pawns and victims of the political power games men play over the use, abuse and mutilation of their bodies. The battles over abortion and over fertility control, which go on today in male-run governments everywhere in the world, are a witness that the motives of men everywhere are, unfortunately, still the same.

The British Government in Kenya failed to provide support at the critical time and watched while the human rights of women were trampled by men determined to gain political power and freedom for themselves. Yet, the same men fought for continuing genital mutilation and the subjection of their sisters, wives, mothers and daughters. Thus, these men assured for themselves undisputed leadership after Independence and most Kenyan and African males continue to support FGM to the present time.

The one who had the most to gain, Kenyatta, not only spoke for the issue but also blamed the Scottish Church Missionaries for the political unrest which he and other ambitious Kikuyu men had planned and organized:

> "It is the Church which first took steps to excite the people of the country,' he said. 'It was the Church that took the initiative in this matter and was the cause of all the unrest among the people.'" [18]

Kenyatta was a consummate politician and was also quite familiar with British life. He had been first educated by the British missionaries he later vilified, and then educated in London by the British Government, which he later fought. No doubt he observed, while living in London, the women's suffrage movement.

It did not escape Kenyatta that, given a chance, women in Kenya would demand freedom for themselves from the heavy burdens of patriarchal rule. With the achievement of self-rule for Kenya, women would no longer tolerate their servile positions vis a vis men and especially not the continuation of polygamy. Kenyatta vigorously promoted polygamy in his book and practiced it himself, demanding polygamy as the absolute right of African men and the "natural" order of the Kikuyu. Indeed, he did not recognize the Moslem limitation to four wives, but he advocated an unlimited number of wives and lived his own personal life accord

Male supremacy had to be reinforced, especially with the struggle for freedom which might put wrong ideas into women's heads, such as demanding freedom from exploitation and oppression by men. Hence, a vigorous support for traditions especially those affecting women went up in Kenya and all over Africa. Traditions are still promoted by male politicians all over Africa today as the surest means to maintain the quite unjustifiable and damaging exploitation of women: this despite the fact that Kenya, as well as every other African constitution, claims that all citizens have equal rights.

The contradictory policies of the Kikuyu Central Association (KCA) prior to Independence can be easily explained. The KCA opted for modernization when it was to the advantage of the male Kikuyu leadership, but they supported tradition when it came to keeping women under control. Indeed, they allied themselves readily with the most reactionary forces to keep women in their traditional subservient place.

The Memorandum by the Mission Council of the Church of Scotland covers all the events in Kenya at the time the missions played a key role in the circumcision controversy. In this document, the background of the issue is discussed, which developed into a political crisis in 1929 after female circumcision was officially prohibited, first by the Church of Scotland Missions, and then by the British Administration.

The origin of the prohibition goes back to the early part of this century. Systematic teaching against the practice by the Church of Scotland began in 1906, based on the observations of the effects of the mutilations by medical missionaries in the mission hospitals. Gradually a number of the African converts who had formed their own African church joined in opposing this practice, and various methods were tried to enable girls, especially those in missionary boarding schools, to escape the practice.

By 1916, several European and African missionary societies working together in the Kikuyu area (Central Province) discussed the female circumcision question and tried to arrive at a joint resolution. However, due to World War I (1914-1918), the matter was postponed until 1919, when a "unanimous recommendation was made for the abolition of the practice and for disciplinary measures to be taken against all Christians who should countenance it." [19] Later, a pamphlet was prepared and printed and widely disseminated among the African Christians of all missions. A number of conferences were held starting in 1920 where the objections to the practice were discussed.

In 1929, at a special meeting of the All-Kikuyu Native Conference at Kambui, this statement was recorded:

> "The elders regret the accusations being made throughout the country that it is only the Europeans who want this custom removed and not the Kikuyu; as Kikuyu, they desire to record in these minutes that the decision is their own free will and not a matter of compulsion by the Europeans. "[20]

In 1926, local action was taken in line with the resolution of the Governor's Conference to limit the extensive operations practiced among some tribes, especially in the Kikuyu Province , "to remove no more than the clitoris". It was the practice in some areas to make additional incisions in the vagina and to remove all soft parts of the female genitalia.

The local resolutions by several Native Councils, limiting the operations, became legal and binding involving penalties in case of disobedience. In April 1929, the first prosecution took place and two women were fined in Kiambu for performing the major operation. There was much indignation on both sides. On the one side against the conviction, and on the other side about the lightness of the sentence. The memorandum of the Church of Scotland Mission nevertheless reports that general progress had been made in limiting the operations.

After 1929, various steps were taken to enable girls unwilling to undergo the operation to avoid it. An increasing number of marriages of uncircumcised women showed that they not only had children but also were as prolific as circumcised women. It had been widely believed that an uncircumcised woman could not have any children at all, or else that her children would die or that she would be less fertile.

Following the Resolution by several local Native Councils to limit the operations under penalty, several more cases involving girls who had been forcibly circumcised were tried in 1929. One went to the Supreme Court and was written up in a lead article in the **East African Standard** pleading "for liberty of conscience for African women". [21]

In the meantime, the Kikuyu Central Association (KCA) was busy organizing resistance against the missions. The Kikuyu Central Association representatives, at an open meeting held in Nyeri at Provincial Headquarters in 1929, stated that they stood for the preservation of all tribal customs, including female circumcision; and they demanded compliance by every Kikuyu girl, in defiance of both the missions and the African church.

A week after the above-cited article on behalf of African women's freedom of choice appeared, the President of the KCA circularized ten Kikuyu chiefs with a "Lament on Abolition of Circumsision". 22 In this "Lament" K .K. Joseph, the President, states, "It is with great sorrow that all the Kikuyu are thus prohibited from circumcision", and then he wrongly accuses two missionaries including Dr. Arthur for being responsible for the prohitition.

The battle in the press continued until the Progressive Kikuyu Party, joined by several chiefs, published a letter the following week expressing its abhorrence of the practice of female circumcision. The issue was also discussed by the East African Women's League Convention, which passed two resolutions. One urged the goverment to protect those girls who wished to break away from this custom, providing information as to what steps were being taken. The other one (issued several months later) asks that legislation should be initiated immediately. Christian elders of the Kikuyu also joined this initiative by asking the government to protect girls and their parents who wished to resist the practice; for this the elders were later abused by the members of the KCA.

The KCA spread rumors of all kinds against the Europeans, using the prohibition against circumcision as a means to raise all kinds of fears and opposition.

In a case tried in 1930, the father of a 14-year-old schoolgirl, who was forcibly circumcized on his initiative, was sent to jail for two weeks and the circumcizer was fined. In another case, a 13-year old girl was seized by her brothers and abducted to a nearby river where she was severely mutilated, despite her strong resistance. The girl lodged a complaint against her two brothers, implicating five more people who had planned the assault for political purposes. [23] The circumcision issue thus was politicized and cleverly used by the KCA who never showed the slightest concern for their girls and women.

The situation between the people and the missionaries worsened. Finally a woman missionary was brutally murdered but the murderer was never found. Others connected with the mission schools were threatened.

The British Administration's position similarly was full of contradictions and inconsistencies. The British Administration for a long time tried to maintain its position of neutrality in this controversy and stressed that it was strictly up to the people to decide what they wanted. This created more confusion and led to the resignation of Dr. Arthur from the Executive Council of the Government, which was interpreted by the KCA as a victory, as Dr. Arthur was the most vigorous opponent of circumcision.

The Government began to waiver with the political impact of the KCA and published a report stating that "the custom is of very ancient origin . . . The policy of the government is not to attempt complete prohibition" but "to get the people to see the evils of the operation. . . in its severest forms. " [24] The Church of Scotland Mission was accused of being the cause of political dissent. The mission, in turn, was critical of the Government, stating that it was being attacked by a political organization and that the mission could not "abandon a principle taught and maintained for many yers on spiritual grounds." [25]

Finally, the matter reached the British Parliament in London.

In a "Dispatch from the Secretary of State for the Colonies to the Officers Administering the Governments of Kenya, Uganda Protectorate, Tanganyika Territory, Nyasaland, Northern Rhodesia and Zanbibar", dated March 8, 1930, concern for women is expressed: the status of women "is in some places scarely distinguishable from that of slavery". The Dispatch asks how the bad health conditions which had been reported, especially of mothers and children, might be improved. The suggestion is made that local women should be trained in maternity work and child welfare. The Dispatch finally urges: "most serious consideration should be given whether it would not be possible to take steps toward the complete abolition of this (female circumcision) and similar practices. . ."[26]

A Dispatch dated April 10, 1930, from the Secretary of State for the Colonies to the Governor of Kenya included a report by "The Committee for the Protection of Colored Women in the Crown Colonies". It refers to the deputation consisting of the Duchess of Atholl, Colonel Wedgewood, Miss Rathbone, and the Select Committee that had been set up with the purpose

> "to enquire into those matters and in especial to lay stress on the need for action to be taken regarding the practice of circumcision, especially in the form in which it exists among the Kikuyu tribes in Kenya. We were convinced that it was there inflicting grave suffering and injury to the health and life among women and causing much infant mortality. " [27]

Several remedies are recommended - "whether legislation be found possible or not".

> "The first need . . . is for a more adequate protection for girls who desire to escape from this custom.
>
> We should be glad if the Governor of Kenya could be asked to consider whether steps should be taken to give the girl the right to avoid the operation by affording her adequate opportunities to express her wishes in the matter. " [28]

Other recommendations made include the extension of health services especially for midwifery and the training of girls for such services selected from Missionary Boarding Schools; also the organization of traveling dispensaries to extend health services and to spread knowledge about the harmfulness of female circumcision.

And, to lay to rest the accusation that the British Administration wanted to abolish African Tradition, it was urged that "great care should be taken. . . to insure that when members of the tribe are being urged to abolish the operation, they are not led to believe that they are being asked to abandon the whole of a series of customs which constitute entry into tribal membership." [29]

And finally, it was recommended in the same report:

> ". . . that an impartial enquiry should be made 'into the effect of the practice on maternal and infant health'. . . conducted with the aid of the natives themselves. . Persons to conduct the investigation should be neither connected with missionary effort nor in the service of the Government of Kenya. " [30]

The report is signed by eleven members of the Committee, as well as four women, including Katherine Atholl,Vice-Chair, who was one of the people most actively involved in this initiative.*

It is interesting to note that up to the present time, more than thirty years after Independence and more than a decade after the death of Kenyatta - the chief proponent of FGM in Kenya, and indeed, Africa - no survey or investigation into the effects of the mutilations on the health of women has ever been made. No research has been published to establish even the most basic facts such as what type of operation is practiced by the different ethnic groups or how many children continue to be mutilated in a country that has the highest birthrate in the world and certainly has quite adequate health facilities to conduct such an investigation. Instead, Kenyans concerned with health on the Governmental and non-Governmental level, as well as the influential national women's orgainzations of Kenya still attempt to avoid the issue and refuse to do any research in order to claim "female circumcision no longer exists" or when challenged, "it is no problem". Nothing could be further from the truth - as is documented here.

It also must be stated that the real concern for the status of African women shown by both missionaries and the British Administration in the field and in numerous dispatches and reports was in no way shared by the KCA or by the male African leadership, which never consulted women at all. Yet, these events of more than fifty years ago still affect the lives and health of millions of girls and women who continue to be victimized by the men of their own familes tribe and country.

An analysis of the issue from a woman's view is long overdue.

African women never took part nor were they asked to participate in the discussions on FGM that so greatly affect their well-being and health. Kenyatta cleverly used the anthropological argument provided for him by his teacher Malinowski to secure his political power and the supremacy of men by taking a stand on this issue, which had enormous emotional ramifications. Kenyatta knew he could count on the support by the world-wide Anthropological Fraternity, which is listened to by political decision makers. Anthropology, a field dominated by men, usually ignores women or discusses them as objects to establish academic theories of male superiority - as this once more demonstrates.

The report was signed by Josiah C. Wedgewood, Chair; Katherine Atholl, Vice-Chair; Eleanor F. Rathbone; Ethel Bentham; W. Ormsby Gore; Ronald Ross; D. Graham Pole; R. W. Hamilton; Edith Picton-Turberville; Victor A. Cazalet; and R. A. Butler, Acting Secretary.

Kenyatta also succeeded to rally both men and women in Kenya to his cause and against the British administration. The British had nothing to gain politically from getting involved in this issue and pleading for women - quite the contrary.

African women remained throughout as the voiceless pawns used by both sides. Female circumcision gained international political notoriety and was labeled with "keep off". Ever since it has been associated with African Independence, with imperialism, conialism and interference. Kenyatta also managed to strike a basic chord of the universal male brotherhood over the issue of sexual control of females and thus enlist the tacit, yet strong support by the vast majority of men which the ruling world patriarchy regards as their untouchable right. There is no doubt that female sexual mutilation greatly enhances male control over females; it serves as the underpinning of polygamy and assures absolute male sexual domination.

Kenyatta cleverly used the sexual implications of the medically indefensible mutilation of the women of his own society to gain attention for himself and as a basis to build his own personal political power and eventually his own supremacy as President for Life in Kenya.

In all this, African women were never heard from at all. For the most part, they knew neither the facts nor the politics involved and no women were sent by the British to study in London as Kenyatta did. The elders who make local decisions by definition are men. There was no way that women could form an independent opinion, let alone speak for themselves. In fact, they were not consulted by either side.

Kenyatta, by propagating female mutilation, also accomplished the consolidation of power of the Kikuyu as leaders of males over all females in Kenya. Women in rural Africa control the essential economic production of food, as women do the subsistence farming. Women also produce children, the other means of establishing wealth in traditional rural societies. Kenyatta made sure that the cause of women's freedom was squelched in Kenya before it could even get started. Women had to remain in their subservient position, working for men. Insisting on observing all "traditions" was the means to that end. Predictably, he persuaded the majority of the women, who were illiterate and had no access to any outside information, to follow his personal leadership, as Champion for Freedom and Independence from the British.

Kenyatta had made sure, by linking the powerful issue of traditions with female genital mutilation and in turn with Independence, that women had no choice: it is doubtful that women at the time really understood what was being done to them. Even now, the issue is overshadowed by the powerful emotions of nationalism that are continuously encouraged by the male leadership. Even now women in leadership in Kenya, most of them Kikuyu and influenced by Kenyatta, refuse to work against FGM in order to keep their positions.

As in so many other freedom fights and revolutions, women were and are used by the politically ambitious men who know that women's help is essential. But once the political goals have been achieved, women are sent back into the kitchen to serve men who divide up the spoils - including the women - among themselves. The lives of women where it matters most - in their families - are rarely changed: patriarchal domination of family life continues all over the world while revolutions come and go.

It is tragic for girls and women of Kenya that Independence meant for them a reaffirmation of genital mutilation, with all the health impairments, the sexual traumas, and the psychological damage these practices entail. While modernization was invited and eagerly pursued in every area, women were relegated to the past and to observe "African tradition" - that is to serve of men.

What are the traditions and what especially was the status of women in the traditional society, which Kenyatta so strongly defended? Perhaps an examination of his own writing will provide a clue as to why he took such a pro-tradition stand. To quote Kenyatta's own description of the relationship between the sexes:

> "The Gikuyu are taught from childhood that to be a man is to be able to . . . keep a homestead with as many wives as possible. . ."

> "Gikuyu male children are brought up to cultivate the idea and technique of extending their love to several women. . . The idea of sharing everything is strongly emphasized. . . Gikuyu custom provides that each wife must be visited by her husband on certain days of the moon, particularly on the three days following menstruation. The wives, knowing that this is the best time to have children, see to it that the husband does not neglet his duty. . . such conjugal relationship is the only way in which a polygamous homestead could be kept in harmony. The three days after menstruation are considered as the most likely for a woman to conceive." [31]

Of course, Kenyatta is entirely wrong about a woman's fertility. Considering that the Kikuyu are very prolific, it is doubtful that this rule was observed. However, "the idea of sharing" seems to be one-sided indeed, considering that women do not have access to other men.

Kenyatta informs us that if friends of the husband come to call, the wives are expected to join the company in the husband's hut; and the husband then distributes them for the night to each friend. This means in effect, that the women are obligated by the husband to prostitute themselves. Kenyatta points out that a wife cannot refuse such hospitality offered by her husband.

However, if a woman chooses to sleep with a man, she is severely punished, and so is her lover. Kenyatta states that it is tabu for a wife to have sexual intercourse outside the homestead.

It appears that the "sharing" described by Kenyatta as one of the important traditions of the Kikuyu simply means that the males are free to take as many wives as they can afford. What a wife earns belongs to her husband, which he then uses to buy more wives. Land is freely distributed by the village chiefs to each man, according to the number of wives he has. The more wives, the more fields a "family" can till, the more children and food are produced, and the wealthier the head of the family becomes. While Moslems are limited to four wives, Kenyatta stresses that there is no such limit set for the enterprising Kikuyu male.

Ester Boserup describes this system in "The Economics of Polygamy" [32] which works for the advantage and enrichment of males in a subsistence farming economy such as Kenyatta describes. Polygamy exploits women whose productive and reproductive capacities are used by men for their own benefit. Under the "duty of wives" the list of tasks that Kenyatta states each women must fulfill, spans almost every activity related to farm life. But there is no list of duties of husbands. The only duty of a man, Kenyatta cites, is to have sexual intercourse with each wife.

While masturbation for boys is considered "right and proper", so Kenyatta states, masturbation for girls is wrong; and therefore,"the practiceof homosexuality is unknown among the Kikuyu." [33] In case of divorce, after all attempts of reconciliation have failed, particularly if the wife was "unfaithful", the parents have to repay the brideprice with interest, while the children are kept by the husband as they are used as field labor.

A Kikuyu who has come under European influence is condemned as "unacceptable" to his family. But Kenyatta himself got his education in London very much under European influence, and he was taught to read and write by the missionaries whom he thanked for their services by condemning them throughout this book.

"No proper Gikuyu would dream of marrying a girl who has not been circumcised," is the cornerstone of his views, and he adds "female circumcision is an essential part of the morality of. . . the Gikuyu" - opinions he politically pursued all his life.

Always with his British audience in mind, Kenyatta claims that it is the wife who, after one year of marriage, asks the husband to take a second wife. And Kenyatta boasts: "If the family. . . is prosperous, after some time. . . the number of wives increases from one to fifty and even more." [34] Nor did Kenyatta limit the number of wives he personally acquired, since he was by any standards, a very rich man: "The husband is the head of the family. . . all belong to him. . . this brings. . . the collective ownership under his guidance." [35] Needless to say, Kenyatta frequently criticized the missionaries' strong objection to polygamy.

This remarkable arrangement of family life by the Kikuyu makes the patriarchal system practiced in the West insignificant by comparison. Polygamy continues to this day in Kenya and most of Africa with no limitations on the number of wives. But what is even more remarkable is that there is no obligation by men to support their wives or children. Just the reverse is true. Women are required to feed the men from what they grow in the fields they do not own. According to African Tradition - as explained by Kenyatta himself - the land is controlled by men as well as the labor force - that is, women who are acquired by men. The bride-price is nothing more than the purchase price for a woman, and what is more, men continuously buy more women from the money or goods realized from the labor of the wives who have no rights to either land or the fruit of their labors.

This certainly is a much superior arrangement than slavery as the African male owner of women had no responsibilities for their upkeep at all. No wonder African men praise "tradition" and try to institutionalize it in modern legislation - as for instance the Kenyan Members of Parliament demanded recently when new family legislation was discussed (see below). But it is discouraging to note that time and again African women are persuaded to praise "tradition" when in fact African Tradition is the means used by men to mutilate and exploit them and deny them all human rights.

Kenyatta in his book - which should be required reading for all women - not only praises all African traditions but he built his political following and party and the new independent Kenya on institutionalizing traditions for women - that is, female exploitation, subservience, polygamy and the exclusion of women from all decision making and even control over their own bodies and lives. And throughout his long life he proudly praised this African kind of female slavery - which has terrible consequences as the continuous civil wars, violence, tribal attacks and failure of governments all over Africa show. All this is the result of a dysfunctional traditional and exploitive male dominated family system.

A story which Kenyatta relates in the beginning of his book about the origin of the Kikuyu provides some fascinating psychological insights into the behavior of Kenyan and African men. He relates that it was said that originally, women were the leaders of the family, and matriarchy was the custom. But then, by a clever ruse, the men overturned the rule of the women. The men, it seems, were dissatisfied because, as Kenyatta tells it:

> "The women became domineering and ruthless fighters. They also practiced polyandry. . . many men were put to death for committing adultery."

He says that the men planned to revolt, but the women were physically stronger and better fighters. Therefore, the men "embarked on a campaign. . . to have sexual intercourse with them." The women were deceived by the flattery of the men. About six months later, the men saw that their plan had succeeded in getting most of the women pregnant and unable to fight due to their condition. Thus, the men took over the leadership of the community and "immediately steps were taken. . . to establish polygamy." [36]

Fear of women by the men who established patriarchy by tricking women is constantly mentioned in that story. Kenyatta then emphasizes that "the father is the supreme ruler of the homestead. . . he is respected and obeyed. He is the owner of practically everything. . . he is the custodian of the family property." [37]

Kenyata's constant stressing of male power throughout his book is suspicious. What is he so afraid of? He also claims that women cannot control their sexuality; therefore excision is necessary. Is the fear of women's sexuality the real reason why African men attack women's genitalia?

Kenyatta describes the controversy between the Kikuyu and the Church of Scotland Mission in his book quite differently from the records cited above, claiming that "a large section of people broke away from the main Christian body. . ." [38] In fact, as Kenya's own statistics show, more than half the population is Christian. And he states again and again that the missionaries were out to destroy African society by attacking clitoridectomy and that his society was "soiled" by the white man.

The British government became involved in the issue of women's health only long after it had been raised by the missionaries. No one had ever before spoken for women anywhere in Africa. Politically, this was a disastrous move for the missionaries and for the British Administration.

The experienced colonial administrators must have been aware of the pitfalls involved. Yet, some of them continued to speak for women. This was a unique situation in international political history and the first time that freedom of choice for a woman was discussed as a political issue in Africa.

The background and the dilemmas of the growing political strife in Kenya are described in great detail by Jocelyn Margaret Murray in her doctoral dissertation about the Female Circumcision Controversy. [39] She records all the events leading up to the prohibition, the height of the controversy in 1928-30, and the aftermath. Jocelyn Murray is the only person who looked with compassion at the situation of girls and women in Kenya who were caught up in this controversy and what it did to their lives - being used for political purposes by both sides.

Murray relates stories of girls in their early teens being captured and recaptured, of families split, of police actions against parents, of missionary schools and hostels serving as sanctuaries for girls rejecting the mutilation. The young girls involved were pushed in both directions, exposed to relentless taunts and threats by their own relatives as well as pressured by their missionary schools, who wanted "to save them and protect them."

Suspension from communion and a whole series of prohibitions were brought to bear on those who insisted on continuing to circumcise "their girls." In turn, girls were perceived as having to be protected "from those heathen ceremonies" and the abuse to which they were increasingly exposed in their villages and communities.

All kinds of derogatory language and songs ridiculing girls for not being circumcised were circulated to intimidate the victims. Resentment against the Europeans and the missionaries as symbols of European oppression was taken out on schoolgirls and young women who dared to opt for change. That the prohibition against circumcision was based on the qualified opinions of physicians and was for the benefit and the future of the Kikuyu - indeed for the whole African society by protecting the health of young women and their yet unborn children- got entirely lost in the political acrimony.

Murray analyzes these issues in her dissertation and shows that the vacillation on the part of the British Administration, but also by some influential members of the Church Missionary Society, was the main reason for the failure of the prohibition legislation, as well as the basis for the popular resentment. Murray adds that "Encouragement of a modified operation became the government policy."

The issue dragged on and was never resolved until finally "no further attempts were made to suppress the custom until 1956-1958, when in Meru and Embu Districts by-laws were passed on FGM which had later to be withdrawn because of popular opposition." [40]

The failure to arrive at a unified policy, the failure to prohibit the operations outright, and the failure to take a strong political stand opened the door for the opposition to twist the cause to suit its own political purposes, quite unrelated to the initial humanitarian intention, and to use it for their own political goals.

As a compromise, Murray informs us, "Christian circumcision" was permitted in some areas. That is, the physical operation was performed without all the "heathen" rites, the feasting and ceremonies. As one missionary observed, it was "very much more painful to the girls than circumcision performed during the course of an emotionally-charged ritual." Murray adds, "it would seem that the institution of 'Christian circumcision' actually led to prolonging the custom. . ." [41]

During the 1930s and 1940s, the circumcision issue simmered on. Cases of illegal circumcision were occasionally prosecuted, so Murray states including some prison sentences (never more than a few months) and fines. In 1952, a state of emergency was declared on political grounds due to the ongoing agitation for Independence. The last document in the file which chronicles the latest and abortive attempt to abolish female circumcision is dated January 1959, Murray states. [42]

The attitude of the missionaries was anti sex and anti polygamy ("sexual excess"). To approach sexuality, so important in the lives of the Kikuyu, with typical Christian hypocrisy and puritanism only damaged the missionaries' cause.

The issue of health, the most important concern in the struggle aginst the mutilations, was lost or hidden by Christian morality. Health, however, is a direct concern of every person, especially in Africa and most of all of women because of their frequent childbearing. The powerful argument for better health for the Kikuyu society, which could have been convincingly presented by teaching about personal health, hygiene, reproduction, and human biology with immediate positive results, was quite ignored. By teaching preventive health care, and about childbirth based on biological facts and education on infection and hygiene a convincing case could have been established, reaching all the people on the level of their own personal health needs.

Basic biological information and education in reproduction, sex and personal hygiene are still quite neglected in Kenya today and by missionaries everywhere quite aside from schools which are still influenced by the religious groups who started schools in Africa.

In 1976, upon my inquiry at a girls' school in the Kikuyu area concerning what was taught about reproduction and women's health, this answer came back: "We teach everything else, but unfortunately nothing about what all the people need to know most urgently: the biological facts of reproduction and sexuality" - this in the now government-organized Kenyan school system, where education has ceased to be under missionary control.

Jocelyn Murray went back to Kenya in 1972 to investigate the situation pertaining to circumcision at the present time. As the daughter of missionaries and herself a member of the Church of Scotland, she had lived in Kenya as a child. She went to the same locations which had been in the limelight of the controversy in the 1920s and 1930s. The girls who were defended by the missionaries then are grandmothers by now.

To make a valid test, Murray obtained permission to conduct a questionnaire with students in seven secondary schools, five in Central Province (the homeland of the Kikuyu) and two in the Embu District of Eastern Province. She describes that the schools were chosen to provide a cross section of districts, origins and religious affiliations. A total of 385 girls responded to the questionnaires, which were concerend first with establishing the basic facts: who was operated on, who not and why. Questions about mothers and female relatives were also included. A staff member in each school introduced the questionnaires which then were filled out by students. Murray states:

> "After the questionnaire papers had been collected. . . I spent the remaining time available discussing the subject with the girls. . . the possible origins of the practice and something of the historic controversy. Though at first taken by surprise to have a European initiate discussion on a tabu subject, the girls responded eargerly to the opportunity of openly discussing an important but usually ignored topic. The girls main reaction was of gratitude that they had been able to discuss openly a subject so important to them but usually repressed." [43]

Murray summarizes: "41 percent of the responding girls described themselves as circumcised, as against 59 percent uncircumcised." The lowest percentage of circumcised girls she found in Kiambu, where contacts with Nairobi were frequent and strong. Closeness to an urban center and exposure to the Western culture are strong factors inhibiting circumcision. Murray's findings confirm that those who are more prosperous and Westernized are the most likely to discard a custom like female circumcision. But it is not true in each case.

She adds: "The figures obtained from the questionnaire reflected in a striking manner the historical situation in each district." [44]

Her findings show that two thirds of the Roman Catholic girls were circumcised, which directly reflects the stand of the Roman Catholic Church "not to interfere;" two thirds of those affiliated with the Salvation Army, as well as those from traditional religious backgrounds, were similarly circumcised; but where the Presbyterian Church is strong, the lowest percentage of circumcision was found. And she adds:

> "All in all, the situation from district to district is very much what one would have predicted from knowledge of the historical facts alone. In Kiambu, where Presbyterian and Anglican alike legislated against female circumcision, less than one-quarter of the girls are circumcised." [45]

These findings not only vindicate the activities of the Scottish and other Protestant missionaries, but they also show that the claims which continue to be made, that opposition to FGM only reinforces the practice, are quite wrong. Indeed, where the greatest pressure had been applied the practice has decreased the most. And Murray writes:

> "There has never been any pressure by the Roman Catholic Church to give up the practice. All this is very clearly reflected in the statistics obtained from the questionnaire. Sixty-eight percent of the Catholic girls declared themselves circumcized, as against a general total of 41 percent." [46]

Murray also asked some questions of the girls who were circumcized about the circumstances of the operation. It appears that all of them were operated at a younger age than in the past, and only half of the girls had recéived some teaching, which is traditionally part of the initiation. During the recovery period from the operations, the girls are taught their duties towards their husbands and how married women must behave. It appears that such teaching now is from older girls, contrary to the belief that experienced women instruct the initiates. A quarter of the girls had been circumcized alone, without any ritual or education.

Of the girls who were not circumcized, Murray asked the reasons why giving it up. The most commonly given reason was church influence (more than half). Other reasons were: dangerous to health (about one-third), and family reasons. The girls were asked if their mothers and older sisters were circumcized. In a few cases, girls were not circumcised while their older sisters had been; but mostly, the same practices prevailed for all family members. Almost every girl who herself was circumcized, knew that her mother had been circumcized, while those who were not, did not know about their mothers.

Murray notes that the answers show a very ambivalent attitude towards female circumcision, and she states: "it is still recognized that in a certain sense the circumcized Kikuyu woman is the 'real' adult woman. . . although exposure to education in Western life has played some part in giving up the custom, acceptance of church teaching on the subject has been far more important. [47]

Summing up the situation in the areas she investigated, Murray states that the ritual accompaniments of circumcision for girls as well as boys are disappearing - including most other traditional Kikuyu ceremonials — except for the physical operation. This survey by Murray is especially important now as the 1982 prohibition of FGM by President Moi makes it very difficult to get any facts or conduct any surveys - though the practice obviously continues. There are no teaching or information programs on FGM sponsored by the government. Some people in remote rural areas may not even know about this prohibition. Where FGM continues it is with this difference: girls are no longer brought to hospitals in case of uncontrollable bleeding or other mishaps, but are left to die and the newspapers no longer report deaths due to FGM.

Kenya, has accepted modernization and western life styles, despite the dire predictions of Jomo Kenyatta that their society would perish if they abandoned traditions. Kenyans also have one of the highest birthrates in the world, despite the on-going mutilations - or more likely bcause of it.

The pressure by Kenyan men — indeed by most African males — to father as many children as possible as a means to legitimate their existence and heighten their self-esteem, is growing in proportion to their failures in other areas. Women, especially when excised, are easy prey to the sexual domination by men and to their demand for children, which men fail to support.

For a long time after Independence, nothing more was said in Kenya and FGM was a tabu subject in Nairobi until 1982 and the prohibition of President Moi (see above). Almost absolute silence has been preserved, especially by all international organizations concerned with health and family planning working in Kenya. Visitors - and tourism has become a major source of income - could never guess the reality, so carefully are the facts concealed. But the mutilations contined with the collusion of those responsible for health, including the health ministry until the prohibition.

In 1975, in connection with International Women's Year, I made an inquiry about maternal health and circumcision at the Ministry of Health. My letter was answered by the Chief Nursing Officer, Mrs. E. M. Kiereini, stating that "There have been no studies conducted in this country on this subject because we do not consider it as our priority as far as our health problems are concerned." [48]

Inquiries concerning any research on the subject of female circumcision addressed to the University of Nairobi's Department of Sociology and to the Medical School produced little information. "Nobody has taken this question seriously as a research topic" stated one reply.

Most people did not answer or replied only after repeated letters that they knew nothing about circumcision or that "female circumcision does not exist anymore except perhaps in a few, isolated rural areas."

The UNESCO Regional Officer, who signed the letter as Communication Adviser/ Population, replied:

> I have not come across any recent literature on the subject (female circumcision). Although the practice seems to have died on its own, occasionally one does hear of isolated instances from various parts of the country." [49]

Though these and other letters provided no factual information, warnings about "cultural values", about "the people's beliefs" and the "importance of traditions" are gratuitously added, to replies on the subject even when the writer pretends to have no information, or states that FGM no longer exists. The same warnings accompany most personal communications on this subject in Kenya, in an attempt to conceal the truth.

Most often, no matter whom one asks, the reply is "this custom is vanishing", or "I don't know anything about it; ask someone else", and the subject is abruptly changed.

The Child Welfare Society of Kenya, one of the best-known charitable organizations under the guidance of the late President Kenyatta's most prominent wife Mama Ngina, responded to an inquiry about children's health in relation to female circumcision in October 1975:

> Quite a few people have posed the same question in the past. . . the practice which was not carried out by all tribes in this country anyway, died a natural death. If there are some girls who are still being circumcized, they must be very few indeed, and in the remotest parts of Kenya." [50]

But Jocelyn Murray only a few years earlier had found that even among secondary school girls up to two thirds were excised. And the vast majority of rural girls do not even finish primary school while many girls do not go to school at all.

A midwife working in rural Kenya replied to an inquiry on FGM in Spring, 1975, as follows:

> Circumcision on females is going on in the rural areas, especially among those who are still believers of our traditions and cultural customs. This is still strongly carried out by the tribes like Kuria, Kisii, Masai, Suk, Nandi, Kipsigis, and Kamba. Their reason for circumcising women is that if a girl is circumcized, the sexual urge will decrease. . . since the sensitive organ is cut off. . . therefore, she does not have sexual relations with a man before marriage. . . The circumcized girl when married does not practice extramarital sexual relationships. . . thus keeps moral behavior in the society.
>
> I would also like to point out that through my experience as a midwife working under the Ministry of Health recently, I have seen some mothers especially primigravida (mothers having children for the first time) having complications such as delay in second stage of labour; because of the scar formed the perineum cannot stretch to give room for the baby's head to be born. In this case an episiotomy has to be performed each time the woman gives birth, if not there is a serious tear to both perineum and the muscles and this involves also the rectum. Sometimes these women end up with V.V.F. (Vaginal Vesicle Fistula) which is very hard to repair. . .

> "Babies born of these women, if premature usually die or have brain damage. Some babies are born dead because of delay in second stage if born at home without supervision of a qualified midwife. Haemorrhage is profuse in case of a tear on the scar. . . the scars always form haemotoma when bruised and it is very painful.*
>
> Although the Ministry of Health has tried to enlighten people. . . a majority are still going on with this custom in rural areas. . ." [51]

This gives rather a different picture of the situation - as seen by a midwife who is involved in women's health and childbirth on a daily basis.

In March of 1977, while in Nairobi, I visited the Department of Obstetrics and Gynecology at the Kenyatta Hospital to inquire about women's health problems. I also talked to Professor J.K.G. Mati, then Chairman of the Department, to learn what the incidence of FGM is among hospital patients. [52] Professor Mati told me that "circumcision" was no problem; but that as editor of **WIN NEWS**, I could do a great service, by attracting attention to another problem they faced - that of fistula operations.* Professor Mati stated that the hospital had a waiting list of more than 300 women who needed these operations, which require careful management and supervision by specially trained nurses and bedrest for several weeks. The hospital does not have enough beds or trained help for this purpose: They were raising funds around the world with the assistance of the African Medical and Research Foundation to start a special 40-bed fistula unit. [53]

This was the priority of Professor Mati. But to prevent FGM, which is the chief contributing cause of fistula formation, seems to have no priority at all. When I visited the African Medical Research Foundation, the Director of Information told me: "It is difficult to exaggerate the human misery from which these poor women suffer." But when I inquired about any education programs to prevent FGM, the Director called in their resident anthropologist, who gave me a lecture on the importance of all African customs and traditions he claimed must be preserved. To this day the African Medical Research Foundation has ignored FGM. Neither the University of Nairobi nor the Health Department or its medical and nursing schools or any private organization concerned with health has done the necessary basic research as to how many people in Kenya today are practicing genital mutilation though it is a major health problem. Basic clinical investigations that, for instance, have been done in the Sudan and many other countries to establish the facts are still entirely missing; instead, the results of FGM are deliberately concealed.

Medical professionals prefer to ignore and even deny the far-ranging damage done by genital mutilation, which is a public health problem of major proportion wherever the operations are practiced. Not even death in childbirth due to genital mutilation is recorded anywhere. The recommendations of the WHO Seminar in Khartoum, to which Kenya sent one delegate, have not been publicized or implemented (see "The World Health Organization Seminar"). The reluctance in Kenya to face facts about genital mutilation, even on the part of medical and health professionals, is greater than anywhere else due to the influence of Kenyatta - with terrible results for women and girls.

Occasionally, the newspapers in Nairobi report some tragic mishap in connection with "female circumcision" or a group of influential persons make statements that this practice should be abolished. But no effective action ever results. For instance **The Nation**, Kenya's leading paper published in Nairobi, reported in January 1978 that a Kanu (the government party) branch meeting passed a resolution calling for a stop to circumcision of girls:

> "This is not the first time we have heard such calls to end circumcision of females. Sad reports abound of young women who bleed to death after the ceremony. Last September, an unconscious girl was admitted to the hospital in Embu for an emergency blood transfusion.

---

* A fistula is the rupture or tearing of the internal divisions between the vagina and the bladder and/or rectum. This results in incontinence. Such women continuously dribble urine and/or feces - which makes them outcasts of their families and society. Such injuries occur due to obstructed labor, which is the result of FGM, because the hardened scars prevent normal dilation. (See "Health Facts".)

"Hospital sources had remarked that each August or December they must treat such cases. . . The incident occurred only a few days after a tragedy in Meru, where a girl died five days after her 'operation'.

Meanwhile, a number of our politicians, health officials and citizens have joined the bandwagon over the years. . .

Their reasons for doing so might be sound. But calling for a sudden halt to an ancient tradition. . . is. . . likely to prove an impractical one." [54]

And the paper goes on to suggest that a better method might be for the hospitals and local clinics to join the government and the clergy to form a working committee on how best to tackle the problem. The article asks:

"Will this mean making the people aware to the point where they, themselves, will decide to ban the custom? Or will our medical authorities. . . launch a grass roots education programme to inform people just what is it about female circumcision that is harming younger women?. . . Let the people know why it might be hazardous, or at times fatal; enlighten them." [55]

In May 1978, The Nation, in a feature article, raised the question "Circumcision or Mutilation?" and reported on the health facts concerning FGM published in **WIN NEWS.** In a "Kenya Diary" published next to the article, the highlights of recent local reports on the mutilations from the newspaper files are chronologically listed:

"January 1967: YWCA national general secretary and Maendeleo ya Wanawake* president, Mrs. Jael Mbogo, plead for a commission to scrutinize female circumsion. They want a united force of Government, religious bodies and women's clubs to work hand in hand on circumcision.

"February 1967: At the National Council of Women of Kenya's annual general meeting, the Minister for Co-operative and Social Services, Mr. Ronald Ngala, says women in Kisii dislike circumcision and they want the Government to make a ruling. He says he would be interested to know what the council feels about the issue.

"March 1970: A Bungoma man is fined for forcibly circumcising his wife after she refused.

"April 1970: A woman in Kapenguiria is alledged to have caused the death of a young girl after circumcision.

"January 1971: Eastern Provincial Commissioner, Mr. E. M. Mahihu, warns a Sunday congregation at Choria that circumcision carries many risks.

"September 1977: A Meru girl is rushed to Embu District Hospital for a blood transfusion after being circumcized.

"October 1977: Bishop of Mt. Kenya East Diocese condemns female circumcision and Kenyatta National Hospital matron Mrs. W. Nyoike supports the Bishop.

"December 1977: Embu medical chief Dr. Omondi calls for an immediate halt to circumcision for girls, as he says it causes severe pain and medical complications.

"March 1978: Five people are jailed forcing a twenty three year old woman in Baringo to be circumcized with a razor blade." [56]

The Kenyan newpapers continue to report on FGM regularly but nothing is done by those who are responsible for health. In Kenya FGM is a preventable public health problem. Due to the very high population growth more children are mutilated now than ever before.

VIVA, a new, independent women's magazine of Kenya, in 1978 published an article entitled "Cultural Oppression", where the subject of FGM was discussed:

---

* Maendeleo Ya Wanawake (which means 'Women's Progress'), is the largest national village women's organization of Kenya with affiliates all over the country.

> ". . .At puberty she undergoes an excruciating painful operation. In often totally unhygienic conditions, without anesthesia, her sexual organs are modified so that her sexual pleasure is dramatically diminished. . .At home she is regarded as an economic asset to be exchanged for wealth at marriage. In marriage, she becomes the property of her husband to be used, misused, and mistreated at his will." [57]
>
> "There are. . . aspects of our own culture which are unacceptable to us. Female circumcision, infibulation, much of the Islamic treatment of women, marriage, property, and inheritance laws are some of them. It has become common for people, especially men, to excuse injustice to women with the phrase 'it is African'. There is nothing African about injustice. . ." [58]

The August 1978 issue of **VIVA** featured "The Neglected Question of Female Circumcision" in large letters on the cover. "The Silence Over Female Circumcision in Kenya" is the heading of the inside story where a diversity of opinions of women and men who were interviewed is explored. Conflicts and differing views about circumcision split families, generations, and communities.

"The circumcised women regard me as a child", says Rachel, a young woman of a large family, who has chosen to remain uncircumcised. She had the support of her parents, though several of her sisters went behind their parents' backs under pressure of their peers to undergo the mutilation. "Among her people, Rachel sees no chance that female circumcision will come to be seen as harmful. . . if something goes wrong, it is believed to be due to. . . evil spirits." [59]

In Kenya, so the article explains, female circumcision still is a potent political issue, due to the controversy of more than 50 years ago. And the magazine states: "The central question really is: What are the effects of female circumcision on the women who undergo it? Are those effects compatible with steps now being taken to improve the position of women generally?" [60] In Kenya today, "development" has been made into a national goal and creed. Are not the physical risks and the health damage inflicted by those unnecessary operations completely incompatible with the commitment for development?

Yet the fact that circumcision damages women's health is still regarded by some Kenyan men as an invention by the West, so **VIVA** reports. Dr. Simeon W. Chilungu, an anthropologist at the University of Nairobi, claims that infections or physical damage, including childbirth problems, have never been proved, and he states that the notion that clitoridectomy removes a woman's source of sexual pleasure arises out of Western perspectives. Evidently Dr. Chilingu has never discussed the operations with his colleagues in gynecology who are qualified to make statements on medical facts, while he is not. The **VIVA** article states:

> "Once again, the argument is used by certain Kenyans that objection to female circumcision is based on Western notions. Hardly. The current objections to female circumcision are based on the fact that medical evidence proves conclusively that the practice threatens women's health and also degrades them. . . Our people readily accept Western 'notions' such as medicine and technology; how can we oppose ideas just because they are Western?" [61]

But the vast majority of Kenyan women in rural areas are still illiterate and don't read articles in **VIVA**. Citing examples of the sophisticated Western educated leadership in the nation's capital could be misleading. What happens in Nairobi and what goes on in the villages are two different things. A health worker from the rural areas in Western Kenya writes:

> "In the Central part of Kenya, the practice of excision is decreasing, but in the Rift Valley and some Districts in Nyasa Region the practice is still quite popular.
>
> The girls are circumcized at the age of eight to ten when they still can't make decisions of their own and, therefore, must follow the parent's decisions." [62]

Formerly, sixteen to eighteen years was the age when female circumcision was performed; this has changed because more girls now go to school. Due to education, the age of circumcision changed because parents became aware that when older, many more girls refused.

And the health worker continues: "Yes, girls do run away; but parents track them down and bring them back to be circumcised. . ." [63] However, some girls are eager to undergo the operation due to peer pressure and because they fear being ridiculed. Girls who are not circumcised are publicly mocked by the community: in a village, everyone knows every one else's business: it is hard for young girls to stand up against the community, and to be different from their friends. They are made to pay a heavy price for such behavior. To be accepted, to be part of the group, especially while growing up, during the vulnerable time of puberty is important to every young person in all societies.

The answers to some of the questions Jocelyn Murray asked in the questionnaire on circumcision given in several different schools, provide some information on present attitudes: "Who is the oldest uncircumcised woman in your home area? What do people say about her?" Two thirds of the circumcised girls showed an unfavorable attitude towards those not circumcized. Uncircumcized women are described as lacking in discipline, bad mannered and immature. "She was rejected by her non-Christian parents and was subject to general abuse from the community", one girl stated. "She was married only last year. At the wedding, the old women abused the man for marrying the uncircumised girl, and the bride was sad all day." [64] To find a husband for an uncircumcised woman continues to be a problem in many areas.

Though group ceremonies still continue, a midwife who works in Western Kenya reports: "In certain parts of the area in which I work, for example among the Kisii, Masai, Kuria, Kalenjin, circumcision is done by women at home. . . In urban areas, it is also done as 'private ceremony'. At times, young women who have a job in a town and even in Nairobi, go home to be circumcised in their village with the other village girls." [65] Whatever the type of ceremony, group or individual it is abundantly clear that FGM contributes to AIDS infection which is rampart in Africa including in Kenya, as a result of the sexual behavior by African men.

A recent survey done in a girls' high school in the Tharaka region (East of Mount Kenya), among the 97-strong sophomore class (ages 16-21), produced these results: [66]

a) How many are circumcized? 97 out of 97.

b) Do you think your daughter will be circumcized?

Yes, answered 78 out of 97.

c) Do you think your granddaughter will be circumcized?

No, answered 93 out of 97.

The survey, made by a teacher of the school, continues:

> "In Meru, on the Western side of Mt. Kenya, about 90-95 percent of the girls are circumcised. Here in Tharaka, all the girls are circumcized without a doubt. . . . Most girls would be circumcised between the ages of 11-15. The 'operation' often takes place for schoolgirls during the holiday periods (April/August/December) so that they can rest a full 3-4 weeks. On the books, female circumcision is illegal. .
>
> Circumcision usually takes the form of removing the clitoris and then scooping out, often up to a handful and with a knife, the flesh from the inside walls of the vagina. In some districts, e.g. Tigania and parts of Tharaka (both in Meru District), an object funnel-like might be inserted into the vagina to keep the walls from narrowing. . .
>
> The operation is carried out to clear a path and widen the birth canal for safer deliveries and to remove the clitoris which, it is said, is prone to pick up dirt, disease, or just plain smell, given the fact that. . . people often sit on the dirt floors both inside and outside the homes and. . . undergarments are not worn.
>
> The ritual is to help the young girl about to embark on womanhood (which means having children) to fulfill her meaning in the community. . . Socially, of course, it had other interpretations (preparation for the difficulties of adult life, initiation into the clan, specific preparation for marriage, etc.). The traditional Masai, for instance, circumcise their girls the night before the wedding.
>
> What complications sometimes occur? Besides pain, for no anesthesia is given, there is infection, usually from the knife used or the dirty ground. . .

> "Secondly, sometimes there is stenosis of the vagina or a constriction of the birth canal. Other times and, of course, more serious, is the setting in of septicemia, which can even cause death. . ."

And the report concludes: "If a girl thinks she will be laughed at, no law of Kenya or anyone will stop her from asking to be circumcised." [67]

This candid description also confirms that the drastic and very damaging form of the operation described by the physicians in the Report of the Scottish Missionary Council still continues today.

That circumcision is an extraordinarily lucrative business is confirmed by this report from a Kenyan community health worker and midwife:

> "Though circumcision is always done by women, the circumcisors are particular people who are known in the community to be specialists in this practice. The job usually runs in the families, so the young people learn the trade from the grandmothers, mothers, and so on; and in case of male circumcision, by their grandfather or father. The circumcisors consider themselves to provide an important and respected service to the community. The money paid is considered in appreciation for the service rendered. The current rate for girls is six Kenyan shillings per girl, and during the circumcision period, the circumcisor can perform the operation on 40 girls per day. The rate for boys is 12 shillings per boy. These rates are also affected by inflation, and tend to increase year by year." [68]

The earnings of a circumcisor, it appears, are considerable. There are no other jobs in a village that pay a comparable income. But even here, the price for circumcising boys - paid to a man - is twice as much.

In Kenya, indeed in most Africa, having children and fertility are still of overriding importance: to make childbirth more hazardous and painful through FGM seems contrary to the objectives and desires of the population. But especially in Kenya, the professional health sector has completely failed, for political reasons, to establish the fact the FGM is a public health problem of considerable magnitude; but worse, they have failed to make it clear to the population that these operations are highly damaging and dangerous and are a real threat to both mother and child in childbirth.

Factual information on reproduction and sexuality is one of the best kept secrets in Africa today. The truth about the biological facts is mystified, concealed and surrounded with magic beliefs and all kinds of practices many of them dangerous. How can young people learn about their own bodies' functions and health when all such information is hidden under cover of so-called "morality" imposed by the missionaries and myths.

In traditional Africa, the biological facts are unknown, and reproduction is enshrined in traditional practices and myths that are both dangerous and damaging to health. The schools in the past were run by Christian missionaries; but missionaries who teach the facts about reproduction and what is called "sex education" are rare indeed.

Even though the schools are now run by the government, most of the teachers got their own education in the missionary schools. Education, predictably, continues to be influenced by their values - teaching women what is known in the West as home economics, to be obedient to men and to be meek. Yet these women by tradition are forced to assume the major responsibility for growing each family's food and have all the responsibility for their children's health and well-being. But the schools do not equip girls for those responsibilities, such as teaching about agriculture and certainly not about childbirt or managing family health. Yet in Kenya today eight is the average number of children per woman.

How can young people make a choice when they are denied the information they need? How can a girl learn what affects her well-being and health when the very subject of reproduction is tabu and never mentioned in the schools?

As an educator who runs a girls' school in a rural area in Central Kenya states:

> "Unfortunately, little is being done in the schools in the area of sex education, though the Ministry of Education is making attempts, especially in the upper primary grades, to break down some of the barriers to such instruction. . . Many schools were founded by missionaries or church-oriented groups. . . and as such 'sex' just wasn't discussed in the classroom. . . It is a question of embarrassment, social/religious in nature, that is preventing it from being included in the curriculum, especially in girls' schools . . . "[69]

And, because of this embarrassment by the male moral leadeship, the younger generation continues to be kept in ignorance. But the price is paid by women and girls whose health and lives are damaged and destroyed, not only in Africa: the same "morality" is propagated all over the world, which is increasingly life threatening due to AIDS .

In a research study published by the Institute for Development Studies at the University of Nairobi on the Sexual Knowledge and Practice of Kenyan Youth, 320 young people in teacher training colleges, secretarial schools and commercial schools in Nairobi were questioned:

> "The questionnaire was aimed at collecting information concerning knowledge, attitudes and desires of the young people concerning reproduction, family planning, contraceptives, desired number of children. . .
>
> The knowledge level concerning human reproduction is very low indeed. . .
>
> The conclusion drawn is that there is clearly a need to introduce sex/population education for in- and out-of- school youth. The need is all the more urgent because our under 20 year olds who constitute 50 percent of the Kenyan population have inaccurate ideas about their sexual and social selves. The fact that the parents are as ignorant about these matters as their children makes the situation more serious."[70]

And, parents who are "ignorant about these matters" decide that their daughters must be circumcised to conform to a past that no longer exists. They force the mutilation on their daughters at a much younger age - as long as the girls are still under their control and cannot refuse.

In an article on sex education, **VIVA** investigated the knowledge about reproduction among young girls and women in Nairobi. [71] Early teenage pregnancies, abortions that permanently injure or kill, and baby dumping have become an increasing problem in the modern sector in the towns.

Several schools were contacted by **VIVA** in Nairobi. It appears that "out of five schools contacted, none had any kind of program of instruction regarding reproduction and the female body". Interviews with students revealed that most of the young women did not know when they could conceive. "Young girls are armed with wrong information and very little even of that. . ." ,**VIVA** states. One girl answered the question "When do you think you are likely to get pregnant?" with "I intend to get married after school so I do not have to know anything now". Other young women believed that they could have sex relations with their boyfriends because "You can only get pregnant when you are married." [72]

The majority of the young women interviewed knew about contraceptives, but very few knew how to use them or their information was wrong. Although many young women go for treatment to government hospitals after undergoing illegal abortions, any factual knowledge about abortion was similarly lacking.

The VIVA article states "sex education as a national program does not exist and until recently, young people were left out of the family planning movement." [73]

The emphasis of most Western-designed family planning programs in Africa is to persuade as many women as possible to accept birth-control services; education in personal health and reproduction has not been part of this approach.

Eddah Gachukia, who was head of the National Council of Women of Kenya (NCWK) for a number of years, which coordinates all women's organizations in Kenya, and was appointed by Kenyatta as Member of Parliament, to speak for women's affairs in the government. She stressed the problem of teenage pregnancies:

> "Girls are not allowed to continue in school when they get pregnant, no matter how bright they are. There is a very high dropout rate in the higher grades - we are now fighting for girls to keep on in school."[74]

And Eddah Gachukia added, when I asked about circumcision, that some mothers now have their girls excised to prevent pre-marital pregnancy. But the National Council has never done any investigation on FGM - claiming that the operations are "dying out."

Life is rapidly changing in Kenya's urban areas, especially in Nairobi, but rural areas are left out and left behind. A large number of men have left the villages to seek employment in the towns; women stay behind with their children to do all the argricultural work by themselves. Life is changing, but for the women left behind in the rural areas, it is getting worse - with the social and economic gap between women and men widening.

Village women are too rarely heard. Perdita Huston went to speak with village women in Kenya and many other countries, and recorded what village women told her in a book, **Message from the Village**. She asked the women some basic questions about their lives, past and present, as well as about their aspirations for the future. How did the women in the rural areas of Kenya feel about their families and the changes in living conditions that are beginning to affect village life?

Here is what some of the village women had to say about change and about their lives and families:

> "Life is more difficult now than before // Men have changed - their heads are too big // Women could really run the country much better than men // Men must be taught that we are human beings like them // Women seem to be taking over the work of men // The children sometimes don't know their fathers // What can you do if you have a husband who is always drunk and does not help his wife?
>
> Girls are better than boys because girls help a lot // Sometimes if you get married, he goes out, he drinks, he doesn't even care what you and the children have to eat // You see our men take many wives so that the wives will do everything for the family, then the husband won't have to work hard // Women are starting now to fight for their places in local councils and Parliament and they are defeating men // You'll never see a man going to a family planning clinic - they are not interested // Men don't care much about their children // Men who earn more just go and have more women outside and forget about their wives // There should be a law - one man, one woman // Men are very selfish and jealous - they just think about themselves. . ."[75]

Polygamy is legal in Kenya and still widely practiced. The legal situation within the family and in regard to property ownership is critical for women's development. In a recent study on **Law and the Status of Women**, Kenya is included. The chapter on "Law and the Status of Women in Kenya" was written mainly by members of the Faculty of Law of the University of Nairobi, and it minces no words:

> "Women are legally less privileged than are men and this explains much of their subservient position in society.
>
> Most Kenyan women reside in rural regions, lack the educational advantages enjoyed by their male counterparts, and generally remain under the authority of their fathers or husbands. Although urbanization has wrought radical changes in the status of a fraction of women, it has had little impact on the vast majority of Kenyan women. . .
>
> Kenya, like other former British colonial possessions, has several different systems of laws regulating various aspects of life. There is the imported law which is inherited from the colonial powers; there is the customary law regulating the lives of the various ethnic groups in areas that have not been altered by legislation; and there are also religious laws, mainly Hindu and Islamic. The multiplicity and overlap of these legal systems complicates the task of ascertaining the precise status of women in Kenya. . .

> "Section 82 of the Kenya Constitutionof 1969 prohibits discriminatory legislation, and what is 'discriminatory' is broadly defined; but, significantly, this prohibition does not apply to laws made with respect to adoption, marriage, divorce, devolution of property or death or other matters of personal law. Under the present constitution, therefore, many existing or newly established tribal, religious and common laws and practices that discriminate against women qua women are legal in Kenya. . ." [76]

The report goes on to examine women's rights pertaining to marriage, property, divorce, inheritance, health, education and training, employment and related matters; it points out the confusion that exists, especially in family law, which recognizes both polygamous and monogamous marriages. There is a Christian as well as Hindu Marriage and Divorce Act, and besides that, both tribal and Islamic law are recognized. Though free consent to marriage by a woman is required, such consent is easy to obtain since "the majority of women in Kenya possess little economic power." And the writers add ". . . by their very designation, polygamous marriages function within a discriminatory framework." [77]

Polygamy is of course illegal in most of the world and since the constitution of Kenya states that all Kenyans have equal rights, polygamy is in fact illegal, but no one has ever examined this. What is more FGM is not only criminal child abuse but an international human rights violation. Parents who subject their children to FGM - as has happened among African immigrants in France - would face criminal court procedures in Europe and most of the industrialized world. By law children would have to be removed from any home where they are threatened with physical abuse or mutilations. While President Moi prohibited FGM in 1982, there never has been any follow-up, no indictment or investigation.

Both customary and Islamic law still requires the payment of bride-price, which goes to the bride's father. The bride-price, a tradition which continues to be a requirement for marriage in Kenya and much of Africa as well as the Middle East, is only beginning to be rejected by educated young people all over Africa, but it is still upheld by most male heads of families. Fathers greatly profit from this institution in financial terms, as well as power and prestige, as the male head of the family arranges the marriages to suit himself.

Since excision or infibulation is a traditional requirement for marriage made by the groom's family, a father will insist on having his daughters mutilated; otherwise, he might lose the brideprice. Hence, fathers see to it that their daughters are "done." In turn, the male head of the family requires that the brides chosen for his sons, for whom he usually has to put up the brideprice, are suitably mutilated: this to assure that "morality" prevails and that women do not seek sexual satisfaction outside the polygamous marriage that is forced upon them; the mutilations remove any possibility for pleasurable sexual intercourse, which often becomes a painful duty and ordeal.

The customs of the brideprice, polygamy and sexual mutilation serve to reinforce the patriarchal power and the oppression and exploitation of women by the men of their own families, their fathers, husbands, brothers and sons.

As **VIVA**, in an article on the bride-price in Kenya states:

> "Brideprice, operating in a money economy, has come to acquire the qualities of a sale. . . it is now, more than ever before, the price of a woman. Greed of gain has led some parents to force their daughters to leave school, even when they are still young, and wed rich elderly men for fat bride-prices. . .
>
> It is always argued by protagonists of bride-price that it protects the virtue of girls. . . that it ensures good treatment and care from the husband to the wife. . . that it compensates the bride's father for the loss of her services. . . and ensures stability of marriage. . .
>
> Even a cursory glance at the state of our marriages today, however, shows that bride-price no longer fulfills these functions. . . The brideprice is an anachronistic and archaic custom that reduces the status of women. . . And in an overtly polygamous society, like Kenya, it sanctifies inequality. . ." [78]

Several attempts have been made to formulate new family legislation in Kenya, which, as outlined above, is omitted from the Kenyan Constitution of 1969. Most recently, a new marriage bill was discussed in summer of 1979, in the Kenyan Parliament - which has only four women members. The new bill was concerned with regulating polygamy - specifically, it required a husband to have the consent of his first wife before marrying another one. [79] It was pointed out - correctly - by the male MPs that no wife would ever agree to a second marriage, and thus the MPs rejected this clause.

Other reforms introduced in the bill, drafted by Attorney General Charles Njonjo of Kenya, proposed to outlaw wife beating. The male MPs argued in the Kenyan Parliament, in favor of wife abuse as the traditional right of all Kenyan and African men: "It is very African to teach women manners by beating them," Kimonai Arap Soi, the MP representing the Kalenjin tribal area, said in Parliament: "The husband is the boss of the house". He was, of course, joined by other MPs and no doubt spoke for a majority.

All this was reported around the world including by **TIME** magazine. Needless to say, after several days of debate, the "Marriage Reform" bill was shelved once more "by an overwhelming majority." **TIME** reported.

Men have nothing to lose from shelving family reform, since this keeps in place the discriminatory, traditional, tribal, religious and common laws that condone abuse of women, FGM, polygamy, and that deprive women of property rights, making women into second class citizens in every area, but especially where it matters most: in the family. The status of a woman in the family is, of course, at issue when decisions are made whether or not to mutilate a daughter or to whom to marry her.

Kenya has several very active women's organizations which are coordinated by the **National Council of Women of Kenya (NCWK)**, [80] a roof organization which speaks for women's needs to the national government, as well as representing Kenyan women internationally. For many years the NCWK was headed by Eddah Gachukia, who enjoys a great deal of political influence.

The United Nations "Mid-Decade World Conference for Women" in 1980 in Copenhagen provided the opportunity to heighten the awareness about FGM internationally. Kenya had sent one of the largest delegations to the Conference, led by Eddah Gachukia, that included most of Kenya's women leaders. Several workshops on FGM were held at the "Forum 80", the open, participatory parallel conference organized by United Nations accredited Non-Governmental Organizations. [81]

An international panel discussion on FGM by African women was moderated by Eddah Gachukia with speakers from Egypt, Sudan and Somalia. Eddah Gachukia stated that it is unknown to what extent "female circumcision" is still practiced in Kenya. She claimed since no research had been done, the facts were unknown and she could not speak on this subject. An offer was made from the audience to assist such research, but it was immediately turned down by the Kenyan women. When at the 1985 UN Decade Conference Forum held in Nairobi the Inter African Committee (IAC) arranged a number of discussions on FGM, the Kenyan women leaders stayed away.

Maendeleo Ya Wanawake, [82] which literally means "Women's Progress," reaches most villages and is perhaps the most effective grassroots women's organization in Africa. Under the leadership of Jane Kiano, the wife of a prominent politician, Maendeleo realized its most ambitious dream: building a multistory building of its own in Nairobi, close to the university. It houses its business activities, and has meeting rooms to conduct leadership and training classes, as well as conferences; the building also has much rental office space that provides income.

Maendeleo, due to its large village membership, has real political power and politicians eagerly seek its endorsement. Because of its influence, the national government party KANU took over Maendeleo in 1987, [83] but this was short-lived. Due to international political pressure for "privatization" Maendeleo once more was returned to its previous status. Maendeleo then sent a delegation to participate in the 1990 IAC Conference in Addis Ababa and became interested in taking up the issue of FGM: The research and program they are developing is discussed in the chapter on "Women and Health."

KENYA: ECONOMIC/SOCIAL FACTS & SUMMARY

Kenya: Seven rural provinces.
Climate: From tropical to arid.
Population: 21 6 million. (1987 estimate). Nairobi (capital), 959,000 (1987). Annual Growth Rate: 4.1%.
Life Expectancy: 58.5 years (1985) // Infant Mortality: 59/1000.
Government: Republic. Constitution. Parliament. Independence: December 12, 1963.
Ethnic Groups: Kikuyu 21% // Luhya 14% // Luo 13% // Kalenjin 11% // Kamba 11% // Kisii 6% // Meru 5% // Non African, Asian, European, Arab 1%.
Languages: English // Swalhili // Many tribal languages.
Religions: Indigenous beliefs 26% (animist) // Protestant 38% // Roman Catholic 28% // Muslim 6%.
Literacy: 25% (women less).
Education: Not compulsory. First 8 years primary school free.
Annual/Capita Income: $ 322 (1986 estimate).
Economy: Growth Rate: 4.9% (1986). Inflation 10.7% Agriculture 30%. Industry 13.8%. Trade 16%.

FOOTNOTES

1. "Moi Condemns Girls' Circumcision", **Nairobi Times,** July 27, 1982, p. 3.
2. "Female Circumcision: Educate the Ignorant", **Daily Nation**, Wednesday, July 18, 1982 (Editorial).
3. "Girl Rites Banned in Hospitals." **Daily Nation**, September 1, 1982.
4. Kenyatta, Jomo. **Facing Mount Kenya.** Vintage Books, Division of Random House, New York. October 1965, pp. 128-129. (The book was first published in the 1930s). Note: Jomo Kenyatta was the first president of Kenya after independence and was declared 'president for life' by his grateful subjects who credited him with attaining independence.
5. Bruce-Chwatt, Leonard, Dr. "Female Circumcision and Politics", **World Medicine**. January 14, 1976, p. 47.
6. Ibid, pp. 44-45.
7. Kenyatta, op. cit., pp. 128-129.
8. Bruce-Chwatt, op. cit., p. 45.
9. **Memorandum Prepared by the Mission Council of the Church of Scotland, "Female Circumcision"**, Appendix 1, Section I, pp. i, ii. (Contents: Section I: Introductory // Section II: History of teaching against circumcision at puberty // Section III: The attitude of government to female circumcision // Section IV: Opposition to constituted authority among the Kikuyu // Section V: Causes and history of the 1929 crisis // Section VII: Some general observations and answers to criticisms // Section VIII: Appendices.)
10. Kenyatta, op. cit., pp. 139-140.
11. Ibid., p. 141.
12. Bruce-Chwatt, op. cit., p. 45.

FOOTNOTES (continued)

13. Beck, Ann. **A History of the British Medical Administration of East Africa,** 1900-1950. A Commonwealth Fund Book, Harvard University Press, Cambridge, MA 02139, 1970, pp. 94-5.
14. Ibid., p. 96.
15. Ibid., p. 98.
16. Ibid., p. 100.
17. Ibid., pp. 100-101.
18. Ibid., p. 103.
19. **Memorandum** - Mission Council of Church of Scotland, op. cit., Section I, p. 15.
20. Ibid., p. 17.
21. Ibid., p. 38.
22. Ibid., p. 39.
23. Ibid., pp. 56-57, 61.
24. Ibid., p. 67.
25. Ibid., p. 73.
26. **Papers Relating to the Health and Progress of Native Populations in Certain Parts of the Empire.** No. 1. "Dispatch from the Secretary of State for the Colonies to the Officers Administering the the Governments of Kenya, Uganda Protectorate, Tanganyika Territory, Nyasaland, Northern Rhodesia and Zanzibar". March 8, 1930, p. 9.
27. **Papers Relating to the Health and Progress of Native Populations in Certain Parts of the Empire. Eastern and Central Africa.** "Dispatch from the Secretary of State for the Colonies to the Governor of Kenya." April 10, 1930. Report by the Committee for the Protection of Colored Women in the Crown Colonies.
28. Ibid., p. 12.
29. Ibid.
30. Ibid., p. 13.
31. Kenyatta, op. cit., p. 172.
32. Boserup, Ester. "The Economics of Polygamy", **Women's Role in Economic Development,** St. Martin's Press, 1970 / George Allen & Unwin Ltd., 1970, pp. 37-41.
33. Kenyatta, op. cit., p. 156.
34. Ibid., p. 170.
35. Ibid., p. 17.
36. Ibid., pp. 8-9.
37. Ibid., p. 10.
38. Ibid., p. 17.
39. Murray, Jocelyn Margaret. **The Kikuyu Female Circumcision Controversy with Special Reference to the Church Missionary Society's "Sphere of Influence."** University of California, Los Angeles, Ph.D., 1974.
40. Ibid., p. xi.
41. Ibid., p. 228.
42. Ibid., p. 326.
43. Ibid. p. 358.
44. Ibid., p. 337.
45. Ibid.
46. Ibid., p. 339.
47. Ibid., p. 352.
48. Letter in author's file from Chief Nursing Officer, Ministry of Health, Nairobi, dated March 18, 1975.
49. Letter in author's file from UNESCO Regional Officer, dated April 8, 1975.

FOOTNOTES (continued)

50. Letter in author's file from Child Welfare Society of Kenya, dated October 6, 1975.
51. Letter in author's file from Kenyan midwife, dated April 8, 1975.
52. **WIN NEWS,** Vol. III, No. 2, Spring 1977, p. 35.
53. **WIN NEWS,** Vol. II, No. 4, Autumn 1976, p. 34. African Medical & **Research Foundation** / Flying Doctor Service, Wilson Airport, P.O. Box 30125, Nairobi, Kenya.
54. **The Nation**, Sunday, Jan.1, 1978, "Circumcision: It's time for the Facts", p. 6.
55. Ibid.
56. **The Nation** (Nairobi), May 1978, "Circumcision or Mutilation?" "Kenya Diary", p. 15.
57 **VIVA,** a publication of Trend Publishers Ltd., P.O. Box 46319, Nairobi, See also **WIN NEWS** Vol. IV, No. 2, Spring 1978, p. 44.
58. Ibid., pp. 19-20.
59. **VIVA**, August 1978, p.6.
60. Ibid., p. 11.
61. Ibid., p. 12.
62. Letter in author's file from a health worker in Kenya, dated June 1978.
63. Ibid.
64. Murray, op. cit., p. 348.
65. Letter in author's file from a Kenyan midwife and community nurse, dated July 1, 1978.
66. Survey dated October 17, 1975, in author's file. See **WIN NEWS,** Vol. II, No. 1, Winter 1976, pp. 40-41.
67. Ibid.
68. Letter from Kenyan midwife, op. cit., dated July, 1978.
69. Letter in author's file.
70. Gachuhi, J. Mugo. "Kenyan Youth: Their Sexual Knowledge and Practices:" Paper No. 159, Institute for Development Studies, University of Nairobi, December 1972.
71. **VIVA**, November 1978, pp. 11-12.
72. Ibid.
73. Ibid.
74. Hosken, Fran P. "She Carries the Standard for Women in Rural Kenya", **Christian Science Monitor**, April 11, 1978, p. 21.
75. Huston, Perdita. **Message from the Village**. Sponsored by UNFPA: United Nations Fund for Population Activities, published by Epoch B. Foundation, New York. See also **WIN NEWS,** Vol. IV, No. 3, Summer 1978, p. 48.
76. **Law and the Status of Women, An International Symposium.** Centre for Social Development and Humanitarian Affairs, United Nations; edited by the Columbia Human Rights Law Review, Columbia University School of Law. "Law and the Status of Women in Kenya", by Rose Maini, V.W. Muchai, and S.B.P. Gutto, Faculty of Law, University of Nairobi, Kenya, pp. 185-187.
77. Ibid., p. 190.
78. **VIVA,** January 1979, "Bride Price", pp. 20-21. See also **WIN NEWS** Vol. V, No. 2, Spring 1979, p. 72.
79. **Daily Nation,** July 13 and 14, 1979. See also **WIN NEWS,** Vol. V, No. 4, Autumn 1979, pp. 49-50.
80. National Council of Women of Kenya, P.O. Box 43741, Nairobi, Kenya.
81. **WIN NEWS** Vol. VI, No.4 Autumn 1980. pp 42-43
82. **WIN NEWS** Vol. XIV, No.1 Winter 1988 pp 53-54, and **WIN NEWS** Vol. XVI, No.1, Winter 1990 p.54. **Sunday Nation,** (Kenya) Nov. 5, 1989.
83. Maendeleo Ya Wanawake, P.O. Box 4412. Nairobi, Kenya.

INTRODUCTION: WEST AFRICA

West Africa, which in part is very densely populated - Nigeria has the largest population of any African country - can be divided into Francophone and Anglophone countries: that is, those which were French or British colonies until after the Second World War and whose governments retain not only those languages as official ones but have adopted many of their institutions. Before that, Arab traders coming from the Northeast and the West Coast were active throughout the entire area for many centuries, propagating Islam and conducting extensive trade, including in slaves.

The French began to come to this area in the early nineteenth century and in part conquered, in part infiltrated, large areas of West Africa and organized them into different administrative units which were changed several times during the colonial period. The British proceeded in similar ways, though their zone of influence extended over a much smaller geographic area. Besides the British and French, the Portuguese and Spanish established smaller colonial areas, quite aside from the Belgians, who explored and exploited the region of the Congo.

Female genital mutilation (FGM) is practiced throughout this area though it has not been definitely established how far south the operations extend; there are reports available from northern Zaire that some ethnic groups practice FGM as initiation rituals.

There is little information on FGM available from the sparsely populated, huge region between the Sudan and Mauritania. This area is under the political boundaries of Central Africa, Chad and Niger, including the southern areas of Libya and Algeria. In 1990-91 an extensive study in Chad was conducted by UNICEF and established the fact that excision is practiced throughout the three zones of the country including in N'Djamena, the capital. [1] There young people are beginning to oppose the practice which is still universally accepted in the traditional Moslem areas. The study includes recommendations to conduct information and education campaigns - according to the different needs of each zone. This region also includes northern Mali, the northern part of Burkina Faso and Mauritania; much of it is desert or savannah with very few settlements. A large part of this region was hard hit by droughts in the 1970s. As a result, the few inhabitants of this huge region, many of them nomads, are even fewer and more widely scattered today.

Compared to East Africa, Sudan and Egypt, there are very few publications about genital mutilation of women in West Africa, and hardly any medical research has been done.

The present political boundaries of the countries of West and Central Africa are as arbitrary as those in East Africa. They were imposed by the European powers with little or no regard for the inhabitants or ethnic groups in the area. One can find today the same ethnic groups in several different countries, and customs such as FGM are generally tied to ethnic groups or tribes. Nomadic people following their herds continue their traditional patterns of migration, regardless of present political boundaries.

Trade is one of the activities West African women have traditionally engaged in, especially those in towns. The power of the market women, for instance, in Ghana and parts of Nigeria, is legendary. However, with modernization, the market women are losing ground. Most of them are illiterate and have no access to the modern banking and credit systems or safe storage facilities. In Ghana, for example, the government built supermarkets while restricting the products in which market women may trade. The supermarkets and banks, indeed everything modern, are managed, of course, by men.

While in the past in a traditional setting the market women may have had some power and influence, this is no longer true today as the women lack the education and skills to compete with modern business methods. What is more, as all statistics on education - including those by UNESCO - confirm, the literacy gap between women and men is continuously growing, especially in West Africa.

Much as in East Africa, rural women do most of the subsistence farming and continue to live in traditional ways. They are often bypassed by modernization and what is called "development." Men leave the rural areas in large numbers to work in town - leaving women and children behind to do all the hard agricultural work alone.

The northern parts of Nigeria, Ghana and other Gulf of Guinea countries are Moslem and very traditional. Every year hundreds of these Moslem families make the pilgrimage to Mecca - the Hadj. For instance, the Hausa from northern Nigeria leave from Kano by special flights. In the past the same trip by camel caravan took years. To go on the Hadj is still the dream of every devout Moslem throughout West Africa.

At the present time, the influence of Islam is growing and spreading steadily southward throughout West Africa. Moslemization of the traditional animist village society is growing. The local religious leaders in many areas claim that genital operations for women are a religious requirement. Many local Marabouts, the Moslem religious leaders, teach that female circumcision is a requirement of Islam, though religious scholars always deny this and it also has been denied by the religious leaders of the influential El Azhar University and Mosque in Egypt, which is an arbiter where Islamic rules are concerned.

Genital operations on girls were practiced in West Africa long before the advent of Islam, as is pointed out in historical research. No one has attempted to explain why or how these operations started and spread all over West Africa, or if they were imported from the Middle East.

Awa Thiam, in her book **La Parole aux Negresses,** [2] which mainly deals with the status of women in West Africa, discusses the history of genital operations. But she has no explanation of when or how these practices started in West Africa. Yet, the kinds of operations as well as the rituals involved are frequently quite similar to those in East Africa. Most people in West Africa do not even know that the same mutilations are practiced in East Africa any more than East Africans are aware that FGM goes on all over West Africa.

Arab traders moved along the West African coast for hundreds of years and built settlements to support their trade, much as they did off the coast of East Africa. Wherever they went, they took their customs along. Female genital mutilation may have been one of them. Secrecy accompanies the traditional rituals everywhere and they are concealed from all outsiders, sometimes under threat of severe penalties, for instance, by the secret societies in Sierra Leone and Liberia. The people of a different ethnic group or another village, even though nearby, are often considered to be outsiders and not to be trusted. This rivalry between ethnic groups often results in local raids or even tribal war, as recently happened again in Liberia

A very large number of local languages - few of them written - and the rivalry between different ethnic groups make it much more difficult to draw any conclusions about the origin of FGM, which is so deeply ingrained and widely practiced today all over West Africa.

The reasons given in West Africa - that the operations are necessary for a girl to become a woman and an adult member of her society and that sexual castration of the female is necessary to preserve the family - are quite the same as in East Africa, though many elaborate stories are often added, which vary with ethnic groups. In the towns and especially the capitals, FGM is done on ever younger children, often by trained health workers without any traditional rituals. But the reason is the same everywhere: Men require that the girl they marry is mutilated, or they do not pay the bride-price.

In the areas where excision is compulsory, polygamy is also practiced. Polygamy could not be maintained if women were normally sexually active. Polygamy in a traditional rural environment means that a girl, after she is excised just before reaching puberty, is sent to the household of the husband-to-be as soon as he has paid the bride price. There, the older women take charge of her and she is integrated into the household labor force. As soon as she menstruates, she is impregnated - even if she is not fully grown. Childbearing and child care become part of her duties aside from helping in the household, which is under the control of the first wife.

In Sierra Leone, this system still functions in rural areas, reinforced by the secret societies which claim to bestow power on women. But in reality the rural household, though women are in charge and do all the hard labor, works for men who own what the women produce as well as the land. And the secret societies, while claiming to give the excisors special powers, in fact mutilate girls to make them pliable wives to become property of polygamous men.

Polygamy was the subject of a recent article in **Famille et Developpement,** [3] a West African magazine concerned with social issues, which described the lives of women in polygamous families. The reality of women's lives, stated by the women themselves, is far different from academic discussions on this subject. Based on a survey, the report shows that the vast majority of women responded: "Polygamy means too much pain and uncertainty."

But the real victims in a polygamous marriage are the children: Jealousy and rivalry between the children are constant problems. The father has too little time for his many children and often hardly knows them. Today, to adequately support several households, which in Africa often means more than a dozen children and their mothers, is impossible, except for the richest men.

In traditional rural life the economic advantages for a polygamous man are obvious, since wives and children are his wholly owned labor force; they work for the benefit of the male head of household. But under urban living conditions, the economic situation is quite different. Nevertheless, African men who are unable to provide for one wife and her children often have several wives and large numbers of children. In urban areas many women live in abject poverty in the miserable squatter settlements that form ever-larger parts of the rapidly growing African cities. Often the only way to support themselves and their children is by prostitution, which is rampant throughout all West African cities - while AIDS is spreading ever more rapidly. According to WHO, more people in Africa are infected than anywhere else in the world.

West Africa as a region has the fastest growing cities; their growth rate is matched by rampant corruption, which affects all business enterprise and development. West Africa also has the highest infant and childbirth mortality rates. The highest illiteracy rates - especially for women - can also be found in Francophone West Africa. Growing food shortages now beset many countries that were self-supporting in the past, for instance Mali and Sierra Leone and much of the budget of Senegal is paid by France.

Population growth rates are still increasing all over West Africa. Though most of the women are sexually mutilated, they are pushed into continuous childbearing by men who believe that fathering numerous children is the way to validate their own lives. Child marriage is practiced especially in Moslem areas, for instance, by the Hausa in northern Nigeria. (See Case History: Nigeria.)

Despite recent claims about the success of family planning around the world, in Africa this is not true. In demographic terms not only are the number of living children/woman increasing - until recently most children died in infancy - but the rate of population growth is increasing as well, despite recent droughts and constant civil wars.

The reason family planning is failing in Africa is really quite obvious: Every African man seeks to confirm his ego and his manhood by fathering as many children as possible, and male sexuality is completely out of control - not female sexuality as claimed by proponents of FGM.Nowhere is it mentioned that family planning is a responsibility of males. African men have been ignored by internationally sponsored family planning programs.

Men are not held responsible for the support of their children in most traditional African societies, and this has not changed in the modern sector or in urban areas. The enormous burdens and responsibility for children rest on women everywhere in Africa. The failure of men to support the many children they father is entirely ignored by the male dominated governments and by the international family planning programs, that are still almost entirely directed toward women. Men - the real cause of the rapid population growth - are never made to face the reality of their obligations. As some midwives who give out contraceptives to women in the hospitals in Bamako told me, if a man finds that his wife is using contraceptives, he often not only beats her but also may divorce her.

Everywhere in the world a correlation can be made between the education of women and the reduction of pregnancies. It would seem more productive for family planning organizations to finally address the education of women and especially health education.

West Africa continues to have the highest illiteracy rate in the world, and, the gap between the education of women and men is growing. As is known and all statistics confirm, there is no hope for change where a large majority of women are illiterate, and that is the case in most of rural West Africa.

The basic facts about reproduction continue to be entirely unknown to most African women while childbearing and fertility are surrounded by many damaging myths, traditions and tabus. Family planning organizations, which now are active all over West Africa as my recent investigations confirm, have done almost nothing to lift this ignorance that keeps women in bondage and destroys their health.

Women can be helped to understand reproduction and how their bodies function, as well as the terrible damage done by FGM, through **the Universal Childbirth Picture Books.** [4] These books are addressed to the community health worker for use in teaching the basic facts of reproductive health, regardless of language or literacy. They are designed as flexible, graphic teaching aids that can be readily adapted to local needs. Their objective, in summary, is "to make the human story of how we are made available to the largest number of people all over the world."

Recurring droughts in the Sahel area and the steady, southward advance of the Sahara are creating enormous economic and environmental problems and dislocations of people who have to leave their traditional lands. In addition, there are many frictions and local incursions between ethnic groups that at times flare up with full-fledged civil wars such as in Liberia recently, quite aside from Angola and Zaire.

To these natural and man-made disasters, a blind adherence to damaging traditions is added - traditions that seriously impair and restrict the health and lives of women and children, that is, the majority. Yet, they are promoted by men including the political leadership despite the fact that these traditions jeopardize the proclaimed national objectives of development. Female genital mutilation often in the most severe and damaging forms - including infibulation - is practiced throughout West Africa. A physician who works in Francophone West Africa and who often travels through some very remote areas, relates from his experiences among the very traditional inhabitants:

> "There are many variations of genital operations practiced, which depend on how the local circumcisers carry out their cruel trade . . . Many of the old women cut off as much as possible, the clitoris, the small and large lips, and the surrounding flesh. Then, with the help of pins or thorns they close the wound, leaving only the smallest opening . . .
>
> The number of girls who die, victims of the overly conscientious circumcisers, is apparently quite large . . . When I recently had to travel cross-country through a remote area, we stopped near a group of huts. A woman, seeing I was a doctor, came out and asked me to come and see some patients. Inside a hut, two girls about eight years old were stretched out, naked on a mat on the ground. Between the legs of each child was a deep cut of 8 to 10 centimeters (about three inches) with gaping edges over a bloody hole. The area of the wound was swollen and covered with abcesses and pus. I tried to examine the little girls but I could not touch them without making them scream . . .
>
> After I managed to clean at least the outer area of the operation, I put some disinfectant powder on the festering wounds and gave some more to the old woman as well as some sulfa tablets to take by mouth. That was unfortunately all that I could do . . . it was impossible to take the children along in the jeep in their condition - on a trip of hundreds of kilometers with hardly any roads. I was sure they would soon die in any case.
>
> When one speaks to the men who require these operations about the danger of these practices, they say it is the custom . . . Sometimes they add it is necessary to do this to protect the girls from temptation . . . The women are completely fatalistic . . . they know neither hope nor change. But it is a shame that those of us concerned with health and from a different world have done so little . . ." [5]

In West Africa, as in East Africa, in the traditional environment it is the decision of the local village chief whether or not and when the initiations take place. Most of the time the operations are performed on a group of girls. Connected with this initiation is a village feast.

A teacher from West Africa relates the story of his sister; his father was the village chief and had a large family:

> "I am the youngest son of my mother - she had 13 children, only three remained: my older sister, my older brother and myself. My older sister was loved and respected throughout our village.
>
> It is our custom that at the age of eighteen, when the girls want to get married, they have to go through excision. The time came for my sister to be excised. One day, very early in the morning, my sister, with other village girls, was taken outside the village to the place where these procedures are usually conducted. After some time, one of the old women who take care of the operations came to our house and said that there were some complications. The other girls had come back to the village accompanied by tam tams. In our society, excision is an occasion for a great festival, with no expenses spared by the parents of the girl and the parents of the boy the girl is promised to marry. In the evening, my sister was carried back to our house very ill. We called the medicine man who tried to stop her bleeding from the operation.
>
> My sister continued to bleed throughout the night. The news had been passed around in the village and everybody was worried, as she was the oldest of her group and her accident ruined the festival. After a night of great pain, she died the next morning.
>
> My mother, who had lost her 11th child, collapsed and wanted to kill herself. It was necessary to watch her for a month to keep her from committing suicide. Even today, after many years, she speaks to me about it.
>
> In all the surrounding villages, the news of my sister's death spread because my father was the village chief. Since this time, excision - which formerly was an important occasion for people to show their wealth and social status - has lost its prestige in the entire region. Other girls died from excision before my sister but because of the status of my father and because my sister was so well liked, her tragic and unnecessary death made the people in the whole region realize the danger of these operations.
>
> To be sure, excision has not yet vanished from our area, but it has lost the magic of former times. The traditionalists still continue with it, but everybody knows that it will eventually be given up. I shall be the first one who will celebrate its abolition. I do not want that others lose their sisters or their daughters whom they love, in this terrible way, like a lovely flower that was destroyed for no reason at all." [6]

In the modern sector, it appears that due to education, the operations are abandoned by some. But, most often, they are performed on much younger girls, as, for instance, Assitan Diallo in her study of excision in Bamako states [7] and as the midwives in Bamako relate. (See "Case History : Mali") The grandmothers are often the most vocal advocates of continuing the operations. They have been socialized to believe that the family structure and their own prestige would collapse without the operations. A woman's only security, especially in a Moslem environment, is the family, and each woman is taught that the operation is essential "to preserve the family."

Though traditional rites have been abandoned in the towns, the mutilations are now performed most often individually or on sisters at a very young age. Assitan Diallo calls the practices "a caricature of the traditional rites." In Nigeria, which has a highly trained, sophisticated medical sector, the operations are now also performed by surgeons in the hospitals - for educated wealthy families and paid for by the fathers. (See "Case History: Nigeria") This is often seen by African men as an easy solution to the problem - and it also makes sure that the daughter will not die, so her father can collect a hefty bride-price.

But Nigeria also has a very active National Committee on Traditional Practices Affecting the Health of Women and Children, affiliated with the Inter African Committee (IAC), [8] which by now has training programs all over the country. In addition, the national midwives and nurses assocoation has taken up the issue all over the country. (See Case History: Nigeria).

Though Liberia and Cote d'Ivoire are not specifically examined in this report, almost the entire female population in both countries is excised. In Liberia, secret societies quite similar to those of its neighbor - Sierra Leone - function. Though Abidjan is replete with prestigious ultramodern skyscrapers and features an enormous concrete Catholic cathedral, the women who come to deliver in the local hospitals are excised, so the maternity in the University Hospital Center of Abidjan in Treichville confirms. In Odienne in the northwest of the country and in other towns, excision is similarly practiced so medical sources confirm, and excision is universal in all rural areas.

In other West African countries - all along the Gulf of Guinea including Ghana, Togo and Benin - excision is practiced much as in the other countries of West Africa with some of the same ethnic groups involved. In Ghana, FGM is practiced mainly in the northern part of the country, rather than on the coast. FGM is an ethnic practice and the same ethnic groups often live in several countries - indeed they lived there long before the political borders were drawn. In Cameroon some northern areas adjoining Nigeria are involved and on the Atlantic coast FGM is practiced in both Guineas.

In Guinea an IAC affiliate has been actively fighting against excision in a country where it has been widely practiced as long as anyone knows. But very little research has been done, especially in Francophone countries - as the French colonial administration never concerned itself with the mutilation of almost the entire female population in the countries France colonized. Probably more women are mutilated in West Africa than in East Africa though until quite recently there was no communication on this subject between East and West Africa.

Even now the practitioners in different regions of Africa don't know that it is practiced anywhere else. Until I published the article on the epidemiology of FGM in the **Tropical Doctor,** [9] the facts had never been surveyed Africa-wide. A year later I was asked to present this information on the spread and distribution of FGM at the 1979 Khartoum Seminar called by WHO. But the real dimensions of FGM in West Africa were not clear until sometime after the seminar as there was practically no research available from the Francophone countries and no medical survey of FGM was ever published in France. The health of African women is still ignored by the French development agency which is active in its former colonies.

Some women are beginning to perceive and understand the damage done by the operations but the traditional belief structure does not allow for cause and effect. Evil spirits, or jinns, or the victim herself is blamed for any accidents resulting from FGM

Fatalism and a belief in the supernatural prevent a rational approach to health. Though immediate problems, such as bleeding and/or infections, may be sometimes recognized as linked to the operations, the fact that many girls survive and only some die makes it more likely in the minds of the people that some evil spirits are at work, spirits who bewitched the girls who die - a statement that parents often make. Childbirth problems, obstructed labor, even death of both mother and child are never related to an operation that took place years earlier; nor are any of the many other pathologies, from painful menstruation to fistulae or cysts and urinary infections, ever related to their real cause. Rather the women seek help from "traditional healers" that offer them dangerous or useless remedies - as they are similarly ignorant about anatomy and the concept of germs is quite unknown.

Factual information about women's bodies and health, about reproduction and sexuality is especially difficult to get in West Africa and quite unavailable in a form that would make such information accessible to women. More than 90 percent of the female population of West Africa cannot read. Most of the traditional information and myths surrounding sexuality and reproduction are damaging to women but they enhance the power and sexual control exercised by men: Hence these myths are supported by the male-dominated society and leadership, regardless of the damage they do.

The Christian missionaries in West Africa as elsewhere have utterly failed to introduce any health education about human biology, which - given the great importance Africans attach to fertility and the very large numbers of women who die in childbirth - would certainly be what families need most. Though for instance in southern Nigeria a large part of the population is Christian, polygamy and FGM continue, ignored by all Christian groups and missionaries.

Damaging misconceptions about women and female sexuality exist everywhere in the world, fostered by men, as the continuing admiration and propagation of Freud's misogynist misconceptions in the West show, despite the fact that Freud was a cocaine addict which no doubt affected his mind and reasoning. [10] But his theories about women bolster the male superiority complex; hence they are discussed.

In West Africa the oppression of women is multiplied: traditions relegate women to be subservient to and the chattel of men, and that is the real reason why the anthropological brotherhood speaks for all traditions, no matter how damaging to women and children - traditions always support the male power structure.

The colonial system reconfirmed the traditional system and worsened the situation of women by excluding them from education; Christian missionaries reinforced women's servility and dependence, and the apostles of growing Moslemization proclaim that excision is a religious command. Modernization and development have recently added to the plight of women by denying them modern technology and tools, while admonishing them to keep the traditions - traditions that make women the chattel of men.

The case histories document this summary.

FOOTNOTES

1. Nabia, Prof. Ache. **FEMALE EXCISION IN CHAD - Report of an Investigation,** published by Ministry of Planning and Cooperation and UNICEF, August 1991. See **WIN NEWS**, Vol.18, No. 2, Spring 1992, p. 43.
2. Thiam, Awa. **La Parole aux Negresses.** Denoel Gonthier, Paris, 1977.
3. **Famille et Developpement,** January 1977, article on "Polygamy." "La Polygamie: est-elle un mal necessaire?", pp. 23-31.
4. Hosken, Fran P. , **The Childbirth Picture Book** / Program - "A picture story of reproduction from a woman's view," pictures by Marcia L. Williams. Published in English, French, Spanish, Arabic and Somali, with Additions to prevent Excision and Infibulation, by **WIN NEWS**, 187 Grant St., Lexington, MA 02420.
5. **WIN NEWS,** Vol. 3, No. 3, Summer 1977, p. 24.
6. **Famille et Developpement,** op cit., April 1975, p. 17.
7. Diallo, Assitan. **Excision at the Bambara.** Bamako Teachers College thesis, 1978. See also **WIN NEWS**, Vol. 4, No. 3, Summer 1978, p. 23.
8. Nigeria National Committee on Traditional Practices Affecting the Health of Women and Children in Africa., P.O. Box 6051, Lagos, Nigeria.
9. Hosken, Fran P. "The Epidemiology of Female Genital Mutilation." **Tropical Doctor,** Royal Society of Medicine, Vol. 8, 1978, pp. 150-156.
10. Thornton, E.M. **The Freudian Fallacy - An Alternative View of Freudian Theory.** Dial Press/Doubleday, New York, 1984.

CASE HISTORY: NIGERIA

Nigeria is the most populous country of Africa with a multi ethnic population estimated to be at least 115 million - though for political reasons this figure is contested. Nigeria's population is growing at about 3.5 percent annually despite the recent introduction of government supported family planning programs. The country has been recently re-organized as a federation of 30 states - following the United States model - with considerable autonomy for each state. There are great differences between ethnic groups - with the people following very different religious teachings, mainly Moslem in the North and Christian in the South, as well as various traditional beliefs. Yet despite these differences a Ministry of Health survey established that in every state of Nigeria, Female Genital Mutilation (FGM) is practiced. (See below.)

Polygamy is also widely practiced especially by the Moslem majority. Pushed by the desire of each man to boost his self-esteem by having as many children as possible, the already huge population is growing rapidly. Nowhere else in Africa can one see as many pregnant women as in the streets of Lagos and other Nigerian towns.

A new, planned capital Abuja in the center of the country is being built to replace the overcrowded traditional federal capital in Lagos, located on the coast on a series of overcrowded islands connected by overcrowded highways and ringed by squatter settlements. There are large new high-rise office buildings, stadiums and sports palaces, but adequate sanitation and water systems are lacking, electricity and telephones function intermittently and garbage removal works hardly at all. Personal security is a great problem not only in Lagos but in many other areas of Nigeria.

The recent oil boom, which led to the building of superhighways, highrise-buildings, and projects of all kinds all over the country including universities, as well as the construction of the new capital, started a building boom that was short-lived and ended by plunging the country into deep debt. Inflation and corruption are rampant, affecting life especially in the overcrowded urban areas.

Women in southern Nigeria and in Lagos actively participate in politics and in the busy markets as traders and entrepreneurs. Lagos, with its large port, was the hub of the Nigerian oil boom, while the north - where the Hausa predominate - is the area of Moslem traditions.

Most of the subgroups of the three main ethnic groups in Nigeria - the Moslem Hausa of the north, the Yoruba in the southwest including the area of Lagos and the Ibo in the southeast - subject their female children to genital operations, mostly excision and clitoridectomy. The Yoruba traditionally practice these operations on newborn babies. Among other groups, excision is practiced as a coming-of-age rite. Infibulation is said to be practiced by some groups in the Moslem north, as well as Gishri or Gishiri cuts into the vagina of girls just before puberty. Child marriage and seclusion of women are also widespread among the Moslem Hausa - with terrible results for women's health.

A survey by the federal Ministry of Health gives an overview of the current status of Female Circumcision in Nigeria as FGM is locally called. This official document of March 1981 is signed by Dr. O. A. (Mrs.)Adelaja, Senior Consultant/Medical Statistics and gives an overview of the situation:

> "According to the response obtained from questionnaires completed by most Nigerian states, female circumcision is still being practiced in most states of this country. It is practiced mostly on babies and small girls of Christian and Muslim parents. But certain tribes perform the ceremony when the female is ready to wed or when the first pregnancy is about seven months. Very few tribes perform the ceremony after marriage and in such tribes, it is the duty of the husband to perform the operation. . . "[1]

Next, the circumstances of the operations are described:

> "The ceremony is usually performed on a group of girls, though some report that individual girls are circumcised in their respective homes. A token fee is paid and ranges from two naira to ten naira.
>
> The operator may be a man or a woman. Male operators usually perform it as a business and circumcise male children as well. Tools in use vary and include a small knife, a sharp blade, or a razor.
>
> Post operative management also varies, some report hot fermentation with charcoal daily and feeding with roasted meat and some gruel. Snail juice and palm oil are poured on the incision by some. Native soap and native medicine are also used by another tribe.
>
> **Complications:** Some deny any complications. But among those who admit complications, bleeding is the commonest problem reported. Other complications include tear, septicaemia, fistula, stenosis, delayed second state labor, tetanus, urinary obstruction, and dyspareunia.
>
> **Reason for Circumcision:** The majority attribute the operation to age-old custom, culture and tradition. Some claim that circumcision will prevent promiscuity and reduce sex urge, while others believe that if the newborn baby's head touches the clitoris, such a baby will die.
>
> **Conclusion:** There is no doubt that female circumcision is still being performed in present day Nigeria. . ."[2]

A questionnaire sent by **WIN NEWS** in 1976 to the federal Ministry of Health was answered by the Ministries of Health of Bendel State and Cross River State, giving much detailed information on local practices.

The Bendel State Ministry of Health, located in Benin City, stated that almost the entire population of the state observes this tradition, though it is dimininishing in urban areas. The operations are carried out usually on the eighth day after birth. However, traditional healers advocate the operation as a cure for infertility for adult women who are not circumcised. Since so many deaths have occurred as a result of the operation, the Ministry of Health reports that in some places, instead of cutting out the entire clitoris, it is now just nicked with a sharp instrument.

The reasons given why the operations are done in the area of Bendel State are:

> "- As mentioned above on sterile women, and it is believed that an uncircumcised female is less prolific than a circumcised female;
>
> - It is believed that female circumcision reduces sexual promiscuity in females;
>
> - It is also strongly believed that an uncircumcised female always has difficulty at childbirth. . ."[3]

The reply from the Cross River State Ministry of Health, also from the summer of 1976, states that "female circumcision was widespread"[4], but the specific information provided refers to the Efik Tribe, which has a population of about half a million people who live near the town of Calabar.

The reasons given by the Efik for the operations are that "circumcision is the first step to control waywardness in girls" and "uncircumcised girls are considered to be abnormal since, according to the belief, they have both male and female organs. . . These girls. . . are regarded as unclean and are always subjected to public ridicule and abuse. The members of their families too are subjected to this same ridicule." [5]

The traditional circumcision procedure is described in this way:

> "Very early in the morning, the local woman who performs the operation puts fresh plantain leaves on the floor of the backyard. . . Only herself and the girl's mother and one or two senior women in the family are allowed to help and also witness the operation.

> The girl is then put on top of the leaves in a lithotomy position with two people, one on either side, helping to support the legs and expose the field of operation. The woman then holds the clitoris and pulls it, using the already prepared soft ash to rub it and massage it, thus making it soft and elongated to make the excision easy. When it is found to be very soft, it is tied at the base with some strands of raffia (usually white). With a sharp razor, the clitoris is then cut off at the base, making sure that no portion of it is left out.
>
> Some quantity of hot water is poured on the operated areas to clean it and water squeezed out of the (Nwebeb) leaf is poured into the bleeding area. . . or some quantity of native gin. . . The wound is treated by applying palm oil as often as the face of the wound is dry. . ."[6]

The question about any indication of change is answered with "the practice is not dying out as fast as one would wish", and a recent case history is cited. It appears that a young woman of about 30 years was recently rushed to the hospital in shock. It was found that she had undergone excision of the clitoris to cure her infertility. She had lost a lot of blood but was resuscitated by tranfusions after the severed blood vessels were repaired in the operating room.

Of course, in the rural areas where no such facilities are available, the girls or women usually die. Though since that report was made, more families in urban areas may have stopped operating on their daughters, in the rural areas, as all over Africa, traditions are still deeply entrenched and continue to this day.

Dr. Lawrence Longo spent from 1959 to 1962 in Nigeria as a gynecologist and physician among the Yoruba, in Ile-Ife, which Dr. Longo states is considered to be the spiritual center of the Yoruba. Fertility is most highly prized and all-important for the women, and this is still true today all over Nigeria:

> "Since a man's wealth is often evaluated on the basis of the number of his children, the inability of a woman to conceive is considered a major catastrophe. Fertility rites play an important role in the community life. . . In many villages an annual festival is celebrated with thousands of young women participating in the ritual, which they believe will insure pregnancy. . ."[7]

And according to traditional beliefs, FGM assures and enhances fertility. That in reality girls and women die from the operations or have serious health problems as well as great difficulties in childbirth somehow is not recognized or is blamed on other causes. Dr. Longo reports from his experience in Nigeria: "The most common cause of maternal death in West Africa is obstructed labor. . . Unfortunately, most patients are not brought to the hospitals until treatment at home has failed."[8] A frequent cause of obstructed labor is the hardened scars of excision operations that prevent dilation and often result in tears and injuries of the mother and sometimes death of both mother and child. Often, fistulae develop due to the obstruction of the opening; that is, the vagina ruptures. Women with fistulae are incontinent and become outcasts of their families and communities.

Many traditional practices during pregnancy - though this is the preferred state for all women in Nigeria - are often incompatible with a positive and healthy outcome. Dr. Longo explains:

> "Yoruba sanctions prohibit the ingestion of meat, eggs, beans or other protein-containing foods during pregnancy, and these tabus militate against an optimal state of nutrition.
>
> In the Yoruba culture a large portion of the family farming is the woman's responsibility. This strenuous work is usually continued until the last weeks of pregnancy and is resumed within several days after the delivery. . ."[9]

A survey made in 1990 on food tabus in Nigeria by Ms. E.M. Alabi, a midwife and Project Coordinator of the Nigeria National Committee of the IAC (Inter African Committee), confirms that damaging beliefs on what pregnant women should eat continue to be widespread:

> "Pregnancy is attended by many food tabus and other cultural practices. For no reason tabus are passed from generation to generation, and pregnant women are made to suffer in the midst of plenty.
>
> There are many food items prohibited for use by pregnant women. It can clearly be seen that pregnant mothers are deprived of most foods rich in proteins, calories and other nutrients. For instance, in the Western areas of Nigeria, various fruits and vegetables are prohibited for fear that the newborn babies would be jaundiced, and because of worm infestations. . ." [10]

Many traditional childbirth practices and the treatment of the newborn infants, no doubt, result in many unnecessary deaths of the babies and of the mothers as well:

> "Upon delivery the infant is put on a mat and no attempt is made to stimulate it or cut the cord until the placenta is delivered. . .
>
> Traditionally, the baby is exercised by throwing it into the air several times and swinging it by its extremities. The infant is then forced to swallow a mixture of herbs. The amount of this feeding is usually determined by the amount of abdominal distension that develops. . ." [11]

These traditional treatments of the newborn are not only dangerous but also jeopardize the baby's survival. Dr. Longo explains:

> "Until the placenta is delivered, the infant is not stimulated. . . If the child survives this neglect it may be traumatized if it is violently exercised. Further hazards include the possiblity of septicemia or tetanus from the application of contaminated dressings to the umbilical stump and the danger of aspiration from forced feeding. . ." [12]

Circumcision at the Yoruba is done early - usually on the sixth day after birth; the baby is named at the same time. Dr. Longo describes the operation:

> "Circumcision is performed by the local doctor shortly after sunrise. Scissors or two small pieces of bamboo used in a scissor-like action remove the anterior portion of the labia minora and the clitoris in a piece the size of a 'date stone'. In some instances, the entire labia minora and majora are excised. No anesthesia is used. Bleeding is controlled by placing moistened cotton over the area of excision and pressure is applied by holding the legs together. . . Occasionally this operation is complicated by haemorrhage or the development of infection or tetanus. . ." [13]

Other traditional gynecological treatments such as the insertion into the vagina of all kinds of herbal and other preparations believed to either enhance fertility or alternatively cause abortion of unwanted pregnancies often result in severe damage to the genitalia, such as stenosis - the narrowing of the vagina. This in turn leads to obstructed labor and may cause permanent inability to conceive. Yet such treatments by local traditional practitioners - who have no medical training and often are illiterate - are eagerly sought by women especially in case of infertility. The excision performed by a surgeon in London on a Nigerian woman in the early 1980s which resulted in the British law against FGM was done because her Nigerian husband brought her to the British physician to cure her infertility by excision. (See "The Western World".)

In the November 1977 issue of **Drum,** a Nigerian magazine that is distributed all over the country, Esther Ogunmodede, a Nigerian journalist, published an article with the title: **Female Circumcision: How Much Longer Will We Allow Our Girls to Be Brutalized in This Barbaric Way?** [14]

First, Ogunmodede inquires as to why these operations continue to be performed:

> "No one to whom I spoke could tell me why, though the easiest and commonest answer is that it is our 'custom and tradition', the shield behind which we hide the more hideous and inexplicable of our practices.
>
> But the world now knows the reasons, just as our forebearers knew. Our ancestors were no scientists but they knew where and what was the seat of sexual pleasure in a woman - so they chopped it off. . ." [15]

And she adds that the usual reasons given all over Nigeria and Africa are that the operations are done to prevent "waywardness of girls" and to keep married women "faithful". "Since discussions about sex and sexual organs are not proper subjects for polite conversation in African society, the adverse effect of genital operations on girls has remained hidden for generations. . ."

Next, Ogunmodede describes the procedure as carried out among the Moslem Hausa, the largest population group in Northern Nigeria. Ogunmodede states the operations are performed by barbers. The only other place where barbers are recorded to do the operating is Egypt. In most Moslem areas, the operations are an all-female affair. Many devout Moslems from Northern Nigeria take part in the pilgrimage to Mecca and thus are familiar with the practices of the Middle East, especially Egypt. This may explain why the Hausa use barbers as operators.

Ogunmodede describes the procedure and its results candidly:

> "Most children become so uncontrollable with bewilderment and panic that 'accidents' occur, resulting in serious mutilation of the girl's genitals. . . Why then do we subject our own daughters to the same horrors?
>
> We now shrink from tribal marks. Girls who have been badly scarred are ashamed all their lives of the results, and the embarrasment of circumcision can be far worse."
>
> By pretending that anything to do with sex is not a topic for conversation, it is little wonder that so much ignorance exists about the true effect on girls of circumcision." [16]

The results in childbirth are equally damaging: "The labour is unnecessarily prolonged for hours and even days until both mother and baby die of exhaustion. . ." In many cases, serious tears result or the baby may be injured or brain damaged.

At the Yoruba, the operations, as Ogunmodede explains, are an inherited trade. The Olola families are the traditional operators who have done this kind of surgery for centuries and also do tribal marks - the deep scars and markings that many older Africans have on their cheeks.

The recently made movie and videotape on traditional practices for the Inter African Committee which they distribute to educate people all over the world about damaging traditions, were photographed in large part in Nigeria. They show how such traditional practioners, who are highly respected locally, operate and mutilate large groups of small children inflicting terrible agony and permanent damage by cutting off the external genitalia and slashing bodies and cheeks with tribal marks - one child after another. These mass mutilations continue to this day in many parts of Nigeria. [17]

Esther Ogunmodede also relates the personal stories told to her by two young women who were subjected to these operations as children:

> "The story of Jumai: 'I wondered what all that boiling water was for. Nobody said anything but by 6 a.m. our local barber had arrived; the elders in our house gathered.
>
> 'I was getting scared as I was only ten years old. My elderly aunt undressed me and blindfolded me with a scarf. I was then forcibly held down and my legs were pulled apart, while the barber/surgeon did his work. I was screaming until I could scream no more and passed out. When I came round I could not urinate for hours. It was sheer hell when I did.'" [18]

The other story is from a young law student who vows that none of her daughters will be subjected to this terrible and useless ordeal:

> "'It took five people to hold me down and I was only eight. All the neighbors had gathered and were shouting advice to the Olola and jeering at me for lacking courage. In the struggle the Olola accidently cut the wrong section, which has left me mutilated. It is a nightmare that still remains with me today. . .'" [19]

After enumerating all the dangers and problems resulting from the operations, Ogunmodede who does not beat about the bush, asks the people directly:

> "Who is responsible for making sure the message reaches every family? You, women's organizations, hospitals, health centers, our ministries of health, our churches and mosques. Let us all mount a campaign against the evil that impairs the health of our women and puts their lives in danger, as well as their babies' lives." [20]

This article made a remarkable impact in Nigeria, where the reactions of the people in the form of letters to the editor of **the Drum**, opened up a national debate on the subject. For the first time in any African country, this article provided people from all backgrounds and ethnic groups, both women and men, with the opportunity to be heard on this tabu topic. Once the ice was broken - which Ogunmodede's skillful article accomplished by providing the critical health facts - the reluctance to speak was gone.

In fact, any inhibitions to discuss sex and sexual practices are far greater in Western countries. In Nigeria and elsewhere in Africa this artifical embarrassment was introduced by the Christian missionaries - some of whom opposed FGM and especially polygamy, which is widely practiced throughout the country. But Christian missionaries never taught about reproductive health or even the biological facts, keeping women ignorant about their own bodies and what they most urgently need to know, especially since fertility is so very important in all African societies.

The variety of opinions voiced in the letters that were printed in many subsequent issues of **the Drum**, is as great as the diversity of people who wrote them. Here some samples:

> **"End This Barbarism" by Olu Babajide, Principal, School of Nursing, Ife:**
>
> "Our forefathers practiced what I term 'facial decoration' with tribal marks as part of their cultural components. How many of you advocates of female circumcision for reasons of 'culture' would want to mark the faces of your children? I agree with Esther Ogunmodede: The act is brutal and barbaric. It should be stopped."
>
> **Miss Nigeria, 1977, Toyin Monney:**
>
> "'Biologically, the clitoris is the most sensitive woman's organ, and that was why parents of past days made sure they cut off this sensitive part in order to stop their girls from being wayward. . . The act is cruel and it should not be encouraged. As for me, I will never have it done to my daughters.'"
>
> **"How Esther Got It Wrong" by David Irogbe, Calabar:**
>
> "The ultimate aim of a girl is to grow up and become useful to her husband and the society to which she belongs. . . Taking a closer look at women in. . . the United States for example. . . women there are very impetuous and. . . in their desperate drive for sexual satisfaction. . . cause irreparable harm to their husbands.
>
> Even in Nigeria, the few uncircumcised women tend to be brutal and wicked in dealing with their husbands."
>
> **Circumciser, Alhaji Jimoh Ala-Bede:**
>
> "Circumcision is the profession of my family. I have built two houses with the proceeds from circumcision and I have several children in different schools. I circumcise both males and females, and inscribe tribal marks on people who want them. I have dealt with almost all ethnic groups in Nigeria.
>
> On the question of circumcision for female children: Our forefathers believed in it, and there must always be tradition. What damage does it do to the female organ? As far as I am concerned, it does no harm. Even the Quoran supports circumcision for both males and females."
>
> **"An Unhealthy Archaic Tradition" by Jenyo Aladejeibi:**
>
> "Reading the opinions of fellow Nigerians on this matter, one is bound to conclude that most of us either do not know or do not understand the evil effects of female circumcision. Apart from the pain that women suffer from the crude knives of the so-called native circumcisers, they are subjected to nothing but agony whenever they dare get close to their loved ones. This itself leads to frustrated sexual as well as married lives.

It is beyond my comprehension how a man or a woman could postulate that a woman has no right to enjoy sex, if that is what they mean by women being 'too sexy', and that her clitoris should be removed. To male chauvinists who argue that only men have the right to enjoy sex, I say what is sauce for the goose is also sauce for the gander. . .

Let us ask ourselves how much men would like it if the case were reversed, if men were castrated by the native 'circumcizers' so that they would not be 'too sexy' and run after women. . . It is high time the African women claimed their rights as human beings, not as second-class citizens, brainwashed to accept that sexual pleasure is restricted to men only."

Businessman, Michael Ayilara:

"In the Yoruba tribe, circumcision is just like tribal marks. It is part of custom and tradition left for us by our fathers. I have heard that some tribes in Nigeria don't circumcise their girls, but in my own tribe in Kwara State we do circumcise our girls. Naturally, uncircumcised girls are more sexy and if they are in such a state they may lose interest in more important things like their education and other things which they have to do."[21]

Unfortunately, neither the state health ministries nor the Department of Health of the federal government took up the issue or organized health education campaigns following this public debate and the great interest shown all over Nigeria. Many people kept writing to **the Drum** for more than two years after the article had appeared.

Dr. Bertha Johnson, chief consultant of the Neuro Psychiatric Hospital of Yaba, Lagos, was one of the delegates from Nigeria to the WHO (World Health Organization) Seminar in Khartoum in 1979 (see " The World Health Organization Seminar"). Her research prepared for this meeting provides important insights into the motivations and values of the multiethnic Nigerian society vis a vis women; these values support the mutilation of many thousands of female children annually and also support rapid population growth.

A doubling in population in the next 20 to 30 years is predicted in Nigeria, a country that is already densely populated. How is it possible that in this very patriarchial society which so strongly emphasizes childbearing and fertility, women - who are the source of what is so highly prized, offspring - are at the same time regarded as inferior and often treated with contempt.

In a conversation in Lagos shortly after the WHO seminar, Dr. Johnson shed some light on the situation:

"As a psychiatrist, I am aware that people here in Nigeria have an obsession about children. Infertility is a terrible problem for women who become very depressed if they cannot have children. If you are infertile, you are useless and the only purpose of an African woman's life is to have as many children as possible. For men also, to have a child is essential as his manhood is involved. A woman who does not want children is considered mad.

As far as circumcision is concerned, among the Yoruba who live in this part of the country (Lagos), it is believed that circumcision is necessary to dampen the sexuality of women, and to prevent stillbirths because if the clitoris touches the head of the child during birth, the child will die." [22]

The importance attached to childbearing is overwhelming in Nigeria, indeed, in most African societies. A woman who does not produce children is divorced and sent back to her family. In the paper Dr. Johnson wrote for the WHO Seminar, she explains:

". . . No African male (maybe all males) can tolerate any doubt about his manhood, especially his ability to father children. He is anxious and preoccupied with his potency and must have visible signs to prove this. He rarely accepts that his wife's 'barrenness' (or tendency to produce only girls) may be due to him. . ." [23]

Whatever the cause, in Africa it is always the woman who is blamed for failing to produce offspring. "A child is the only ticket to a woman's security", Dr. Johnson states. In her practice as a psychiatrist, she has plenty of occasion to observe the results of these pressures on women, from anxieties to severe depressions. Women who fail to have children are accused of everything from adultery to witchcraft. And Dr. Johnson adds: "A woman is held responsible if she has daughters, as men want sons. Men refuse to acknowledge that it is the male who is responsible for the sex of the child." [24]

In Nigeria, as most everywhere else in Africa, marriages are arranged between families, and the brideprice represents a considerable source of income for the father of girls; nevertheless, the birth of a daughter is not welcomed as is the birth of a son.

> "... Brideprice is paid by the groom to the bride's parents and serves a dual purpose; it grants the bridegroom and his clan the right to the children of the union. In some places, if the wife fails to bear children, she is returned to her parents and they pay back the brideprice. . .
>
> Brideprice also can be regarded as an indemnity or compensation to the bride's parents for the care and expense they have incurred in nurturing her, as well as for the loss of their daughter. . .
>
> But in some societies, the birth of a girl may be received with mixed feelings. . ..At the worst, it may be outright rejection of the girl and her mother. . .who is blamed, reprimanded, cast off and rejected for giving birth to a girl when having a son and heir was almost mandatory. . .
>
> Child rearing practices obey the rule of division of labour; girls are expected to be with their mother and learn 'feminine' trades, housework - laundering, cooking, fetching water, cleaning, pottery, basket work, weaving mats and textiles, petty trading and street hawking. In other words, most of the heavy work, in spite of their being thought of as the weaker sex. . .A girl may be denied formal education altogether, or stopped after a certain class in deference to her brothers. . .There is a genuine fear that too much learning is detrimental to being a good wife. . ." [25]

Dr. Johnson then describes that a girl who conforms to these standards and limitations of her education poses no problems; but girls who are ambitious and like to study and are interested in what are called 'masculine' pursuits are "considered abnormal and often pay a heavy price, sometimes ending up on the streets."

It goes without saying, as Dr. Johnson also stated, that all girls are expected to marry and have children and spend their lives taking care of the household and serving their husbands, which is considered the purpose of their existence. Marriage traditionally is regarded as the union of two families - not of two people. As a result, "Traditional families have the right to settle quarrels between couples, but this creates worse problems. There is a lot of wife beating, yet the beaten wife gets no help from her own family." And Dr. Johnson adds: "If a man would try to beat me, he would not do it twice. If all women would feel that way, wife beating would disappear in Africa."[26]

Circumcision of girls is practiced in different ways and at different ages by most Nigerian ethnic groups: Yet it is done in literally all parts of the country, including cities as well. Dr. Johnson states:

> "Circumcision of girls. . .may be done from the ninth day of life or delayed until puberty, or in preparation for marriage. . .It is also possible that the operation may not be limited to clitoridectomy but extended to excision of the labia minora. There is also risk of excessive scarring and keloid formation, possibly resulting in difficulty during delivery. . .
>
> In many Nigerian societies (such as the Yoruba) the traditional 'bringing out' and naming ceremonies with its rituals take place on the seventh day for girls. . . and may be combined with circumcision by traditional healers or anyone with the expertise. . . [27]

Polygamy is widely practiced in Nigeria, despite the brideprice and despite the inability of the men to support even one wife and her children or that they are Christian. The results of polygamy are often traumatic for a woman and her children.

> "Often the men do not have even the financial means to maintain one wife and her children, let alone three to four wives. The wives then have to fend for themselves and for their children, as well as shoulder the resonsibility to keep and feed him, and entertain his guests. Sub-nutrition and malnutrition. . . are the natural result . . . (for the women and children).
>
> The woman's health may be adversely affected if she resents or lives in fear of the husband chosen for her, as may happen in cases of child brides, or worse still, if she is not getting on well with her in-laws, or co-wives. . . She has to be on guard to protect herself and her children. She may be starved of funds as well as of affection. . .
>
> Her condition may be worsened if she cannot be independent, nor is able to return to her parents who usually insist that she stays (with her husband). In the extreme, some women feel so bad that they resort to/or have frequent abortions rather than bear the children of a husband they detest. . ." [28]

One would think that menopause whould be welcome after a life of constant childbearing and the exhaustion - both physical and psychological - that this entails, especially in this society where all the burdens of heavy household labor and child care as well as procurring enough to eat and all necessities are borne by women alone. But, a woman at menopause in Nigeria - and in most of Africa - ceases to be a woman, in the view of society. All sexual relations are stopped. For a woman who has no children or only a few or only daughters, severe depression may result.

When visiting Nigeria repeatedly in the seventies and eighties, besides meeting with Dr. Johnson, I visited other physicians and a number of hospitals concerned with women's and children's health.

In Lagos, I also met with Dr. Nike O. Grange, a pediatrician at the University of Lagos, who investigated some of the traditional practices affecting children in her country, including genital operations. Dr. Grange sums up these traditions as "the ritual of the knife. The knife is worshiped in the community, we see the end results in hospitals." [29]

Scarifications of all kinds are made on the bodies of babies and young children "as protection against evil spirits" - including cauterization (burning by hot irons) to cure disease. Since in Nigeria many ethnic groups subject their female children to circumcision while very young, often a few days old, pediatritions are often called to deal with the adverse results - if and when the children are brought to hospitals, often too late. But only a few people in urban areas have any access to hospitals and modern health care.

Many of the traditional health practices have devastating results, especially for mothers and babies as they are most vulnerable. Since there is no health education, damaging traditions continue, causing much unnecessary suffering and even deaths, especially of children. Dr. Grange, when we met and talked together about these problems, stated:

> "Adolescents need to be educated regarding their own health and bodies; this will change their attitudes. It is important that young girls are taught about themselves; but men also have to be educated as they still control women's lives. Legally, and on paper, they do not; but in realtity, women accept too much. They are not aggressive, and so they are exploited everywhere. Of course, the women in rural areas and the urban educated women are very different. Many of the professional women are socially aware and aware of their lack of privileges.
>
> We have a Constitution now and legal backing (for our rights), access to. . . divorce and child support; but the question is how to make more women aware of this. In the urban areas, women are exposed to communication, and there women are coming along. But where there is no communication, women accept their inferior position and are exploited.

> For instance, the brideprice is a practice that is very damaging. It is maintained by the parents. Ibos do it and the Yoruba do it. Yet in Lagos, even poor men manage to acquire several wives, although they cannot support them. They give the women some money so they can start to trade and support themselves by buying and selling. Prostitution is very widespread, and women change their husbands frequently." [30]

I asked Dr. Grange about my observation that there seemed to be many more pregnant women in the streets of Nigerian towns than I had seen anywhere else in Africa.

> "Children are a status symbol for men. They are not aware of the needs of children. . . . It is believed that polygamy is necessary so that women are looked after, but polygamy is very bad for children. It is expected that every woman must get married and have children. Other than that, she is not respected as a full person.
>
> A man takes a new wife simply by telling the parents of the woman, or writing to them. There is a great deal of competition between women because of polygamy. As a result, women do not trust each other. . ." [31]

From Lagos, which is very hot and humid, I went to Kano in the north of Nigeria on the dry plateau of the African savannah. It had not rained for more than six months. The heat in the middle of the day was oppressive and the air saturated with dust. No rain was expected for another four months.

In Lagos transportation is by automobile and during the now defunct oil boom, many expensive cars were imported. In Kano and rural areas, motorcycles, bicycles and mopeds are widely used. Many men drive motorbikes dressed in their traditional robes with motorcycle helmets on top of the traditional, colorful headdress, followed by clouds of dust. Women mostly walk or are passengers, but few drive themselves.

The maternity of the main city hospital of Kano is a very busy place and so are the midwives. The hospital keeps mothers for about a day after delivery - that is all. Child marriage is the custom among the Moslem Hausa of this region. Most of the new mothers I saw at the Kano maternity all seemed incredibly young.

I asked the doctors and midwives about genital mutilation. They told me that they do not see much excision, but that another operation is practiced. Many mutilated little girls, often very young - only about 10 or 12 years old - come to the hospital with infections and bleeding, their vaginas cut. Incontinence frequently results, quite aside from infections. The doctors said since child marriage is widely practiced and the girls are too small for sexual intercourse, they are cut open to make penetration possible. These gishiri or gishri cuts, as they are called, are performed by local practitioners.

In the hospital, such mutilated children are brought in often when infections have taken over and they are beyond help. However, most of them never come at all, as the local people are very suspicious of hospitals and modern medicine. The physicians said they see all kinds of terrible genital injuries which often are fatal, the result of traditional practices; but the people refuse to tell about their practices and the young girls, often barely teeenagers, do not know what was done to them or why.

The situation of women who are used as breeding machines in this strict Moslem society is very difficult to assess. I watched in the maternity at Kano a row of very young mothers who had delivered the night before, their new babies on their laps, wrapped in the same colorful fabrics of their dresses. It was early in the morning, and they were waiting to be taken home by their families. Their young faces were drained and incredibly sad - not at all what one would expect from a new mother; none of them looked at the tiny packages on their laps containing their babies. They sat on a long bench near the door of the one big room full of iron beds (none of them with sheets), where other women in labor were lying often moaning in pain surrounded by women relatives. Only some screens separated them from those in the final stages of giving birth.

I was taken right through the labor room to talk to the head midwife, who ruled her flock of young nurses: Each one came into the office and curtsied before the matron to get her assignment for the day.

The women start childbearing at the earliest age; they go through a dozen or more pregnancies unless they die in childbirth; and many do. At least half of the children die, but no statistics are kept. The obsession by men to have as many children as possible to prove their manhood is so great that girls are married before they even menstruate. The gishri cuts the doctors talked about, are the local way to initiate girls into their life of constant pain and childbearing.

In Kano, I also went to the private clinic of Dr. A. Iman at the Mustapha Memorial Hospital located on the outskirts of town. Dr. Iman confirmed what I was told at the city hospital. He said that the gishri cuts are practiced all over this area "in order to make a girl marriageable so the father can collect the brideprice." Many are not even teenagers when sold to a man. Sometimes the girls become incontinent because the urethra is cut, and others become sterile as a result of the infections, quite aside from the injuries resulting from forced sexual intercourse. In Lagos also, the doctors in the hospital maternities I visited told me of the many genital injuries they see of very young girls, their vaginas and genitalia torn as the result of forced sexual intercourse. Girls are often married to men twice their age. "Many young women are injured because of lack of gentleness on the part of their cohorts," is the way one Nigerian physician in Lagos put it. Sexually injured young wives can be found in hospitals all over Nigeria and in all other parts of Africa as well. The same problems are reported by physicians, for instance, in Ethiopia. (See "Case HIstory : Ethiopia.) Only the most fortunate ones are brought to the hospitals. In most of Africa death rates of women as a result of sexual violence by men and childbearing are higher than from all disease.

Venereal disease and prostitution are rampant despite of or perhaps because of these traditional marriage and sexual customs. To this now has to be added the spread of AIDS. Nigeria for a long time refused to acknowledge that AIDS was an issue and officially Nigeria claims (1992) 184 recorded cases registered by WHO in their worldwide AIDS/HIV statistics. This figure obviously is entirely unrealistic and only will accelerate the inevitable spread of this fatal disease for failure to warn the population, given the prevalent sexual practices as documented here. The widespread practice of child marriage by the Moslems, quite aside from polygamy practiced throughout the country as well as prostitution and rape, greatly contributes to the spread of AIDS. WHO estimates there are 7.5 million AIDS/HIV infections in sub-Saharan Africa. Considering that Nigeria is the most populous country with a very mobile population, AIDS/HIV infection is a very great threat to the people unless sexual customs and practices are drastically changed and all female mutilations prohibited. Because of the sexual customs in Africa as many women as men are infected - according to WHO statistics - and as a result many newborn babies are infected as well.

Since having more and more children is an obsession with each man, it therefore also is the goal of each woman. For that reason, she undergoes often damaging and painful traditional treatments in the belief they will enhance her fertility - often with tragic results. In Nigeria even today the belief that excision is a cure for infertility is very widespread. Health and sex education should be a priority in a country where educational resources are available.

But neither the highly educated, sophisticated Nigerian intellectuals including physicians nor any of this country's powerful leaders have publicly spoken against the ongoing mutilations of most of the female children, many in their own families. Excision is practiced by all the major ethnic groups. The majority of Nigerian men still consider the sexual castration of females imperative for their manhood, despite the new universities and research institutes, computers and cars, and electronic gadgets of every kind that are readily available in Nigeria.

A European physician who must remain unnamed wrote me after visiting Nigerian universities and medical schools:

> "I asked my colleagues at one of the medical schools about female circumcision, so it was arranged for me to witness an operation performed that day at the University hospital on a three-year-old girl by the staff surgeon. From a medical point of view, the operation - excision of the clitoris - was uneventful. Judging from the skill of the surgeon, he must have done the operation many times before." [32]

Child marriage, which in truth is gross sexual assault and abuse of children as well as sexual mutilations of the worst kind, is practiced with impunity by the men of this society under the label of "our cultural traditions". This goes on with the full knowledge of the intellectual and especially medical elite who write reports on the "cases histories" of raped and mutilated children, who are brought to the hospitals with their genitalia torn apart. All the physicians I talked to in Nigerian hospitals related such experiences.

How can one have any respect for Nigerian men who, despite their wealth and education, lack all responsibility to teach their own kind the basics of human behavior and self-discipline? Do these men enjoy raping helpless, bleeding children - screaming in fear and pain - as a proof of their 'manhood'? Yet this goes on all over Nigeria as hospital records document and newspapers occasionally report.

To impress the rest of the world, Nigeria has staged international arts festivals and huge sports events that have attracted thousands of people from all over the world, to the tune of many millions of dollars. But in the back streets of Lagos and alongside the new skyscrapers, thousands of little girls continue to be mutilated and violated with the full knowledge of Nigeria's male intellectual elite and leaderhip and all health professionals, men who are recognized all over the world.

Yet these men are unwilling to protect the health and future of their own female children - the future mothers of Nigeria - who are mutilated, raped, abused and exploited by their own fathers and husbands - the men who by using force and violence are in control of this corrupt male dominated society.

Family planning, despite the pro-natalist attitudes by the male population, was finally officially introduced by the Nigerian government in 1987 in the wake of the collapse of the oil prices as "the Government has realized that the population growth rate is a major obstacle to economic development":

> "The program is tentatively scheduled to cost $100 million for the first five years with the money coming from the Nigerian Government, the World Bank and the United States Agency for International Development. Nigeria's decisive move toward family planning comes as Africa leads the world in population growth. Across the continent the population is growing at 3 percent a year, which means a doubling every 20 years. . ." [33]

"In Nigeria", **the New York Times** reports, "from 19 million in 1931 the population is now estimated at 105 million" (1987). "Population experts forecast that in 30 years there will be more Nigerians on the globe than Western Europeans".

At present (1992/93), after extensive public debates in Nigeria on the effects of family planning, internationally financed programs, many developed and funded by the US, are being implemented all over the country though their effectiveness is not yet visible. It will take years for results to show in the Nigerian economy, which has been in a steady decline since the collapse of the oil boom.

Though women's health was cited as one reason for introducing contraceptives by the Government nothing was said about the damage done to women's health by child marriage and genital mutilation - which still continue throughout the country, despite education and despite the fact that some states have passed laws against early marriage, penalizing parents who arrange it - as **the New York Times** reports:

> "To attack child marriage, three northern states - Borno, Bauchi and Kaduna - have passed laws recently imposing fines on parents who take their daughters out of school for marriage. In a test case, 16 parents were convicted recently in Bauchi state for this practice. . . Despite the outcry, the campaign against child marriage runs against strong cultural traditions in Nigeria's predominantly Moslem north. People believe that there is something immoral about a girl over 14 who is not married. . ." [34]

Women's organizations in Nigeria have recently begun initiatives to speak for women's concerns more forcefully; for instance the group Women in Nigeria, at Amadu Bello University in Zaria held a conference on women's health in 1990. The lack of women's political power and their lack of education were cited as reasons for the lhuge maternal mortality, claiming that "75,000 women's deaths each year come under the heading of 'maternal mortality' which is to say that one Nigerian woman dies every 10 minutes". [35]

While the conference report cites research findings on traditional practices such as the gishiri cuts and child marriage among the abuses that affect women's health, little is said about excision, which is still practiced by a very large part of the population throughout Nigeria. A telling statistic reported at the conference is that the average life expectancy of Nigerian women is 52 years - which is 4 years less than men while in most of the rest of the world the life span of women is considerably longer than that of men. This lower life span of women is due - the research presented at the conference states - to the very high maternal mortality, "the highest in the world".

One of the health problems resulting from too early marriage and childbearing is vaginal fistulae - tearing of the vagina - which was cited by the above women's conference and is cited in all hospital reports - leading to incontinence and virtually destroying a woman's life at an early age. A report from Maiduguri Teaching Hospital in Northern Nigeria states that there, as well as in other hospitals, the number of deliveries is steadily increasing; hospitals are more and more overcrowded - which is both due to population growth but also more and more women come to deliver in hospitals rather than as is traditional, delivering at home.

> "Among the Hausa, early marriage is practiced with pregnancy before the girl is fully grown, resulting in vesico-vaginal fistulae (VVF). Circumcision may result in a tight introitus which delays delivery of the head. Another common result is severe tearing. . .
>
> About gishiri cuts, this is a traditional Hausa form of treatment, also done by certain ethnic groups influenced by Hausa customs, e.g. Fulanis. . .
>
> The reason most often given for gishiri cuts is prolonged labour. . . 'to let out whatever evil is holding up delivery' and make the cervix dilate. The traditional birth attendents, theTBAs, emphasize that this is not blood letting, as with other gishiri cuts. Some. . . will do a 'prophylactic' cut at 36 weeks to ensure an easy labour. . . In Zaria, we had two deaths from blood loss from 'prophylactic' cuts which divided the artery to the clitoris. . ." [36]

These cuts into the vagina are, according to various medical reports, done for a variety of ailments by practitioners of traditional Hausa medicine to deal with evil spirits and include animal sacrifices. But the results often are fatal as blood vessels are severed. The report concludes with the hope that through the spread of education girls may begin to question the treatment that is imposed and will be taught to think for themselves as well as take jobs - rather than being married at 10 or 12. But "it will take 10 to 20 years before any such changes take effect" the writer concludes. Can we really - indeed should we-wait that long, the writer asks.

One of the Nigerian traditional practices that is especially dangerous and is reported only in Nigeria is to excise pregnant women in their seventh month when the pregnancy is well developed, which makes the operation especially dangerous. The Nigerian nurses association alarmed about this practice, which is prevalent especially in Bendel state, made a survey that was reported in a national newspaper to warn people about these dangerous interventions.

> "'The practice has led to the death of many women because it is often unhygienically performed, and can cause bleeding, extreme pain, shock and infection,' said Mrs. Adebayo, General Secretary of the National Association of Nigerian Nurses and Midwives. Quoting from the association's survey in all the states, she also disclosed that some parts of Yoruba-speaking states practiced post-birth circumcision, usually between seven days to three months after birth.

> She revealed that female circumcision is practiced in 13 of the nation's 21 states, and that it is more predominant in Ondo, Oyo, Kwara, Bendel, Imo and Cross River States, where about 90 percent of the females are circumcized.
>
> Mrs. Adebayo added that the association, through its 'national campaign for the eradication of female circumcision', will ensure that the practice is eradicated and called for government support. . ." [37]

The National Association of Nigerian Nurses and Midwives (NANNM) organized a major national campaign after conducting this survey. A project entitled "The Eradication of Female Circumcision" was developed by the 60,000 member organization and funded in 1987 from international sources. [38]

A two-day national workshop on "The Damaging Effects of Female Circumcision and Other Harmful Traditional Practices and Their Eradication" was held in November 1987 in Ikeja (Lagos) with the collaboration of the Inter African Committee (IAC - see below) where female genital mutilation (FGM), Gishiri cuts, early childbearing, nutritional tabus, damaging childbirth practices and traditions and their effect on health were discussed. Strategies were developed for eradication, for raising community awareness and for mobilization on the grass roots level, and plans were made to implement change. [39]

The NANNM produced all kinds of local programs and initiatives as well as leaflets and informational material, booklets for grassroots mobilization in local languages with appropriate illustrations. Some short plays were produced, as well as local videos and puppetry shows representing the risks and health consequences of FGM and other damaging traditions. Nigerian media were involved including radio and TV. The reactions to the campaign were very positive on many levels due to the extensive network of the NANNM, which reaches throughout the country. The NANNM will continue to use their skills acquired through this campaign to implement their objectives and to reach local families and community people.

The influence, standing and prestige that midwives have in their local communities in all traditional societies certainly contributes to the immediate impact of such a campaign. The evaluations made by the program developers show mostly positive results. This campaign provides an excellent example that should be followed in other countries and should be widely and internationally supported by the World Health Organization, UNICEF, US Agency for International Development and other internationally funded agencies as well as private organizations - especially those concerned with family planning, which is now gaining acceptance in Nigeria.

The results of the NANNM campaign, which will have to be continued for years to be really effective and reach the very large, diverse and traditional population of Nigeria, can only be fairly evaluated in years to come. Many more local campaigns will have to follow to finally persuade the male leadership of Nigeria to take action on this issue and provide governmental support to eradicate these mutilations that involve every father of every family: because decisions of whether or not daughters are excised and when and to whom they are married are made by men in Nigeria. Everywhere in Afica men are responsible for the ongoing mutilation of their own children.

The Childbirth Picture Books (CBPB) [40] which I developed following the World Health Organization seminar in Khartoum in 1979 to implement the recommendations, are widely used in Nigeria and sent to local health centers, hospitals, teachers, midwives and health workers and all who write **WIN NEWS** for free copies. A growing correspondence, especialy with health workers, nurses and midwives shows that the books are circulated from person to person and that they are well understood and widely used.

Each book includes a section on excision or infibulation - showing graphically the damage done by the mutilations - after teaching about normal reproductions. The **CBPBs** are easy to understand regardless of language or literacy and each book with the additions on FGM includes a message to the recipient to send **WIN NEWS** a note that they will not have their daughters excised -- now that they have learned about the damage done by FGM -- and they will be sent more books. The response has been very positive and the requests for these teaching materials are continuously growing not only from Nigeria but from other African countries as well.

For such a grass roots campaign to be really effective, the **CBPBs** would have to be distributed in large quantities in a given area. To test the effectiveness of these books, questionnaires "before" and "after" could be easily administered. This method of teaching positive health and preventing damaging traditional practices is very inexpensive and does not require any experts from abroad or professionals to spend time on training. Most people can readily understand the drawings of the books with a minimum of guidance, that is always available from local midwives. The subject matter - reproduction - is certainly of very great interest to this pro-natalist society, as the experience with the **CBPBs** has shown.

The **CBPBs** go directly to the people and often are circulated from person to person and family to family. They cannot take the place of efforts such as the ones outlined above by the NANNM or any other professional health organization whose services are very much needed and must be greatly expanded, especially to the rural areas, where any trained health services for women are rarely available - as outlined above. What is more, the leadership in each community must be mobilized to address these problems in each region and state and finally the whole nation..

The Inter African Committee of Nigeria is doing just that. It cosponsored the two day national workshop in 1987 with the nurses and midwives on the damaging effects of FGM and other traditional practices and the organization is active all over Nigeria. The IAC of Nigeria is headed by Dr. Irene Modupeola Thomas, the first woman physician of Nigeria who is very influential in medical affairs in her country. The Nigerian IAC was organized following the 1984 NGO Conference in Dakar on traditional practices affecting the health of women and children, which in turn was based on the 1979 Khartoum seminar and its recommendations. [41] Dr. Thomas is also vice president of the IAC and directs regional activities for West Africa.

The IAC of Nigeria as soon as it was organized was joined by many influential women's organizations including the Medical Women's Association, the Women Lawyers, the Nigerian Red Cross Society, the National Council of Women's Societies and many more. They participated with a presentation in the two day IAC workshop at the United Nations Decade Conference in Nairobi in 1985. The first issue of their biannual health magazine, **Your Task**, reports first on the development of the IAC in 1984 and then the organization of the Nigerian IAC affiliate. The plans, activities and accomplishments of the Nigerian IAC are reported in this publication as well as the many meetings, training programs and local actions to educate people about health and encourage them to stop the many damaging practices.

The emphasis of the Nigeria IAC is on TBA (traditional birth attendants) training and workshops to train trainers who in turn will go to teach all over the country. Mrs. E. M. Alabi, project coordinator of the Nigeria IAC and a health professional with impressive credentials, is contributing to the extensive training programs that have been held all over Nigera. The IAC magazine not only provides an overview of the many positive actions that are being organized but also documents the many devastating traditional practices that so far have been ignored that inflict great damage on girls and women.

In a summary Ms. Alabi reviews the health situation of women and reaches the same conclusion as the Women in Nigeria Conference cited above: The rate of maternal mortality and morbidity is alarming; there are 15 maternal deaths reported for every 1,000 live births (though many more deaths go unreported). But for every death there are at least five mothers who are permanently physically handicapped due to birth. Many of these deaths and permanent injuries related to childbirth occur - so Mrs. Alabi states - due to traditional practices shrouded in customs that people are often reluctant to admit. Most of the deaths occur in rural areas where no hospitals or clinics exist nor any trained health workers and midwives. The training of midwives and expansion of health services, therefore, are of special concern to women who, due to frequent childbearing and exposure to damaging traditions, are most vulnerable.

Despite the oil boom, which initiated a vast number of building and modernization programs of every kind including huge road building and agricultural schemes, high-rise construction and import of large numbers of cars by men who profited from this boom, it appears that very little has been done to expand essential health care services.

Given the large numbers of births, one would think that the men who are so concerned with having more and more children also would care enough to make sure that both mothers and children are safe and have adequate care. But that obviously is not the case, as the maternal mortality figures show.

Nowhere else in Africa is it so obvious that neither poverty nor lack of education is the cause of FGM, maternal mortality and great suffering by women that could be easily prevented quite aside from stopping such medieval practices as child marriage, widespread rape and sexual assault - much of it sanctioned and hidden by "tradition". Nigeria has no lack of highly educated professionals and brilliant intellectuals as well as many wealthy men judging from the large numbers of expensive imported cars that create enormous traffic jams in Lagos and all other towns.

But this gross abuse of women and children goes on with the full knowledge and collusion of the male leadership and male professionals including large numbers of physicians, many of whom profit from FGM; the rest are too corrupt to stop these mutilations. Many male leaders sell their own immature daughters into marriage out of greed. There is no excuse for such behavior or for tolerating it by the men who run the government. These men must be held responsible for human rights violations before the whole world and for the violation of their own women and children. The leaders of this patriarchal society have the power and the education, the skills and the money to stop this abuse. One can but wonder where this violent phallocratic society is going - that is faster growing larger than any other in Africa - especially now with AIDS spreading ever more rapidly throughout this troubled continent - AIDS that is transmitted by the violent, reckless sexual practices of African men.

NIGERIA: ECONOMIC/SOCIAL FACTS & SUMMARY

NIGERIA:	30 States and Federal Capital Territory
Climate:	South, tropical swamps to tropical forests; open woodlands, grasslands, and semi-desert in far north.
Population:	115 million? (estimate disputed). Greater Lagos (former capital), 8 million; new federal capital Abuja, 850,000. Ibadan, 4-5 million (estimate). **Annual Growth Rate**: 3.5%
Life Expectancy:	51 years.
Government:	Military, transition to civilian system started in 1992. Constitution: took effect '92. Independence 1960. Civil war 1967-1970
Ethnic Groups:	Hausa-Fulani, Ibo, Yoruba (largest). About 250 tribal groups.
Languages:	English (official); Hausa, Ibo, Yoruba.
Religions:	Muslim (majority), Christian, Indigenous African (Animist).
Literacy:	30-40% (women much less).
Education:	6 years compulsory. Attendance primary school 40-50% (estimate).
Annual/Capita Income:	$250 (1989 estimate).
Economy:	Growth Rate: 4% (1989). Inflation: 40% (1989). Resources: petroleum, tin, iron ore, coal and other minerals. Agriculture products: cocoa, palm oil, yams, cassava and millet and other grains. Livestock. Industry: textiles, cement, food products, footwear. Oil boom of late 1970s collapsed 1980s with severe economic problems resulting.

FOOTNOTES

1. "Final Report on Position of Female Circumcision in Nigeria", signed by Dr. O. A. Adelaja, Sr. Consultant, Medical Statistics, Federal Ministry of Health, Federal Secretariat, Ikoyi, Lagos, Nigeria (dated March 1981). See also **WIN NEWS**, Vol. 7, No. 3, Summer 1981, p. 41.
2. Ibid.
3. Answers to questionnaire in author's file from Ministry of Health (Administration and General Division), Benin City, Bendel State of Nigeria, dated June 1, 1976, signed by Dr. V. B. Giwa-Awu, Director of Health Services for Permanent Secretary, Ministry of Health.
4. Answers to questionnaire in author's file from Ministry of Health, Administrtaion Division, Government of Cross River State of Nigeria, Calabar, dated June 11, 1976, signed by Dr. E. U. Ukpong, Director of Health Services. Reasons given were written by Chief Mrs. I. E. Ekanem, Matron in State Ministry of Health.
5. Ibid.
6. Ibid.
7. Longo, Lawrence, MD. "Sociocultural Practices Relating to Obstetrics and Gynecology in a Community of West Africa". **American Journal of Obstetrics and Gynecology.** Vol. 89, No. 4, pp. 470-5, 1964. A film is available from Loma Linda University, Audio-Visual Service, Loma Linda, California 92354 USA. (Dr. Longo was part-time lecturer at the University College Hospital in Ibadan and Staff Obstetrician at the Ile Ife Hospital in Nigeria. Dr. Longo is now at Loma Linda University).
8. Longo, Lawrence, MD. "Obstetrics and Gynecology in a West African Community". **Medical Arts and Sciences**, Loma Linda University, Vol. 18, 1964, pp. 116-24.
9. Longo, op. cit., "Sociocultural. . .Africa", p. 471.
10. "Food Tabus Affecting Pregnant Women", (Ms.) E. M. Alabi, Project Coordinator, Nigerian National Committee of the Inter African Committee on Traditional Practices Affecting the Health of Women and Children, P.O. Box 60511 Lagos, Nigeria. See also **WIN NEWS,** 17-2, Spring 1991, p. 31.
11. Ibid, pp. 471-72.
12. Ibid, pp. 474.
13. Ibid, pp. 471-72.
14. Ogunmodede, Esther. "Circumcision: How Much Longer Will We Allow Our Girls to Be Brutalized in This Barbaric Way?",**the Drum**, Nigeria. November 1977, pp. 15-16.

    NOTE: This article, the first time the subject was discussed in such a candid way by a Nigerian woman journalist, not only made a remarkable impact in Nigeria but has also an interesting international history. According to Esther Ogunmodede, the article, some time before it was published by **the Drum** in Nigeria, was submitted to IPPF (International Planned Parenthood Federation) in London to John Rowley the editor of **People** - the IPPF magazine which is distributed worldwide. He turned it down, though he had asked for it. Then, when the World Health Organization (WHO) Seminar was scheduled for 1979, John Rowley went back to Esther Ogunmodede and got permission to republish her article from **the Drum,** where it had appeared in Fall of 1977. Prior to that, IPPF had refused to publish any information about excision and/or infibulation, not even factual medical reports which I had sent them since 1975 including all my research published by medical journals. **WIN NEWS** published the article by Esther Ogunmodede before it appeared in **the Drum** in 1977, as Ogunmodede made the manuscript available to **WIN NEWS** after it was turned down by IPPF. After the article appeared in **People** in 1979, it was picked up and reprinted in part by many publications that had previously refused to mention the subject, or like IPPF, had for years suppressed all information on genital mutilation (see "The Politics of FGM").

FOOTNOTES (continued)

The Esther Ogunmodede's article was also reprinted in part by the **Development Forum** - a United Nations-sponsored newspaper published in Geneva; by several feminist magazines and numerous other establishment and feminist publications - following its publication by IPPF- which evidently, was the signal that it is acceptable to make known some of the facts - but only when written by an African journalist.

In the original article in **the Drum,** Ogunmodede had given me credit for supplying her with information about genital mutilation in other parts of Africa,

> "Fran P. Hosken, publisher and editor of **Women's International Network News,** visited many African countries, collecting information on girls' circumcision. Her report is of major importance, for never before has such a detailed study been carried out on this problem."

It is interesting to note that not only IPPF (International Planned Parenthood) publications but also ISIS (an international feminist journal published in Geneva) who had the original article from **the Drum** by Ogunmodede, omitted the above paragraph and the credit that was given there for the Africa-wide research cited as background in the article.

The true importance of the article, however, is that it succeeded in stirring up a great deal of discussion in Nigeria, where there is by now a larger reading public than in other parts of Africa. However, though an extensive discussion of female circumcision followed - in the form of letters to the editor of **the Drum** - no substantive action such as a health education campaign by the Ministry of Health or Education or by the magazine itself followed Ogunmodede's urgent plea "Who is responsible for making sure the message reaches every family?" It still goes unheeded today.

15. Ibid., p. 16.
16. Ibid.
17. Inter African Committee on Traditional Practices Affecting the Health of Women and Children, 147, rue de Lausanne, CH-1202 Geneva, Switzerland; c/o Economic Commission for Africa, ATRCW, P.O. Box 3001, Addis Ababa, Ethiopia. A 40 minute film/videotape on "Traditional Practices" introduced by IAC President, Berhanne Ras Work. (Available from IAC)
18. op. cit.
19. op. cit.
20. op. cit., p. 16.
21. **WIN NEWS**, Vol. 5, No. 2, Spring 1979, pp. 57- 58, as reported in several issues of **the Drum** (Nigeria), 1977-79.
22. See also **WIN NEWS**, Vol. 5, No. 2, Spring 1979 pp. 28-29. Interview with Dr. Bertha Johnson, Lagos, Nigeria, March 1979.
23. Johnson, Bertha, Dr. "Traditional Practices Affecting the Health of Women", paper prepared for the World Health Seminar: "Traditional Practices Affecting the Health of Women and Children", February 10-15, 1979, Khartoum, Sudan, pp. 3-8.
24. Ibid.
25. Ibid.
26. **WIN NEWS**, Vol. 5, No. 2, Spring 1979, p. 28.
27. Johnson, Bertha, Dr., op. cit., pp. 6-8.
28. Ibid.
29. **WIN NEWS**, Vol. 5, No. 2, Spring 1979, p. 30. As reported in the **Nation** (Feb. 25, 1979) Kenya/speech by Dr. Nike O. Grange at the International Pediatrics Association First Regional Pediatric Congress for Africa, Nairobi, Kenya, February 19-23, 1979.
30. **WIN NEWS**, Vol. 5, No. 2, Spring 1979, p. 29. Interview with Dr. N. O. Grange.
31. Ibid.
32. Letter in Author's file.

FOOTNOTES (continued)

33. **New York Times**, March 27, 1987. See **WIN NEWS**, 13-2, Spring 1987, p. 30.
34. **New York Times**, August 17, 1987. See **WIN NEWS**, 13-4, Autumn 1987, p. 44.
35. "WIN - Women in Nigeria". Theme for 1990: "Women and Health" Amadu Bello University, Zaria, Kaduna State, Dept. of Sociology - Reported in **West Africa**, UK (21-27 May 1990). See **WIN NEWS**, 16-4, Autumn 1990, pp. 49-50.
36. Report from Maidiguri Teaching Hospital. See **WIN NEWS**, 10-2, Spring 1984, p. 38.
37. **The Vanguard** - National paper of Nigeria, Dec., 2, 1988. National Association of Nigerian Nurses and Midwives, National Secretariat, 66 Oduduwa Way, GRA Ikeja, Box 3857 Ikeja PO, Lagos, Nigeria. See **WIN NEWS**, 15-2, Spring 1989, p. 37.
38. National Association of Nigerian Nurses and Midwives (NANNM) Project: "The Eradication of Female Circumcision and Other Harmful Traditional Practices". Technical support from PATH - Program for Appropriate Technology in Health (Final Report), funded by Population Crisis Committee, Washington DC.
39. "National Workshop on the Damaging Effects of Circumcision and other Harmful Traditional Practices and their Effective Eradication", Nov. 16-17, 1987. Ikeja, Lagos Nigeria. See: **WIN NEWS**, 14-2 Spring 1988, p. 33.
40. **The Universal Childbirth Picture Book/ Program** - "A Picture Story about Reproduction from a Woman's View " with additions to prevent **Excision** and **Infibulation**. Published by **WIN NEWS**. Used in Africa on the grassroots level to teach about healthy reproduction and to stop FGM. Available in many languages. Free books are distributed to community health workers, midwives, teachers, health and family planning programs, midwifery schools and others in Africa .These teaching materials are useful regardless of language or literacy and are sent free to women and men in Africa who write for the books. Each book contains a message asking the recipients to send a note, stating that their daughters will not be operated on, when writing for more books. For excerpts of letters received, see **WIN NEWS** - section on FGM - or write to **WIN NEWS** for copies of letters and to sponsor distribution of books.
41. The Inter African Committee of Nigeria : Mandilas Motors Complex 9-13, Atitebi Str. (Off Apapa Road) Ebute - Metta (Lagos) Nigeria. Dr. Irene Modupeola Thomas MD. President. **YOUR TASK** - Health magazine of IAC Nigeria.

CASE HISTORY : MALI

In the book **Women of Mali,** [1] Danielle Bazin-Tardieu, who has lived a number of years in Bamako, the capital, analyzes the situation of women in Mali's very traditional society. Her study and descriptions provide a good view of the status of women, not only in Bamako and Mali but also in much of Francophone West Africa. In this region strong Moslem and French influences are superimposed on African traditions. Polygamy is the rule, as it is both a traditional African practice as well as the custom of Islam.

"A woman in Mali", Bazin-Tardieu states, "has many duties, but also rights. The first duty is to obey her husband and to respect his first wife (if she is the second, third or fourth one)." [2] She must get along with the other wives. She is also obligated to respect the customs of the ancçstors of her husband's family and must take part in the extensive household work shared among all the wives including growing of food for the large family. She has the right to have a certain amount of independence; in most cases, she has a dwelling to herself, where she keeps her things and which is shared by her children up to the age of puberty. The hut or house usually belongs to her husband - the wife is only the user - though among some ethnic groups, where the woman builds her own house, it also belongs to her.

Marriages are arranged by the father, who decides to whom he gives his daughters for marriage in return for a brideprice - paid to the father. Adultery is severly punished for women, but not for men; according to tradition women were excluded from public life. Today, the traditions are still strongly followed in the rural areas; but they are changing in the towns under outside influences. Marriage means the alliance of families; a decision by the father, as in all patriarchal societies, is practically absolute. Divorce is easy and can be initiated by the husband as well as the wife, in which case, the woman must return to her father's family who must be willing to accept her, as in other Islamic societies. It does not exist that a woman lives alone.

Bazin-Tardieu explains that each wife has the right to the favors of her husband at specified times. That is, the husband must observe certain rules among his wives and spend a night with each one in turn. He eats with the wife with whom he spends the night; that is, the wife whose "turn" it is to be the recipient of his sexual favors is also obligated to feed him.

With ethnic groups where each wife owns her house, for instance with the Sonrai, the husband has no dwelling of his own, as he spends each night with a different wife. With other ethnic groups, the husband also has a house as part of the family compound.

In the towns, Bazin-Tardieu explains, as the houses are built closer together, lack of room makes it necessary to find some other solutions; however, the same principles prevail. At times, the houses of the wives are arranged around a common court, or each wife has a room of her own in one house, which is divided up in various ways. In situations where women have jobs outside the home in the modern sector, which recently has occurrred in the towns, they also have their own place to live where the husband comes to visit them on certain days. In rare cases, when the husband is very wealthy, he provides a separate house for each wife.

The children of such unions do not belong to the mother. They belong to the family of the husband, which the woman has entered through her marriage.

If the marriage is dissolved, the children stay with the father and his family. The father makes all the important decisions for the children such as education, where they are to live, and in the case of girls, whom they are to marry as well as when they are excised, which traditionally is a puberty rite Though almost every girl in southern Mali is excised, which obviously is a traumatic experience that influences the rest of her life and may cause her permanent suffering and health problems, Bazin-Tardieu says nothing about that - nor do almost all other books about women in Africa.

Bazin-Tardieu explains the different variations of the family rules that are practiced by different ethnic groups in Mali, but the principles are similar. The mother has no right to her own children, though she is obligated to support them, take care of them and feed them as well as feeding the husband when it is her turn. Divorce can be initiated by the husband any time. Usually, children stay with their mother until the age of seven - especially the girls - also when the wife is divorced. Since young children in polygamous households spend most of their first several years very close to their mother - the first two years mostly on her back - very strong bonds develop between them.

In **La Parole aux Negresses**, Awa Thiam gives some examples of how this system functions from a woman's point of view. She relates several personal histories - as told to her. Here is the story of a first wife, married to a wealthy, influential man, describing what polygamy really means to a women even where no economic problems beset the family relationship.

MOUNA: (Married to a Moslem religious leader)

> "I have been married since I was 16 - I am now 43. I have given my husband 12 children, two died as infants. I am the first wife of my husband and have had 13 co-wives - over the years - of all different ages. The youngest one is only 20 - my husband is in his fifties. Some of the wives did not live in the same house or even town. But at present, all four of us live together, according to the wishes of my husband. He travels frequently.
>
> Since I have been with him longest, though I hardly see him now, I know all that has happened. Each time a new wife comes, she is the center of my husband's attention. After a while, she finds herself neglected, either because of the arrival of another wife, or because of another voyage. This kind of married life is impossible, no matter how we try to please, how well we behave. . . my co-wives and I are always abandoned in favor of another woman. I did not dare to do what some of the others did - take a lover or get a divorce - because I was afraid for my children.
>
> Often when my husband left, one of his wives would take a lover, and then he divorced her when he returned. The second to the last wife had a child by another man after my husband married yet another woman. He took her child as his own. I do not speak against my co-wives. They are young and they cannot stand being neglected and ignored when another woman takes their place. I am already a grandmother. My oldest son is quite a bit older than the most recent co-wife.
>
> When one cannot get a divorce, there is nothing else to do but to be resigned to one's fate. The Moslem religion is strict in this respect. There is no solution. My oldest child is 26 and the youngest only three; what would become of them if I divorce their father? The situation of the wives who have divorced is just as bad." [3]

Neither men nor women seek love in marriage; rather it is an association from which a man expects to get his offspring and an alliance between families of influence as well as for the man satisfaction of his needs for sex and food. It provides him with stability and status in the male community. Marriage takes care of women's material needs and her need to have children. Fertility, the production of many children, is her only way to legitimate her existence as part of her husband's family. All women are considered minors before the law and only after her first marriage does a woman have some independence, though a divorced woman cannot live alone.

The legal rights of women in Mali seem to depend largely on customs that differ with each ethnic group. According to some ethnic groups, a woman can neither own property nor inherit; in other ethnic groups, the income from what she sells in the market is her own. In Islamic societies, boys generally inherit twice as much as their sisters. Compared to the customs of pre-Islamic African societies, which are still observed in many areas in West Africa including Mali, the Islamic inheritance regulations mean an advance for women - as is often pointed out by Moslems.

In many traditional African societies, women not only cannot own anything but upon the death of the husband, a woman is part of the inheritance and becomes the property of her husband's brother or any other male member of his family. That is, rather than owning property, according to African tradition, a woman **is** property, which is also confirmed by the brideprice.

Mali and much of the surrounding territory is inhabited by some of the most traditional societies anywhere in the world. Many ethnic groups are still bound by a feudal caste system that has hardly changed for hundreds of years and is quite incompatible with any notion of development: according to tradition where you are born, there you stay for your life - following your ancestors. The idea that you can improve your status by work or that upward mobility is possible or desirable is quite foreign to this traditional view of life. The Moslem religion furthermore teaches that whatever happens is the wish of Allah and cannot be changed because Allah knows best.

That these traditions are totally incompatible with "development" as introduced by the West and the United Nations does not seem to have occurred to the highly paid experts - almost all of them men - who come to Mali and other African countries to introduce development programs. They all support "tradition" and encourage all customs without examining the terrible damage done by the blind adherence to traditional practices, for example, Female Genital Mutilation (FGM) and without any rational examination of the facts which show that traditions are the main stumbling blocks for development. Indeed most traditions oppose all change, yet change is the very objective of development.

In Mali, as in many other parts of Africa, "traditions" are strongly emphasized by the male leadership in the modern sector and government because this is the way to protect male privilege and keep women subservient. Such claims by African leaders are often accompanied by strong nationalistic overtones. Women are socialized and politicized to join in, proudly stressing the importance of their tradtions and heritage: traditions that disenfranchise them legally and make them into chattel, as the wholly owned work force of men, besides robbing them of their children and castrating their sexuality.

Men, not only in Africa, for obvious self-serving reasons, support the traditions that put women "in their place", that is as dependents of men to do with as men please. Everywhere in the world, tradition is made out to be the greatest good entrusted to women, and women are praised and charged to perpetuate traditions. Thus women are made to endorse and support their own exploitation, disenfranchisement and exclusion from decision making.

Some African traditions which go back hundreds of years are quite similar to what was practiced in the past by feudal peasant societies in Europe and in other parts of the world. One only needs to read European medieval history about the conditions of women in Europe about 800 or more years ago: The status of women in many of Europe's peasant societies in those times was quite similar to that of traditional ethnic rural groups in Africa today. Women were posessions of men with no rights, with one important exception: Sexual mutilation of females was never practiced anywhere in Europe by the indigenous peasant societies. Yet, in Africa, these mutilations seem to have been a custom generally practiced by a majority of ethnic groups from prehistoric times to the present.

Illiteracy of women in Mali and the surrounding areas of Francophone West Africa is the highest in the world. Only a few percent of the female population can read and write. Yet these illiterate women are used by the educated male leadership to clamor for preservation of "their traditions" as a nationalistic good, traditions that deprive women of even learning to read. The damage done to women's lives and status by tradition is never examined or explained.

The French colonial system which ruled over all of West Africa, never stressed education. Learning was only for the selected few men the colonial administrators needed to implement their rule and keep order. Women were not needed; therefore they were excluded from this system. All but a very few, who became wives of men employed by the French, remained illiterate and bound by their inherited medieval traditions.

It is no accident that today Francophone West Africa has the highest infant and maternal mortality and the highest female illiteracy in the whole world. In Francophone West Africa, FGM is still practiced much as it has been for many hundreds of years and in drastic forms - including infibulation - except for the relatively few who moved to Bamako or other towns: There they have some contact with new ideas, with education and with present day ways of life.

A new family law was passed in Mali after Independence in1962 by the socialist government, including a new marriage code. Bazin-Tardieu explains that this new legislation in this traditional society was indeed, a "revolution". Nevertheless, polygamy and the brideprice, the two most damaging traditional institutions for women, were preserved, quite aside from FGM, which was not even discussed.

The very first article of the marriage code states that marriage is a civil act,, and that such a union is not legal unless both partners consent before an officer of the law; no traditional religious or caste impediments are recognized, though the marriage prohibitions of the Koran are accepted. The man must be at least 18 and the woman at least 15 years old to get married . The money that may be paid for the brideprice is regulated, because "the brideprice has become in our times simply a purchase price for women and the occasion of scandalous speculations on the part of the family head". [4]

The high cost of buying a wife was discussed in an article in March 1979 in **SUNJATA**, a monthly publication of the Information Service in Mali. Some of the points made show that little has changed, even among the limited number of people who can read and live in Bamako, despite the new family legislation that was passed 17 years earlier:

> "If you want to create equality between men and women you must first of all abolish the brideprice; the price for a woman is constantly increasing, this is becoming a great handicap for marriage. The brideprice by now has lost all its social and cultural significance and has become a menace for the young and a source of enrichment for the parents (= fathers). In traditional society of the past, the brideprice simply meant to be a compensation for the parents of the girl, since they lost the work she did in the fields. Polygamy was a means to increase the field laborers and to assure plenty of help in the house.
>
> Article 3 of the Marriage Code of Mali stipulates that the brideprice may not be more than 20.000 Francs for a young girl and no more than 40.000 for a woman - including all presents. There is a prison sentence between three months to two years and a penality of 20.000-40.000 Francs for breaking this law. But nowhere has anyone been prosecuted for breaking it.
>
> Enormous amounts of money are wasted on weddings that are the height of foolish snobbery. Certain fathers, instead of being concerned about the happiness of their daughters, are only looking for the richest merchant they can find as a son-in-law to improve their own financial condition. The girl is given no choice and she is told that if she does not obey her father she will be damned and thrown out of the house." [5]

Many provisions of the new marriage code, despite the fact that they are unlikely to be enforced, are nevertheless important as they define the customary situation and break with it. Women for the first time are provided with full civil rights. Another unique innovation is that, at the time of the first marriage, a man must choose either monogamy or polygamy; but the bride is not at all consulted. The law provides that an adulterous man can be punished the same as an adulterous woman. One-sided repudiation of the marriage is prohibited, and divorce must be before a civil court.

Bazin-Tardieu points out that these changes in the Mali family code break entirely with many traditions; for the first time, specific rights are vested in a person - a married woman - vis-a-vis the patriarchal family groups who control all individuals in traditional societies.

Despite all the new legislation, only about one man in three chooses to enter a monogamous marriage, according to a survey Bazin-Tardieu conducted in Bamako. Tradition also seems to prevail where caste rules apply that prohibit marriage outside one's station in life, thus preserving a medieval caste system that prevents economic development. In Mali, as well as in many other areas of West Africa, a caste system still prevails whereby occupations and trades are inherited from father to son in the rural economy and stay with certain families who perpetuate occupations such as blacksmiths or medicine men or chiefs or midwives - one of the few influential occupations for women. In the same way, excisors or those who do the traditional mutilations also belong to a caste: In West Africa they often are the wives of blacksmiths who make their knives.

Labor legislation, including rules for maternity leave and social security, were also put on the books, though only a tiny percentage of women work in the modern sector. Traditionally, women do not engage in any salaried work. Bazin-Tardieu questions the significance of such legislation in Mali, or indeed in any country where more than 90 percent of the population, both male and female, live in rural areas from subsistence farming.

As in other African and Moslem societies, the worlds of women and men in Mali are quite separate. The division into two parallel traditional societies, one male and one female, continues today, each according to its own rules made by the familygroup or the caste. Some attempts have been made by legislation and by a series of official proclamations circulated by the government to bring the two worlds together and to endow all persons with individual rights (both men and women).

This means a complete break with the traditional collective, hierarchical society, where the individual is strictly subservient to the patriarchal group. Decisions for the family groups are made by the village chief and for each family by the patriarchal male head. The individual person has no rights, and takes no responsibility for his or her life, which is directed by the group and subject to Allah's or the Ancestors' wishes.

Bazin-Tardieu polled the opinions of educated groups of men and women in Bamako concerning the relationship between the sexes and family life. She found by asking adult men, that many of them are against all change in their relationship vis-a-vis women. However, they express a keen interest in their own new-found personal freedom and individuality, which they claim is exclusively for men. Most men favor polygamy and they state that there is a "great danger for the family, for themselves, and also for the women" by giving women a greater voice.

One of the important changes is that men and women in the modern sector now eat together and talk together. In traditional African and also Middle Eastern societies, men eat first, served by women; women and children eat later what is left by the men. Conversation traditionally is between men alone - women never join a group of men or sit with them and talk. However, in the modern sector men and women share many activities, which they never did in traditional society, where work as well as all other activities is segregated by sex.

The men in Bamako - that is in the modern sector - whom Bazin-Tardieu asked, note that women have changed; but most men are convinced that such changes are for the worse. "Women lack respect for their husbands. Traditionally, the role of a woman is to be on her knees before her husband. That is the role that God has assigned to her."[6]

Women in turn complain that men neglect the needs of their family and abdicate their responsibilities vis-a-vis their children. "The men cheat, they don't respect marriage, they drink excessively and they run after other women" sums up the women's opinions of men. It is of course impossible for men to really know and guide their children in polygamous families and there is often fierce competition for attention between the many siblings.

The statements of the women from Mali about men are much the same as what women say in other parts of Africa, for instance Kenya (see "Case History Kenya"). The reactions of men pertaining to how women are changing and the "danger for the family" which is supposed to result, are certainly universal. The exact same statements can be heard today almost anywhere in the world by men of literally all societies including Europe and the US. The same patriarchal system bent on preserving male privilege even at the price of women's and children's lives exists everywhere in the world, as this report documents

Bazin-Tardieu, as other sociologists, only briefly mentions the existence of excision for girls in Mali. But she quite omits all explanations as to what the operations entail, and she fails to state the devastating physical and psychological influences that genital operations have on the lives of women. And noone has examined the actual costs of these mutilations as more and more women seek help in the hospitals for the devastating problems caused by these interventions. The healthcare and hospital costs in every African country have to be paid by the government. (See Health Facts and Overview)

The vast majority of female children in Mali and almost all who live in Bamako continue to be subjected to excision, and infibulation is also practiced by some ethnic groups. These mutilations have drastic consequences for the health, the well-being, and the daily life of the women. In Mali, except for two population groups in Timbuktu and the northern part of the country, every ethnic group mutilates their female offspring. Even in Bamako, more than 95 percent of the women coming to the maternity of the Gabriel Toure Hospital are excised and infibulation also can be found.

The situation of an excised woman in the modern sector who gets an education is especially tragic when she becomes conscious of herself and the life long deprivation inflicted on her by her parents, often as a young child. Dr. Jean G. Taoko, who as a physician, has direct experience with this situation, states:

> "One of the most dramatic and cruel consequences of excision is frigidity. . . many women also experience pain during intercourse and, therefore, can never enjoy normal sexual relations because of excision. . .
>
> From a psychological and social point of view, the results are similarly serious. For a woman who has been educated and who begins to be emancipated, excision - to which she was subjected as a child - is resented as deep humiliation. . . It is the visible sign. . . of her inferiority. It is a psychological wound even deeper than the physical one. "[7]

And Dr. Taoko adds: "It is imperative that this practice must be abandoned."

In a letter to the editor, in response to the article in Famille et Developpement quoted above, where Dr. Taoko also describes all the damaging health problems that result from the mutilations, an educator from Mali claims that excision is a necessary protection in his society. He argues that since polygamy is not practiced, for instance in Europe and the US prostitution, debauchery and venereal disease are the rule. [8] Apparently, this educator does not know or wish to acknowledge that prostitution is rampant throughout African urban areas and venereal disease is now being spread by men into the remotest villages. According to the World Health Organization, it has assumed epidemic proportions all over Africa and so has AIDS - with more than 7.5 million Africans infected or more people than in any other region of the world.

Awa Thiam, from Senegal, traveled all over Francophone West Africa to talk to women; she relates many of their stories as told to her. Here one, from a woman who grew up in a Malian village where she was subjected to the customary sexual mutilation as a child of twelve:

> "I remember every detail of the operation. In our village, several girls of the same age are operated on at the same time by a special 'excisor' in her house. The village people come together to celebrate this occasion. The night before the operation, the drums were beaten until late.
>
> Very early the next morning, two of my favorite aunts took me to the house of the excisor. . . an old woman from the blacksmith caste. In Mali. . . the women from this caste traditionally do genital operations, both clitoridectomy and infibulation. . .
>
> Once inside the house of the operator, I became terribly frightened, though I had been assured that it would not hurt. . . I was told to lie down on a mat on the floor. Immediately, some big hands fastened themselves on my thin legs and opened them wide. I raised my head, but two women held me down to the floor and immobilized my arms. . .
>
> I felt something being sprinkled on my genital area. Later, I learned this was sand, which is supposed to make excision easier. I was terrified. Suddenly, some fingers pulled on my genital organs. I tried to escape but I could not move. A searing pain pierced me through and through. The excisor cut. . . and cut: it took an interminable time. . . I felt as if I were being torn to pieces. The rule says that one must not cry during this operation. . . But I screamed and cried, and I was bleeding all over. Finally, the operator put a mixture of herbs and butter on the wound to arrest the bleeding - I have never felt any pain as overwhelming as that.. . .

"Next, the women who had held me down let go of me; but I couldn't get up. The voice of the operator called "it is finished. You can get up. You see, it didn't hurt much.' With the help of two women, I was put on my feet. I was forced to walk to where the other girls who also had been excised were waiting. Then they made us dance. Under the orders of the women in charge, I was forced to join a group of people who had gathered for this occasion to see us dance. I can't tell you how I felt. I was burning all over. In tears, I jumped about a little, together with the other girls who all were forced to hop about, bleeding and hysterical from pain. I remember this monstrous affair of bleeding girls writhing in pain, being forced to jump up and down in a cloud of dust surrounded by gleeful shouting and clapping villagers. Then everything began to reel about me. I remember nothing more

When I came to, I was stretched out in a hut with several people around me. Later, the most terrible moments of my life were those when I had to urinate. It took a whole month before I healed. When I was well again, I was ridiculed by all the villagers because they said I wasn't courageous." [9]

A professional woman from Mali with a French university degree relates from her experience:

"The practice of infibulation and excision is deeply anchored in our society. Though today young women and girls are in revolt against it, older people resist any change. What happened in my family is an example: After I became conscious of all the trouble and problems that result from genital operations, my husband and I decided that we would not allow our children to be either excised or infibulated. My children were born in France, where both my husband and I finished our studies. When we returned to Mali my mother asked if I had had the girls operated. I said no and that I am opposed to it.

During the children's vacation, after I had found some work, I left them with my parents. One day, coming home from work, I stopped by my mother's house. . . 'Where are the girls?', I asked my mother. 'Oh, they are in their room', she said. They were lying on the floor on some straw mats. Their swollen eyes and faces took my breath away, and I screamed: 'What has happened to my children?' But before they could even answer, my mother replied: 'Don't trouble yourself about my little girls. I had them excised and infibulated this morning'.

I cannot say what I felt at this moment. What could I do against my mother? I felt revolt rising in me, but I was helpless against her. My first reaction was to cry. She said: 'You should be very happy. Everything went very well with the girls.' Rather than being disrespectful, which is very badly taken in our society in Mali. . . I quickly left the house. I believe nothing can be done unless the women who are concerned organize and discuss openly their objections against these practices." [10]

This story, unfortunately, is not at all unique. Respect for the wishes of grandparents and the older generation comes before everything else in Africa and so the lives and health of countless children are sacrificed. While Western societies are accused of lack of respect for their elders, the results of such respect often entail the sacrifice of the future of their own offspring as this example illustrates.

Respect for one's elders is important; but it is also important for older people to continue to learn and accept change. However that is an idea which has not reached Africa where "the Elders" (all men of course) in every village make all the decisions for the young without ever consulting them and on the basis of what their forefathers in turn did.

In Africa the future of the most vulnerable but most important members of each society are sacrificed - the lives and health of young girls. Since they will become the mothers of future generations, the health of the entire society is, therefore, diminished and compromised. For instance, food tabus that are widely practiced all over Africa against young girls and pregnant women (see also Case History : Nigeria) do not only deprive them and ruin their own health, but babies born from mothers who are mutilated and deprived of essential nutrients are often saddled with permanent deficiencies, inabilities, retardation and birth defects.

African men, who dominate their societies and impose genital mutilations, nutritional tabus and many other burdens such as chronic overwork on women, may think they gain from such exploitation by guaranteeing their own superiority in this way. But the real long-range results are that all Africans are gradually diminished and becoming less and less able to compete with other societies and especially with young people who are born of women who are healthy, able and well fed.

Infibulation is still widely practiced in Mali sometimes on very young children. Another personal story, as related to Awa Thiam, shows the appalling situation that one young woman faced when she discovered her own condition. Unfortunately, her situation is not unique. A Malian woman of 29 with a degree in literature told this to Awa Thiam:

> "I have no memory of my own excision and infibulation as I was operated when I was very young. I only became conscious of my condition when I was twenty, just before my marriage. I have lived in a traditional environment where sex and sexuality were tabu subjects. When I became aware that I was excised and infibulated, I was appalled and revolted. I wondered what to do. I would not allow myself to be opened with a knife the day of my marriage, as is the custom. . . I wanted to get the operation done in a hospital.
>
> I went to see some physicians. But each time my request was refused. It seems I faced a complete social barrier. Everybody I asked was against doing this operation. Those in the hospital looked at me as if I were out of my mind. One of the doctors. . . told me 'You want to lead a life of debauchery, and for this, you are asking for my complicity?' He almost threw me out of his office. I got angrier and more frustrated every day. . . The day of my marriage approached. My chances to escape the knife decreased. In the end, the evening of my marriage, I had to submit and suffer my misfortune." [11]

How many young women are caught in this situation? No one knows, Awa Thiam states. More and more young women in West Africa oppose the mutilations, but usually too late. Fathers, in order to assure getting a high brideprice, have their daughters done at ever-younger ages. Universal silence perpetuates these traditions especially among the male leaders of each ethnic and social group. Most women do not want to talk about it, as they are ashamed or they believe the many myths that they are told and are totally ignorant about the basic biological facts of reproduction. Nowhere in Africa, where women often go through twelve or more pregnancies, is any information on childbirth or reproductive health care available. Most of the women are quite unconscious that there is even a possibility to question the damaging traditional practices.

With the Dogon, one of Mali's ethnic groups, excision is obligatory. The Dogon believe that each girl has male and female characteristics, and the same is true of boys. It is necessary to extirpate the male characteristics in a girl before she can become a woman, and in turn, all female traits must be removed in a boy before he can be a member of the adult community of men. The clitoris is said to be a male characteristic; therefore, girls must be excised. In turn, boys are circumcised to remove the prepuce, which is said to be a female vestige. The operations are necessary so that a young person can become a responsible, adult member of society and sure of his or her sex.

The Bambara practice both infibulation and excision, Awa Thiam relates. "The Islamic leaders whom I questioned all declared that excision is practiced because it is a religious requirement." When Awa Thiam pointed out that nowhere in the Koran is it stated that excision is required, the Moslem leaders told the story of Mohammed, who said to a woman excisor - UmAtiya - she should not cut too deep. But he did not say: Do not operate.

Therefore, in the eyes of the Moslem leaders, the operation is not forbidden. On the other hand, those who are against the practice can claim that Mohammed never spoke for the operation. However, no religious statement of any kind can be cited by anyone to justify infibulation. Infibulation is an obscene cruelty invented by men to control and debase women.

A physician, Dr. Pascal James Imperato, who worked for several years in Mali and adjoining countries, describes the excision operations he saw performed among the Bambara and the Malinke in traditional village environments:

> "Bambara girls are excised by the women of the blacksmith caste, who are also the pottery makers. The operation is performed on the outskirts of the village in the presence of the assembled adult female relatives of the candidates for the operations. In some villages, the operation is done at the site where the women make pottery. Each girl is seated on an earthen jar, which is turned upside down. Three adult female relatives stand behind her and hold her. With the legs spread apart, the operator takes hold of the clitoris and amputates it with a swift cut of a knife or razor. The amputated clitoris is buried or thrown into a rat hole. There is considerable variation in the disposition of the amputated clitoris. . .
>
> Often animal feces are placed over the wounds. . . Such practices frequently lead to the development of serious secondary infections. . . Complications such as tetanus, gangrene and hemorrhage are not uncommon. Some of the children die from these operations, but precise statistics are not available. It was my impression that most deaths occurred. . . from hemorrhage. . .
>
> Circumcision and excision ceremonies among the Malinke of Mali are held about every three years. Among the animists, the average age of those operated on is 16 years. But among the Islamized people, most girls are from eight to twelve years. . .
>
> The girls are excised in their mother's house or else in the house of the blacksmith's wife, who performs the operation. . . Some are excised in the enclosure surrounding the family latrine. The girl sits on a flat rock with her legs spread apart. Her mother, older sisters, and the family's praise-singer surround her. Nowadays, razor blades are frequently used; but formerly knives were employed.
>
> The operator seizes hold of the clitoris with the index finger and thumb. Occasionally, she stimulates it with her fingers if it is difficult to get hold of. The operator then pulls on the clitoris and amputates it at its base. It is then given to the girl's mother who traditionally places it in a rat hole. . ." [12]

Dr. Imperato worked for the World Health Organization Smallpox Eradication Program, which took him all over Mali. No effort was spared by the WHO team to convince the nomadic groups to let themselves and their children be vaccinated, though most of them had never had any contact with modern medicine and were very suspicious. This remarkable preventive campaign has succeeded - smallpox no longer exists: Mali was one of the countries where smallpox persisted to the end.

However, nothing was done to persuade the same population groups to stop the mutilation of their own children, though many continue to die from the genital operations and many others suffer all their lives. Medical teams, with the guidance and support of WHO and UNICEF, immunize children against infectious diseases and teach the people why this must be done; but they look on and do nothing about the mutilations of little girls as the above description documents. Dr. Imperato spent many months in Mali and surrounding countries and gained the trust of the people; but he did nothing to stop the mutilations. The people are kept in complete ignorance about the biological and sexual facts, and that genital operations are damaging, are dangerous and do not increase fertility as is often believed, though UNICEF and WHO have representatives and offices in all African countries.

Assitan Diallo, a student at Teacher's College of Bamako, wrote her thesis in 1978 on "Excision at the Bambara". In this extensive study, she documents the traditional coming of age rituals that surround the operations, including the songs that were sung by the initiates. She describes that the Bambara excise their girls in the cool season (November/February) in a group ceremony as a puberty rite. Women under the influence of Islam are considered "impure" unless excised.

When the country was Islamized, the Bambara already practiced excision of girls and circumcision of boys in order to confirm each individual's sex and make her/him acceptable in adult society. It is also believed by the Bambara that according to tradtiion the clitoris and prepuce are the seats of an evil spirit called "Wanzo"; this Wanzo prevents a young person from having a union with a member of the opposite sex; therefore, it must be removed. [13]

Traditionally, excision was performed on girls just before puberty, between eight and thirteen years of age. Generally, each girl was already promised to a man. Therefore, the family of her husband-to-be took part in the festivities.

Assitan Diallo's description of the operation is almost identical to that cited by Dr. Imperato (above) and performed on a group of girls. Diallo states that traditionally during the recovery period, the girls stay together in a room, and are taken care of by an old woman who has special powers to keep the evil spirits away. The girls are secluded for about three months; during that time they are taught to sing various songs, and their wounds are taken care of mainly by applying butter. Finally, a big fire is made at a crossroad, where all the objects with which the excised girls had contact are burned. It is believed that the Wanzo - the evil spirit - is thus destroyed.

Each girl emerges from this seclusion a completely changed person. During this retreat, the girls are taught about marriage and their role in the family. Each girl is instructed that she must submit to her husband in all matters. Her relationship to his parents is defined. The traditional way a household is organized at the Bambara - and it is similar among many other ethnic groups - requires that she accepts her inferior position vis-a-vis her husband and all men, including her sons. When the father of the family is absent, the oldest son takes his place as head of the family and makes the decisions for the entire family.

Diallo asks: "Does excision today in our society still have any functional value as initiation or as social education? And does it continue to be practiced as widely as in the past?" [14] To find out, Diallo developed a questionnaire and asked these questions of women and men in Bamako, people who by virtue of living in the capital have contact with a new way of life.

The responses, which are analyzed in her thesis, show that though excision in the past was a puberty rite, by now more than a third of the people in her survey in Bamako had their girls excised before they were one year old. Most of the others were excised while small children long before puberty. The results from the questionnaires also show that most traditional rites connected with initiation have been abandoned by the people living in Bamako.

Most people in Bamako were unable to identify any positive social values of the operations. However, they are continued by traditionalists because "it is the custom". Though many seem to be aware of the damaging health results, custom is the most frequent justification given why the operations are done; religion is another reason that was often emphasized.

Typically, more men than women still attach social values to the operation. A majority of both men and women stated the operations are done for "hygienic reasons". Seventy percent of the women in the modern sector believe that excision makes childbirth easier. This shows that in Mali also, there is a great lack of health education and specifically education in reproduction, though methods of communication are plentiful and relatively inexpensive, and people can be reached by radio even in the remotest areas.

Diallo also states that most people she asked did not want to talk about excision, especially not women; and she often had to rephrase her questions to get replies. She adds that, "In the urban environment, excision has become a caricature. All socialization and education have disappeared, and the operation itself is often performed in the hospital." [15]

In March of 1979, on the return trip from the WHO Seminar in Khartoum, I visited with the midwives of the Gabriel Toure Hospital, the largest general hospital of Bamako. Male doctors do not take care of deliveries and only are called for help in special cases where surgery is needed, which is similar in all Moslem countries. The average number of births in Mali is nine per woman, but infant mortality is also one of the highest in the world.

The two midwives in charge, Madame Sy Sokoma and Madame Ly Mama, invited me to watch a delivery. There were no sheets, no linen at all, not even paper towels and no anesthesia is given. The young woman writhing on a table had no exterior genitalia at all; no clitoris, no small lips, and only the front part of the large lips were left.

It was a premature delivery of a tiny, malformed fetus. The woman was lying on her back with her street clothes pushed up, on a table covered with black oil cloth. A round bowl was pushed under her genitalia to catch the product of her labor. A midwife wearing rubber gloves told her when to push. There was nothing clean to wipe her off in the oppressive heat; she was sweating profusely, pushing and moaning. [16]

All the women who come to the hospital look like that, the midwife told me, pointing to her genitalia; nearly all of them are excised with nothing left of their exterior genitalia. In rural areas, girls are operated on usually at fourteen or fifteen years of age, in a group. They are married a month after they come out of seclusion - after the operation. In some areas one of the midwives said women are operated after their first baby to keep them faithful to their husbands, as polygamy is the rule. There is a special group of people who do the operations, it is an inherited trade. The midwives said: "The blacksmiths make the special knives for the operations; they operate on boys, their wives operate on girls." To be an excisor is an inherited trade that pays very well.

I asked about infibulation. The midwives explained that infibulation is not done by sewing or clamping, but the wounds, due to the extensive cutting, often grow together closing the vagina. Sometimes, the legs of the girls are tied together in order to create a closure of the vagina, as virginity in this Moslem society is very important. In some areas, cuts into the vagina are also added after excision. Episiotomies have to be done most of the time because the scars are so extensive.

In Bamako and in the cities, the operations are done on newborn babies because, the midwives said. "The younger one does it, the easier it heals". Some do the operations on children several years old, but most knowledgeable people do it to even younger girls as it is said that there is less risk of hemorrhage. One of the women who worked in the hospital lost two of her daughters as a result of the operations, the midwives said.

The women who deliver in the hospital have their daughters excised by traditional excisors as soon as they come home - often accidents happen and the babies get infections, the midwives told me. The hospital now has a traditional excisor on the premises who does the operations on the newborns when the parents demand it, as there is less danger of infection in the hospital and when something goes wrong there is somebody to help. [17]

The Moslem leaders in Mali claim that excision is a religious requirement - if a woman has a clitoris she is unclean and then her prayers are not accepted by Allah. Before praying, all men must wash - "perform their ablutions" - the midwives related. Similarly to be proper and clean, a girl must be excised. Virginity is highly prized among all ethnic groups but especially those who are Moslem.

Animists, the midwives informed me, say it is necessary to reduce a girl's sexual urge so she does not make any "mistakes". A woman who is excised behaves better; if a girl is not operated on before she is married, the husband says, "you are not a proper woman if you are not excised". In polygamous households - most men have several wives - the women who are excised often force the co-wives who are not operated to have the operation by teasing them and making their lives miserable. Girls who go to school are usually operated on during their vacations. And upon my questions the midwives said:

> "There are some excisors who have exceptional magic powers, they are able to operate without any bleeding at all. They are very much in demand. But the people who live in the northern part of the country do not excise their girls; the Songhai, the Moors, and those of Arab or Berber origin don't practice it. The Moors, the Peuls and the Saracole marry their girls very young. Sometimes women come to the hospital who are barely fourteen and already have several children." [18]

Rape, despite the fact that each man has several wives, is frequent; so is wife abuse. The hospital gets many cases of rape, as many women are badly injured. Some of the victims are only seven- or eight- year-old girls, or even younger. When a rape victim is brought to the hospital (most are not, unless they are too badly hurt), the parents may go to the police and press charges, but usually the rape is covered up because it may affect the parents' ability to find a husband for her.

The maternity also gets many cases of abused and injured women; many are pregnant and so badly beaten by their husbands that they have to be hospitalized. Polygamy, the midwives said, is one reason for wife abuse. There is great tension and rivalry between the wives in a polygamous family and there are frequent quarrels. The husband then beats all of his wives. A woman, even if she is badly injured by the husband and comes to the hospital, is reluctant to press charges because she is afraid of divorce. Divorce is very frequent; a man in this Moslem society can divorce a woman anytime - that is throw her out of the house and then get another one. Women are economically totally dependent on men. "We earn our own living", the midwives said; "we don't accept being beaten".

In the traditional animist society, men are not limited to four wives as their Moslem brothers are and can have many more - and some do. The traditional trousseau of a woman includes a leather strap, the instrument used to beat a wife. "A woman must kneel before her husband to receive chastisement from her husband, who beats her because he loves her", is the popular justification for wife abuse which is very widespread in Mali. It is also said (by men) that a woman who is beaten and maltreated will produce sons who will become "great men". The more a woman suffers, the better will be her children, it is claimed. And if a woman dies in childbirth, the people believe she will go to heaven - so the midwives said.

I asked about family planning, which has been recently introduced in Mali: all maternities give out contraceptives and teach women about birth control. The midwives replied, "All men are opposed to family planning. It is a scandal to use contraceptives, the men say. What else are women good for but to make children? If a woman is not pregnant, she will run around." And the midwives continued:

> "The men have to be taught if anything is to change! Men must be re-educated; they must be made conscious of the real role of women. Women must take part in the decisions in every area and must be actively involved in politics. The woman is the basis of the state and a stable government. The whole mentality of men must be changed. A man should have only one wife. At present, a woman who is not married is not respected, so men claim, because they want to dominate women.
>
> A woman has to ask permission of her husband for whatever she does; some men still demand that their wives be veiled; it is a matter of male pride so that only he can see her. He controls everything she does and even what clothes she wears. To change these conditions, you must educate the men; only then will things change."

"Not until women have a share in all the decisions will anything change in our society", the midwives claimed, "and change we must. It is not possible to just fight against excision or against polygamy or illiteracy - look what is happening. . . Women are needed everywhere and men must recognize the true position, worth and contributions of women. . . Without women being involved in decision making, we shall never be able to improve our lives. . . Everything must change and most of all men, who still think that they can own a woman. Polygamy must be abolished. It is an evil institution, it pits woman against woman and it creates suspicion and hate between children who live under constant pressure." [19]

Nowhere else in Africa have I heard the urgent need for change pressed so strongly; nowhere else did I find women so conscious, so critical and so aware of the needs of their own society. I stayed in the small office of the maternity wing in the Gabriel Toure Hospital for a long time, talking with different midwives who came and went, adding their ideas and eager to answer my questions.

At the Point G. Hospital, built with French assistance on the outskirts of Bamako, Madame Keita Fatimata, the midwife in charge, confirmed what the midwives at the City Hospital had said; Madame Fatimata was in her office on the second floor of the long maternity wing, surrounded by galleries that serve as corridors. As elsewhere in Africa, the families of the patients were camped on the grounds alongside the hospital buildings and were just preparing their morning meal. To get to the maternity, I had to pass by the Nursing School - most of the trainees are men. Nursing, as in other Moslem countries, is largely a male profession. The only female trainees are those who will become midwives or are planning to work in maternities.

Health care, as well as all other occupations in traditional Moslem countries such as Mali, is strictly segregated, starting with training. This usually results, especially in poor countries where the health budgets are very limited, in the least money being spent on mother and child health and maternity services. All this was clearly visible in the many hospitals in Africa which I saw and is confirmed by the staggering childbirth and infant mortality death rates, which are the highest in the world in Francophone West Africa, as is documented by the World Health Organization.

"All the women coming to this hospital are excised", Madame Fatimata said. "To say 'you are not excised' is a great insult. The women are constantly teased about this; therefore, they continue to do it to their children, mostly out of ignorance of the real consequences. A woman who is not operated on is not 'serieuse' - she is not considered to be a mature person", Madame Fatimata told me. [20]

"Many women have their vaginas almost closed", she added, "because after the operation, the legs of the girl are tied together or crossed so the two sides where the labia are cut adhere, closing the entrance to the vagina except for a tiny hole: this is done because of the importance attached to virginity. A bride must be cut open for intercourse and in childbirth this practice creates great problems in delivery. Our midwives are trained to do the necessary cuts."

The genital operations are done by the traditional birth attendants, usually on babies before they are 40 days old. Madame Fatimata informed me. The women cut the babies very quickly; they don't know what they are cutting. Often they do terrible damage. "A two-month old baby was brought in recently, bloated with urine; she was completely closed."

The women who come to the hospital to deliver get anti-tetanus shots. The babies, therefore, have some immunity when they are excised early. "In the rural areas where deliveries are at home and no shots are given, many baby girls die from exicision due to tetanus or infection or they bleed to death; but it is hushed up."

I asked if the operations are done here in the hospital. "No, I certainly don't permit that", Madame Fatimata firmly said.

As in other Moslem societies, tradition requires that on the marriage night, blood must flow; a bloody cloth or sheet must be shown in the village. If there is no blood, the mother of the girl is blamed and the honor of the father is irreparably damaged.

The Moslem religion teaches that a man should support his wives; in fact, as all the midwives confirmed again, most of the men do not. Women have no choice but to support their own children, mostly by trading in the towns or by their labor growing food in the rural areas. There also is a great deal of divorce. Each woman and her children are regarded as a separate family group. The husband goes from one wife to another and spends each night with a different one. Religion requires that all men and women be married, but many don't want to and this creates problems.

"Rape cases are also frequent at the Point G. Hospital", Madame Fatimata said in answer to my question concerning rape. "Many of the victims are children or very young."

This is the reality of the lives of women in this society, as described by the midwives, who are in a good position to know. Mali is one of the poorest countries in Africa, with growing food shortages and widespread malnutrition. Yet, up to 1965, the country was self-sufficient in food: since then, harvests have diminished while the population increases, and recurring droughts in the 1970s and 1980s have created enormous problems throughout West Africa.

In the middle of March 1979, when I visited Bamako, the city along the huge, slow-moving Niger River was enveloped in dust clouds that blotted out the scorching sun. Everything was dry and sandy; yet, wherever the river water touched the earth, bright green vegetation sprouted. Why is the water not used to grow vegetables along the wide flat riverbanks around Bamako? Surely they would sell easily in the city market, but no one I asked could answer that. Huge sand storms were reported throughout northern Mali, a frequent occurrence at that time of the year. The Sahara is slowly but relentlessly moving south covering more and more land with sand.

Added to the oppressive climate is the oppression created by the people who live under the inflexible rules of a medieval class and caste system that is utterly out of tune with modern life, and that opposes all change and denies the very concepts of personal achievement and economic development. Many of the people live on the edge of starvation much of the time. Women in this society bear the brunt of the social burdens of petrified, cruel customs that do not recognize a person as a person and an individual endowed with rights.

Yet, talking to the midwives in the hospitals of Bamako was a revelation: Seldom have I met women so conscious of the needs and worth of women and so realistic about the necessity for change. The midwives are forced every day in their work to deal with the terrible, physical mutilations that are imposed on all females by this patriarchal society where men oppose all change in order to preserve their traditional privileges and control. Without much contact with the rest of the world, the midwives of Bamako arrived at the same ideas and aspirations that are shared by feminists all over the world, indeed, by women from all societies. This is one great hope - despite the terrible revelations about the corruption and violence of men, that is documented in this report.

As the midwives said, "Change cannot be accomplished piecemeal. We must change our whole society - every part of it, and men must be made to recognize that nothing will get better until women take their rightful place and have a voice in all the decisions. . ."

But since these perceptive statements were made, which evaluate the situation not only in Mali but in most of the other African countries that are cited in this report, the economic situation in Mali has gotten worse. While in the past Islam was an accepted background of everyday life, it now has become an active escape from the hard reality. The call to prayer by the muezzin rings out over Bamako - broadcast by loudspeakers starting at dawn. And all over the city, one can see several times a day, men by the side of the road kneeling on their prayer mats, much like in Khartoum.

Bamako is overcrowded with immigrants from rural areas who squat on every available piece of land, and whole families with children can be found camping under the huge mango trees planted by the French many years ago at the side of all roads leading to the now terribly overcrowded bridge over the wide Niger River - the lifeline of the country.

The Gabriel Toure Hospital, the main hospital of the city, was in even worse shape in 1988 than when I had visited it before, and the maternity, predictably as in other African countries, is the most neglected area of all. Due to the stringent austerity measures by the World Bank/IMF (International Monetary Fund), all health care has been drastically cut - and as always what little there is for women is cut most of all. "We need everything," the director of the hospital told me, "We have no drugs, no instruments, no pharmaceuticals", and he gave me a long list of the most urgent needs for the maternity.[21]

One of the surgeons told me that the other day in the middle of an operation the electricity suddenly went off - and that was not the first time. Essential services are often disrupted due to a variety of reasons, most of them related to poverty. There were few nurses or midwives in the huge empty hospital hallways and open galleries built by the French many years ago, as the government is unable to pay their salaries.

The same is true of school teachers and so many schools and clinics, especially in rural areas, don't operate anymore. One can but wonder about the objectives of the international financial institutions - directed and financed by the US and Europe and the West - of depriving people of the most basic life-sustaining resources in order to force repayment of government debts, that were incurred by men who ran the country without representation of the people and who now have been removed from power.

Is it responsible for the men who run the World Bank/IMF to make women and children pay - often with their lives - for the loans these institutions made voluntarily to governments run by African men who took power by force, mismanaged their countries into deep debts. Many of them are gone - accused of corruption. Why did these international institutions support military dictators providing them with the means to oppress their own people - and many still do ? Why are women and children made to suffer to repay these ill-gotten loans made years ago without their knowledge or consent.

This situation is especially drastic in West Africa and Mali where women had no say in the governmental decisions that now victimize them most of all. By cutting back all investment to pay back past loans which forces the economy to shrink, these international financial institutions make sure that debtor countries will stay permanently in debt and dependent - as the only way to repay the huge debts is with an expanding economy.

The World Bank/IMF - who do not even maintain local offices but operate from Washington - oppress and squeeze the people and especially women in more devastating ways than any colonial power dared to do - with the collusion and as an arm of the United Nations. And health is always the area which is most affected: It is ironic that UNICEF - yet another agency of the United Nations - recently pointed out a dramatic increase in infant mortality especially in West Africa, which is most adversely affected by the World Bank/IMF "structural adjustment policies" - that is, the forced cutbacks of all government services (see "The Politics of FGM" and "Women and Health: Actions for Change").

It is ironic that in 1987 the World Bank held a "Safe Motherhood Conference" by organizing a midwinter safari for their staff to Nairobi's luxury hotels - to deplore the staggering and increasing maternal mortality rates for which their own policies are largely responsible. The damaging effects of these policies in West Africa I had occasion to see for myself in Mali and the other countries I visited in 1988 again. [22]

In Mali I contacted again all those concerned with women's health whom I had met before and tried to follow up on any actions organized to stop FGM or who were using our **Childbirth Picture Books** in French with the Additions to prevent Excision and Infibulation.

The government of Mali had already been invited in 1979 to send a delegation to Khartoum to the WHO Seminar on Traditional Practices Affecting the Health of Women and Children. Because of transportation problems due to drastic oil price increases at that time, they were unable to come. In 1985, the UNFM - the Union National des Femmes du Mali - the national women's organization supported by the government organized their own seminar inviting delegations from neighboring countries. [23]

Benin, Burkina Faso, Cote d'Ivoire, Guinea and Senegal sent participants and UNESCO as well as UNFPA (United Nations Population Fund) sent representatives. Besides excision, abortion, teenage pregnancy and infanticide were on the agenda. Both the Minister of Health and Minister of Social Affairs presided at this meeting and the Ministry of Public Health was also represented.

The seminar featured a report on a research project carried out in seven administrative districts as well as Bamako on the subjects discussed at the Conference. Excision which is a deeply anchored tradition in Mali, is also practiced by a large majority in all the other countries that sent delegations. Here are some of the findings:

> "In **Mali**, 60% of the people questioned were in favor of the practice; in **Benin**, excision is considered a rite of passage; in **Burkina Faso**, excision is considered to remove a male element from a woman, which also is dangerous for the child at the moment of birth and is a danger for the man during intercourse. Excision is deemed important for the faithfulness of wives as it reduces the sensibility of the woman and protects her virginity until marriage. In **Guinea**, excision is believed to purify women and has been practiced throughout the country for centuries. In **Cote d'Ivoire**, excision is considered important to integrate the girl into her traditional group."

The Seminar participants concluded that "despite the social and cultural considerations excision is a very damaging method to convince women of their inferiority. It is an attack on each woman's physical integrity, her freedom and capacity for development." The health effects and the terrible suffering resulting from excision were also discussed extensively and religion was debated again as it is still used locally by some religious leaders as incentive to continue this tradition.

> "In some countries, those who practice the operation claim that excision is a religious act introduced by Islam. However, the seminar established that in the participating countries, which are mostly Islamic, the Islamic scriptures reveal that excision is not obligatory. In fact, it was stated that research in **Mali** shows that in the most Islamized regions of the country, **Gao** and **Timbouctou,** excision does not exist."

Next, the seminar dealt with the medicalization of FGM in the modern sector.

> "It has been claimed that many lives can be saved by carrying out the operations in hygienic ways. However, this also opens the door to the institutionalization of this practice and, therefore, medicalization must be rejected."

Infibulation, which is also practiced in some areas of Mali, was vigorously condemned by all seminar participants who demanded its abolition wherever it exists. The other topics of the seminar - abortion, teenage pregnancy, and infanticide - were discussed next, and public education was recommended as a means to inform and educate people about these social problems. It was especially recommended that girls and divorced women should have access to family planning.

As with other seminars, recommendations were made. Indeed two commissions were organized, one specifically to work on excision, the other to deal with the other subjects of the seminar.

The seminar specifically recommended that those in leadership positions, especially religious leaders, should "demystify" the practice and that information campaigns should be organized. Some of the specific recommendations are:

> - "A large mass media information campaign to sensitize the population and to make people aware about the problems resulting from the practice
>
> - The seminar condemns the medicalization of the practice
>
> - The seminar appeals to all political authorities, as well as administrative and religious bodies and all other organizations to join this information campaign
>
> - The seminar condemns infibulation without reservation and demands that the competent authorities take measures to deal with its eradication." [24.]

The medicalization of FGM was specifically cited and condemned - which is especially important as this issue continues to be raised in many other parts of the world. Due to civil wars and political upheavals, more and more African families from countries where FGM is practiced go to live in Europe as well as North America and bring their customs along. In most of Europe and North America where these mutilations are classified as criminal child abuse, prevention and education programs have been initiated. (See "The Western World")

In the summer and autumn of 1992, the issue of medicalization was vehemently debated in the Netherlands due to a misguided proposal by health professionals to introduce FGM into hospitals (see "Health Facts and Overview" and "Women and Health"). It is significant that in this seminar in Mali - with participants of many other Francophone African countries - medicalization of FGM was thoroughly condemned and rejected by all the African participants, who by all definitions are most knowledgeable on the subject.

It is a fact, however, that in the Gabriel Toure Hospital in Bamako, as the midwives also readily reported, FGM was performed on newborn babies by an excisor who works in the hospital and operates on the newborn female infants by request of the parents. This, as the midwives explained, would reduce the large death toll due to uncontrolled bleeding which often results when blood vessels are severed and which cannot be repaired by traditional medicine. As the midwives stated, there is hardly a family group who has not lost a female child at some time due to excision. But records on deaths of newborns are not kept anywhere in Mali or most of Africa.

The UNFM, which organized the above seminar in 1985, also adopted the Action Plan of the Inter African Committee on Traditional Practices [25] which is an extension of the WHO (World Health Organization) Seminar of Khartoum recommendations and has been adopted by all their affiliates to provide guidelines for action.

The UNFM, which was government supported, was the only national women's organization and had set up a special committee on FGM. But with the change in government due to the recent elections, the UNFM no longer exists and instead numerous local women's groups are being organized as well as a National Council of Women (see below).

In1988 during my visit to Bamako I went to "Centre Djoliba" as I had been contacted by one of their Catholic sisters asking for copies of our **Childbirth Picture Books** (CBPB) to use as teaching materials for their program to stop FGM. [26] Women's International Network has sent many hundreds of the French CBPBs with the Additions to prevent Excision and Infibulation to Mali in support of this program and to distribute to the participants as well as to the midwifery schools to give to all their new graduates, most of whom go to work in rural areas. [27]

This program of the CentreDjoliba is run by Mme. Sidibe Kadidia, who herself is from Northern Mali where FGM is not practiced. Mme. Sidibe took me along to a meeting with local women on the outskirts of Bamako where she held one of her regular discussions and demonstrations on FGM by invitation of the local women. The meeting was held in the empty ground floor room of a house with a large porch - used for local meetings of all kinds. When we arrived with a small truck that was able to negotiate the very bumpy dirt roads, a large crowd of women was already assembled in the bare room.

The older women were wearing the local printed dresses, most of them with the traditional wrapped turbans as well as loose head scarfs, as is the custom of Moslems. A few of the younger ones were in sleeveless T-shirts and skirts as the heat was oppressive. The discussion on excision was in progress; our arrival was hardly noticed. Many women talked, especially the older ones, explaining why excision was practiced and why in their view it was necessary.

The women, most of whom spoke in Bambara, a few in French, talked about tradition. One claimed, "A woman has to be excised to be a woman - otherwise she is like a man." Another one stated that many women thought "You have to be excised to have children", but one added, "But now it is different - it is no longer necessary."

The religious argument was discussed at length. Is there a religious requirement? "The Koran does not say so." One woman said, "It is done because the clitoris is dirty." Another claimed, "It is done because the clitoris closes the vagina when the woman has sex with her husband." Yet, another one said, "It is done so that girls keep their virginity."

It is the Caste of the Forgeron - the Blacksmith Caste - that do the operations. The wives of the blacksmiths are usually the excisors, as they have access to sharp metal tools. This occupation is hereditary, as the caste system still prevails in Mali today.

Infibulation was also discussed. "It is done by closing the legs of the girl after excision and tying them together - then a scar forms and closes the vagina, showing that the girl is 'intact'". "If the girl is not operated, she will run after men" one woman stated. "That is why it is done."

Next, the discussion turned to where excision comes from and how it started. "It goes back to ancient times", the women said. "Ibrahim's first wife demanded that his second wife, whom he took to have children, must be excised because she was jealous. Thereafter, excision was practiced." The many children in the hot stuffy room were amazingly quiet. Some of the older ones were playing outside on the open porch of the room.

Then a nurse who had come with Mme. Sidibe explained the damage done and the difficulties that often result in childbirth due to the scars. "Did you not have problems" she asked the women, all of whom were excised. Some readily admitted it.

Finally, the leader of the meeting Mme. Sidibe stepped forward to provide some information. By then, a number of women had left and others had joined the meeting. There was an average of 50 women in the small room. Mme. Sidibe had a flip chart of flannel with movable parts in the form of female genital organs to visually demonstrate what happens as a result of excision and why bleeding occurs which is life threatening. Mme. Sidibe explained the medical facts in detail, answering many questions.

Then a three-dimensional model of the female genital organs was shown demonstrating what happens during childbirth. The model, donated to the program by the IAC, has movable parts and first shows the expulsion of a baby of a normal woman showing how the elastic tissues expand. Then an excised woman is shown and how her scars impede the birth and finally tear with much loss of blood.

The women in the audience were very quiet during this demonstration and said very little afterward, though everyone strained to see the model close up. The model clearly shows in three dimensions and, therefore, in a most effective way the problems, changes and damage resulting from FGM.

The meeting took a long time and many women who were there in the beginning, when all the advocates of FGM were heard, did not stay for the presentation of the models, showing the adverse effects, and the discussion by the nurse and Mme Sidibe. By giving the stage first to the very persuasive advocates of FGM, who furthermore have tradition on their side and are leaders in their communities, the views of those who support FGM were reinforced, especially for those who left before the second half of the presentation.

Though it is important to provide an exchange of views and to encourage all women to speak freely, by giving so much time especially at the beginning of the meeting, which set the tone, to the very eloquent promoters of FGM, this kind of program may not have the positive results anticipated. In all meetings on FGM or on any other damaging traditional practices, it is important to establish the objectives first. This can be done by outlining the ideas and facts that are to be communicated: The damage done by FGM and how to prevent it. By giving the stage to promoters and traditionalists first, especially in a local setting that reinforces such views, it may happen, as in this meeting, that the traditionalists who are very eloquent, take over and there is little time left to explain the real objectives.

Large numbers of Malian immigrants live in France, especially in the region around Paris and from time to time various French magazines write extensive articles on excision. The mutilations by now are well-known in France and the health damage is discussed each time and detailed. In addition, there have been several lawsuits by now against immigrants - parents and excisors - who continue to practice the mutilations in France. After three Malian baby girls died from the mutilations performed in France, the lawsuits were moved into criminal court. After several suspended sentences, the authorities finally had to incarcerate some African culprits: According to French law, FGM is criminal child abuse. The only program to prevent FGM in France is organized by a private women's group working with African immigrant women in the suburbs of Paris where most African immigrants, especially those from Mali, live. (See "The Western World").

The "Cooperation", the French international assistance agency, that is part of the government, has extensive programs in Fracophone Africa and other former French colonies. But the Cooperation has ignored FGM and has done nothing to support any local programs by African women in Mali or anywhere else in West Africa to stop FGM. Visits to French embassies in West Africa as well as to the offices of the Cooperation in Paris showed that there is no interest in the subject and very little interest in women's development in general. A meeting in Paris with the Cooperation after the third edition of this Report was translated and published in France by a well-known publisher produced no action, no interest and no preventive education programs on the part of anyone of the French Cooperation. [28]

Other international assistance programs, for instance the ones sponsored by the US Agency for International Development (US AID), have similarly ignored FGM, especially in Mali - despite many efforts on my part and despite the fact that USAID finances now a large family planning program in Mali. Neither UNICEF nor WHO - both have offices in Bamako - have made any effort over the years to initiate any education or prevention activities, though they have all the facts - as I established by visits to their offices in Bamako each time I was there.

The political change in March 1991 in Mali resulted, among other changes, in the abolishment of the UNFM (Union Nationale des Femmes due Mali), the government supported national women's organization that had adopted the IAC (Inter African Committee) Action Plan and had set up a committee to work on the issue. The IAC in their 1991 Activity Report states that in October 1991 an "Association pour le Suivi et l'Orientation des Pratiques Traditionnelles" was registerd as a nongovernmental organization and has been promised assistance by the new Minister of Health, Social Affairs and Status of Women as well as UNFPA (United Nations Population Fund.).

In 1991 a young Malian woman, Aminata, fled to Paris, as she had been thrown out by her family after refusing to be excised. This event managed to attract a great deal of attention by the international press. Though she is only one of many young girls who try to escape from these terrible traditions, most others are ignored. In African towns and capitals one can find many such unfortunate young women who escape from the brutalities of traditional village life and, cut off from all family support, have no choice but to support themselves as prostitutes. But none of them get to Paris.

Aminata, born in a village near Sikasso in the southeastern part of Mali, was sent to school in Bamako, where she lived with relatives. But when it became time to get married - her marriage had been arranged years ago by her father - she first had to be excised as tradition demands. In the area where her family lives, it is the custom to excise all girls just before they are married usually in their early teens - and none of them can escape.

Aminata's best friend had recently died from excision after suffering terribly for days. Therefore Aminata refused to undergo this torture after returning home to get married. Her father insisted and called in the Marabout, the local Moslem leader, to persuade her. But she still refused, went back to Bamako and finally fled to France with the help of a friend who was a stewardess at the airlines. All her relatives with whom she had lived while going to school in Bamako shunned her and she had no place to go.

In France with the help of some Malian immigrants, she found a lawyer, Linda Weil-Curiel, an expert on human rights. Weil-Curiel had argued several excision court cases and had established that FGM is not only a criminal offense according to French law but also an international human rights violation. Linda Weil-Curiel got Aminata's status as political refugee accepted so she can stay in France temporarily. Her case does not qualify under the Geneva Convention, but recently she was granted special permission to stay. [29]

The status of a daughter in Mali who is repudiated by her family in a country that recognizes no independent life for women outside the family means that no one will marry her or employ her, and she is cut off from all social and community life. The only way she can earn a living is by prostitution. She has no protection from anyone and can never return to her family or community. She is no longer regarded as a Moslem, as in her community the Moslem leaders claim that excision is a religious requirement. The same claim is made by the religious leaders all over West Africa, though it is not in the Koran. And in traditional communities religious leaders are all powerful.

But Aminata is lucky; she is in France and has found new friends and many supporters in her plight. She can look forward to a new life, certainly better than what was prescribed for her by her father, as one of several mutilated wives of a villager in a remote area of Mali, working from dawn to late at night to feed her many children.

Aminata is getting an education in Paris and she has become a cause celebre. It is her mother who is the real victim of this situation yet no one anywhere speaks for her. As the senior wife she has been thrown out by her husband who kept all her children. She has no place to go. It is the mother who is always blamed if a daughter does something "wrong" - that is, wrong from the view of the men who run this society. Women are used as slaves, with no rights of any kind, mutilated at an early age to make sure they are faithful and pliable.

The lives of the women in rural areas of Mali - one of the least populated regions of Africa - are regulated by traditions made by men for their sole benefit and practiced for as long as anyone can remember. Being female means you are subservient to men in all things, according to tradition. "You must kneel before your husband" so the midwives related. Your master - that is your husband or before him your father - literally has your life in his hands. If you don't please or serve your master according to his requirements, you can be put out of his house and no one will take you in and no one will help.

Life for the female half of these traditional societies is short, brutal and terribly hard. Most women die in childbirth or as a result of the relentless hard work, mutilations, lack of food and proper nourishment, lack of all education as well as constant abuse by men. That is the "female lot" - Allah knows best - so the all powerful Moslem men of Mali assert.

But the real result of these traditions that are vehemently defended by all men, because they will not give up any of their privileges or recognize that women have any rights, is that Mali is one of the poorest countries of the world. And Mali is steadily getting poorer, more isolated and ignored, dependent on handouts and quite unable to even feed itself.

Lest we are taken in by romantic accounts of traditional life and the stunning pictures in travel books or videotapes of colorful village life in Mali and the rest of West Africa, the reality is quite otherwise. It is claimed that slavery in West Africa, which was widely practiced by Africans in the areas where nomadic populations still abound, no longer exists. But the real question is: how is slavery defined?

If a human being is mutilated at an early age in such a way as to damage her normal physical and psychological functioning, creating recurring excruciating pain and programmed to work to the limit of her strength under constant threat of abuse - should that not be called slavery? And if a human being is cut off from all communication with the outside world, deprived of education and mobility, forbidden from owning anything while living in fear that her children may be taken away unless she serves her master's every wish - is that not a valid definition of slavery?

And that is still today the reality for too many women in Mali, in much of the rest of rural Africa and unfortunately also in other parts of our one world, a world of instant electronic communication and advanced technology that has quite forgotten these women or pretends they do not exist.

MALI: ECONOMIC/SOCIAL FACTS & SUMMARY

Mali: Seven regions.

Climate: Semi-tropical to arid, Savanna, Northern half of country is desert.

Population: 8 million. (80% rural). Bamako (capital), 800,000 (1986). Segou, 75,000. Annual Growth Rate: 2.7%. Majority famers and nomadic herders.

Life Expectancy: 47 years // Infant Mortality: 173/1000.

Government: Newly elected Democratic government took over June 1992 after 22 years of one man rule. National assembly (French model). Independence 1960.

Ethnic Groups: Mande (Bambara or Bamana, Malinke, Sarakole) 50% // Peul 17% // Voltaic 12% // Songhai 6% // Tuareg and Moor 5%.

Languages: French (Official) and Bambara (spoken by 80% of the population).

Religions Islam 90% // Indigenous 9% // Christian 1%.

Literacy: 10% (women less).

Education: Primary attendance, 21%. Secondary, 9%.

Annual/Capita Income: $200 (1987 estimate).

Economy: Growth Rate: 2.9% (1977-87). Inflation 4.4% (1987). Agriculture 50% of GDP. Industry 15%. Imports are more than double exports. Trade: cotton and cotton products, animals, fish, tannery products, ground nuts.

FOOTNOTES

1. Bazin-Tardieu, Danielle. **Femmes du Mali**. Editions Lemeac, Inc., Ottawa, Canada, 1975.
2. Ibid., p. 86.
3. Thiam, Awa. **La Parole aux Negresses**. Denoel, Paris, 1978, pp. 56-58.
4. Bazin-Tardieu, op. cit., p. 101.
5. **Sunjata**, March 1979. Published by the Information Service of Mali. (B.P. 141, Bamako, Mali) - excerpts translated from French. See also **WIN NEWS**, Vol. 5, No. 2, Spring 1979, p. 74.
6. Bazin-Tardieu, op. cit., p. 220.
7. Taoko, Jean G., Dr. "L'Excision: Base de la Stabilite Familiale ou Rite Cruel?" (Excision: Base of Family Stability or Cruel Rite?), **Famille et Developpement**, Spring 1975, Dakar, Senegal, p. 16.
8. **Famille et Developpement**, October 1975, Vol. 3. Letter from Minmin N'Ji Doumbia, Director of Elementary School of N'Gara-Segou (Bamako), Mali, in answer to Taoko article, printed in "Letter Column" (in French).
9. Thiam, op. cit., pp. 81-84, 94. See also **WIN NEWS**, Vol. 4, No.3, Summer 1978.
10. Ibid.
11. Ibid., p. 86.
12. Imperato, James, Dr. **African Folk Medicine: Practices and Beliefs of the Bambara and Other Peoples**. York Press, Inc., Baltimore, MD, 1977. See also **WIN NEWS**, Vol. 3, No. 3, Summer 1977, p. 25.
13. Diallo, Assitan. "Excision at the Bambara", Bamako Teachers' College Thesis, 1978.
14. Ibid., Chapter 2.
15. Ibid.
16. **WIN NEWS**, Vol. 5, No. 2, Spring 1979, p. 33.
17. Ibid.
18. Ibid., p. 34.
19. Ibid., pp. 9-10.
20. Ibid., p. 35.
21. Hosken, F. "Austerity's Human Toll: Why are international agencies ignoring the devastating human costs of World Bank and IMF cutbacks?" **The Humanist**, Jan./Feb. 1989, published by the American Humanist Association, 7 Harwood Drive, P.O. Box 146, Amherst, NY 14226-9982.
22. "Safe Motherhood" conference sponsored by the World Bank, 10-13 February 1987; and cosponsored by WHO (World Health Organization) and UNFPA (United Nations Population Fund). See **WIN NEWS**, Vol. 13, No. 2, Spring 1987, pp. 23-26. World Bank President, Barber Conable, at the conference promised to set up a fund for safe motherhood: To start it, he promised that the Bank would donate one million dollars. This fund never materialized, the one million dollars (for which the **NY Times** praised Conable in an editorial) vanished and Conable recently left the Bank. The one million dollars - as **WIN NEWS** computed - means less than 1/2 a cent per woman counting only those in the poorest countries with the most urgent need of health care.
23. Seminar by L'Union Nationale Des Femmes Du Mali (UNFM) on Excision, Abortion, Teenage Pregnancy and Infanticide, 21-25 January 1985, Bamako. See **WIN NEWS**, Vol. 11, No. 2, Spring 1985, pp. 38-39.
24. Ibid.
25. Inter African Committee (IAC) on Traditional Practices Affecting the Health of Women and Children, 147, rue de Lausanne, CH-1202 Geneva, Switzerland; c/o Economic Commission for Africa, ATRCW, P.O. Box 3001, Addis Ababa, Ethiopia.

FOOTNOTES: (continued)

26. Centre Djoliba, B.P. 298, Bamako, Mali. See also **WIN NEWS**, Vol. 14, No. 3, Summer 1988, p. 36.
27. **The Universal Childbirth Picture Book/Program** - "A Picture Story about Reproduction from a Woman's View" with Additions to prevent **Excision** and **Infibulation.** Published by **WIN NEWS**. Used in Africa on the grassroots level to teach about healthy reproduction and to stop FGM. Available in many languages. Free books are distributed to community health workers, midwives, teachers, etc., health and family planning programs, midwifery schools and others in Africa. These teaching materials are understood regardless of language or literacy and are sent free to women and men in Africa who write to **WIN NEWS** for the books. Each book contains a message asking the recipients to send a note, stating that their daughters will not be operated on, when writing for more books. For excerpts of letters received, see **WIN NEWS** - section on FGM or write to **WIN NEWS** for copies of letters and to sponsor distribution of books.
28. **LES MUTILATIONS SEXUELLES FEMININES** by Fran P. Hosken. **Denoel**, October 1983. EDITIONS DENOEL, 19, rue de l'Universite, 75007 Paris, France.
29. "Honte a toi, Aminata!". **Le Nouvel Observateur**, 14-20 March 1991. See also **WIN NEWS,** Vol. 17, No. 2, Spring 1991, p. 39.

CASE HISTORY : BURKINA FASO

Most of the population of Burkina Faso depends on subsistence farming and herding. In the past twenty years, this very poor, landlocked country was repeatedly hit by devastating droughts that decimated the herds and worsened the problems that face a subsistence economy dependent on rain. The Sahara is steadily advancing southward into the savannah region that covers the northern half of Burkina Faso. Even in Ouagadougou, the capital, which is located in the center of the country, dust and sand-laden clouds often obscure the broiling sun and make breathing difficult during the dry months of the year. The rain when it comes, often in short downpours cools the atmosphere only for brief intervals. As soon as the sun comes out, it is as hot as before. But with the rain come the mosquitoes that proliferate in all the puddles and open ditches by the side of the roads. The dry season starts in November, and the Hamadan - the hot, sand-laden desert wind - begins to blow in March. But when the rains don't come during the four-month wet season in summer, all is lost.

Most of the population lives in the southern part of the country; livestock, cotton and nuts are among the main products. Women do a substantial part of the subsistence farming. Many men leave the countryside in search of jobs mostly in neighboring Cote d'Ivoire or Ghana. Their families are left behind in the villages, dependent on what women can grow using traditional ways. Some population groups still follow their herds as they have for centuries with little contact with the rest of the world.

From an early age, girls must help with the housework and in the fields - very few ever go to school. Illiteracy is very high, more than 90 percent of the women cannot read or write, with the gap between men's and women's education steadily growing. The importance of women, who do a substantial part of the subsistence farming, has gone unrecognized by development experts who swarmed all over the country during the recent droughts, and so have women's needs.

The health statistics are dismal; infant and maternal mortality rates are among the highest in the world. No doubt the customs that dictate that practically all girls must be excised contribute to the poor health conditions of women. But until quite recently no one mentioned that.

The plight of women in this very traditional society, which strictly divides work according to sex - with women doing all the heavy household chores besides much of the food growing - was for the first time ever addressed in a UNESCO-assisted program, "Equal Access to Education for Women and Girls", which was started in 1967. This program not only was the first time a development program dealt with women and their education but it also continued for many years.

The French colonial system made little effort to reach the people with education; but in all the countries of West Africa, the French trained a small elite of men, mostly at French universities, to be able to fill administrative posts, while the vast majority remained untouched by education and modernization.

The education of women was neglected, except for a very few of the politically involved families. This is reflected in the education statistics today. Illiteracy in Francophone West Africa is the highest in the world, with the greatest gap between men and women, a fact that is also due, in part, to the Moslem influence.

For all these reasons the UNESCO program was especially important as it not only dealt with the obstacles women face to get an education and tried to deal with them but also tried to improve the socio-economic conditions of women in general. More and more villages opted to join the program, which had bcome known all over the country.

In Burkina Faso, which was called Upper Volta then, the US Agency for International Development (USAID) planned and implemented two of the most comprehensive development programs for women, as it was recognized that women held the key for the betterment of the rural economy. "Strengthening Women's Role in Development" was the first and larger program that started implementation in 1979 and was designed to help women subsistence farmers by developing a network of trained women agricultural extension agents throughout the country.

A revolving loan fund for women farmers was set up because all existing credit facilities refused to lend to women. In addition, technical services in agricultural production and subsistence farming, in home economics, in health and hygiene, as well as in functional literacy, were included in this program. The introduction of intermediary technology and labor-saving devices such as small mills for grinding millet, carts for transportation of firewood, and improved water supplies was a priority. "Training of Women in Sahel",[3] a similar program by USAID, was added later to cover the northernmost, dryest and poorest region of the country.

These innovative programs in rural areas were assisted by international governmental and non governmental organizations to reach women through an organized system of local women paraprofessionals (animatrices) and to introduce women to new ideas, new methods of agricultural production and new foods.[4] This in a society where the lives of the rural people have hardly changed for hundreds of years.

Both programs were among the largest women's programs ever developed by USAID and were designed to support the rural women directly in order to achieve economic development. Perhaps because the programs tried to do so much all at once and deal with too many problems, they failed. The implementation was overwhelmed by difficulties in the field and finally the programs had to be withdrawn. This was the first time that any programs tried to deal with women's needs directly and in a comprehensive way.

Health and hygiene were included, and midwifery training was one of the specifically cited skills to be taught. But there was no mention anywhere of excision, though it is practiced throughout the country, including by the Mossi - the dominant ethnic group. Female Genital Mutilation (FGM) does terrible permanent damage to women's health and is responsible for the highest maternal and infant mortality rates. The mutilations also have a debilitating effect on women's productiveness in essential subsistence farming.

A medical advisor who worked in Burkina Faso describes the traditional mutilations and what is done to the young girls - who have no way to escape this torture which is accompanied by all sorts of magic and witchcraft that still is widely believed:

> "The age at which excision is performed varies, but the girls are accepted for the operation as soon as they begin to grow pubic hair. No girl may refuse. The Wizard or Medicine Man of the village determines the date and the place of the operation (usually an area outside the village early in the morning). In order to prevent 'accidents' certain rites must be followed and sacrifices (chickens and lambs for instance) are made, and banishments against evil spirits are pronounced.
>
> The excisor digs a hole in the ground over which each girl must sit to be operated on. The girls are told they must not cry because this can cause the death of their mothers. The operation takes place with many women 'helpers' who shout as loud as they can - to cover up the screms of the victims."

A woman who witnessed one such a procedure in a village describes it as follows:

> "The operation consists of an incision made the length of the small lips up to the clitoris with the special knife of the excisor. A piece of wire is then hooked into the clitoris to pull it out completely and cut it off at its root. The girl is then forced to get up and made to jump twice over the hole which is full of blood and the pieces of flesh cut out of the girls. Afterward each girl is made to sit down and watch the others while they are operated on. The girls must then eat some millet while various ceremonies are performed. Then the girls are taken to a house where a woman applies to their wounds some ointment made of cinders and butter."[5]

In some areas itinerant excisors go from village to village to operate on the girls aged about 8-10 years - usually about six or more girls are operated on at a time - each girl is held down by several women so she cannot move.

> "After the operation the wound is washed with hot water and soap and then a salve of earth or cinders and butter is directly applied to stop the bleeding. The evening after the excision the operator applies a liquid made with several plants, and this treatment is repeated on the following days."

From a medical point of view, these dressings of earth, cinders and plants cannot stop the bleeding, and they greatly increase the chances of infection and tetanus. The only way to save a bleeding child is to take her as quickly as possible to a hospital to repair the injured blood vessels and for blood transfusions before shock sets in. Shock also results from the extreme pain. The aftercare is explained next - if the girl survives:

> "During the following two weeks or the convalescent period, a strict feeding schedule is observed - the excised girls are not allowed to eat meat or peanuts nor sesame or eggplant - all foods that are in the usual diet.
>
> When some girls die, either from hemorrhage or infection, this accident is variously interpreted: Mostly it is blamed on fate or on the presumption that certain customs have not been properly observed. But it is never the responsibility of the operator. During their convalescence, the girls are taught what they need to know as future wives and are given both sexual and social education. Most of all their absolute obedience to their husband is taught and that they are required to be faithful to him. They are also taught about medical plants and how to take care of the most frequent maladies and to consult the medicine man.
>
> At the end of 5 or 6 weeks, the girls who have survived go back to their village where a big festival is arranged: Many chickens and goats are slaughtered and eaten. The men celebrate the return of the girls who are promised to them as wives and who have now become 'real women' ready for marriage.
>
> According to women questioned, the psychological consequences of the operations represent a terrible ordeal in their lives, which they are forced to suffer under the threat of even worse punishments. No matter at what age the operation is performed, due to the traumatization of the sexual area and the removal of the clitoris, most or all sexual pleasure of the woman is eradicated. It can also happen that all sexual intercourse becomes very painful for a woman. For a man the sexual satisfaction from intercourse with an excised woman is less than with one not operated - as a result, he seeks other partners than his wife.
>
> Women remember the acute pain of the operation throughout their lives, and this memory is evoked with each sexual intercourse. Permanent psychosis may result from the torturous sex life." [6]

Very few women in the capital and towns have access to physicians. Midwives who know the reality and effects of excision in a country where all deliveries are handled by women describe the situation of women:

> "The girls are often married at seventeen, many have great pain during intercourse; but they hope to be free of this torment when they become pregnant. However, the birth process often creates worse problems and even greater agonies that the women are unable to face. So they become depressed and psychotic and lose their minds. One also encounters among the women who have access to the hospital services a number of suicide attempts.
>
> The means presently used to commit suicide are an overdose of anti-malaria drugs or barbiturates by the educated. In some villages some of the women try to electrocute themselves or use local methods. These suicides are frequently caused by the problems women have with their husbands, problems they cannot escape any other way. In the villages in Burkina Faso nothing has changed; most of the people have not been reached by education and the women are quite unconscious that any other way of life is possible for them." [7.]

In the towns - so the midwife relates - questions are beginning to be raised for instance in the schools about sex education. And she describes how some teachers call in physicians to answer the questions of teenagers. She cites a meeting of 13-and 14-year-old students where a lot of questions were asked about excision, but only the boys asked the doctor; the girls sat silent.

In Burkina Faso, as in other African countries where FGM is practiced, some people have their daughters mutilated in clinics and hospitals. Sterilized instruments are used and the wound is dressed according to modern methods with antitetanus shots and antibiotics given. All rituals are gone; no mystery surrounds these sexual castrations, which are very lucrative for the midwives or trained health workers, who do them.

The only purpose of women, according to this polygamous traditional society, is childbearing. Girls are married as early as possible and often promised long before reaching puberty. The brideprice is arranged between the male heads of the two families, which is a business transaction and as elsewhere in Africa represents an alliance between families. The young people, neither the groom nor the bride, are not consulted. Given the importance attached to childbearing, it is strange that the connection is never made between FGM and the many problems or death in childbirth or that the operations often result in infertility.

That obstructed labor - one frequent cause of death in childbirth - is the result of excision is not understood by any of the traditional societies that practice excision. Talking to trainers in health ministries, I found this is not understood even by trained health workers. Invariably the reaction of those who see the drawings of the effect of excision on childbirth in the **Childbirth Picture Books (CBPBs)** is one of amazement. [8] Though many of the traditional midwives and birth attendants may have great skill and experience in delivering, most of them have no knowledge of anatomy or comprehension of what causes infections. As a result their services often make birth even more hazardous.

Not only in Burkina Faso, but also in most traditional societies in Africa the belief in evil spirits and witchcraft, the evil eye and all other kinds of supernatural influences is pervasive and often has devastating results for health.

In 1977, when I first visited Ouagadougou, I went to the maternity at the Yalgado Hospital to talk to its director, Dr. Joseph Kabore, a gynecologist. He reconfirmed from his experience all what is stated above. Dr. Kabore asked me to meet him very early in the morning at the hospital. The maternity is in a separate wing. The relatives of the hospital patients usually camp outside in the yard of the hospitals where they also prepare their meals, as they often are a long way from home. When I arrived at the hospital, several families were just beginning to cook breakfast over some open fires on the ground.

Dr. Kabore was in a small office opposite the entrance door. He invited me to ask him anything I wanted to know.

> **FPH:** "My first question is, what is the health situation of women now, and what do you suggest should be done concerning excision?"
>
> **Dr. Kabore:** "Excision is practiced universally because it is the custom. Almost all women who come to this maternity are excised, usually all external genitalia are cut off. Frequently the size of the opening to the vagina is drastically reduced by the scars - creating many health problems.
>
> Last year, we did a radio campaign against excision on Radio Rurale, Ouagadougou. I spoke about the medical and health aspects; Lale Naba, the Chief of the Province, spoke in Mossi, the local language, about the customs; and the religious aspects were discussed by a Catholic priest. We explained the reasons why excision is dangerous and should not be done from our points of view and experience. We got lots of letters. You can see them; they are still at the radio station."
>
> **FPH:** "What about the Moslem leaders? A large part of the population after all is Moslem. Did a Moslem leader join your talk?"
>
> **Dr. Kabore:** "No. The Moslem leadership supports this practice. Many Marabouts advocate it, and say it is necessary and a religious prescription."

FPH: "How old are the girls when they are operated?"

Dr. Kabore: "In the towns, especially here in Ouagadougou, it is done to very young children, sometimes only a few months old. The parents know if they wait until the girls reach puberty, they will refuse. In the bush, it is done at puberty, as initiation. After the operation, earth and dirt are put on the wound to stop bleeding. This guarantees infection, but the bleeding continues. A girl was brought in just a few days ago, she had to have several blood transfusions, she had lost so much blood. But most children are never brought to the hospitals.

There are many other problems. I get girls who cannot urinate; and there are other complications. Although the girls are not sewn up or deliberately closed, the wound frequently adheres and closes most of the vagina. Some women cannot have intercourse. One husband brought his wife - he was her third husband - because he could not have intercourse with her as she was almost completely closed. Both the other men had sent her back to her parents."

FPH: "What are the results in childbirth?"

Dr. Kabore: "There are many women who conceive even through a tiny opening. The scars obstruct childbirth. The women cannot give birth normally. They need two episiotomies; that is, they have to be cut open in front and back of the vagina because they cannot dilate. Without help, they die in childbirth as well as the baby. Vaginal fistulae - that is, ruptures of the vagina - are another frequent result." [9.]

The maternity is a long, two-story building with a concrete floor and a dark corridor running the length of the building with cubicles on both sides. There are open shower rooms next to the entrance. The midwife in charge of the delivery room came to call the doctor. A woman about to have a child had been brought in during the night. She had not yet delivered, so the doctor took me to see her. The woman - this was her first baby and she was very young - was lying on her back on a table, completely naked, with an enormous belly.

It was plain to see why she had not delivered: Her vagina was closed. A small incision made by the midwife evidently had not helped. She did not seem in pain but was frightened. She had no external genitalia at all. There was a solid bridge of skin between her legs, except for the small cut recently made, much too small to allow the baby to emerge. The doctor spoke to the midwife, and told me that he might have to do an extensive episiotomy or even a casarean if she could not give birth any other way.

Back in his office, I asked the doctor: "What do you suggest should be done to persuade people to stop these operations?"

Dr. Kabore: "The problem is the people are completely steeped in traditions; but we are now beginning to have schools also in the bush. After the radio talk, I got some threatening letters; we need legislation so we can speak for change without being threatened. If we have the law behind us, it is another matter.One campaign like the radio speeches does not help; it needs a continuous educational effort.

For instance, it was forbidden by law to put tribal marks on the face. Tribal marks are scars, another form of mutilation. Not all people did it. The parents decide. Now they have stopped it as a result of the legislation. We need similar legislation about excision; that is the first step. Then, we need to have an education campaign with explanations concerning health, andwith visual aids because most people cannot read. First, a record should be made with photographs to show the problems visually and explain also to the men what the results are of these operations. Then the Minister of Health and Minister of Social Affairs should be involved to develop the legislation." [10.]

The midwife called Dr. Kabore; she needed his help in the delivery room. The young mother-to-be was going into labor now. Dr. Kabore left with the midwife. From the dark bare concrete building, I went out into the bright morning sun. A group of children, girls and boys, were running about and playing happily together under the large tropical trees, carefree and enjoying themselves. I stopped to watch their fun. What, I wondered, could possibly compel people to so grieviously torture and mutilate their own children, and why? Why inflict this needless suffering and pain on their own young?

Two years later in 1979, on the return trip from the WHO Seminar, I stopped again in Ouagadougou and visited with Dr. Kabore. Nothing had changed, he told me when we met once more at the maternity. Dr. Kabore still wants to do a multimedia education program teaching about health and showing the damage done by excision. But this takes money, and in Burkina Faso as elsewhere in Africa there are other priorities.

In an article on excision published in **Famille et Developpement** [11], written by Dr. Jean Taoko of the Yalgado Hospital in Ouagadougou, he describes the situation in this country and provides an insight into the local customs and beliefs.

Dr. Taoko relates that among the Mossi, the largest and dominant population group, it is believed that a woman who is not excised is unable to have children as the clitoris is a dangerous organ which kills a baby at birth; and it is also believed that the clitoris can cause impotence in men. The parents see to it that all their daughters are excised: The operations are obligatory.

Dr. Taoko adds that among the Bambara who live in this region and other ethnic groups as well, it is claimed that a man who has sexual intercourse with a woman who is not excised risks death because the clitoris, like a dart, will sting him. And Dr. Taoko also relates that the reason why only women do the operations is that when a male circumcisor first did the operation on a woman, he became blind. Since then, only women can operate on girls. Circumcision of boys is one of the most ancient trades inherited from father to son; male circumcision is obligatory among almost all animists in Africa and a traditional rite universally observed. It is an absolute command by Allah, according to Mohammed, his Prophet.

The actual date and time of the operation, Dr. Taoko states, is set according to the wishes of "higher powers", made known through the village chief. Usually some sacrifices are made to prevent accidents and prevent any evil magic by enemies. "The most favorable day for the operations is usually Saturday", states Dr. Taoko.

> "The operations traditionally take place outside of the village under a tree. A variety of instruments is used, including razors and knives. Usually the clitoris and the small lips are cut. Sometimes the operations are very radical, with terrible consequences for the girl." [12]

The women who help with the operations must themselves have been excised in the past: They shout and make a great deal of noise during the operations to cover up the screams of the girls who are supposed to bear their terrible torture without making a sound.

Dr. Taoko answered some of my questions from his research and his clinical experience as a physician in the Yalgado Hospital:

> **FPH**: "What reasons do the people give for continuing these operations?"
>
> **Dr. Taoko**: "Tradition is one of the most frequent answers. People say because it always has been done! Objective reasons are added such as it controls the sexuality of women, and they are, therefore, faithful to their husband. The practice is correlated with polygamy. Keeping virginity until marriage is another reason both parents and bridegrooms are interested in."
>
> **FPH**: "What are the results on women's health from your experience in the hospital?"
>
> **Dr. Taoko**: "In my practice, I have had the occasion to encounter numerous haemorrhages; also difficulties in childbirth, the death of the fetus, and many infections, the worst of which is tetanus. Then there are the psychological and social consequences for the young women involved. Once they become familiar with modern life, they understand that they have been victims of a brutal mutilation and everybody knows it. . ."
>
> **FPH**: "Does the Health Department take notice of these practices? Is anything done to educate families about health care and the biological facts of reproduction?"
>
> **Dr. Taoko**: "The Health Department is interested in these problems, but it must be stated that it is not their priority. . . Women's organizations are campaigning against this practice. But I am not optimistic because alone, they cannot manage an education campaign in the rural areas. They need active support by men.

As far as I am concerned, an information and health education campaign is necessary. The suppression of excision comes under the heading of preventive health care. Though this is the work of women, the participation of men cannot be neglected. These customs are continued due to the jealousy of men and their insistence on following customs."

FPH: "Is the government making any attempt to prohibit these operations?"

Dr. Taoko: "It would be necessary to have a large information and education campaign first to get such legislation accepted: It might be successful if the many accidents of the operations are publicized. The government, the women's organizations, health professionals including myself, and others battling against the practice are convinced education is needed. It must be said that reproductive and sex education is very limited, especially as far as young people are concerned because of the educators and the limited materials that are available to young people. There are too few people able to deal with such a task.

FPH: "Are those operations now also practiced in the cities, and do educated men demand the operations for marriage?"

Dr. Taoko: "Yes, excision is also practiced in the cities. . . The ceremonial part of the initiation has been abandoned; however, the physical operations continue. Today, few educated parents accept the responsibility to send their daughters to be excised; however, they do not oppose it and in fact, they often suggest it. There is a great deal of hypocrisy about this practice. Educated men fail to raise their voices to refuse or to suppress the practice. In the public health sector as well as the hospitals, the practice is opposed; but the problem is not a priority.

I want to emphasize that excision is just one of many problems that we face in the medical and politcal world. . . You must realize that complications due to excision comprise several hundred cases a year that come to the hospital; but we have to deal with many diseases, malnutrition, and parasites that kill thousands of people every year. We are confronted every day with a great many problems in public health that are often overwhelming." [13.]

This unfortunately is the same answer that many other thoughtful health officials give. So far in Burkina Faso only a tiny fraction of girls and women who suffer and die from the operations seek help in the hospitals; hence the caseload is low. In the vast rural areas there is little medical assistance available and tradition often forbids that help in the modern sector is sought. But why add man-made problems to the many health hazards that abound in the African environment and that are costly and difficult to treat? Why not concentrate on eliminating the man-made mutilations that everyone knows must be stopped before any real development can start. Yes, it is a question of priorities; but what affects the life and health of every family must come first!

While in Ouagadougou in 1979, I also went to the Ministry of Health to see the WHO (World Health Organization) representative to tell him about the WHO Seminar Recommendations formulated in Khartoum which had not reached him yet via the bureaucratic route. Dr. Martin Samos, the WHO representative at that time, asked his local assistant to join our meeting. Mr. Paul Halidou Ouedraogo, a Mossi, explained that excision was universally practiced among his ethnic group. He added that he and some like-minded young families - all the men were working for the government - are refusing to submit their children to excision, which is done by the urban population at a much younger age than in the rural areas. "We refuse to have our girls excised", he said. "But the problem is the grandparents. They will not change."

"Many girls are excised when they visit their grandparents in the village. This has happened to some of my friends", Mr. Ouedraogo related. "But I have solved this problem", he said. "You know with us here in Burkina Faso all the decisions are made by men. I tell my wife what to do." Mr. Ouedraogo had told his wife that if something happens to their daughters when she visits her family or her in-laws, then he will hold her responsible. "I told my wife if she does not watch the children and the girls are excised, I don't want to see her or the girls ever again."

With this threat, Mr. Ouedraogo may have solved his personal family problems, but this does not change the problems of his society.

There are more young couples now in the capital, according to Mr. Ouedraogo, who refuse to excise their children; but they are still very few. "Old people cannot change", he insisted, "that is hopeless. They stick to the customs no matter what." [14]

From conversations with many other health officials, present-day conditions became clear; in the villages, nothing has changed. The people accept traditions because that is all they know. The women are overwhelmed by the demands of the daily work and the needs of their children - they have no time to think about their lives and they have no control over what is done to them. They have little contact with the outside world and no access to education. The daily struggle to survive is still all consuming, dominated by traditions that put women last with no rights over their own bodies or lives and no room or time for change.

That is why the two women's programs described above were so important; they addressed some very basic needs such as access to credit, which is essential to women farmers to improve agricultural production, and access to basic resources especially land ownership, which women are still denied. But the programs evidently tried to do too much too fast in this very traditional environment.

When I visited again in 1988, Burkina Faso had emerged from devastating droughts, from drastic changes of government as well as changing its name from Upper Volta to its present one. But the status of women had not changed, except for the few in Ouagadougou working for the government.

At the maternity of the greatly enlarged Yalgado Hospital, nothing had changed. The old gray concrete building was much the same except that there were women waiting in line in front of every door. I met the midwife in charge who took time from her very busy schedule to talk to me. I showed her the French edition of our **Childbirth Picture Books** - we have sent many hundreds of them every year to the midwifery school and for the training programs of the Health Ministry. Mme Traore, the midwife, who had a long line of patients waiting, agreed to meet with me later that day.

Midwives in Burkina Faso, and indeed in most of the rest of Africa, are in charge of women's health and especially all matters relating to childbirth. Midwives handle practically all deliveries, except where major surgery is required. In West Africa, except in strict Moslem areas for instance in northern Nigeria or Mali, women are not prevented from being treated by male physicians as they were traditionally in the Sudan. Midwives enjoy great respect in their communities, and in the maternity hospitals they are in charge and responsible for all deliveries as well as treatment of maternity patients.

The conversation with Mme. Traore covered many issues. Almost all women who come to the Yalgado maternity are excised - some in drastic ways. More and more women in Ouagadougou are seeking help in the hospital while in the past they went to traditional midwives and healers. The maternity is desperately short of equipment and drugs due to the austerity measures imposed by the World Bank/IMF (International Monetary Fund). Under threat of canceling all present and future loans by the WB/IMF, the government is forced to cut back in all areas . Education and health care - especially maternity services - are cut back most, as women lack political power.

Practically all health services and hospitals are run and financed by the government. For the many women who are now seeking modern health services in Ouagadougou and other towns, there is less help available in the publicly financed modern health sector due to demands by the WB/IMF to pay back loans made by past governments. [15]

Mme. Traore, who as a midwife worked every day at the hospital, told me she had three children - two girls and a boy ages 12, 10 and 8 - whom she supported alone. Her husband who had worked for the government for 15 years had died the year before in a car accident on a trip related to his work. But surely, as widow of a government employee she was entitled to a pension or insurance, I asked. It turned out that according to traditions, that are apparently still very much in force, her husband's family took everything her husband owned and threw her and her children out of their house.

The family claimed her and her husband's house and everything in it, including all his papers and documents. Without these, she could not claim government support. This since she had refused to marry the man in her husband's family, whom the elders had picked out for her. According to tradition still observed even in the capital, a widow has no right to anything - even her children. But in the city, children, who are an asset as agricultural labor in rural areas, have become a burden. Hence the family elders got rid of them.

> "If I tried to oppose my husband's family, this would not be well regarded and people would make life impossible for me and my children. I do not know how I shall manage and pay for the schooling of the children; the family took everything. They don't care what happens to the children - now that I refused to accept the man they decided I must live with." [16]

Mme. Traore is now living with her parents' family which is headed by her younger brother, as her father is dead. But the young man is afraid to speak for her or make demands on the family of her husband. He wants no trouble with the powerful elders of her husband's family. She knows her rights, but the social pressure is too great, and as a widow she has no one to speak for her. She cannot go to court, as there is no modern family law to protect her from these African traditions that make women into property owned and disposed of by men.

Such family action is accepted as quite normal - women are not persons in this traditional society - and similar traditions still prevail in most of sub-Saharan African rural areas. As a direct result, African countries are sinking into ever greater poverty, as all international economic statistics show. Though the present government of Burkina Faso has set out on a course of modernization, family legislation has lagged and was passed only quite recently. But experience shows that there is a great deal of difference between legislation and practice or implementation.

Mme. Traore as a midwife fortunately has a profession that enables her to earn a living, but to earn enough to bring up and educate three children is very difficult. She also is a Christian and a Catholic. But the local Catholic parish to which she belongs did nothing to help her and her children or protect her rights against the greedy family or the marriage which the elders tried to force on her.

In the capital, educated women are aware that there are alternatives and that women have rights. But they are unable to assert them against the terrible burden of tradition and the heavy hand of patriarchy. In rural areas women are treated like the property of men whose land they must work and whose children they must bear and raise.

The idea that women have any rights is still quite foreign to the thinking of this society where the majority of families depend on subsistence farming. Some families are supplemented by the limited wages earned by men who work in neighboring countries since they can't earn any money at home. But women have no way to earn anything at all and are overburdened by heavy labor - serving their families. Development programs financed from abroad mostly ignore women. Development experts from overseas talk to the men in the ministries in Ouagadougou and tell them "African traditions must be preserved". But tradition and development are mutually exclusive: They go in opposite directions. As a result, most development programs fail.

In May of 1988, a national seminar on "Traditional Practices Affecting the Health of Women: The Case of Excision and Proposals for Elimination" was held in Ouagadougou, sponsored by Action Sociale, a ministry of the government that then was headed by Secretary of State, Alice Tiendrebeogo. In 1979, Alice Tiendrebeogo was the lone participant from Francophone West Africa at the WHO Seminar in Khartoum - which she attended as an observer. She headed the National Women's Organization of what then was Upper Volta. and even then was working for the eradication of FGM.

The 1988 three-day conference included delegates from all over the country. It was held in three local languages besides French in order to reach as many people as possible. Posters, leaflets in different languages as well as radio programs took the information all over the country. The conference was organized to develop a campaign and raise the consciousness of participants: They were encouraged to spread what they had learned all over the country and to help organize a national network to stop excision.

> "In order to abolish this practice, active opposition has to be organized and everyone must be made to understand that excision is bad for women, bad for families, and bad for society.
>
> It is important to involve everyone, women and men, grandparents, and all other family members, to start discussions in villages and urban centers. Women especially must make the men of their families aware of the suffering involved.
>
> This will be a long and extensive battle that requires tenacity and continuous actions to break through the indifference. . ."[17]

Specific strategies were outlined and agreed on by the conference participants. They urge all concerned people to:

- Mobilize all forces and resources that can be useful in the abolition of practices that damage the health of women and invite religious authorities to participate in actions against damaging practices.
- Propose legislation and specific measures to stop excision.
- Develop research studies and assure follow-up of all actions started.
- Organize and institute provincial committees and develop all kinds of information and education programs.
- Introduce the subject of excision into national education programs and schools as well as women's health and sex education.
- Initiate the printing of educational materials and use television, radio, film programs and all other media as well as involve the talents of writers, poets, etc.

The provincial committees that participated in the conference all were instructed to follow similar actions. The campaign is supported by the government as there are no private organizations able to undertake such comprehensive national initiatives which require the active participation of all governmental bodies.

This conference took place almost at the same time as the one in Mogadishu, Somalia (see Case History : Somalia), which similarly was a broadly based, government supported initiative held at the Somalian Parliament. However the seminar in Somalia had financing and organizational support from Italy and AIDoS - the Italian Association for Women in Development. (See Case History : Somalia.) The conference in Ouagadougou depended on local efforts and had little or no support from France or the French government or French women's organizations and the same goes for the campaign.

The French government has failed to show any concern or provide any assistance for programs to eradicate FGM anywhere in Francophone Africa. France ignored FGM and the needs of women when they administered West Africa as governing colonial power. The extensive development programs currently financed by France in all their former colonies similarly fail to support women's programs and continue to ignore the existence of FGM - though it now has been brought to France by African immigrants. (See: "The Western World")

While extensive research on FGM was sponsored in East Africa under the British colonial system and many attempts were made to curtail or stop FGM - for instance in Sudan and Kenya (see: Case Histories) - the French completely ignored the damage done to women's health. There are no clinical or any other medical or health studies by French physicians, except for a recent survey by a woman-doctor; and there are no medical publications on FGM by French trained African professionals. The French health system which was introduced in West Africa under the French colonial regime, has resulted in the highest maternal and infant mortality rates anywhere in the world at the present time.

The support of all traditions by French anthropologists has led to the perpetuation of FGM and the disenfranchisement of women in Francophone Africa, for instance in Burkina Faso, as the story of the midwife above confirms. The highest illiteracy among women - recorded by UNESCO - is in West Africa; this must be attributed to the French colonial system and French institutions introduced into West Africa. The governments of Burkina Faso since the 1983 revolution are strongly committed to the eradication of FGM. But they lack the necessary financial support and financial means to implement change.

In autumn 1989, a 72-minute film "My Daughter Will Not Be Excised" [18] was launched in Ouagadougou by the Minister of Information and Culture together with the Secretary of State of Action Sociale, under whose guidance the film was made, together with the Committee on the Eradication of Excision. The film made in the rural areas of Burkina Faso is also available in Europe. Its main purpose is to persuade the people in Burkina Faso to stop these damaging traditions by creating an awareness of the physical and moral consequences of the mutilations - raising questions among the audience about the problems in their own environment. It is used to start the discussion at meetings all over the country and as a basis for education.

Given the strained economic conditions worsened by the World Bank imposed, austerity as well as the constant threat of drought, it is difficult to organize and finance the kind of national campaign that is needed to eradicate FGM. Literacy is essential for change and for contact with the world outside the village in order to introduce new ideas to replace damaging traditions. While the government leadership is committed to change, the village chiefs and local leaders must be persuaded, and that is a formidable task.

In spring of 1991, the United Nations Center of Human Rights held a regional seminar on "Traditional Practices Affecting the Health of Women and Children" that discussed excision as well as other damaging traditions. Representatives from other African countries participated including Benin, Cameroon, Central African Republic, Chad, Cote d'Ivoire, Ethiopia, Gambia, Ghana, Guinea, Kenya, Mali, Mauritania, Nigeria and Senegal. The objective of the seminar was to assess the human rights implications of FGM, son preference and traditional birth practices that often damage both mothers and children.

The participants, sent by the governments from the different countries, described conditions and research on FGM in their countries; but the seminar did not report on any grass-roots or action programs. Most participants agreed that while FGM was declining in urban areas, there is little change in villages - as has been observed in Burkina Faso. It was also noted that health personnel including physicians, midwives and nurses were performing the mutilations in hospitals or homes for financial reasons and that greed was one factor behind the continuation of the practice in the modern sector.

Discussions and research on FGM have become increasingly "accepted" at international meetings since the subject was introduced by WHO in Khartoum in 1979. Until then, total silence prevailed. While such conference discussions certainly are effective in spreading information on FGM among those working at United Nations agencies and governments or international organizations, they have not resulted in effective actions for change on the grass-roots level where real change must be implemented. Burkina Faso certainly is an example. Though the government supports change, neither United Nations agencies nor international development organizations have so far been ready to effectively support what is needed to implement this important campaign that could set a precedent.

It is easy to talk about FGM at international meetings but to effectively work for change on the grass-roots level over many years is quite another matter. In Somalia a national effort was initiated which now has been wiped out. In Burkina Faso the national education effort to stop FGM has a program and governmental support, though it faces great problems such as lack of infrastructure, lack of transportation and communication as well as illiteracy in rural areas and a very difficult climate.

More extensive distribution of visual teaching materials such as the **Childbirth Picture Books-CBPBs,** which are already widely used by the health department in Burkina Faso, may be helpful and have been offered to the campaign. For several years **CBPBs** have been sent to the midwifery school in large enough numbers so that each trainee can get some copies to take along upon graduation to use with the families and women she serves. Experience with the **CBPBs** shows that they are understood with very little explanation, they do not require literacy since the drawings speak for themselves.

Many changes have taken place recently - such as the passage of a new family law which came in force in August 1990. It applies to all people and does away with the dual system of traditional law and modern law. It makes brideprice illegal, gives women equal rights in marriage and equal jurisdiction over children - the interests of children coming first.

Family planning as national policy was adopted already in 1986 and is gradually being implemented all over the country. The Ministry of Basic Education is implementing literacy campaigns. Major political changes also are taking place. The military government has relinquished power, and the former head of the military government has been elected president and is continuing his work for changing this very traditional society and country to improve the standard of living and health.

The National Committee against Excision headed by Mme. Mariam Lamizana [20] is coordinating the activities of the provincial committees - but the problem is financing. A budget has been developed for the next several years covering educational materials as well as training. Indeed the official documents speak about a "revolution for the liberation of women" - which is very unusual language for an African country. In the program various money-making activities for women are included to strengthen women's economic base and to enable them to claim their rights, which the new family law provides.

According to the report submitted to the United Nations Committee on the Elimination of Discrimination Against Women by the government - that is the Ministry of Health, the Secretariat of the Action Sociale and Directorate of the Promotion de la Famille, numerous initiatives on behalf of women have been organized by the government. [21] The activities of the National Committee Against Excision are outlined, including radio programs that are broadcast all over the country and many other information and education actions. These activities also include meetings all over the country showing the film "My Daughter Will Not Be Excised" (see above), which was made specifically to use at such occasions to raise the consciousness of rural decision makers.

A training program of more than 500 traditional birth attendants as well as hundreds of community workers organized by Action Sociale is also cited. The National Committee collaborates with the IAC (Inter African Committee on Traditional Practices Affecting the Health of Women and Children), which works throughout Africa on the eradication of FGM and is developing various programs to inform, sensitize and educate the people. Support of international agencies such as UNICEF, UNFPA and UNESCO has been sought. It is clear that there is not only a committment for change on the part of the government but numerous actions have been initiated and plans have been developed to guide such activities.

The question now is who will assist these plans, who among the international community of donor agencies and especially the many international non governmental organizations will assist this campaign with cash and resources? FGM has been discussed on an international level now since 1979, when the issue was first brought up at the Khartoum Seminar which opened the problem not only for discussion but also for action. In Burkina Faso the government has done everything possible to provide a framework and plan for such action. But where are the donors and where are the agencies, both governmental and private - to provide the urgently necessary support for this initiative that could change the whole country and set an example for all of Africa? WHERE ARE THEY?

FOOTNOTES

1. UNESCO Project "Egalite d'access des femmes et des jeunes filles a l'education" (1967-1976). Report available from: United Nations Development Programme, B.P. 575, Ouagadougou, Burkina Faso.
2. For a description of the "Strengthening Women's Role in Development (SWID) Project" see **WIN NEWS**, Vol. 4, No. 2, Spring 1978, pp. 61-63, and **WIN NEWS**, Vol. 5, No. 2, Spring 1979, p. 32. Program Plan: U.S. Agency for International Development, c/o U.S. Embassy, B.P. 35, Ouagadougou, Burkina Faso.
3. For a description of the "Training of Women in Sahel (TWIS) Project," see **WIN NEWS**, Vol. 5, No. 2, Spring 1979, p. 32. Program Plan: U.S. Agency for International Development, c/o U.S. Embassy, B.P. 35, Ouagadougou, Burkina Faso.
4. Taylor, Ellen. **Women Paraprofessionals in Upper Volta's Rural Development,** published by the Rural Development Committee, Center for International Studies, Cornell University (New York), 1981.
5. See **WIN NEWS**, Vol. 5, No. 3, Summer 1979, pp. 29-30.
6. Ibid., p. 29.
7. Ibid., p. 30.
8. Hosken, Fran P. **The Childbirth Picture Book**/Program - "A picture story of reproduction from a woman's view", pictures by Marcia L. Williams. Published by **WIN NEWS**, 187 Grant St., Lexington, MA 02173. USA. Books, flipcharts, color slides in English, French, Spanish, Arabic. Additions to prevent excision and infibulation.
9. Author's interview with Dr. Joseph Kabore, Chief of Maternity at Yalgado Hospital, Ouagadougou, Burkina Faso, See **WIN NEWS**, Vol. 3, No. 2, Spring 1977, p. 40.
10. Ibid.
11. Taoko, Jean, M.D., "L'excision: Base de la Stabilite Familiale ou Rite Cruel? (Excision: Basis of Family Stability or Cruel Rite?)". **Famille et Developpement**, Dakar, Senegal, No. 2, Spring 1975, pp. 13-17 (in French).
12. Ibid., pp. 13-14.
13. From a questionnaire in the author's files, answered by Dr. Jean Taoko, Yalgado Hospital, Ouagadougou, Burkina Faso. See also **WIN NEWS**, Vol. 3, No. 2, Spring 1977, pp. 38-39.
14. See **WIN NEWS**, Vol. 5, No. 2, Spring 1979, p. 31.
15. Hosken, Fran. "Austerity's Human Toll: Why Are International Agencies Ignoring the Devastating Human Costs, **The Humanist**, American Humanist Association, 7 Harwood Drive, P.O. Box 146, Amherst, NY 14226-9982, pp. 17-19 and 44.
16. See **WIN NEWS**, Vol. 14, No. 3, Summer 1988, pp. 48-49.
17. National Seminar on Traditional Practices Affecting the Health of Women: The Case of Excision, Proposal for Elimination May 26-28, 1988. Sponsored by: Action Sociale B.P. 515, Ouagadougou, Burkina Faso; Contact: Alice Tiendrebeogo, Secretary of State. See **WIN NEWS**, Vol. 14, No. 3, Summer 1988, pp. 34-35.
18. Film "Ma Fille Ne Sera Pas Excisee" made in Burkina Faso by Boureima Nikiema. See **WIN NEWS**, Vol. 16, No. 1, Winter 1990, p. 30. For the film write to: La Mediatheque des Trois Mondes, 63, rue du Cardinal Lemoine, 75005 Paris, France.
19. Report: United Nations Seminar on Traditional Practices Affecting the Health of Women and Children, April 29-May 3, 1991, Ouagadougou, Burkina Faso. Sponsored by the UN Commission on Human Rights Sub-Commission on Prevention of Discrimination and Protection of Minorities: E/CN.4/SUB.2/1991/48 12 June 1991; United Nations Center for Human Rights, CH-1211, Geneva 10, Switzerland. See **WIN NEWS**, Vol. 17, No. 2, Autumn 1991, pp. 29-30.
20. Comite Natinal de Lutte contre la Pratique de l'Excision, 01 BP 515, Ouagadougou.
21. Report to the UN Committee on the Elimination of Discrimination Against Women, submitted December 1990, by the Government of Burkina Faso, Ministry of Health and Action Sociale.

BURKINA FASO: ECONOMIC/SOCIAL FACTS & SUMMARY

Burkina Faso:	Former name: UPPER VOLTA. Changed August 4, 1984. 30 Provinces. The name BURKINA FASO means "Country of Upright People".
Climate:	Sahelian, wet and dry seasons. Semi arid North, green/forest South. Savanna plateau.
Population:	8.7 million (estimate 1988). Ouagadougou (Capital) 500,000. **Annual Growth Rate**: 3.3%
Life Expectancy:	48 years. **Infant Mortality**: 134/1000.
Government:	Multiparty Elections May 1992: President Blaise Compaore elected, head of Organization for Popular Democracy (headed military government from 1987 to '92). Independence 1960. Constitution 1977; abolished 1980.
Ethnic Groups:	Two main cultural groups: Voltaic and Mande. Mossi, Bobo, Mande, Fulani, others. Emperor of Mossi, the Mogho Naba holds court in Ouagadougou.
Languages:	French (official); Mossi and local languages.
Religions:	Traditional African (animist): 50-55%. Muslim: 35%. Christian: 10%. (mostly Catholic).
Literacy:	27% (women much less).
Education:	Attendance (1985) 32%. Few have formal education. Only higher education institution founded in 1974 - University of Ouagadougou - one third of students female.
Annual/Capita Income:	$300 / year (1992 estimate).
Economy:	Growth Rate: 4.3% (1982-1987). Inflation: 4.4% (1988). Exports (Less than half of imports.): cotton, livestock, nuts, other agricultural products. Gold (limited). Subsistence agriculture, 80%. Many men work in Cote d'Ivoire or Ghana.

CASE HISTORY : SIERRA LEONE

In Sierra Leone, women, as a group, have been more politically active in traditional rural and village life than women in most other African countries. Women have enjoyed considerable political and personal power in the past, for instance as chiefs, especially locally. But also in Sierra Leone - much as in other African countries - women are quite underrepresented if one looks at the modern government. The traditional position of political influence of women, furthermore, is eroding with modernization: This is one reason why women of Sierra Leone are often strong advocates of tradition, for instance in international meetings. They feel that what personal status of leadership they have enjoyed in their own country is threatened by the introduction of change.

"Within the Mende/Sherbro area, there are 81 chiefdoms, 10 of them are headed by women,"[1] writes Carol Hoffer, who looked into this situation.

Hoffer goes on to describe that women are chiefs, heads of descent groups and key officials in the secret societies. These secret societies, much like their male counterparts - including those existing today in the West - are held together by secret initiation ceremonies, the events of which no one is allowed to reveal on pain of expulsion from the group. It is, however, known that clitoridectomy and excision are part and parcel of the secret initiation rites of women, to which no male and no outsider has access. Women chiefs derive their considerable political influence from the secret societies which they control and where magic is said to play an important part.

A strictly hierarchical system that depends on the personal power and political skills of the chiefs continues today in many parts of rural Africa. The chiefs and their village elders, by definition, are men with the exception of some ethnic groups in Ghana and in Sierra Leone, where women participate politically and successfully compete with men for leadership. Women chiefs exercise absolute control over their subjects, just like male chiefs, and they received a tribute until quite recently. Now, chiefs are allocated salaries by the central government, Hoffer relates, and are no longer allowed to command contributions of labor from their subjects.

"Women chiefs seeking higher office employ the same strategies male candidates use . . . both stress loyalty due to them from kin, clients and friends." Hoffer states:

> "High status women often ally themselves through marriage to men who are chiefs or prominent administrators.They begin to build their political network in early adulthood in relatively wealthy and influential households filled with kin, clients, wards and guests.
>
> Polygamy is a common marriage form in the Mende/Sherbro area. Within polygamous households the first or 'big/wife' is a formidable figure. She is responsible for training junior wives and for organizing them, older children, wards and clients into an agricultural work force. Much of the wealth of the household, then, is of her creation. In Mende/Sherbro society, a head wife is a recognized authority figure, and in some cases, access to a chief can only be gained through her. Predictably, it is not uncommon in both the Mende and Sherbro areas for a wife to succeed her deceased husband in his chiefly office, even though she usually has no genealogical right to rule in the villages of her descent group."[2]

The rivalry that usually arises between women in polygamous households, especially where direct political influence is derived from access to the chief, is overcome in part by the secret women's initiation societies called "Bundu."

> "At puberty, the initiates are separated from the larger society for weeks or months, while in the Bundu bush, a clearing in a sacred grove. There, in a liminal state, they are intensely trained to womanly responsibility by older Bundu women. They are made vividly aware of their incipient womanhood and their value in the larger society. . ."[3]

Hoffer further explains that Bundu women in provincial towns often form neighborhood groups and that they may return to the Bundu bush to participate in initiation ceremonies or to give birth, at which time they are given the full support of the group. Membership in the group serves women well; they acquire political know-how, and they profit from the authority held by their leaders.

The solidarity of women - no male is allowed to even get a glimpse, let alone attend, any of the secret Bundu meetings - enhances the status of women and gives women in Sierra Leone a unique position in their society, quite different from women in the rest of Africa. The Bundu women obviously also play an important role in modern political elections, as they support their candidates with great loyalty.

Hoffer states that "in the modern nation of Sierra Leone . . . approximately 95 percent of all women in the provinces are Bundu women . . . [who] present a formidable block of political support and actual votes." [4]

Men have similar secret initiation societies called "Poro," which revere and enforce the laws of the ancestors, writes Hoffer. Some men of course claim that they and their secret societies are the ones who really hold power - including power over the women's group. But since men are entirely excluded from all women's activities, it is hard to tell who is or was in control as modern communication and Western influences increasingly undermine and take over this traditional world which is often based on beliefs in supernatural powers, witchcraft and irrational fears.

Several women paramount chiefs became famous figures in the past, using marriage to strengthen their political alliance and influence. Today, some women chiefs are members of the House of Representatives. [5] Thus, in Sierra Leone, the political power of women has been traditionally linked to the secret societies, which, in turn, base their influence on secret initiation rites. These rites traditionally have included excision, though that aspect is never discussed, and it is absolutely tabu for all women in Sierra Leone to even mention, let alone discuss, what is done at the secret initiation gatherings.

When the subject of excision is brought up at an international meeting and a woman from Sierra Leone is present, she will instantly cut off all discussion. Oblivious to the health damage involved and disregarding the fact that excision is not only practiced in her country but all over the rest of Africa, a woman from Sierra Leone usually interprets the mere mention of excision as an attack on her political status, that is, an attack on the secret Bundu societies.

Secrecy also conceals the health damage and help is rarely sought. In turn, the Creoles, who represent only a few percent of the population living in Freetown - the descendants of the freed slaves who were resettled in Sierra Leone - and who do not practice excision, refuse to discuss it on political grounds. They are in the minority and are held in contempt because they do not excise their daughters. They do not join the secret Bundu societies that practice excision and therefore do not share in their political influence.

That the operations continue today in all areas of the country is confirmed by a report provided by "Kankaylay," the Sierra Leone Muslim Men and Women's Association. Kankaylay responded in 1976 to a questionnaire of **WIN NEWS**, which was sent all over Africa. Its response is mainly concerned with the customs of theTemne and the Mende, the two largest population groups who inhabit the northern and southern area of the country respectively and speak languages of their own:

> "The Temnes and Mendis*, like all other inhabitants of the Republic of Sierra Leone, have their secret societies called the 'Bondo.'* Girls who have reached the age of puberty and are ready to be given in marriage, must of necessity be initiated into the society. Boys who have also reached the age of discretion are circumcised. It is during the initiation of the former that clitoridectomy takes place.

---

* Throughout the Kankaylay report, the spelling "Mendis" is used, though in the ethnographic literature, the spelling is "Mende." Mende are 30 percent of the inhabitants of Sierra Leone; Temne are also 30 percent. Similarly, the name "Bondo" used here has the same meaning as "Bundu" used above and in other publications.

> According to our customs, the girl or girls initiated into the society are kept in a secluded place usually reserved for that purpose for a period not less than two weeks, or more than two months, and only on rare occasions these girls are kept or confined for any longer period.
>
> No specific reason has been advanced for circumcision of either boy or girl in this country, but custom has it that any girls who fail to be initiated in the secret society will become a liability in society and will not be permitted to enter into the secluded place reserved for the Bondo girls or have any dealing with them.
>
> The initiation of young boys and girls is practiced by most of the indigenous ethnic groups in the Republic of Sierra Leone, chief among whom are the Temnes, Mendis, Lokos, Limbas, Konos, Kurankos, Susus, Fullah and Mandingos. The only ethnic group who does not initiate its girls into any secret society before and after marriage is the Creoles.* These people are in the minority, and according to history, their ancestors were liberated slaves, who came to settle in this country when Britain pronounced the abolition of slavery.
>
> I think that initiation and circumcision are on the increase in the Republic of Sierra Leone, despite the impact of Western influences. Even those children of the highly educated class have begun to realize the importance and necessity of circumcision. These are occasions of great feasting and merriment during and after the period of initiation.
>
> The majority of the people who are active in initiation and circumcision live on subsistence farming. A few live on herding and rearing of domestic animals and production of cash crops . . . The majority are illiterate." [6]**

Reports about the great secrecy and importance of the initiation rituals practiced in Sierra Leone are already recorded in historical texts. Remondino provides such a description from the past and writes:

> "At the appointed time the maids are gathered together and conducted to the river-bank; they are placed under the care of expert matrons . . . they are maltreated, punished and abused by the old women with a view to make them hardy and insensible to pain; they are also schooled in the science and art of African household duties. Among the Galinas of Sierra Leone, in addition to the other observances, the clitoris of the young maids is excised at midnight, while the moon is full, after which they receive their name by which they are known through life. The initiation of each sex into these mysteries is exclusively for the sex engaged and it would be as fatal for a man to steal into the camp of the women during these ceremonies as it would be fatal for a woman . . . to enter . . . where the young men are going through the ordeal. After their initiation into womanhood, the maids live by themselves, similarly to the young men, until they marry." [7]

Zaborowski [8], in his extensive and historical research published in 1896, also reports that the Veis or Gallinas of Sierra Leone practice circumcision of both boys and girls.

An exact and detailed description of an actual secret ceremony in the Bundu bush is given by an eyewitness in a book that was published in Paris in 1957. The eyewitness, Dr. Ruth, evidently participated in the whole proceedings in a village in Sierra Leone, though this was and is against all the rules of the secret societies. Her description provides a unique account of the proceedings:

> "The girls had been prepared for several days ahead of the ceremony . . . and were decked out with most of their family jewels. They wore skirts . . . decorated with colored ribbons and belts with all kinds of fetishes and charms.

---

* Creoles are two percent of the population of Sierra Leone most of them live in Freetown.

** The overall literacy of Sierra Leone, according to the latest official figures, is about 15 percent of the population; for women, that usually means far fewer can read - estimated to be about 8 to 10 percent. Yet, Sierra Leone has one of the oldest, most prestigious universities of West Africa: Fourah Bay College in Freetown, which was founded in 1827, by the British.

"On the morning of the long awaited day the arrival of the head woman of the Bundu organization was announced with prolonged soundings of a large horn.

The matron was entirely covered in a long robe made from black leaves . . . and multicolored straw braids. Her head was encased in an enormous red mask which had slits for the eyes and mouth. She did not talk outside of the Bundu woods but she transmitted her wishes to her assistants with signs.

The girls selected to go to the Bundu wood were carried by their brothers or the men whom they were promised to on their shoulders in a procession preceded by a diabolical Bundu dancer clad, as the matron, with a black mask and four assistants following.

The Bundu woods is an area of about one acre, protected by a high fence. There were two long buildings with thatched roofs, one for the matron of the Bundu and her entourage and the other for the girls. At a distance from the entrance . . . the men put the girls down who then proceeded on their own. The Bundu matron received them, her assistants took the skirts off the girls and rubbed their bodies with white lime paste. The Bundu matron then gave each one a new name and they got new skirts.

The goals of the Bundu organization were explained: These were first of all to assure them fertility and to acquaint them with all their conjugal duties . . . all the girls knew that unless they passed through the Bundu initiation they would be unable to get married and a woman in Africa who is not married practically does not exist. Thus they were under considerable stress.The girls seemed very tired, perhaps because they had been up the entire night dancing. The initiation was to take place under a big tree in a special area, with some benches made of bricks.

The astonished Dr. Ruth then saw a young man come toward her surrounded by four assistants. They carried amulets on strings around their necks and arms and in each hand they carried short sticks, which served to chase away the devils. When the young man proceeded to go to the brick bench Dr. Ruth saw that he was almost blind. He lay down on the bench with his face up . . . His gestures were those of a woman but his body that of a man, his hair cut very short. Dr. Ruth learned later that he was a hermaphrodite who was considered to be female and had been retained by the rulers of the Bundu as a member of the organization.

Then a tom tom was beaten and the Bundu matron and the devil dancer followed by four of her helpers proceeded to the hut of the girls and returned with one of them. They went to the stretched out figure on the bench and the two helpers made the girl lie down with her back on top of the body of the hermaphrodite. The girl's eyes remained fixed on the black mask of the dancer. . . The Bundu matron came forward, wearing black gloves, her face covered with yellow powder . . .

The stretched out body of the hermaphrodite on the bench became an operating table. He took the arms of the girl into his and the two assistants opened the legs of the girl and entwined them with those of the hermaphrodite - she was thus rigidly held. The Bundu matron advanced towards her. The girl still had her eyes fixed on the dancer's black mask.

The two helpers who carried a small drum started to beat it . . . and the helpers began to sing in an even monotone. After a moment the body of the girl who still had her eyes open began to relax. The devil dancer retreated, the eyes of the girl no longer followed her. The tom tom became louder and so did the chanting. The Bundu matron knelt down in front of the girl. She held a small knife with a long handle and a curved steel blade that was no bigger than a nail of a man . . . With the greatest care the Bundu matron then cut off the labia minora and the skin surrounding the clitoris.

One of the helpers took the legs of the girl and lifted them up toward her belly while the 'operating table' held her arms. Now the Bundu matron cut out the entire clitoris and the soft parts of the vagina until her knife met firm tissue. A big piece of the brown material which had been previously used to wipe off the girl was then drenched in oil and powdered salt and used as an ointment while the rag itself was used like a tampon. The brown material was made from some tree bark and branches.

"Then the Bundu matron got up. The 'operating table' released the girl and the assistant raised her up on the seat. Evidently she had been hypnotized the whole time. The devil dancer came back, then stood in front of the girl, and waved in front of her eyes some pieces of black material. The girl slowly recovered consciousness, sighed and then screamed from the pain. The girl then was . . . carried to the Bundu matron's hut, her legs were tightly bandaged up to her thighs. She was laid down while the ceremony resumed with the next girl.

The girls were then left lying to rest for 24 hours after which time the bleeding stopped. The tampon was left in place for another 24 hours. After that the excised area was rubbed twice each day with oil to prevent the wound from adhering. A small piece of wool soaked in oil was inserted in the lower incision so that when the wound healed an enlargement of the vagina would result which is supposed to make childbirth easier . . . It is from that cut that most of the disasters in childbirth occur because the hardened scars do not allow stretching of the orifice.

As soon as the girls were well enough they were instructed in their duties as wives and mothers and were continuously encouraged to sing. Many of the songs are concerned with sexual questions. The villagers hear them sing and so they know they are happy. When a girl dies from the operation while she is in the Bundu bush, she is buried by the Bundu matron's assistants. The parents are informed by the helpers of the matron, but custom requires that the family does not grieve . . .

The day before the girls are released from the Bundu bush the matron sends a message to the village chief. Then the Bundu matron leads all the girls back to the village wearing new skirts of dried straw, their bodies and faces covered with white chalk. They form a circle around the house of the chief who receives them. The Bundu matron then is given some presents and money from the families of the girls and their husbands-to-be. Their families provide the girls with a complete set of new clothes and sleeping mats as their trousseaux.

The Bundu matrons continue these initiation operations up to this day as they derive status and power from them as well as financial gain." [9]

In her thesis on the effects of Western education on the Themnes (or Temnes) and Mendis (or Mendes) for the Department of Education of Fourah Bay College, the most prestigious institution of higher learning in Sierra Leone, A.M. Kamara writes:

"Before acquiring an education, I was a great admirer of the Bundu society. At one time, before my relatives could afford the expenses to have me initiated, I almost ran into the bush when I heard all the beautiful singing there. In which case I would have been initiated immediately. Yes, I was very proud of being a member of the society. I did not then realize the danger to health incurred by having the clitoris cut out without surgical precautions.

When I came to college, the student Christian movement had a discussion called 'Man-Woman Relationship.' At this discussion, I learned that this operation had several bad effects which can complicate childbirth. The immediate effect is sometimes so dangerous as to be fatal. When I was initiated, one of the girls almost bled to death. I see no reason why women should join this society and one day I was bold enough to tell my mother that if they had waited until I got to secondary school, before they decided to have me initiated, I would never have joined. I have sworn that none of my daughters will suffer what I had to suffer due to ignorance.

Western education has almost eradicated the practice of forcing women, especially the Creole women, to join the society. The illiterate members of the Bundu society sometimes pick a quarrel deliberately with those who are against this evil practice, and when they berate the practice, they are dragged into the Bundu bush and initiated by force.

Nothing was done about this until 1953. Then, a Creole woman in one of the villages near Freetown was treated thus. Her relatives took the case to court. The Bundu women were sent to prison and, above all, the initiation rites and especially the operation, which is supposed to be secret, were exposed in the local newspaper, the **Daily Mail**.

> "In March of 1964, there was another article in the same newspaper: 'Nine Bundu women of Hastings Village have been sent to jail by a Freetown Supreme Court for initiating into their society and detaining against her consent a 36-year-old housewife.'
>
> Although some people might feel that the Western type of education is doing something wrong in trying to abolish the only society which brings the women of the Provinces together, yet I and many other educated Mendes and Themnes feel that it should die out and die out it will as education spreads more and more." [10]

Unfortunately, this young woman, who by virtue of studying at Fourah Bay College is a highly privileged member of her society, takes the unrealistic position that these mutilations will be abandoned with education and without any further efforts. But only a small fraction of women in Sierra Leone even now are literate. It takes an organized effort, so experience shows, and continuous information campaigns to change the attitudes and convictions of the families. In Sierra Leone, the political and economic incentives that promote these mutilations are very powerful. They are further supported by the self-interest of women leaders and chiefs who derive their power from the secret societies and their initiations - which always include sexual mutilations.

In a letter dated May 1982 from the Sierra Leone Muslim Men's and Women's Association 'Kankaylay', their earlier report (see above) is updated and amplified: "It can be said that 90 percent or more of the Temne and Mende, with a population of two million, practiced female circumcision." [11]

The report states that the Mende operate on girls at puberty (average age about 15) and the Temne girls are circumcised at 12 years. Usually a group of girls is operated on together and initiated into the 'Bondo society.' They are kept in the 'Bondo bush,' where the operation takes place, from two weeks to two months, so the report states. "Both the Mende and Temne traditions have it that female circumcision is a prerequisite for marriage. A knife or blade is used by the operators known as 'soways' in Mende and 'digba' in the Temne language."

The average fee for the operation is 40 leones.* This is a very large payment for the Bundu matron and society, when one considers that it is multiplied by the number of girls operated at the same time. In a country where the average annual per capita income is less than $200, this fee represents an enormous economic incentive.

It is interesting to note that the Kankaylay report again claims that "Fortunately, only an insignificant number of cases of damages do come up, or are forwarded to the hospital - the majority of which are hemmorhage . . . "

This claim is made regularly everywhere in Africa and wherever FGM (Female Genital Mutilation) is practiced by people who do not visit the maternities of hospitals, or don't talk to midwives and physicians. This account, as well as most others made locally, quite ignores the problems that arise in childbirth due to the scars that obstruct normal delivery. Many thousands of women die as a result and most of the time their babies die as well. As the report below written by a woman physician from Sierra Leone shows, the operations also take a terrible toll of physical and mental suffering and result in health damage and psychological trauma that are often lifelong.

A **"Proposal for the Eradication of the Practice of Female Circumcision in Sierra Leone"**[12] was developed as a thesis by Dr. Olayinka Koso-Thomas, a physician from Sierra Leone, who in 1982 got a public health degree at the University of California in Berkeley. This 52-page program is the first of its kind to propose the eradication of the operations throughout a country. A detailed and staged budget is included to gradually reduce the operations over a 20-year period. The author shows the costs (0.776 leone per year/per person) are small compared with the real costs of the operations that are detailed and described in this comprehensive program. Every sector of the country is to be involved, though the direction is to come from the health care sector.

---

* One leone at the time was equal in value and purchasing power to about U.S.$1.00 - a very great expense for the parents

Dr. Koso-Thomas states in the abstract:

> "The proposal has two main areas of impact: **Health Eduation**, to increase knowledge of the dangers of circumcision and to correct wrong religious doctrines, and **Health Care**, to provide early diagnosis, treatment, and complete rehabilitation of the victims of circumcision . . .
>
> The purpose of this proposal is to bring about the complete elimination of the practice of circumcision of females . . . and to rehabilitate all those circumcised so far, who are still alive but suffering from its aftereffects . . . " [13]

First, the problems due to the operations, that are faced by girls and women of Sierra Leone today are outlined:

> "Female circumcision in Sierra Leone has been allowed to go unchecked for generations . . . The practice continues as a requirement for marriage in many ethnic groups in the country. In many districts, it is associated with the traditional religion and is performed with a strong, ritualistic flavour.
>
> The excision is usually carried out without any form of anesthesia. Victims struggling through pain and fear are held down by brute force. Occasionally, dislocation of the shoulder joint and fracture of the clavicle, upper arm or femur occur during the operations. The practice is a national tragedy . . . " [14]

A survey made at a clinic in a village outside Freetown serves to document the dangers and health damage: Of 100 girls, one died, 12 had to be sent to the hospital, 10 were bleeding heavily and up to five had tetanus infections. Without medical assistance, many more would have died. Only 17 of the girls showed no obvious clinical symptoms. Yet, it is claimed again and again, including in the above-cited report by the Kankaylay society, that accidents are rare and hospitalization is seldom needed. Accidents and even deaths are usually concealed, as the above-cited eyewitness account confirms.

Dr. Koso-Thomas states: "This record shows that 83 percent of those undergoing circumcision are likely to be affected by some condition requiring medical attention . . . Without modern medical facilities . . . a child developing uncontrolled bleeding or infection after circumcision may die within hours of the operation . . . " [15]

But the damaging aftereffects of the operations do not stop with the healing of the flesh wounds, as Dr. Koso-Thomas explains:

> "It has been observed that as girls grow older, some of the symptoms first identified after circumcision recur in their adolescent life. New symptoms also come to light. The most common of these is dyspareunia (difficult or painful coitus in women). This leads to frigidity and to serious mental upset. Some working women tend to worry over the disorder to the extent that they lose their concentration at work and eventually lose their jobs.
>
> Housewives in this category, particularly those in polygamous communities, tend to lose interest in life as they realize that they can no longer hold the interest of their husbands, who may transfer their affection to other wives. Such cases add further to existing mental health problems in the country . . . " [16]

The very high maternal and infant mortality in Africa is never related to FGM, though the statistics show that especially in West Africa, where FGM is practiced almost universally, maternal and infant mortality is the highest in the world, including all Francophone countries. That the cause of childbirth problems is FGM is not admitted especially by western professionals working in development, including physicians dealing with health programs:They never talk to midwives, as many Western physicians consider this below their dignity and only talk to men who do not attend births.

For instance, at the "Safe Motherhood Conference" [17] organized in Nairobi in February 1987 by the World Bank and cosponsored by the World Health Organization (WHO) and the United Nations Population Fund (UNFPA), FGM was never mentioned at all by any speaker or health professional despite the fact that FGM is also widely practiced in Kenya. It is this kind of hypocrisy and corruption by the male dominated health sector that costs thousands of girls and women their lives every year; unfortunately, the hypocrisy and corruption continues today.

The Safe Motherhood Program of the World Bank to this day completely ignores FGM. Its director, Barbara Herz, refuses to acknowledge even the existence of FGM and does not respond to information on the subject. (See: "The Politics of FGM")

Dr. Koso-Thomas documents the facts from her medical practice in Freetown in her thesis:

> "Women who are expecting their first delivery fall into a high risk group, who may develop urinary fistulae after delivery, as scarred vulva tissues narrow the external opening of the vagina and make labour prolonged and more difficult. This condition is extremely distressing to women. . . They smell of urine wherever they go and become social outcasts even among the traditional folk protecting the system that caused their predicament. Some of these women are never able to produce a live child at term; others suffer from frequent miscarriages during the first trimester as a result of infection contained in urine escaping from the urinary tract into the uterus. Yet others, overcome by the hopelessness of their condition, take their own lives.
>
> There are no statistical data available for Sierra Leone, but data collected by the Family Planning Clinic in Freetown indicate that 25-30 percent of women seen annually suffer from this condition. In addition, it has been found that the incidence of obstructed labour is quite high in some areas of the country due to the prevalence of circumcision in this area. . ." [18]

A table given by Dr. Koso-Thomas shows that in the Northern Province of Sierra Leone, where the practice of FGM is most widespread, 95 percent of the women surveyed suffered obstructed labor. This must be compared to about 5 percent on the average, under normal conditions. Dr. Koso-Thomas also deplores the loss to the community which results from the operations:

> "It has now come to the nation as a rude shock that this practice is reducing the proportion of young fertile females in the population who could contribute to the developing society or take positions as social reformers, policy makers, industrial workers, or administrators. . .
>
> A population consisting of so large a proportion of unhealthy women can never make the progress expected of it towards economic and social development. . . Modern Sierra Leone needs all the hands she can mobilize for taking her out of her underdevelopment into a future of prosperity. All the women, not just a small proportion of them, must contribute to the fullest extent and with a healthy and sound body and mind. . ." [19]

An assessment of the economic loss - due to the operations - shows that it is a strain on the whole community:

> "Although 87 percent of the girls who undergo circumcision may require medical treatment, not all will have access to it. It is known that about 40-45 percent of people needing medical attention. . . get it from recognized medical centers and units at which they or the government has to pay for the treatment. . . Therefore, the economy of the country will have to bear the cost of treating a large percentage of all girls undergoing circumcision. . . and this is quite a significant proportion of the health budget. The cost of treating older women is even greater. When this is added to the cost of reduced output due to circumcision of those in the productive sector of the economy, the economic repercussions of the problem become obvious. . ." [20]

Dr. Koso-Thomas then states that the only action taken in Sierra Leone up to that time came from a small group of doctors whose "work has been directed towards improvement of the surgical procedure so as to reduce the risk of infection. Nothing has been done to eradicate the practice itself. . ."

Dr. Koso-Thomas then describes that this misdirected effort to medicalize FGM proved to be quite unsuccessful even on its own terms and did nothing for the victims. She states: "Instructions should have been given on the anatomy of the organs being operated upon, and on the risks and futility of the operations, using living examples of those suffering from mutilation and various disabilities caused by the Digbas (the matrons who perform the circumcisions)."

As noted earlier, most of the thesis by Dr. Koso-Thomas is devoted to a program to eradicate FGM. It describes what to do as well as outlines a timetable with specific results to be achieved at the end of each four-year cycle. Evaluations are scheduled at regular intervals. The other part of the program outlines health care for women who have been operated and will continue to suffer from the results of FGM; they need rehabilitation and care for their many health problems for years to come.

Under the Health Education part of the program, a task force is proposed led by the "fox squads" to work directly with and inside the circumcision societies, with a view to changing their role in the community and to stopping the operations. Instead of the operations, positive aspects of womanhood training are to be substituted, including training in childcare and nutrition, thus improving the high infant mortality rate.

According to the proposal, a National Council for the Welfare of Women will take on the administrative functions, with headquarters in the capital and with a staff from the Ministry of Social Welfare and Health. The country will be divided into four administrative areas, each of which will have similar Health Education and Health Care programs. The regional programs are planned to be set up in intervals of several years, following the model and experience of the first one in the Northern Province. A Community education Committee and a Health Care Committee in each case will take care of the Education and Health Care programs respectively, with specially trained "fox squads" helping with the execution of the Education program.

Sub-groups formed in each of the provincial areas will work at the grassroots level and will take on the task of contacting personally specific sectors of the population such as market women, women farmers working in the fields in rural areas; some will visit homes; others will go to patients at the hospitals; others will go to schools or visit with Imams in the mosques and the community leaders. That is, an intensive educational effort by personal contact is planned - reaching all sectors of the population.

The **Health Education Program** depends on special educational materials, booklets, and visuals developed by the research group in keeping with the local needs. A special education program is planned for the Digbas - the women who perform the operations - and other circumcision society officials.

The **Health Care Program** is designed to help those recently circumcised who are suffering from different complaints, as well as those who have sustained birth injuries or fistulae, as a delayed result. Both physical and emotional support in the form of community groups, is planned. The overall execution of the program is planned to be in the hands of the **National Council for the Welfare of Women**, which in turn is assisted in each of the four regions by a similarly organized Provincial Council.

A detailed budget is divided among local contributions and those made by the government or internationally; it covers every part and phase of the programs. Dr. Koso-Thomas concludes that the cost per patient which, at the time this was written, was estimated at leones 15.52 per person for the whole program for the 20-year period. The average cost per year/person was estimated at leone 0.776. (At the time this was written, one leone was approximately $I.00 in purchasing power.)

This is a very small price to pay for the eradication of a custom that severely damages the health, well-being and productiveness of the vast majority of the female population of the country. What is more, this custom, as Dr. Koso-Thomas shows, must be considered a serious drain on the national economy and damages the national development of Sierra Leone. Since the late 1980s, the national economy of Sierra Leone has steadily deteriorated. This program could be adapted for many other areas and countries, as it provides a remarkably thoughtful and practical example for tackling FGM in a coordinated way in a large area.

The situation in Sierra Leone is unique with many economic and social factors reinforcing genital mutilation, which has been practiced there ever since anyone can remember. The special pressure to preserve secrecy exerted by the initiation societies and their powerful women once more confirms the importance of discussing the facts of reproduction openly and frankly everywhere.

The mystification of these traditional practices in Sierra Leone endows them with a special power and influence and veils their real dangers and purpose, which in Sierra Leone as elsewhere is quite the same: to deprive women of their sexuality and keep them under male control. Indeed, as Dr. Koso-Thomas states, traditionalists claim "circumcision confers virtue and loyalty on females"; therefore it is a requirement for marriage. Without marriage, life for a woman in Africa is still unthinkable.

The influence of the men-only secret societies called Poro (the spelling often differs) is visible in family life where all decisions are made by men. Men also claim that the secret groups of men have the real power in the community and tell the women's societies what to do; but all these transactions are carefully hidden from outsiders. Beliefs in witchcraft and supernatural influences of all kinds are very widespread and these support activities like FGM. Literacy throughout the country is officially only 15 percent, which means that the literacy of women especially in rural areas is much lower.

The thesis of Dr. Koso-Thomas was published in 1987 in book form, **The Circumcision of Women - A Strategy for Eradication,** [21] which also includes a study of 300 women in Western Sierra Leone to establish the health facts with a statistical analysis of the affects of FGM on women's health. The plan for eradication of FGM and the health care program for mutilated women are outlined. Dr. Koso-Thomas is uniquely qualified to propose these programs due to her experience treating women suffering from the results of FGM.

The FGM eradication plan outlined in this book is backed up by a realistic budget and a phased implementation. The costs of the plan are juxtaposed with the real and increasing costs of FGM in terms of women's health damage and the resulting hospital costs, time lost from work and decreased productiveness, all of which are paid by the government and affect the national economy. (See "Health Facts and Overview/ Economic costs of FGM".)

The economic situation of Sierra Leone has been worsening in recent years. The participation of women in the national economy is very much needed especially in food production. Until a few years ago, Sierra Leone was self-sufficient and even exported food. Recently the rice production on which the people depend has decreased so much that rice is now imported in ever greater quantities.

In 1986, the first workshop was organized by the Sierra Leone National Committee of the Inter African Committee on Traditional Practices Affecting the Health of Women and Children and headed by Dr. Koso-Thomas. At that meeting held in Freetown in the form of an open forum discussion, the "Negative Aspects of Our Cultural Heritage" were discussed. [23] Subsequent meetings were held - most recently a one- day workshop for youth in 14 secondary schools in Freetown. Other activities by the IAC are training of TBAs (Traditional Birth Attendants) and many other programs and seminars also with rural women all in collaboration with the Health Ministry according to the IAC.

In Sierra Leone as in other African countries where FGM is practiced, the **Universal Childbirth Picture Books** (CBPBs) with Additions to prevent Excision have been distributed following my visit in 1983. I discussed FGM prevention with Health Ministry representatives, the Midwifery Training School, Dr. Koso-Thomas, Peace Corps volunteers and many others. The **CBPBs** provide information on healthy reproduction and graphically show the severe physical damage of excision. In Sierra Leone they have reached people in many rural areas according to the letters received by **WIN NEWS** in response to leaflets inserted in all books asking the recipients to write if they find the books useful and why, or what changes should be made, and would they like more. These evaluations of the users of the **CBPBs** contribute to revisions made with each printing.

With the requests for more books increasing from the grass-roots level, a leaflet was added - first on a trial basis - asking the recipients to send a statement that they will not have their daughters excised now that they have learned from the pictures of the **CBPBs** how damaging these operations are. This leaflet has resulted in a large positive response, and therefore it is now included in all books sent to areas affected by FGM. In Sierra Leone, where the **CBPBs** are widely circulating locally, they are most successful with dozens of letters arriving every month from the interior of this country and from small towns.

For instance, from Kenema, a market town in the center of the country, letters come every week from many different people - men and women - from local health centers, from school teachers and principals, nurses, midwives and more. Excerpts of these letters are reprinted in **WIN NEWS** once or twice a year, as they provide direct information on the way the local community leaders and people think about FGM. Their attitudes are critical for the eradication of FGM. It is encouraging to hear how very interested most of the letter writers are in learning the biological facts of reproduction and how many are opposed to FGM and use the books to teach their neighbors. (See: "Women and Health".)

To be sure, women and men who write for more books must be regarded as leaders in their communities because they can read and write and because of their initiative. This extensive correspondence shows that many people are anxious to help eradicate the mutilations in their own communities. Many people on their own initiative and without any salary or payment, go out to teach their neighbors and people in their own communities - as photographs they have sent confirm.

Many more women and men from Sierra Leone write for books than from any other country; most of them are from the health or education sector. They strongly support the eradication of these traditional mutilations. The largest number of letters are coming from the area of Kenema. The Kenema Female Circumcision Project [23] was organized by a secondary school principal, Mr. Sei, using the **Childbirth Picture Books (CBPBs)** and other teaching materials designed for health professionals. This program, which was locally developed without any development experts from abroad involves the whole community. It demonstrates that people are ready to organize on the local level in their own communities. Many internationally funded health programs never reach the people they are intended for or don't involve them in the planning; as a result they fail.

The **Childbirth Picture Books** are designed in such a way that it does not take experts to teach with them. Anyone who can read can teach others, using this teaching program based on pictures. The people living around Kenema and other aeas of Sierra Leone have written more often for **CBPBs** than those from anywhere else. In other African countries similar initiatives and contacts with community people have been started - for instance Nigeria and Ghana. Requests for the **CBPBs** come from all over Africa - indeed from all over the world.

This kind of local project, which is based within a community and involves local people, can accomplish a great deal with very little financial support. In Sierra Leone the people now seem to be quite receptive to change because it is evident that traditional ways only lead to more poverty as the economic problems that beset the country clearly show. But for such local initiatives to make a real and lasting impact would require that they are replicated in small towns and villages all over the country. Such local community programs could effectively support regional and national eradication programs such as the one proposed by Dr. Koso-Thomas.

Border conflicts and invasions from Liberia, where a civil war has devastated the country, have recently spilled over into several areas of Sierra Leone, with people forced to flee A military government took over Sierra Leone in the spring of 1992: at this writing the political as well as economic future is not clear.

Finally this must be said: It is difficult for an outsider to understand why people would subject their own children to such devastating and senseless suffering in a country which seems to have everything anyone could wish for. A beautiful coastline of white beaches meets a cloudless blue sky fringed by palm trees of all kinds that bear rich fruit. The warm tropical ocean is full of fish; no one needs to go hungry in what looks to any observer like a tropical paradise with everything necessary to sustain life plentiful and free.

Why and how is it possible to build up a sinister secret culture of torturous practices that devastate the health of women, the truly productive half of a rural society that depends on the children they bear? Why? And why do those who go to this country's outstanding university in Freetown, who know the truth and who by virtue of their education and contact with the rest of the world, understand the results of these traditions for their country and their own society - why do these educated men and women fail to stop these horrendous practices on their own young?

FOOTNOTES

1. Hoffer, Carol P. "Mende and Sherbro Women in High Office," **Canadian Journal of African Studies**, VI, ii, 1972, pp. 151-164.
2. Ibid., p. 158.
3. Ibid., p. 159.
4. Ibid., p. 161.
5. Steady, Dr. Filomena. "Female Power in African Politics: The National Congress in Sierra Leone," **Africana Library Notes**, No. 31, VI, 1975-76.
6. Response to Questionnaire by Kankaylay-Sierra Leone Muslim Men's and Women's Association, P.O. Box 1168, Freetown, Sierra Leone; document in author's files.
7. Remondino, P.C. **History of Circumcision from the Earliest Times to the Present**. F.A. Davis Publishers, Philadelphia and London. (1891) pp. 43-44.
8. Zaborowski, M. "La Circoncision ses Origines et sa Repartition en Afrique et a Madagascar." **Anthropologie Par**. 1896, vii, p. 659.
9. Gervis, P. **C'Est Arrive Dans la Sierra Leone**. Albin Michel, Paris, 1957, especially Chapter XII, "An Initiation Ceremony in the Bundu Bush," pp. 266-275. See also **WIN NEWS**, Vol. 4, No. 3, Summer 1978, pp. 27-28. Translated from French and summarized.
10. Kamara, A. M. **Traditions and Superstitions Among the Themnes and Mendes, and the Effect of Western Type of Education Upon Them**, Freetown, Fourah Bay College, 1964, Dept. Ed. Thesis No. 97.
11. Response to Follow-Up Questionnaire by Kankaylay-Sierra Leone Muslim Men's and Women's Association, P.O. Box 1168, Freetown, Sierra Leone; dated May 10, 1982; document in author's file.
12. Koso-Thomas, Olayinka, M.D., M.P.H. **Proposal for the Eradication of the Practice of Female Circumcision in Sierra Leone**, dated March 16, 1981.
13. Ibid., "Abstract," p. i.
14. Ibid., Part I, p. 3.
15. Ibid., p. 5.
16. Ibid.
17. Safe Motherhood Conference, February 1987, Nairobi, Kenya, organized by the World Bank, 1818 H St., NW, Washington, DC 20433; cosponsored by WHO - World Health Organization and UNFPA - United Nations Population Fund. See **WIN NEWS,** Vol. 13, No. 2, Spring 1987, pp. 23-26.
18. Koso-Thomas op. cit.
19. Ibid., pp. 7-8.
20. Ibid.
21. Koso-Thomas, Olayinka, M.D., M.P.H. **Circumcision of Women: A Strategy for Eradication**. Zed Books Ltd. 57 Caledonian road, London. N1 9BU, UK. 1987, See **WIN NEWS**, Vol. 13, No. 3, Summer 1987, pp. 34-35.
22. Sierra Leone National Committee of the IAC (Inter African Committee), Dr. Koso-Thomas, President, P.O. Box 1069, Freetown, Sierra Leone; IAC, 147, rue de Lausanne, CH-1202 Geneva, Switzerland.
23. Kenema Female Circumcision Project, c/o Mr. M. K. Sei, SLMB Secondary School, P.O. Box 165, Kenema, Sierra Leone. See **WIN NEWS**, Vol. 16, No. 2, Spring 1990, pp. 42-43. Kenema Female Circumcision Project: Progress Report. See **WIN NEWS**, Vol. 17, No. 3, Summer 1991, p. 33.

SIERRA LEONE: ECONOMIC/SOCIAL FACTS & SUMMARY

Sierra Leone:	Republic of Sierra Leone. 12 districts, including Freetown. (Northern, Southern, Eastern and Western areas.)
Climate:	Tropical: mangrove swamps / wooded hills / upland plateau.
Population:	3.7 million (estimate 1985). Freetown (capital), 500,000. Kenema, 340,000. **Annual Growth Rate**: 2.3% (1985 estimate).
Life Expectancy:	46 years.
Government:	Military government, Spring 1992. Republic. Independence 1961. Constitution (1978) suspended. Local Government: Paramount Chief and Council of Elders.
Ethnic Groups:	Temne: 30% // Mende: 29% // Creole: 2%.
Languages:	English (official). Mende // Temne // Krio (lingua franca) and others.
Religions:	Muslim: 60%. Traditional (Animist): 30%. Christian: 10%. (1985 estimate).
Literacy:	15% (women much less).
Education:	Fourah Bay College established 1827.
Annual/Capita Income:	$120 (1985 estimate).
Economy:	Growth Rate: 0.5% (1985). Inflation: 76% (1985). Agriculture: coffee, cocoa, ginger, rice, etc. Industry: diamonds, rutile, bauxite, etc. Imports exceed exports. Work force, subsistence agriculture, 75%.

CASE HISTORY : SENEGAL

In no other city of Africa is the contrast between modern life and African tradition more glaring than in Dakar. A distinctly French atmosphere pervades the handsome, tree-planted avenues and squares, the sidewalk cafes and the colonial office buildings that are now increasingly being replaced by modern high rise concrete blocks. They all come to life every morning under the call of the muezzin, which is broadcast at sunrise all over the city from the mosques.

Dakar was the seat of the French government in exile during the Second World War, something that has left a permanent imprint on this city. Before that, Dakar was built by the French as the center of their colonial administration for West Africa. Today the beautiful coastline of Dakar is the winter playground for wealthy tourists, mostly from France, with European women sunbathing topless around the pools and beaches of the luxury hotels.

The African women who flock to Dakar from all over the country are wrapped in long, flowing traditional printed robes: Most of them were excised before puberty to preserve chastity and guarantee their faithfulness as wives.

The sophisticated, intellectual aspirations of the urban elite are in stark contrast to the widespread illiteracy in rural areas. Among women, illiteracy is especially high, but very little is being done by the government to change this situation. Illiteracy is a major handicap for women, since it prevents their participation in the job market and in the government. Women's organizations in Dakar hold literacy classes, but there is little publicly financed support for the education of women.

In the rural areas, as elsewhere in Africa, women do much of the agricultural work and are overburdened with heavy daily chores. For many of the village women, learning to read would be a luxury for which they would have little practical use. Ninety-four percent of the population is Moslem, and polygamy is widely practiced in the rural areas, where life follows traditional lines and has hardly changed - this in total contrast to Dakar. Dakar also functions as seat and communication center for regional business interests as well as headquarters for Non Governmental Organizations active in Francophone Africa - much like Nairobi in East Africa.

In the capital and other towns, women have few opportunities, as they lack the education for modern jobs. Women are engaged in petty trade and countless street vendors constantly urge you to buy their cheap wares in the streets of Dakar. Yet, a few outstanding women who have succeeded, against enormous odds, to get a good, professional education are accepted: Such women also manage occasionally to get important positions in the government or the media. They are the exceptions that prove the rule; there seems to be no ladder for upward mobility.

Excision is practiced by most of the smaller population groups of Senegal. But the Wolof - 43 percent of the population of Senegal - who live in the area of Dakar and hold most of the political power, do not excise their daughters. As a result, Female Genital Mutilation (FGM) is entirely ignored. At a meeting with Professor Paul Correia, [1] the Chief of the maternity section of the Hospital Dantec in Dakar, and Madame N'Diaye Bineta, Deptuty Chief of the School of Midwives, at my visit in March 1977 stated that about one-quarter of the women who come to the hospital's maternity are excised.

Dakar, as all other African capitals, is a magnet for ambitious people from all over the country. These newcomers look for jobs, for change, and for an escape from the hard work and monotony of rural life. Recent droughts have increased this influx, and squatters build shacks wherever they can, though city authorities periodically evict them and bulldoze their ramshackle abodes, calling them a health hazard and eyesore.

A mixture of all different population groups can be found in Dakar, much as in all other African capitals. In the maternities of the largest city hospitals, therefore, one can learn about what kind of genital operations are practiced by which ethnic groups.

Madame Bineta, the chief midwife in charge of the maternity, stated that circumcision of boys is, of course, mandatory according to the beliefs of both the Moslem and animist population groups. The government now urges people to have the circumcision of boys done at an early age in a hospital or a clinic under sterile conditions to prevent infections and accidents. The operations on girls are far more drastic and dangerous, she said. Madame Bineta wondered why no precautions concerning girls are advocated or taken. "Boys are well taken care of", she said, "but no one says anything about girls who continue to be operated on by the old women with their dirty hands and knives and on the ground."

Madame Bineta and other midwives at our meeting said that most of the ethnic groups of Senegal, except for the Wolofs and the Serer, excise their children. It is practiced all over the rural areas and especially along the Senegal River, where the Toucouleur live. The Toucouleur also practice infibulation, they stated, and added that they are the most traditional ethnic group. In the western part of Senegal, the Mandingo, including the Soce or Casamas, excise their female children and so do the Peulhs or Fulani. The midwives also noted that all the people who come from Mali to Senegal - mostly Bambara - practice excision as well.[2]

Professor Correia, in response to my question, suggested that to effectively prevent the operations on girls, it would be essential to have political support; that means prevention of FGM would have to be supported by the government as the health care system and hospitals are funded by the government - as in most of Africa. Therefore, any actions to stop FGM would need governmental support. An information campaign would have to be organized, including radio talks. The Moslem religious leader of Senegal, the Great Marabout, would have to back such a campaign, Dr. Correia asserted, and the Ministry of Health should be in charge.

Professor Correia pointed out that some people used various products to bleach their skin. This created all kinds of health problems. The government forbade the practice and prosecuted those involved in the distribution of these damaging products. Genital mutilation should be treated similarly, he thought. The first step would be to contact the Director of Medicine at the Ministry of Health.

The actual chances of persuading the religious Moslem leadership to speak out against the operations on girls in Senegal might be realistically assessed as nil, judging from the fact that the Moslem religious leaders all over West Africa's rural areas speak for the practice, indeed they claim it is a religious requirement.

Awa Thiam, who is from Senegal, describes in her book **La Parole aux Negresses,**[3] her conversations with Moslem leaders in West Africa who advocate excision of female children and claim it is a command by the Koran. Scholars of the Koran state that there is no such command; but there is no prohibition against excision either. Therefore, different interpretations can be made.

In rural areas the followers of the local Moslem leaders have no way of knowing the facts, as most of them cannot read and it would be sacrilege to dare to question their leader's views. The Moslem leaders speak for the men and the village chiefs in each community: They uphold the traditional order, including polygamy and excision. Women are neither asked nor heard.

The contrast between the sophisticated life of Dakar's modern government area, with the handsome white villas surrounded by lush tropical gardens, and the reality of the daily struggle in the many self-built squatter shacks is very great. But the contrast between the village life, which has not changed for centuries, and urban living conditions, is even more extreme.

Women in the rural areas do all the daily household chores of pounding grain (often millet), preparing food and hauling water, despite the scorching heat. Women start their day before dawn, while men still sleep. The role of the village woman continues to be that of childbearer and servant to men - her traditional role in Africa for centuries.[4]

She is acquired by a man from her father for a bride-price: This is a commercial transaction. The wealthier the man, the more women - that is servants - he can buy. The agricultural production of each woman is the property of the man who owns her. He sells what his wives produce in the market, enabling him to buy more wives. He discards the older women. That is he divorces them the Moslem way while keeping their children as agricultural labor force. Then he buys more young women always limiting their number to four at one time as his religion demands.

In due course each new young wife produces more children - a useful addition to his estate: the more farm workers, the more they produce and the larger his fortune. After all, in the rural economy it costs him next to nothing to rear a child - indeed his wives do all the work of rearing and feeding them. But, of course, the children are his property alone.

Women accept their life without question. How could it be otherwise, as they have never known anything else. Even the possibility of another kind of life is yet beyond the imagination of the rural woman who is struggling to survive under an overwhelming burden of heavy work, for which she lacks all modern tools.

The reality of life in rural Senegal as opposed to Dakar is a huge infant mortality rateas well as child malnutrition - the result of the neglect of education for girls and women who remain illiterate and under the spell of damaging traditions. All of which is ignored by the government in Dakar. [5]

In 1984, it was Professor Correia, whom I had asked about excision at my visit to Dakar in 1977, who gave the opening speech at the Dakar Seminar on **"Traditional Practices Affecting the Health of Women and Children"**. This meeting was organized by the Working Group on Female Circumcision of the non-governmental organization Sub-Committee on the Status of Women, Geneva, Switzerland. It was cosponsored by the Ministry of Health of Senegal, the World Health Organization (WHO) and UNICEF. [6]

Professor Correia in his address provided an overview of the medical aspects of FGM and he reconfirmed the recommendations made at the WHO Seminar on "Traditional Practices Affecting the Health of Women and Children" in Khartoum in 1979. (See "World Health Organization Seminar") These recommendations provided the basis for the expanded version adopted at Dakar by the Inter African Committee (IAC), which was organized at the same meeting. And the expanded recommendations are now used for guidance by the more than twenty IAC-affiliated groups all over Africa. At the Dakar seminar, mostly Francophone West African countries were represented, except for reports from Egypt and Sudan. Berhane Ras-Work, who hails from Ethiopia but lives in Geneva, took over as leader and president of the IAC.

The WHO Seminar in Khartoum was for government representatives, sent by their respective health ministries; but the Dakar Seminar was by and for non governmental organizations. Already at the Khartoum Seminar the hope was expresed by WHO and the Conference Secretariat - which is included in the official paper - that another follow-up meeting for West and Francophone Africa would be held to discuss traditional practices. For a variety of reasons only one West African country was represented in Khartoum - that is Nigeria. The only representative of a Francophone country was an observer from Burkina Faso (which was called Upper Volta at that time): Alice Tiendrebeogo was not in the government then and therefore could not speak.

It took from 1979 to 1984 to finally fulfill what all participants of the WHO seminar in Khartoum had urged. Some months after that seminar the WHO Regional Office for Africa and the Middle East that sponsored this fateful meeting invited me to a consultation at their headquarters in Alexandria, Egypt, as I had been a member of the WHO Secertariat. It was suggested that I should organize a meeting for NGOs as follow-up to the Khartoum Seminar to be held in West Africa.

I pointed out that it was essential that such a seminar must be organized by African women if it was to have permanent results. It took five years, but the seminar finally was held in Dakar with WHO and UNICEF support, hosted by the Health Ministry of Senegal. Non governmental groups and delegations from a large region of sub-Saharan Africa where FGM is practiced were represented, with Berhane Ras-Work from Ethiopia presiding.

It is significant that Senegal was hosting this groundbreaking meeting which no doubt in part was due to the influence of Professor Correia. Since then and because the dominant population group - the Wolofs - does not practice FGM and therefore is not affected by the health damage resulting from the operation, very little has happened in Senegal concerning actions to eradicate the mutilations. Indeed, it took until the 1990s before even the basic research was done in Senegal to establish unequivocally by local surveys who - that is, what ethnic group - practices which type of FGM, as well as other pertinent information.

The first systematic survey and report on FGM in Senegal was researched and written by Marie Helene Mottin-Sylla and published by ENDA (Environmental and Development in the Third World) of Dakar. [7] ENDA occasionally publishes some research on women in Senegal, but most of its work is on environmental issues. This very thorough report, **"Excision in Senegal - Information for Action"**, is in French, as are all publications of ENDA; it provides detailed information on the different ethnic groups of Senegal and to what extent they practice FGM. The report concludes that some twenty percent of the inhabitants of Senegal are involved in the practice. But as far as the geographic distribution is concerned, it is evident that FGM is practiced in most of the country's rural areas but not in the Dakar region, where the largest part of Senegal's population is concentrated.

According to the research of Mottin- Sylla published by ENDA, excision in Senegal is a "village rite" that is performed, depending on the ethnic group, on girls anywhere from two to eleven years of age. In a few areas infibulation is also practiced among the most traditional groups. Though in Senegal many different ethnic groups live in the rural areas, most of them practice FGM as a puberty rite. Many of the Marabouts, the Moslem religious leaders, support excision claiming it is a religious requirement. But it is also clear that the majority - that is the Wolofs and the Serere or fifty-eight percent of the population, according to ENDA - do not mutilate their daughters and their Moslem leaders obviously don't require it.

Since ninety-four percent of the population are Moslem, it is clear that FGM is an ethnic practice and not a religious one - no matter what the local Moslem leaders who promote FGM claim. For instance, in Pakistan, Bangladesh, Iran, Syria and especially in Saudi Arabia, which is very influential in Moslem religious matters as well as representinmg the most conservative Moslem society, excision or infibulation is not practiced as educated Moslems always cite. But then rural people in Senegal and elsewhere in Africa listen to their own local religious leaders and are not concerned with the arguments by Islamic scholars.

In Senegal, from a national point of view, FGM is practiced in rural areas by a small minority that has no political influence. Therefore, it is especially difficult to persuade someone in Dakar in the government from a different ethnic group to start any significant action. In Dakar FGM only affects a small number of immigrants who continue to mutilate their girls because that is what they are accustomed to do at home.

Immigrants everywhere follow their traditions even more fervently to assert their identity than do their own people at home. Many families from Senegal live in France where the men go first to find work and then bring their wives and families along. Some young people from Senegal and other Francophone countries go to universities in France and live there for years as well as rearing children in France.

Inevitably problems arise regarding excision when they visit their parents and relatives in the rural areas. It often happens that the grandparents and relatives have the girls excised "to follow tradition" even if the parents who live in France or Dakar are strongly opposed to it. For instance in Paris, G.A.M.S. (The Women's Group for Abolition of Sexual Mutilations) is working with African immigrant women many of whom come from rural areas of Senegal. [8] Many immigrant families from rural areas in Dakar continue to mutilate their daughters. However, much as in other African capitals - for instance in Bamako - the operations are performed on much younger children. All the traditions are ignored, only the physical mutilation remains, because otherwise the fathers believe they will not get a good bride-price.

Following up on its research and publication, ENDA organized a meeting on "Excision, Islam and Culture - the Views of the Halpulaar and Mandingue* and the Coordination of the Social and Medical Aspects of Excision." [9] At the meeting, according to the report published by ENDA, the Moslem leaders who had participated in the earlier survey were asked to present their views on excision. Professor Diawo Bah of the Maternity Department of the Hospital Le Dantec was invited to present the medical view. No women were invited to speak nor is a female view included in the ENDA publication.

The objective of the meeting, according to the report, was to present the views of the two ethnic groups as well as the medical one to representatives of development organizations in Senegal to learn about the health and social situations of women and children. But the ultimate objective was to see if the Moslem ideas and the medical view are compatible. Though the subject discussed is of utmost concern to women and girls, ENDA only asked men to speak.

Predictably the Moslem leaders of both ethnic groups who are among the most conservative ones in Senegal insisted that excision was mandatory, that it was required by the Koran and/or the Moslem scriptures and that it was "the dominant and central value in women's lives". ENDA, by giving the word to these Moslem leaders in rural areas of Senegal also bestowed on them enormous influence all out of proportion to the population they represent. Women were entirely ignored.

The publication of ENDA fails to put in context the statements of these isolated Moslem men who oppose and ignore prevailing views of Moslem scholars as established for instance by the highly respected El Azhar Moslem University in Cairo. Moslem leaders and scholars have asserted unequivocally that there is no religious requirement for excision - an opinion that was also confirmed by the Ministry of Religion in Khartoum and was again discussed at the 1988 Conference on Strategies to Eradicate FGM in Somalia, a country which is nearly 99 percent Moslem.

Professor Bah in turn as representative of the medical opinion after reviewing at length the health and medical problems resulting from the mutilations proposed to medicalize the operations by training the excisors in anatomy and how to perform the mutilations in sanitary ways! This eleven years after the Khartoum Seminar by WHO on Traditional Practices Affecting the Health of Women and Children where the medicalization of FGM was categorically rejected and eight years after WHO published and distributed worldwide a specific statement condemning medicalization!

Finally ENDA had to state in their own publication that the views expressed at the meeting they organized could not be reconciled - which had been their objective. It is astonishing that ENDA, as an organization that claims to work internationally, speaking for Africa, would publish such one-sided regressive views in their own publication without any explanation as to the real facts. As an African research organization publishing for an international audience, ENDA failed its responsibility to publish all the facts and also misrepresented the Islamic view of FGM by omission. But what is even worse is that ENDA published this document without giving women any voice at all.

As for the medicalization of FGM, it is fortunately quite unrealistic to think that the Ministry of Health will spend its very limited budget which is subsidized - as everything else in Senegal - from France, on training traditional excisors in remote rural areas.

The research by Mme. Mottin Sylla was recently published in book form, **Excision in Senegal,** [10] with dozens of tables, statistics and maps full of detailed analysis and figures representing hundreds of hours of work. The question is what are all these details good for? Perhaps the time and money spent on such very academic presentations - there are others including a detailed computer analysis on infibulation in the Sudan - might better be used for teaching illiterate women and men about the biological facts of reproduction and to organize women's groups for health.

---

* Halpulaar (Peul and Toucouleur) about 22 percent of the population, Moslem, traditional, living near Senegal River; Mandingue, 3.6 percent of the population, Moslem, traditional, living in lower Casamance area.

The conclusion states: "In Senegal excision is a public health problem which directly involves 20 percent of the population or 700,000 girls and women." But nothing is said based on the experience of collecting the information what might be done to start the necessary work on prevention.

Here some summaries of several women's statements from this publication:

A young Halpulaar who has gone to school speaks about excision

"In Halpulaar excision means purification - because if a child grows up without being excised, she is not only impure but she is the offspring of a polluted mother. She is rejected by the whole community and the very idea that a girl should not be excised is blasphemous! In order to make a girl faithful when she later gets married, it is necessary to amputate a part of herself. Not to excise her implies that she is not respected and this will make her a second-class person. She should remain respectful of her parents and her future parents-in-law. She becomes a member of the adult community only after she is excised and assumes her place in society. The excisor, after the operation, uses all kinds of incantations to chase away the evil spirits; goat dung and nut butter are used for therapeutic purposes. One has to pay the excisor eight pounds of rice and some soap.".

A young woman student in Dakar relates:

"The reason for the operation typically is religious. I was nine-years-old when it was done to me. I remember everything. I was taken to the excisor and told she was my aunt. After entering the house I was amazed when some women held me and opened my legs. The aunt took out a knife which she first put in boiling water and then she cut my clitoris off. I felt a terrible pain all over and thought I was dying. The excisor put some paste that burned between my legs. I was told I must push my legs together as hard as I could and not to move.

I was terrified and I think this practice was invented to dehumanize women. The very thought of it still makes me ill. Under no circumstances will I ever have my daughter excised because it is a permanent handicap for personal development."

Partial infibulation is practiced by the Toucouleur:

"Because virginity is considered sacred, infibulation is added to excision. That is, the flesh on each side of the big lips is held together and fused to form a scar over the entrance of the vagina. When I was excised they also closed the entrance to my vagina because my fiance was away on a trip. I was taken to the excisor who told me I have to open my legs in order to become a woman. And I must not cry too much to gain the respect of my fiance. I was held by two women so I could not move. The excisor wound a string around my clitoris and tightened it like a tourniquet and then she cut it off. Then she held the two bleeding sides and took a needle and string and sewed my small lips together. After two weeks she took out the string and all that remained was a scar formed by the dried blood."

A Serere woman relates:

"With us excision is directly connected with initiation and tradition in an Islamized environment. The girls stay with the excisor for three days. On the fourth day the operation is done early in the morning with scissors while two women helpers hold each girl - one the head and shoulders the other the legs. Afterward the girls are devided up into those who have cried and those who were courageous - one group got white armbands the other red ones and the excisor got a chicken. To stop the bleeding and make the wound heal a concoction of leaves is boiled and put on the wound as well as nut butter and the girls have to sit in hot water."

The Senegalese National Committee on traditional practices affiliated with the IAC held a seminar on "Excision, Religion and Culture" in September 1992 which included ten circumcisers and representatives of youth organizations and women's groups. The participants set up some groups around the theme "Strategies and Prospects", with a special group formed by circumcisers. [11]

The gulf between Dakar the capital and rural Senegal is widening in every area but especially in education and is much greater than in any other African country. All this together with the strong Moslem influence does not look promising for the future of little girls who have the misfortune of being born in the rural areas of Senegal.

FOOTNOTES

1. See **WIN NEWS**, Vol. 3, No. 2, Spring 1977, p. 4.
2. Ibid.
3. Thiam, Awa. **La Parole aux Negresses**. Denoel/Gonthier, Paris, 1978.
4. McBride, Steward Dill. "Senegal: A Day in an African Village", **Christian Science Monitor**, July 11, 1977.
5. Braun, Armelle. "A New Role for Women In Senegal", **Ceres**. FAO Review on Agriculture and Development, Vol. II, No. 4, July-August 1978.
6. Seminar on Traditional Practices Affecting the Health of Women and Children. Contact: IAC (Inter African Committee) for report and recommendations. Address: c/o Economic Commission for Africa, ATRCW, P.O. Box 3001, Addis Ababa, Ethiopia. Or: 145 rue de Lausanne, CH-1202 Geneva, Switzerland. See **WIN NEWS**, Vol. 10, No. 2, Spring 1984, pp. 35-36.
7. ENDA (Environment and Development in the Third World), B.P. 3370, Dakar, Senegal.
8. G.A.M.S. (The Women's Group for Abolition of Sexual Mutilation), c/o Maison des Femmes, 8 cite Prost, 75011 Paris, France. See **WIN NEWS**, Vol. 10, No. 1, Winter 1984, pp. 31-36.
9. **Excision, Islam and Culture: The View of the Halpulaar and Mandingue** (in French). Final Report of a meeting on coordination of the social and medical aspects of excision in Senegal, Dakar, 28 and 29 May 1991. Organized and published by ENDA, B.P. 3370, Dakar, Senegal.
10. Mottin-Sylla, Marie Helene **Excision in Senegal.** Published by ENDA, address above.
11. National Senegalese Committee on Traditional Practices Affecting the Health of Women and Children - Comite National Senegalais sur les Pratiques Traditionnelles Affectant la Sante des Meres et des Enfants-COSEPRAT - c/o ENDA, address above.

SENEGAL: ECONOMIC / SOCIAL FACTS AND SUMMARY

Senegal:	10 regions, 30 departments, 95 arrondissements.
Climate:	Tropical/Sahelian desert or grassland in north, heavier vegetation in south and southeast.
Population:	7 million (1990 estimate). Dakar (capital). **Annual Growth Rate**: 3%
Life Expectancy:	48 years // **Infant Mortality**: 78/1000.
Government:	Republic. Independence: 1960. Constitution 1963. Last revised 1984. President, National Assembly, Supreme Court. Multiparty system. Universal suffrage.
Ethnic Groups:	Wolof 43% // Fulani (Peulh) and Toucouleur 23% // Serer 15% // Diola, Mandingo and others 22%.
Languages:	French (official). Wolof, Pulaar, Diola, Mandingo.
Religions:	Islam (94%). Christian 5%. Traditional 1%.
Literacy:	28% (women much less).
Education:	School attendance: primary 60%. secondary 15%.
Annual/Capita Income:	$630 (estimate).
Economy:	Growth Rate: 6%. Imports exceed exports. Agriculture 22% of GDP: Subsistence peanuts, seafood, phosphates, cereals.

SURVEY OF CONTINENTAL AFRICA

OVERVIEW OF COUNTRIES WHERE FGM IS PRACTICED

The country case histories above provide extensive research on the different traditional practices affecting the health of women and children in continental Africa with emphasis on female genital mutilation (FGM). These case histories include:

MIDDLE EAST AND EAST AFRICA: Sudan, Somalia, Egypt, Ethiopia, Kenya

WEST AFRICA: Nigeria, Mali, Burkina Faso, Senegal, Sierra Leone

Much briefer reports following this summary are given on these countries:

Cote d'Ivoire, Ghana, Chad, Djibouti, Liberia.

---

1 ETHIOPIA / **2** SUDAN / **3** SOMALIA
4 KENYA / **5** EGYPT / **6** UGANDA
7 TANZANIA / **8** DJIBOUTI /
9 CENTRAL AFRICA/ **10** NIGERIA
11 GHANA **12** BURKINA FASO /
13 COTE d'IVOIRE / **14** MALI /
15 GUINEA / **16** SIERRA LEONE /
17 SENEGAL / **18** THE GAMBIA /
19 MAURITANIA / **20** LIBERIA /
21 TOGO / **22** BENIN /
23 CAMEROON / **24** CONGO /
25 GABON/**26** ZAIRE/**27** CHAD/
28 NIGER/**29** LIBYA/ **30** ALGERIA /
31 YEMEN **32** / SAUDI ARABIA /
33 ANGOLA / **34** ZAMBIA /
35 MOZAMBIQUE / **36** SAHARA
37 MOROCCO / **38** RWANDA /
39 BURUNDI / **40**/ MALAWI

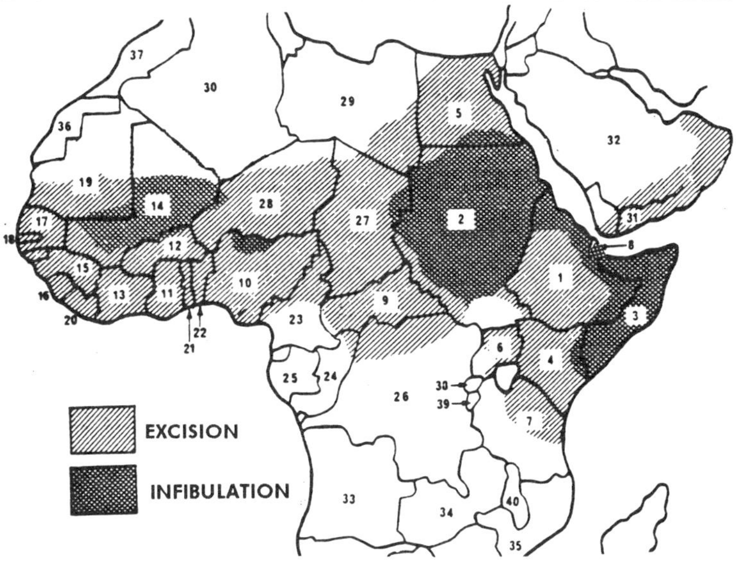

The map shown above - a smaller version of the one in the chapter on Health Facts and Overview - shows where FGM is practiced. For many reasons, it was impossible to include in this report all the countries where FGM is practiced. Space limitation is one; lack of documented information another. Countries where only a minority of the population practice FGM, for instance Cameroon are not included for reasons of space except for Tanzania because of its innovative program to eradicate FGM; this information is under Women and Health, as well as the prevention program of Gambia.

Togo and Benin located between Nigeria and Ghana and inhabited by similar ethnic groups could not be included for lack of documented research. The same is true of Guinea - though it is known that FGM is practiced throughout that country. From Central Africa no research is available, though it is known that FGM is practiced there. In Niger, a few ethnic groups in the south are said to practice FGM. In Uganda only a small minority is involved. Any new information will be published in **WIN NEWS.**

FGM is an ethnic practice. The political boundaries of Africa have been drawn by the European colonial powers regardless of ethnic groups. But these political borders have nothing to do with the traditional practices that existed long before any political lines.

With migration and displacement of ethnic groups due to the many armed conflicts, FGM is spreading to more regions of Africa. While in the past people rarely left their villages, now the migration to urban areas is in full swing all over Africa. Marriage between different ethnic groups which was rejected in the past is increasing. A woman who marries into a family where FGM is practiced is mutilated as a marriage requirement, all her daughters will be as well. It is in this way that FGM spreads, for instance into southern Sudan and to the Egyptian coast and into the cities, for instance, Accra and Dakar.

The following countries have committees affiliated with IAC as of 1993: [1]

Benin, Burkina Faso, Cameroon, Chad, Cote d'Ivoire, Djibouti, Egypt, Ethiopia, The Gambia, Ghana, Guinea, Guinea-Bissau, Kenya, Liberia, Mali, Niger, Nigeria, Senegal, Sierra Leone, Sudan, Tanzania, Togo, Uganda

COTE D'IVOIRE : OVERVIEW

Cote d'Ivoire - the name "Ivory Coast" has been recently officially rejected - was included in the previous edition of this report, and this information is summarized here. No new information is available at present. The research that was suggested by Prof. Agrege Diarra, who for many years headed the maternity section of the University Hospital of Abidjan in Treichville, has never been conducted. But it is known that practically the entire female population of this country is excised. I went to see Prof. Diarra first in 1977 and also on subsequent visits to Abidjan: He stated that excision is widely practiced throughout Cote d'Ivoire including in Abidjan, and this was confirmed by midwives [2]

The maternity section of the Treichville Hospital has complete health records of women delivering there since 1966, so Prof Diarra stated. These records include information of any problems resulting from excision and are available to anyone interested in a serious research study. Since women from all ethnic groups come to the capital, and many of them now have their babies in the hospital, these records provide an overview of what kind of operations are practiced on girls and women by the many different ethnic groups all over the country. But no one to date has undertaken such an investigation. A national committee affiliated with the IAC has been organized [3] and participated in their 1990 IAC Conference in Addis Ababa.

A medical article published by a gynecologist and obstetrician more than 10 years ago records that FGM is widely practiced in the area of Odienne, a small town in the north-west of the country. Dr. Silberstein, who worked in the local hospital sponsored by Belgian medical aid, reported that practically all women were mutilated. The operations are performed on groups of girls usually at the beginning of adolescence and sometimes younger and involve removal of the clitoris as well as the small lips.

The ethnic group living in that area are the Malinke, who are Moslem and are locally called Dioula. Dr. Silberstein in correspondence added that he was called on when several girls were hemorrhaging due to a group excision ceremony; they would have bled to death without his help. He estimates that the death toll is quite high because literally all female children are forced to undergo these mutilations.

But in rural areas there are no hospitals or Western medical help, and the traditional method of dealing with bleeding by throwing dirt on the wound is completely ineffective but results in tetanus which is fatal if the girl survives the bleeding or infection. Dr. Silberstein also observed that all other ethnic groups in the area practice excision including those who are not Moslem. He also observed cases of spontaneous infibulation, which occurs when radical mutilations result in closing the introitus if the legs of the girl are tied together or crossed after the operation and she is immobilized.

At my most recent visit to Cote d'Ivoire in 1988 very little had changed concerning FGM, though a huge new modern concrete Catholic cathedral had been built in Abidjan, and the city was newly resplendent with an array of modern high rise towers including one covered with pink mirror glass. The Catholic president also recently built the largest Renaissance church with a bigger dome than St. Peter's in Rome in his new capital, Yamoussoukro. The Pope came from Rome last year for its formal inauguration. But in the shadow of this huge, new, enormously costly Roman Catholic monument little girls continue to bleed to death due to traditional mutilations that the Pope has not prohibited and that his Church still condones throughout Africa.

Cote d'Ivoire continues to be governed since its independence in 1960 by Houphouet-Boigny who prior to independence represented Cote d'Ivoire in the French Assembly in Paris from 1946 to 1959. The modern appearance of Abidjan with the largest luxury hotels and conference center in West Africa is in stark contrast to an official infant mortality rate of 121/1000 which in reality is much higher and an official literacy rate of 45 percent which means that probably fewer than a third of the women can read.

The education gap between women and men in West Africa is huge due to the legacy of the French plus the Moslem influences. School attendance is not compulsory; official attendance is 76 percent which means less than half of that number for girls. In no other African country is there such a contrast between the very modern and sophisticated image of Abidjan and rural living conditions which, as in most of rural Africa, hardly change.

GHANA : OVERVIEW OF FGM PRACTICES

In Ghana traditionally FGM has not been practiced on the coast or in Accra, the capital, but only in the northern part of the country. But with greater mobility and due to the attraction of urban areas people who move to the capital bring their customs along. The Ghanaian Association for Women's Welfare was formed at the 1984 Seminar in Dakar and joined the Inter African Committee on Traditional Practices Affecting the Health of Women and Children which was organized at that meeting. [4] First of all the association had to research the facts regarding the practice in Ghana, which were not known.

In the official **Bulletin of Nurse-Educators** of September 1985 [5] a survey was published where and why FGM is practiced in Ghana.

> "This practice is prevalent in certain areas in the Northern and Upper Regions, i.e., among the migrant Lobis from Ivory Coast; people who have moved from the Upper East and West and settled in Tamale, but the indigenous Dagombas and Gonjas do not practice it; Upper East, i.e., Bolga, Sandema area, Novorongo, Bawku and the Gambaga Districts; Upper West, i.e., Lawra, Tumu and Wa." [6]

A variety of reasons are given which are quite similar to the reasons professed elsewhere: it is an initiation into womanhood; it is attractive for men and preserves virginity; etc. A family celebration is linked with the procedure. Since circumcisors make money from the operations, they promote them. All kinds of aftercare and treatments of the wound are provided, but of course this does not help if a blood vessel is severed in which case the girl usually bleeds to death.

The article then describes physical and psychological complications resulting from the mutilations and concludes with a series of recommendations to bring about change in the mentality of the people. Finally formulation of a national policy for the abolishment of the practice is proposed. In another study in the upper east region of Ghana by a physician for the Ghanaian Association for Women's Welfare, the above statements of the **Bulletin of Nurse-Educators** are confirmed: FGM is practiced throughout the northern region of Ghana and along the border area of Burkina Faso mostly in the rural areas.

In another study covering southern Ghana also made for the Women's Welfare Association [7] specific areas in southern Ghana, especially those where immigrants from the north settle including in Accra, were investigated. Though FGM traditionally is not practiced in Accra or in the south, the investigators found large numbers of immigrants from the northern part of the country in Accra all of whom continued to practice FGM even after living in town for years though they were from many different ethnic groups.

The reasons given by the immigrants again are similar to the ones cited above and in most other areas in West Africa: because it is the tradition, to preserve virginity, to reduce sexual desire, it is a prerequisite for marriage, it makes childbirth easier: These justifications show again that the respondents have no comprehension of anatomy or physiology. In one ethnic group the Frafra men do the operating, which is unusual. As elsewhere it is claimed that the girl is at fault or evil spirits are at work if she bleeds to death. It is never the fault of the operator or the operation. The study also points out that Islam, which is practiced in the north of Ghana, fails to speak against FGM because it does not conflict with the doctrine of Islam. Christianity however discourages the practice.

As stated before, in Accra and on the coast FGM was not practiced: What goes on in the rural areas is easy to ignore. Due to the above cited research it become known that FGM has spread to Accra now and the south, due to immigration. In this way FGM is spread to ever larger areas. The same goes on in other countries, for instance, in Egypt FGM has spread to the Mediterranean coast and into southern Sudan from Khartoum. African migrants and refugees are bringing along the practice wherever they go.

But there is one great difference: In the Western world FGM is prohibited as a criminal mutilation and classified as child abuse even though some unscrupulous physicians will do the procedure for payment. In Africa the mutilations are being spread over ever larger areas by the bride-price. When a man from an ethnic group that practices FGM wants a wife, he will pay the bride price only if she is mutilated according to what is practiced by his ethnic group; and all their future daughters will be mutilated as well. In this way FGM is spreading all over Africa, as the example of Ghana shows.

CHAD: SURVEY OF FGM AND TRADITIONAL PRACTICES

In Chad FGM is practiced throughout the country as well as other damaging traditional practices such as food tabus and child marriage. A local Committee on Traditional Practices affiliated with the Inter African Committee has been recently formed [8] which found that the infant mortality rate was one of the highest in Africa and in the world - (180 to 210 per thousand) due in part to damaging traditions.

UNICEF supported an investigation of FGM. [9] A country-wide research program was led by a professor of the University of Chad, combining three separate studies made in the three zones of the country. The research was conducted in 1990-1991. In the introduction of the UNICEF report, it is stated that "the problem is being met with openness and tact and that great importance is being attached to the recommendations". Specific recommendations for action are made for each zone, as the study showed that the populations of the three zones have different opinions on FGM.

Predictably, in the area of N'Djamena, the capital, where modern health care is available, the younger generation including younger parents reject the practice. In the southern zone of the country, the Protestant Christians also disapprove of the initiation of girls that includes FGM. But in the eastern and central zones the Moslem religious authorities approve of the practice and social pressure confirms its continuation.

The list of specific conclusions and recommendations which resulted from the research project proposes for the most conservative areas that:

> "In the rural areas it is necessary to start with health care for those excized to limit complications. In the most conservative areas it is necessary to proceed carefully as otherwise the practice will go underground. Information booklets with pictures should be developed in French and Arabic as well as films. The imams need to present a clear position on excision and explain in the mosques that excision is not required by Islam."

In the South and the capital it is recommended to involve the schools and to distribute information at health centers, women's meetings and other public occasions. Radio broadcasts are proposed as well as making a film showing that excision is dangerous. The film should be projected at various public meetings. It is also recommended that the support of health personnel should be enlisted, especially midwives and physicians, and all pregnant women should be taught about the damaging results of excision. Traditional leaders should be involved asking them to explain to their supporters the health damage and risks of the operations; and the same is recommended for the religious leadership. Unfortunately UNICEF in Chad has done nothing about implementing these recommendations and requests for information on any actions have remained unanswered.

These recommendations are quite similar to what has been proposed in many other countries. One important function of the IAC is to exchange such information, but the UNICEF report never even mentions the IAC.

It finally needs to be acknowledged that everywhere in Africa, including in Chad, the Islamic population is most deeply involved in FGM and least ready to change. To be sure, Islamic scholars claim over and over that FGM is not a religious requirement and that the practice pre-dates by many hundreds of years the rise of Islam. Yet in all countries where FGM is practiced, it is the Islamic part of the population that most stubbornly clings to these practices and local Islamic leaders promote them among illiterate people in the rural areas all over Africa, no doubt also in Chad. Islamic intellectuals state it is against the tenets of Islam to hurt or injure another person. But unfortunately these scholars never preach to the people to stop the mutilations because it is against Islam.

The IAC-affiliated Committee of Chad outlined extensive plans already at the 1990 IAC Regional Conference of all IAC affiliates held at Addis Ababa. Their program is specifically concerned with holding a series of training seminars for health personnel and for traditional birth attendants as well as organizing information campaigns. A national seminar is also proposed to reach and raise the consciousness of the public about the damaging results of traditional practices on the health of women and children.

DJIBOUTI: AN OVERVIEW OF FGM PRACTICES

Djibouti, a former French colony that gained independence only in 1977, is inhabited by nomadic, ethnic groups related to the Somalis who similarly infibulate all females. The tiny country of less than half a million people is located in a strategic area at the tip of the Horn of Africa. The French, as elsewhere in Africa, ignored the ongoing infibulation of all female children; as a result nothing has been done about the terrible health problems of virtually the entire female population until quite recently when women in leadership positions, living in the town, began to talk about it. A national committee to stop FGM has now been formed and is affiliated with the IAC. [10]

The United Nations Human Rights Center, subcommission on the prevention of discrimination, recently published a study on infibulation in Djibouti based on a visit to Djibouti by the Special Rapporteur, Halima Embarek Warzazi. [11] At the time of this mission the rapporteur discussed measures to stop FGM with the national committee and also visited the Ministry of Health and Education as well as the Ministry of Justice and Islamic Affairs.

The Union Nationalę des Femmes de Djibout (UNFD) is pressing the government for legislation against FGM. They set up a clinic where girls are taken for a mild form of the operation which is done with local anesthesia. The clinic is designed to sensitize mothers about the danger of FGM. The human rights team, however, was informed that most of the time grandmothers, after the girls were operated at the clinic, had them infibulated the traditional way, claiming that the operation was not complete enough. This unfortunately demonstrates again that any so-called "intermediary step" that is so often advocated especially by physicians, for instance in the Sudan, does not work. The only effective way to deal with the issue is to prohibit all forms of FGM.

Already in spring and summer 1979 the local paper, **Le Reveil**, - which publishes in French - published a series of articles on FGM under the heading "Stop the Sexual Mutilation of Women". [12] This courageous move on the part of the paper was inspired by the WHO Seminar in Khartoum, which had taken place a few months earlier and to which Djibouti had sent a delegation.

The series of articles consisted mainly of letters by readers after an introduction by the editor. It was based - so the editors reported - on a request by a woman asking the paper to provide women with space to discuss affairs of concern to women. She stated: "We live in an Islamic country, should women of Djibouti not discuss what of their traditions they wish to preserve and what to discard"? The editors, after praising the contributions of women of Djibouti, invited everyone to send letters about FGM to the paper and in the following issues printed a large number of them including some editorial comments.

But almost all the letters the paper printed were written by men, including a long one from France. The editor commented that all letters rejected FGM, urging that this practice must be abolished. Once more all the health problems of infibulation were discussed; indeed some of the letters written by Moslem men sound like women's rights advocates. Yet infibulation continues to be practiced by all, as it is a marriage requirement and as everywhere else, it is paid for by men.

Only one man finally had the courage to point out that the vast majority of the people of Djibouti do not read the paper and cannot write; they are illiterate nomads and cling to their traditions, but no one bothers to even talk to them. And he explains that the worst insult is to tell a girl she is open, which means she is a prostitute.The letter writer continues that this whole debate is false as those who practice FGM are left out.

The writer has a point: All too often the debate on FGM never reaches those who practice it. Far too little effort has been made everywhere to reach families on the grass-roots level who do not even know what those who claim to be decisionmakers discuss. Most women are left out of all such debates by men: they cannot be reached by published information because they are illiterate.

In Djibouti - though the traditions are very strong - the country and population are so small that it would be possible to reach the majority and persuade them that it is in their own interest to change. With literacy only 20 percent, which means less than half of that for women - the priorities are clear.

LIBERIA : SUMMARY REPORT ON FGM

Due to the continuing civil war which has been raging intermittently for several years, this country has been largely destroyed with many thousands killed. Liberia had a special relationship with the US as five percent of the population were descendants of freed American slaves who began to arrive in the area of Monrovia, the present capital, after 1822. They united to form the Commonwealth of Liberia in 1838. Most of the rest of the population, at least 12 of the 16 distinct ethnic groups, practice FGM often in radical form.

Secret societies - much as in neighboring Sierra Leone - organize the initiation ceremonies which are obligatory and include excision. Due to the secrecy - society members are sworn not to reveal what is going on in the bush - little is known about the actual practices. The inevitable deaths of some of the initiates are ascribed to bad spirits and supernatural powers, never to the real cause.

Literacy in Liberia is 25 percent officially, which means it is much less for women and therefore the belief in supernatural powers invoked by the secret societies is very strong. Despite the relationship with the US, especially by the elite, nothing has been done to stop this wholesale abuse and mutilation of female children, which continue to this day.

In Monrovia these secret societies have started to advertise in the newspapers announcing their so-called "intensive training programs" for little girls, asking a hefty fee. [13] What this really means is that the children will be excised which is what this "training" of infant girls is all about. The Sande Societies, which maintain special locations in the bush where they "educate girls on the culture of their ancestors", keep them for two months at the time. The children are not told what is going to be done to them.

Recently however, young girls living in Monrovia who have some education are refusing to take part in these initiations. But in the rural areas there is no choice; all girls must undergo the initiation conducted by the secret Sande Societies which operate among most of the traditional ethnic groups.

A research report by the Liberian Health Network [14] surveys the present situation in rural areas which have been difficult to investigate. Most women are afraid to talk as the societies are still very powerful. Mr. Louis Pupo of the health network described the investigation of FGM which he conducted in 1989 before the civil war and which took his team all over the country:

> "In some areas, we were met with strong resistance and with threatening remarks. They said that FGM was a subject no one should discuss or mention in their areas. They placed much secrecy on these activities so that it is difficult to get information. FGM is carried out in the 'Gra-Gra Bush' of the Sande Societies among all tribes in Liberia except the Greboes, Krus, and Sarpos. The procedure is surrounded by secrecy and practiced by traditional midwives called Zoe (older women who are members and instructors in the Sande Societies). The practice is followed by both educated and uneducated women who hold strongly to their traditions. The Zoe is the head of the traditional secret society where many things which are positive in Liberian culture are practiced. The Zoes look after women and children in their area from birth to grave. . ."

Ninety percent of the Zoes have no formal education and have different occupations such as farmers, traders, herbalists; most have practiced FGM for many years. In the absence of any schools in the rural areas, girls are sent to the Sande Bush Schools because, though they learn all the farming and household tasks by practice, they are still considered ignorant and immature unless they go to the Sande Society School, where they are excised.

A young woman in order to establish herself and gain wisdom, get a husband and become a good wife must participate in the Sande Bush School, which is surrounded by mystery with sacred powers ascribed to their leaders. The Sande Societies are regarded as the keepers of culture and tradition regulating the affairs of the female world. The Zoes command considerable influence and prestige in the community; they also deliver more babies than midwives. The Sande women's society headed by a Zoe is supported by a corresponding male indigenous secret society and is the only authentic organization where women exert power in their own right without male interference.

LIBERIA (continued)

There are undocumented cases of infibulation among the Lormas, Belels and Kissi tribes. The tribes that practice clitoridectomy are: Bassa, Kpelle, Gola, Mano, Gio, Vai, Dei, Mende, Krahn, while those practicing excision - removing both the clitoris and labia minora - include: Lorma, Kissi, Belle, Gbandi. FGM of children starts from the age of three years to puberty. Sexual life starts at 12 to 14 years; early marriage is common, and the bride-price is paid to the bride's parents. If it is found that a bride is not a virgin, the husband beats her up and returns her to her parents. Polygamy is commonly practiced and all women live together in the same household.

In addition the women of a number of tribes decorate their bodies with scars. The reason for these tatoos is that this is supposed to arouse the husband. The social pressures to be mutilated and thus become a respected member of society are very great. The penalties for not being excised include lack of respect, refusal by men to marry women who are not excised, persecution and insults by other women. Some girls who are not excised are forced out of their village and are called sinners. And the report concludes:

> "Since the Government licensed and gave permission for the practices to continue it does support the practice and those who adhere to these brutal customs are not ridiculed but keep the information on the issue secret and silent. . . The Zoe pressure people for selfish reasons and financial gain to continue FGM at the expense of the vulnerable. Even the TBAs are involved in the mutilations. . .
>
> The subject of FGM was never open for public discussion and so it does not receive proper public attention by leaders. There is no legislation against FGM in Liberia; it is so strongly entrenched that among the tribes who practice FGM, nearly every woman undergoes the operation. . .
>
> But the excuse that cultural practices are sacrosant is no longer convincing to some Liberians. . . Some women, especially in Monrovia, realize that action must be taken now against female genital mutilation which humiliates and degrades them. They recognize that only women themselves can create awareness in our society . . . and fight against the practice urging its total abolition."

The continuing political mismanagement of this country by the male leadership has obstructed development as the high illiteracy and the economic problems confirm. At the end of 1989 after armed confrontations by men vying for power, the ongoing civil war started which has continued ever since. **The New York Times** reported recently "the conflict grew with a vast tribal war uprooting about half of Liberia's 2.5 million people." [15]

This civil war by now has destroyed much of the infrastructure of this country; women and children as elsewhere in Africa are the victims of their own men who continue to fight over a country that they have all but destroyed. The United Nations, as **the New York Times** reports, is warning the warring factions that it will pull out as mediator, predicting this will make the country ungovernable for the foreseeable future, after three years of continous ethnically based fighting. Gun wielding teenagers, it is reported, roam about the countryside raping and looting villages.

Much as in Somalia, the country has reverted to tribal warfare which was the predominant occupation of men in traditional Africa. But now these men use imported weapons that are far more lethal and devastating than what was used in traditional tribal wars.

This question must finally be raised: Violence - as we have learned by examining the causes of family violence - is learned behavior; it is transmitted in each family from an early age. FGM is the ultimate practice of violence as it is directed against helpless female children. These mutilations in each family socialize boys for lifelong violence, brutality and attacks on the helpless. FGM and other customs such as polygamy, the bride-price, rape, wife abuse, child marriage and the forced subordination of all females are human rights violations. African leaders condone these customs that socialize their own society for destruction at their peril. The civil wars raging all over sub-Saharan Africa have made this continent more violent than any other. The boys in each family are taught by example that violent behavior is the road to success. Unless African leaders learn that human rights are indivisible, African men will destroy their countries by civil wars and AIDS.

FOOTNOTES:

1. IAC - Inter African Committee on Traditional Practices Affecting the Health of Women and Children, 145 rue de Lausanne, CH 1202 Geneva, Switzerland, and c/o ECA/ ATRCW, P.O. Box 3001, Addis Ababa, Ethiopia.
2. **WIN NEWS**, Vol. 3, No. 2, Summer 1977, p. 38. See also "The Epidemiology of Female Genital Mutilation" **Tropical Doctor**, July 1978, p. 153.
3. Comite National du CI-AFM. Ablo Koffi Jean, 01 BP 4377, Abidjan 01, Cote d'Ivoire. -Inter African Committee Cote d'Ivoire.
4. Ghanaian Association for Women's Welfare, Mrs. Gloria Aryee, Chair. P.O. Box 9582 Airport, Accra, Ghana.
5. **NEDUB** - Official Bulletin of Nurse-Educators, P.O. Box 81. Korle-Bu. Ghana. Editor: Mrs. Mavis Akutter. See **WIN NEWS**, Vol. 12, No. 2, Spring 1986, pp. 27-28.
6. A survey report by Dr. John Kadri, M.D. for the Ghanaian Association for Women's Welfare, P.O. Box 9582 Airport, Accra, Ghana. See **WIN NEWS**, Vol. 12, No. 2, Spring 1986, p. 3.
7. From a study by Prof. P. A. Twumasi for the Ghanaian Association for Women's Welfare, P.O. Box 9582 Airport, Accra Ghana. Funded by Population Action International (PAI), 1120 19th Street, NW, Washington, DC 20036.
8. Inter African Committee of Chad: Mme. Adoum Moursal Fatime, B.P. 439 Mairie, N'Djamena, Chad.
9. "An Investigation of Female Excision in Chad," by Prof. Ache Nabia, University of Chad, August 1991. Published by the Ministry of Planning and Cooperation and UNICEF. Sponsored by UNICEF.
10. Inter African Committee of Djibouti. Comite national de lutte contre la circoncision feminine, c/o UNFD, B.P. 127, Djibouti. Mme. Roukya Abdillahi, Director.
11. Study: Traditional Practices Affecting the Health of Women and Children - Final Report by Special Rapporteur Ms. Halima Embarek Warzazi. Commission on Human Rights, Sub Commission on Prevention of Discrimination and Protection of Minorities, Forty-third session, Item 4 of the Provisional Agenda (E/CN.,4/Sub.2/1991/6); United Nations Center for Human Rights, CH-1211, Geneva 10, Switzerland. See **WIN NEWS**, Vol. 18, No. 2, Spring 1992, p. 42.
12. See **WIN NEWS**, Vol. 6, No. 1, Winter 1980, pp. 36-39.
13. Sande Society Advertises "Womanhood Training" by Dr. Patricia Divine as reported in the **Daily Observer** (Monrovia), Jan. 25, 1990. See **WIN NEWS**, Vol. 16, No. 3, Summer 1990, p. 25.
14. Louis Pupo Wiefueh, Liberian Health Action Network, P.O. Box 10-3212, Monrovia, Liberia. See **WIN NEWS**, Vol. 19, No. 2, Spring 1993, pp. 46-48.
15. **New York Times**, November 5, 1993, p. A3, "As Liberia's Factions Talk, Strife and Fear Drag On."

THE ARAB PENINSULA : YEMEN

The present country of Yemen is the result of the union in May of 1990 between South Yemen (capital: Aden) and North Yemen (capital: Sanaa). Yemen, with a population now of about 12 million, is located on the southwestern corner of the Arab Peninsula along the Red Sea and Gulf of Aden. Its population is Arabic and follows Islam. The capital of unified Yemen is Sanaa, though Aden has always been an important port and way station used by the British on the route to India.

Female genital mutilation (FGM) is recorded in the former South Yemen but not in Sanaa and the North - though now due to unification this may change. Besides in and around Aden, FGM is recorded along the southern coast in the Hadramawt (or Hadhramout) area and the Tihama coastal plain but not in the highlands.

A delegate from the former South Yemen, Mrs. Mehani Mohammed Saleh, Maternal and Child Health Supervisor of the Ministry of Health, Aden, [1] participated in the WHO Seminar on Traditional Practices Affecting the Health of Women and Children in Khartoum in 1979, reporting that excision was practiced.

Southern Yemen faces Somalia across the Red Sea, and Somalis, who subject their daughters to infibulation, can also be found in Yemen, including many recent refugees.

Genital operations are recorded throughout the southern part of the Arab Peninsula as Dr. Guy Pieters, a gynecologist, who had occasion to see women from South Yemen when he worked in the hospitals of Somalia, states.[2] The operation, performed by traditional birth attendants, is excision of part of the clitoris of babies between seven days and one month old. The reasons given are "it is the tradition, it does not look nice when a girl is not circumcised" and "she desires sex if not circumcised, which is a shame for her and for her relatives." [3]

Another damaging traditional practice that continues today in the southern part of the Arab Peninsula and along the Persian Gulf is to put salt into the vagina of women after delivery; this induces narrowing of the vagina (stenosis) that may be so severe as to make coitus difficult, quite aside from obstructing childbirth. The purpose of putting salt into the vagina, according to the women who do it, is to restore the vagina to its pre-childbirth dimensions and make intercourse more pleasurable for the husband - because if a woman does not please sexually, she may be divorced.

In 1992 a study on the "Prevalence of Female Circumcision in Yemen - A Compilation of Facts," was prepared by Sereen Thaddeus, an advisor for a family planning project funded by the U.S. Agency for International Development in Sanaa. [4] According to the investigator:

> "All available written and verbal accounts indicate that the practice known as 'khitaan al banaat' (female circumcision) is localized in Yemen. Its prevalence is well documented for the Tihama, widely reported for the Hadhramaut, spotty in other parts (e.g., Lahj, Aden and Abyan) and totally absent from the Highlands and desert areas.
>
> In the regions of Yemen where female circumcision is practiced among Yemenis, it is performed by excising the hood of the clitoris and/or the edges of the labia minora. Infibulation is reported among Somali immigrants and refugees living in Yemen."

The report also states that the birth attendants and the midwives are the ones who excise the female infants. Since FGM is related to Islam in Yemen, the practice, for instance in Aden, is carried out by the most religious and traditional families.

Due to the proximity of Somalia, Yemen - as all other countries within reach of Somali refugees - now has many more Somali immigrants who, as elsewhere, practice infibulation and continue to mutilate their female children born in Yemen. Furthermore, in Yemen there is no prohibition of these mutilations as the above-cited research study also reports, though the practice is diminishing in Aden.

As to who in the family decides whether or not a daughter is to be operated on, the report summarizes:

> "The father appears to be the family member who decides whether his daughters will be circumcised or not. This factor assumes importance in assessing the prevalence of the practice among couples of mixed ethnicities. Their daughters will not be circumcised if the practice is not part of the father's tradition. Cost appears to be another factor affecting decision-making among Yemeni families." [5]

Since circumcision of boys in this Moslem society is a religious command, it has to be done and paid for. But in the case of girls the costs involved sometimes result in sparing baby girls, and in the very large families (the average is more than eight living children per woman) these costs, given the poverty of especially rural areas, mount up and act as deterrent.

In summary the investigator states:

> "There is no indication in written and verbal accounts of health complications resulting from clitoridectomy as practiced in Yemen by Yemenis. When complications such as infection do occur, they appear to be related to negligence rather than to the operation itself." [6]

And in the conclusion of this three-week investigation it is claimed "there are no reported health complications for the infant girl nor the mature woman as a result of this practice . . . . In terms of women's health priorities the practice . . . of female circumcision is not a pressing issue." [7]

The conclusion, that FGM as practiced in Yemen has no reported damaging effects on women's health or sexuality, is of course the same as has been reported in the past in many African countries by official investigations (this one was done in only three weeks), mostly among midwives who are profiting from the practice and other women who have little contact with the rest of the world. Literacy in Yemen is very low, especially among women, and the strict Moslem environment provides very few opportunities for education of women. What is more, FGM is performed in the belief that it is a religious practice - even though it is not a command, which is similar in the Sudan and also West Africa where local Moslem leaders promote the practice on religious grounds.

The operation is performed on newborn babies where infant mortality is very high - but no correlation is made, though is it claimed that "infections are rare." But experience from Africa unfortunately shows that infant mortality in the mind of most people is never related to FGM - rather, many other factors, including witchcraft, are blamed. For instance, severing of a blood vessel in the genital area inevitably results in death unless immediate hospitalization is sought and available.

There is no reason to believe that the mutilations - that is, the accidental cutting of a blood vessel - would not lead to uncontrolled bleeding any less often in Yemen than it does everywhere else, and that is the most frequent cause of death where FGM is performed on infants where no hospitals are available, quite aside from tetanus.

As to the claim that is made again that FGM, as practiced in Yemen, has no influence on sexual satisfaction of the woman, this same claim can be found wherever an outsider has conducted an investigation talking to local women. It is a useless question to ask as it is impossible to get a factual answer. The only way to establish these facts on sexual response would be to compare sexual satisfaction of a large enough sample of women before and after FGM. That is, ask the same group of women about sexual satisfaction before the operation, then have them undergo the operation, and after they are healed to test their reaction to sexual intercourse again. Obviously this is impossible and utterly unacceptable. Yet this would be the way to establish the facts on a strictly clinical basis for those who continue to claim that excision has no effect on sexual response.

However Dr. Salah Abu Bakr did research in the Sudan, examining the skin and tissues cut away during excision under a microscope, which showed large numbers of nerve endings. The skin left in the genital area of women who had been mutilated had hardly any nerve endings; but without nerves there is no feeling. This research unequivocally established the fact that cutting away the skin and tissues of the clitoris - which is what the operations do - results in loss of feeling. (See "Case History : Sudan.")

This surely should have laid to rest the issue of putting any credence in statements by women who are mutilated that the operations do not affect them. Obviously they have no way of knowing the results of the mutilations on their own sexual response or for that matter on their personality, as they have never known anything else.

It is time that researchers finally acquaint themselves with the pertinent medical literature, such as the study by Dr. Bakr cited above which is included in the report of the WHO Seminar in Khartoum and is readily available to all investigators everywhere.

THE ARAB PENINSULA: SULTANATE OF OMAN

In Oman, which adjoins southern Yemen and controls the entrance of the Persian Gulf, excision is practiced similarly to southern Yemen and neighboring Gulf States. The practice of putting salt into the vagina of women after childbirth also is recorded by midwives in the area. [8]

Dr. Layla Jassim Ghulam, the senior public health officer from the Ministry of Health at Muscat, Oman, and delegate to the Khartoum Seminar, contributed a paper on early teenage childbirth and its consequences for mother and child. There is a direct relationship between early teenage pregnancy and mortality of both mother and child. Twenty-seven percent of the women in the study were married before the age of 11; 86 percent were married by the age of 15, according to another study by UNICEF. The entire life of women is spent bearing children - until the women die, frequently from childbearing. Excision contributes to the childbirth problems. Malnutrition, especially of teenage mothers, is widespread due to too early and frequent pregnancy, which in turn results in high infant mortality. [9]

THE ARAB PENINSULA : UNITED ARAB EMIRATES

Due to oil revenues, the per capita income of the population of the Federation of Emirates that make up this country is one of the highest in the world. According to a 1990 estimate, it is $21,335 due to oil. Of the 1.8 million people living in UAR, only 15 to 20 percent are citizens, the rest are guest workers. Literacy, according to official figures, is 60 percent which, in this strict Islamic society, means that it is much less for women.

According to informal reports from maternity clinics in various areas of this country, the status and living conditions of women and female children are ruled by tradition.

All women in the Persian Gulf area traditionally were circumcised (ablation of the clitoris at puberty). Many women from neighboring countries, chiefly from Egypt, Somalia and Sudan, are acquired for a brideprice paid to their parents by the wealthy polygamous men. Frequently, these women are more severely mutilated than those from the Gulf area. Severe tears in delivery often are the result of the operations, so midwives at local clinics report.

It is said that women who are not circumcised cannot pray because they are not pure and clean. Another reason given is that uncircumcised women are so "hot" that they are uncontrollable.

The Arab practice of putting salt into the vagina after delivery, which results in stenosis (narrowing) of the vagina after delivery (see above), is reported in the medical literature to be disappearing, though some claim it is still practiced. Other damaging traditions such as cauterie (burning with red-hot irons), based on the statement of Mohammed, "You shall treat illness with fire," were also reported until recently.

THE ARAB PENINSULA: BAHRAIN

Bahrain, a small group of islands in the Persian Gulf, also has greatly profited from oil, but literacy officially is only 74 percent - much less for women.

A medical source reports that circumcision consists in a cut made over the clitoris. The operation was very widespread until recently but is much less frequently practiced now.

Virginity is all important. After the wedding night, a blood-stained sheet must be shown, or the bride and her family are dishonored (see "Case History: Egypt"). However, medical sources report an increase of venereal disease and out-of-wedlock pregnancies. [10]

There is little doubt that similar practices - excision, child marriage, and putting rock salt into the vagina of women after childbirth - exist in other parts of the Arab Peninsula and around the Persian Gulf. These practices are not subject to political boundaries but are traditions held and perpetuated by ethnic groups no matter where they live.

Some historians claim that the practice of clitoridectomy originated on the Arab Peninsula and was exported from there and spread by Arab traders all over Africa. Arabs have traveled and traded very widely in Africa since antiquity and also engaged in a very extensive slave trade. However, other historic sources claim just the opposite is true: That excision was originally an African custom that was taken up by Arabs and then spread by them. Certainly the earliest confirmed information of the practice is from Egypt where it has been recorded more than 2,000 years ago (see "History").

No firsthand medical records are available at present for Saudi Arabia or from other countries in that region. But due to increased mobility and especially war and civil conflicts that displace large numbers of people, their customs are spread by them. However, due to the huge oil revenues education also has spread, even to formerly remote areas, and health services as well as health education is reaching more and more women who in the past had no access to such information - and this is the yeast for change.

FOOTNOTES

1. Salah, Mrs. Mehani, Maternal and Child Health Supervisor of the Ministry of Health, "The Health of Women and Children in Democratic Yemen", pp. 1-6. Report: WHO/EMRO Technical Publication No. 2, Vol. 2, 1982, "Traditional Practices Affecting the Health of Women and Children", Khartoum, February 10-15, 1979.
2. Pieters, G. "Gynaecology at the Country of the Sewn Women", **Acta Chirurgica Belgica**, No. 3, May 1972 (in French).
3. **WIN NEWS**, Vol. 5, No. 2, Spring 1979, p. 56 "Report from Maternity Clinics in the Eastern Part of the Country - (Arab Peninsula)".
4. The Prevalence of Female Circumcision in Yemen/A Compilation of Facts. Prepared by Sereen Thaddeus, Consultant, and Submitted to the Royal Netherlands Embassy, Sana'a December 1992. Ministerie Van Buitenlandse Saken, the Netherlands Ministry of Foreign Affairs, Postbus 20061, 2500 EB's - Gravenhage, The Netherlands.
5. Ibid., p. 1, "Executive Summary".
6. Ibid.
7. Ibid., p. 14, "Conclusion".
8. Ghulam, Dr. Layla Jassim, "Early Teenage Childbirth: Consequences for Mother and Child", WHO/EMRO Technical Publication No. 2, Vol. 2, 1982, "Traditional Practices Affecting the Health of Women and Children".
9. **WIN NEWS**, Vol. 5, No. 2, Spring 1979, p. 56.
10. Ibid., p. 57

CASE HISTORY : ASIA

In Southeast Asia, the operations practiced on female children can be defined as "female circumcision" and are very different from what is done in Africa in several ways: The operations are performed as a religious Moslem rite and therefore limited to the Moslem population of Indonesia and Malaysia, with no other religious groups involved. The operations are not indigenous in Asia but were imported with Moslemization, while in Africa and the Middle East the opposite is true: Female Genital Mutilation in continental Africa was practiced long before Mohammed, but the practice was adopted and spread by Islam. Inquiries made in other parts of Asia with medical schools and hospitals as well as literature searches all point to the fact that female genital operations are not traditional and are unknown among most of the Asian population.

In Malaysia, only the Malays, who are Moslems, are involved in the practice; large numbers of Chinese and Indians live there as well, but have nothing to do with the religious practices of the Malays. In Indonesia, similarly, the operations are practiced by the devout Moslems and are confirmed at present only on the Island of Java.

According to descriptions from physicians, the intervention most often consists in an incision of the skin above the clitoris; sometimes a cut is made on the clitoris or the labia minora. It is also said that in some cases, no cutting takes place or only a drop of blood is produced by pricking the clitoris.

According to Dr. Haji Ali Akbar of the Yarsi School of Medicine [1] in Jakarta, there are no adverse effects in childbirth; he claims that except for the incision of the clitoris, the genitalia are left entirely intact. However, since the operations, for the most part, are performed by local village women, called 'dukun', there is always the danger of infections, including tetanus.

Dr. Abdul Wahab Ariff from the Faculty of Medicine of the University of Kebangsaan in Malaysia wrote that when he was the Director of Planning and Development at the Ministry of Health, a national plan for a Religious Circumcision Service was instituted for male children to protect boys from infections. But no plan was made for a female circumcision service. [2] And Dr. Ariff wrote: "It is a pity that there has been a conspicuous absence of both official and unofficial information in this country relating to accidents from female circumcision;" and he added: "I strongly believe in the total eradication of female circumcision among the Muslims in Malaysia." [3]

But, in the absence of any action by the Ministry of Health regarding female circumcision the operations continue to be practiced. No one knows how many little girls are injured or infected. No one has done any research if and to what extent female sexuality is impaired by the operation. Yet as a reason given for the operations, it is said both in Malaysia and Indonesia that they are done to prevent "hypersexuality" of women.

INDONESIA

In a book published in 1956, **Guidelines for Health Care According to Islamic Law**, by Ahmad Ramali, this description is supplied concerning female circumcision in Indonesia, which is translated and summarized here:

> "Female circumcision, known as 'chafdh' in Arabic, only involves lifting the 'bazr', which according to several lexicographers is the praeputium clitoridis. An-Nawawi, in the Sahih Muslim, offers the following explanation: 'Regarding female circumcision, it is required to cut a bit of the skin above the vulva.'

> "Therefore, circumcision among Muslim female children involves cutting the praeputium clitoridis, sometimes the clitoris itself or the labia minora. The child lies flat on her back, lifts up her knees and straddles her legs widely. Before that, the child must cleanse herself and urinate as much as possible. Her outer genitals are then washed carefully with soap and water. Above the mons veneris (female genitals) and vulva (vagina), a white cloth is placed by the shaman (healer, medicine man). The cloth is cut so that there is a small hole which is placed against the clitoris. Other instruments include a pair of scissors or a sharp knife and also a slice of Rhisoma (turmeric).
>
> At the time of the circumcision, the shaman fastens his left hand on the genital of the child. The hand is pressed slowly (gently) such that the clitoris protrudes through the white cloth, until the boundary between the glans and the corpus clitoridis is visible. After some words of prayers, the clitoris is cut with a pair of scissors or a small knife, as closely as possible along this boundary. If it is cut by a knife, a slice of Rhisom (turmeric) is placed as a base between the knife blade and the clitoris. It is a very fast procedure, and the child is kept occupied such that she is not aware of what is being done to her. A piece of cotton is placed on the wound to stop or prevent excessive bleeding. When the bleeding stops, the child is bathed again, and the process is thus considered complete.
>
> Some shamans cut a very small part of the praeputium. Others consider making some scarification on the praeputium surface or pricking several times the clitoris sufficient. There are also some shamans who simply touch the outer genitals with a knife, so that the procedure is only considered a symbol of circumcision." [4]

It is interesting to note that this operation is described in a book on health care - though nothing is said how such an operation would contribute to the health of a girl. One can only wonder if the author ever attended such a procedure because of his astonishing claim that the little girl is not aware of a man cutting into the most sensitive organ of her body - an operation that is extremely painful and a traumatic experience for one so young.

Another description of the procedure based on current research by the Population Institute of Indonesia in Yogyakarta was sent by Dr. Valerie Hull:

> "Stricter Muslims have the operation performed in the local Islamic hospital. In this case, a small pair of scissors is used to make a cut, and the wound is cleaned with antiseptic and cotton. The bloodied cotton is shown to the mother of the child as proof of the operation.
>
> Among the urban educated respondents the operation is carried out on girls aged 6-7 (grade 1 of primary school) though in strict Muslim families it is apparently performed on the newborn baby. Ramali's book also cites some variations recorded in Java among non-strict Muslims, ranging from age 2 to age 11. The midwives in our research claim that age 6-7 is most common; however, very poor people might tend to have it while the child is still an infant because then they can combine it with one of two other necessary ceremonies (when the umbilical cord stump falls off or on the 35-day birthday) and it is thus cheaper.
>
> The perceived purpose of the operation also varies according to different information - answers of stricter Muslim informants included to promote fertility and insure virtuousness, help urine or menstruation flow unobstructed. Rural informants who were not strict Muslims tended to be more vague yet - e.g. 'for the well-being of the child.' One midwife stated that a woman who has not had the ceremony (called 'tetesan' in Java) will not be able to cook rice properly; it will always be underdone - a devastating thing for a woman. It was my impression that no one was really sure of the purpose of tetesan, which is the case with most traditional ceremonies here. . .For the vast majority in Java, Islam has been adopted only piecemeal and is combined with Hindu and animistic ideology, which is perhaps the key to the wide variations in practices.
>
> The practice is still widespread in Java, though at least in this area (Yogyakarta) the operation is symbolic only. There is wide variation even within Java, and women themselves have little idea as to what is actually done and for what purpose. This is true even for urban educated informants." [5]

Dr. Haji Ali Akbar of the Centre for Islamic Studies of the Yarsi School of Medicine in Jakarta, wrote:

> "Female circumcision was introduced in Indonesia when the Islam religion was brought in the 8th Century. . .It is a common belief among the Muslims in Indonesia that their daughters have to be circumcised to prevent them from becoming hypersexual.
>
> The operations are performed mostly on small infants by traditional midwives ('dukun') whose knowledge about hygiene and sanitation is almost nil; though many publications on male circumcision are available, almost no information exists on female circumcision and from a religious point of view, it is disputable whether it is obligatory or not.
>
> The circumcision is usually done immediately or not long after the child is born; and it is performed either by a female village healer (dukun wanita) or a midwife. They use a very simple technique, namely by cutting the top of the glans very slightly, or by sticking a needle into the glans and thus produce a drop of blood or by rubbing the glans with curcumae. . .
>
> The village midwife says a few words before the operation and ends it with a short prayer." [6]

Dr. Akbar states that he had never watched anyone performing it, but that the information here supplied by him was gathered from several midwives.

Dr. Akbar also prepared a proposal for "A Research on Female Circumcision and Its Impact on Health in Indonesia", which would be carried out at the Yarsi School of Medicine; it includes a field investigation and evaluation.*

The most detailed description and background information that also links the operation to the Arab Middle East from where these practices were imported is given in a research report by the Indonesian Midwives' Association. In a signed document, Ms. Tuty Mustafa Dangkua, the Secretary General of the Midwives Association, the following information is provided which is summarized here: [8]

> "**Introduction**
>
> Circumcising (to cleanse). . .is a religious rite among Indonesian Moslems. In the Holy Al-Quranul Karim it is written that Moslems should follow the religion of the Prophet Ibrahim. The religion of the Prophet Ibrahim requires circumcising to be performed to all Moslems which is considered by the Prophet Muhammed something clean/pure and to be continued thereafter.
>
> Since almost 90 percent of the Indonesian population are believers in Islam, it is of no wonder that circumcising of female children is apparent throughout the country, even among ethnic groups who do not take Islam as their religion. This tradition is still maintained up to now, probably influenced by their everyday contact with the Moslems in their area.
>
> Circumcising among male children, which is said to have been pioneered by the Prophet Ibrahim, followed by the Jahilyah people who had been present in Indonesia prior to the entrance of Islam to the country, is usually begun and accompanied with a feast affordable by the parents. On the contrary, circumcising of female children is performed rather quietly without much fuss, by a 'dunkun' (traditional midwife), at the presence of the mother and other female members of the family. In reality, not many parents realize the real function of this circumcising, except those faithfuls of Islam who understand the meaning of the ritual. Circumcising is, in fact, one of the many methods of purifying the body, which forms the requirement of prayer to Allah.

---

* This proposal I sent to the World Health Organization, together with the rest of my research giving all sources quoted in this report as documentation of my research for my paper on "Female Circumcision in the World Today: A Global Review". [7]

The Aim of Circumcising in Female Children

- Because Islam considers circumcising an obligatory act due to receive an eternal reward, Indonesian Moslems take faith in it when their children have been circumcised, thus making the latter a fullfledged Moslem. . .

- According to studies, the tip of the clitoris comprises fat, filths from dried urine: all these, if not cleansed thoroughly, will bring forth a nasty smell which will consequently degrade the male's sexual lust for the women. . .it is for that reason the clitoris is circumcised.

- It is one of the requirements for praying that every part of the body should be purified prior to the act.

- To restrain the female libido which is centered on the clitoris, it is necessary to eliminate a little of its tip, which would result in the shifting of the female's 'erogenous zones' from the clitoris to the vagina. . .

Techniques of Circumcising Among Females in Indonesia

- The more devoted the parents in professing their religion, the younger their sons/daughers are to be circumcised. . .

- Female circumcising is done mainly by 'dukun praji' (traditional village birth attendants), but also is widely performed by nurses/midwives and less often by doctors or medical personnel.

- Tools frequently used consist of a sharp knife or a pair of small scissors. . ."

The description of the operation is exactly the same as the one given above from the book "Guidelines for Health Care According to Islamic Law" by Ahmad Ramali. The only difference is that the operator here is a dukun - that is, a woman - while according to Ramali the operator is a medicine man. The use of the white cloth with the small hole for the clitoris is described in identical terms and it is claimed that the cut is made so swiftly that "the child would never know what happened to her".

The report continues:

- "A uniform technique of female circumcising has not been developed yet by nurses/midwives; to a large extent they follow the 'dukuns' way of circumcising, that is only cutting off slightly the tip of the clitoris with a pair of sterile scissors. The genitals are first cleansed, then the child is told to lie down in bed, knees up and legs spread apart as far as possible. After the clitoris is made sterile with alcohol, the child must say aloud the two sentences of the 'Syahadah' and 'Fatihah' prior to the ritual. If the nurse/midwife in charge is also a Moslem, she should do the same. In circumcizing, serious bleeding rarely occurs. . .but should it ever happen the child must at once be transferred to the nearest public health center. . ."

The midwives' report also states that according to Islam in Indonesia female circumcision "is meant as a prerequisite for entering Islam". The following statement concludes the midwives' report:

- "According to experience concerning the ritual, the uncircumcised female has trouble in controlling her lust when encountering the male, thus a saying is produced '. . .this child has a wild behavior and sexual desire maybe because she has never been circumcised'. . ."

In June 1988 Professor Ahmad Watik Pratiknya of the Faculty of Medicine and Faculty of Graduate Studies at Gadjah Mada University in Yogyakarta spoke about Female Circumcision in Indonesia at the International Conference in Mogadishu, Somalia, on "Female Circumcision-Strategies to Bring About Change" (see "Case History: Somalia").[9] Dr. Pratiknya, besides exploring existing publications that are cited above also conducted some interviews and collected information via questionnaires on the present situation of the practice:

"The results of the study showed that circumcision continues to be done by traditional midwives but increasingly medical workers are involved. . .there has been a shift from a mixture of surgical manipulation to non-surgical manipulation."

And the doctor explains the changes: "The practice in Indonesia has undergone changes, especially in its technical execution. Two factors, public health education and religious understanding, have made surgical manipulation the norm in the past, a rarity today." Dr. Pratiknya claims that the change is due to the increased involvement of medical workers and health institutions and that the Islamic reform movement in Indonesia aimed at purifying Islamic teaching of "elements extraneous to the Koran" also contributes to the changes of the physical operation.

MALAYSIA

In Malaysia "everybody of Muslim faith has the circumcision performed" replied the Ministry of Health to my inquiry. The same inquiry and questionnaire was sent to the heads of the largest medical schools. The question on the description of the operation was answered by the Ministry of Health as follows:

> "The traditional midwife recites some prayers. After that she uses a pair of scissors to nip the very tip of the clitoris. For adults she covers the vulva with a betal leaf that has had a hole cut through for the clitoris to be exposed only. This is done so that the women would not feel over-exposed. The midwife then bathes her client. The imam (the head of the local mosque) will then say prayers. There will then be a feast of yellow glutinous rice. The number of people invited and expenses involved will depend on the financial status of the parents.
>
> The main population group that practices this type of operation are the Malays as they all belong to the Muslim faith. Next come the Muslims of Indian origin. There are no other operations on the genital region practiced for other reasons than religious." [10]

The last question of the inquiry was: "What are the reasons given why the operations are done?" The Ministry replied: "Most of the people do not know the reason why. They only say it is traditional. A few say it is for cleanliness." [11]

More detailed information, also in response to the same basic questionnaire, was received from Dato Paduka (Doctor) Abdul Wahab Ariff. In his communication the operations in Malaysia are described:

> ". . .Female circumcision has been widely practiced all over the Peninsula Malaysia, especially among an estimated population of 2 1/2 million Malays. The words 'female circumcision' refer to the excision of a very small portion of the skin covering the clitoris called the clitoral prepuce.
>
> Female circumcision operations are carried out on very young preschool girls aged from 2 1/2 years to 6 years. It is a religious practice among the entire female Muslim population who undergo circumcision operations. The operations are performed mainly by traditional Malay circumcisers, who are elderly women in kampongs (villages), both in the urban and rural areas. Traditional midwives, who do not include government trained midwives, are often invited to perform the circumcision. . .
>
> The surgical technique of circumcision in the kampong is a simple one. A very small piece of the clitoral prepuce is excised using a razor blade. To minimize injury and damage to the clitoris and adjacent structures, the sharp blade is carefully wrapped within a clean white cloth leaving part of the sharp cutting edge exposed for the operation. Aseptic precautions observed during the operations are not to the same level as those practiced in hospital operation theatres. The wound is swabbed with cotton wool which immediately dries it up. No dressing is required. The patient can resume her normal daily activities after the operation without any physical disability.
>
> No male is allowed at the operation. . .The technique of female circumcision is rarely discussed by Muslim women who have seen or performed the operation. . .The situation I think will change when more and more female doctors are available in Malaysia.

> I have not been made aware of any report connected with postoperative infection or complications following the operations during my professional life of 28 years which covered most of the states within Malaysia. It was possible that at least a few postoperative infections could have taken place, though not reported, considering the technique used by untrained people, without a good knowledge of the anatomy and physiology of the area to be operated upon, and in surroundings not conducive for such operations. It is well-known to the medical profession that every operation has its danger.
>
> In the absence of any detailed study, reliable statistics and surveys by the health agencies, family planning departments, medical schools, members of the medical profession, etc., it is difficult to make the interested parties realize the potential. . .health problems. . .as a result of the operations.
>
> When I was the Director of Planning and Development at the Ministry of Health Malaysia my recommendations for the National Plan for the Operation of a Religious Circumcision Service Among (male) Muslim Children was accepted. This was necessary to protect the children from harmful effects of the circumcision operations." [12]

Doctor Abdul Wahab Ariff then goes on to propose the medicalization of the operation: "Sooner or later the female circumcision should be carried out by trained circumcisers, e.g. doctors, nurses and midwives of the Ministry of Health. . ."

Fortunately, the World Health Organization [13] is very influential and highly respected in Asia and they released in 1982 and circulated globally a statement opposing the medicalization of female circumcision, which no doubt also reached the Health Ministry in Malaysia. [13] From a later letter of Dr. Wahab Ariff:

> "Potentially the female circumcision operation, as I had stressed before, has its danger however trivial it may appear to be. It is dangerous to allow such practice in the hands of untrained women. Malaysia has not all the trained personnel for such jobs. In terms of health priorities the country will not be able to produce them in the foreseeable future. . .
>
> Any rough handling of the child in her tender age without the use of any anesthetics, and above all any accident to the highly sensitive areas adjacent to the operative area may bring disaster to the victim both physically and mentally for the rest of her life. . . It is a pity that there has been a conspicuous absence of both official and unofficial information in this country relating to accidents from female circumcision.
>
> I strongly believe in the total eradication of female circumcision among Muslims in Malaysia. This future healthy trend can and should be achieved if an international Islamic organization could declare openly in Malaysia that female circumcision is not mandatory from the Islamic point of view." [14]

Another communication was received from Fatimah Hamid-Don, the Dean of the Faculty of education of the University of Malaya, who has no medical training.

> "Female circumcision, among the Malays, is a purification ritual to give girls a similar ceremonial observance as for boys. . .This practice is very much on the decline among urban lower income groups. For the wealthy and royalty this is a period of minor celebrations and gift giving. Among the rural community this is a purely 'women' get-together. . .
>
> Many people say it is just a ritual so that the sexual urge is lessened, and girls would not be so stubborn.' Many people are prone to believe that 'uncircumcised' females are stubborn! Or if a child is temperamentally unmanageable she is sometimes ascribed to as being 'inadequately circumcised. The practice is not obligatory in Islam, but a practice which stimulates what is 'good in Islam is 'sunnah'. . ." [15]

Recent inquiries confirm what is described above from ten years ago. The coordinator of the Gender & Development Program of the Asian and Pacific Development Program in Kuala Lumpur, Dr. Noeleen Heyzer, answered an inquiry if the Center knew of any recent studies on this subject since they are concerned with all issues affecting women and especially health. Dr. Heyzer wrote that she knew of no reports or studies on this practice which she stated is done "as a religious custom by Muslims."

> "From the personal information I gathered, it is done soon after the baby is born by splicing the skin off the clitoris. Apprarently, by custom it should be done at puberty. But because of the pain involved it now is being done on new born babies. . ." [16]

As a result of additional inquiries with women's groups in Malaysia, a recent study was sent by the Director of the Asian-Pacific Research Centre for Women, Ms. Rita Raj-Hashim, [17] which was made at the Department of Anthropology at the University of Malaya. The findings are quite similar to what is reported above. Dr. Roziah Omar, a medical anthropologist, first states that the field work was carried out in selected villages among rural women who are Malays (53% of the population), all of whom are Moslems-the official religion of the country (there has been a trend toward the resurgence of Islam). Dr. Omar States:

> "Malays interviewed in this research considered female circumcision as **sunnah** or a duty in Islam and it is highly recommended by Islam for a female child. The practice of female circumcision among Malays involves only the removal of the clitoral prepuce. The women and men interviewed in this research offered various opinions in favour of female circumcision. They are:
>
> **Cleanliness**. The removal of the prepuce promotes the cleanliness of the sexual organ of the female.
>
> **Promiscuity**. Circumcision is defended on the grounds that it takes away a part of the female body which can enhance her sexuality and promiscuity. Many argued that it is dangerous if a woman is promiscuous and thus she needs to be circumcised.
>
> **Virginity**. Through circumcision, a Malay girl can preserve her virginity. Virginity in Malay society is a prerequisite and valued highly.
>
> **Tradition and Religion**. It is stated that circumcision is in accordance to Malay tradition and religion. Circumcision is accredited with being the ideal Malay woman and a good Muslim woman. . ." [18]

The field investigator talking to the Malay women - who continue the practice - about the effects of the operation which are done by local village midwives records no adverse health problems as a direct result. However, nearly half the women admitted in private that they sometimes experience no sexual pleasure. Dr. Omar also asked why the women keep practicing this operation on their little girls. Religious tradition - sunnah or religious duty - was frequently mentioned. She reports:

> "However, according to the women respondents there have been significant changes in the ritual. Female circumcision in the Malay society is now often performed well before puberty between five and eight years old, and it is getting younger. Many parents prefer to circumcise their daughters immediately after birth. They said it is easier and less painful for the child. Traditionally. . . the young girl is adorned with gold and beautiful clothing and a feast is held to celebrate the ceremony. Nowadays, according to the village midwives interviewed, the ceremony is much simpler. Often the villagers call the midwife to perform the operation; the parents pay her twenty dollars, and no feast is done.
>
> The government midwife interviewed in this research reported that a growing number of women are bringing their girls to her to be circumcised. She added that with the use of anaesthetics, antibiotics, and better septic techniques the chance of the circumcised girl getting an infection is very little compared to those performed by the village midwife. . ." [19]

While Female Circumcision was introduced with Islamization in Malaysia as a traditional Islamic practice and ritual, it now has become modernized and medicalized. In the process, all rituals that resemble what is still practiced, for instance in Sudan and rural Egypt such as a feast and giving the child special clothes, have been stripped leaving for all to see the real purpose: to deprive women of sexual pleasure which is only for men to enjoy. Apparently, problems do occur according to the Government midwife such as infections or bleeding though the women interviewed did not admit them. And these are the reasons for having the operations done in a medical setting by a trained Government midwife who is also paid by the Government.

That means the Islamic Government is paying for having the Moslem women (about 53% of the women of the country) literally robbed permanently of sexual pleasure and satisfaction: indeed a strange use of taxpayers' moneys. The rest of the women living in Malaysia who are Chinese (Buddhist) and Indian (Hindu) are not Moslem so they are not subjected to the Moslem mutilations of females which are performed as sexual castrations by the medical personnel of the Government.

OTHER PARTS OF ASIA AND THE WORLD

Besides these well-documented practices by the Moslem communities of Indonesia and Malaysia, there is no doubt that in other areas in Asia similar interventions on girls and women are practiced by devout followers of Islam. It is difficult to understand why today this practice is still supported by Islam in Asia - a practice that is essentially African and is nowhere as drastic and as widespread as on the African continent.

Recently an Indian researcher has identified a group of Moslems in the Bombay area - the Bohra Muslims - who circumcise their daughters. Dr. Rehana Ghadially reports that the Bohra, an Ismaili Shia sect in the Bombay area, had been originally converted to Islam in the eleventh century by two missionaries from Egypt, where FGM (Female Genital Mutilation) was and still is widely practiced by the Moslem population. Together with Islam, the missionaries also introduced FGM and apparently it has been practiced ever since, shrouded in secrecy.

> "The Bohras-an Ismaili Shia sect - numbering less than a million and residing predominantly in Western India - practice the **sunna** variety of female circumcision. Known as **khatna** among the bohras, it consists in nicking the tip of the clitoris, about the size of a small bean. The practice is a closely guarded secret and is performed by midwives or **dais, mullanis** (women with semi-religious standing), occasionally by doctors but most often by a woman who has specialized in this function. The circumcision is done when the girl reaches the age of seven.
>
> According to the women interviewed, the most important reason for female circumcision is to curb female sexuality. Other reasons include - sanction by the Shariat (religious authority), a tradition in the community and for purity and cleanliness. In the sample interviewed, 70 percent practice it unquestioningly. . . The most common complaint about the immediate aftereffects of circumcision is difficulty in discharging urine. Cases of infection, swelling, severe bleeding, shock and tetanus have been reported. . ." [20]

It is quite possible that there are other Muslim groups that practice these mutilations in secret as devout followers of Islam: There are persistent rumors that in the Moslem state of Pakistan some groups practice it, but no medical documentation exists.It is also rumored that some Africans in Brazil continue to practice FGM to this day though the practice was never continued by any other Africans forcibly brought to the Americas or elsewhere: indeed the Creoles of Sierra Leone, who went back to Freetown from America and are now two percent of the population, do not practice FGM though all other inhabitants do and the Creoles are ostracized as a result (see Case History: Sierra Leone).

No investigations have been made about whether or not Moslemization has spread the practice to other parts of the world: Islam is rapidly increasing the number of its followers world-wide. Only certain Islamic groups mainly in Africa and the Middle East practice FGM: It apparently depends on where the Islamic missionaries come from - as the example of the Bohra in India shows.

As the above reports from Malaysia show, very little has been done in Asia, including by women's groups, to investigate the facts and document the damage done to girls and women and/or to establish how many women are affected. All this needs to be researched locally and can easily be ascertained by talking to midwives. It is hoped this report will persuade women to finally establish the facts which are of such importance to all women. It is known that many African immigrants and refugees (due to constant civil wars all over Africa) who are now settling all over the world continue to mutilate their daughters no matter where they go to live. This is discussed in the chapters on the Western World and in Women and Health, which includes actions taken to stop the spread of FGM.

FOOTNOTES

1. Akbar, Dr. Haji Ali. "A Research on Female Circumcision and Its Impact on Health in Indonesia". Centre for Islamic Studies, Yarsi School of Medicine, J1. Let. Jen. Suprapto, Cempaka Putih, Jakarta, Indonesia.
2. Ariff, Dr. Abdul Wahab. Doctor Emeritus, Faculty of Medicine, University of Kebangsaan Malaysia, Bagi, Selangor, Malaysia. Letter dated Sept. 25, 1978. From Research Report for the World Health Organization Seminar, "Traditional Practices Affecting the Health of Women and Children", by Fran P. Hosken, Khartoum, Sudan, February 10-15, 1979, p. 20.
3. Ibid., November 2, 1978, p. 21.
4. Ramali, Dr. Ahmad. **Guidelines for Health Care According to Islamic Law**. Dinas Penerbitan Balai Pustaka, Jakarta, 1956, pp. 101-103 (translated from Indonesian). See also **WIN NEWS**, Vol. 5, No. 1, Winter 1979, p. 32.
5. Hull, Dr. Valerie. Indonesian Population Institute, Gadjah Mada University, Population Institute, Bulaksumur H5, Yogyakarta, Indonesia, June 23, 1978. See also **WIN NEWS**, Vol. 5, No. 1, Winter 1979, p. 32.
6. Akbar, op. cit.; WHO Research Paper, op. cit., pp. 15-16.
7. Hosken, Fran P. "Female Circumcision in the World Today: A Global Review". Research Report for the World Health Organization Seminar, "Traditional Practices Affecting the Health of Women and Children", Khartoum, Sudan, February 10-15, 1979, WHO/EMRO Technical Publication Vol. 2, No. 2, pp. 195-214.
8. "Circumcizing Among Female Children of Islam in Indonesia". The Indonesian Midwives' Association, Jalan Johar Baru IV/13 D, Jakarta Pusat, Indonesia. Ms. Tuty Mustafa Dangkua, Secretary of the Association, April 27, 1979. See also **WIN NEWS**, Vol. 5, No. 3, Summer 1979, pp. 30-31.
9. Female Circumcision - Strategies to Bring About Change, Proceedings of the International Seminar on Female Circumcision, 13-16 June 1988, Mogadishu, Somalia. Sponsored by AIDoS (Italian Association for Women in Development) and SWDO (Somali Women's Democratic Organization). Report available from AIDoS, via del Giubbonari, 30 int. 6, 00186 Rome, Italy. Contact: Daniela Colombo.
10. Ministry of Health, Jalan Young, Kuala Lumpur, Malaysia. Letter of November 17, 1978, signed by Dr. Harbhajan Singh, Deputy Director of Health (Family Health) for Secretary General. WHO Research Paper, op. cit., p. 19.
11. Ibid.
12. Ibid.
13. World Health Organization (WHO), 1211 Geneva 27-Switzerland. WHO Position Statement Opposing Medicalization of FGM. June 1982: "WHO has consistently and unequivocally advised that female circumcision should not be practiced by any health professionals in any setting - including hospitals or other health establishments."
14. Ariff, op. cit., September 25, 1978; WHO Research Paper, ibid., pp. 20-21.
15. Hamid-Don, Fatimah. Dean, Faculty of Education, University of Malaya, Lembah Pantai, Kuala Lumpur, Malaysia. WHO Research Paper, ibid., p. 22.
16. Letter in the author's file from Dr. Noeleen Heyzer, Co-ordinator, Gender & Development (GAD) Programme, of the Asian and Pacific Development Centre, Pesiaran Duta, P.O. Box 12224, 50770 Kuala Lumpur, Malaysia.
17. Raj-Hashim, Rita. Director of ARROW (Asian-Pacific Resource and Research Centre for Women), Room 608, 6th Floor, APDC Building, Pesiaran Duta, Off Jalan Duta, 50480 Kuala Lumpur, Malaysia.
18. Omar, Dr. Roziah. "Female Circumcision and Malay Women". Department of Anthropology and Sociology, University of Malaya, Kuala Lumpur, Malaysia.
19. Ibid., pp. 3-5.
20. "The Practice of Female Circumcision Among the Bohra Muslims of India." Dr. Rehana Ghadially, Department of Humanities, Indian Institute of Technology, Bombay 76, India. See also **WIN NEWS**, Vol. 18, No. 2, Spring 1992, p. 45.

CASE HISTORY : THE WESTERN WORLD

The notion that female sexuality is dangerous and has to be controlled exists in the heads of men in all patriarchal societies. Female sexuality is perceived as a threat to masculinity; therefore, many different measures are taken by men in different parts of the world to control the sexual behavior of women. This control by men over the bodies and lives of women takes different forms in different societies.

Family law, as devised by all patriarchal societies, is the means to that end: Husbands almost everywhere are given control over the sexual behavior of their wives, but wives have no control over the sexual activities of the men to whom they are married. What is more, wives in most of the world are forced to submit to the sexual demands of the men to whom they are given in marriage; that is, men have the license - by law - to rape their wives as well as seek sex outside of marriage.

Family law has been found to contradict specific clauses of the Convention Against Discrimination Against Women - also called the "Bill of Rights for Women" - which by now has been ratified by more than 120 countries. [1] But instead of bringing their laws - including family law - into line with the convention, as governments are bound to do by adopting it, some governments have opted to exempt certain sections, for instance family law in Egypt. And such exemptions recently have increased.

The real objective of all measures known as family law is to control female sexuality and to give men formal jurisdiction over women's behavior, especially their fertility and sexuality. The list of specific practices designed by men to control the "dangerous" sexuality of females is almost limitless and varies with each society. It includes seclusion or purdah, which means the imprisonment of women in their father's or husband's homes; all kinds of economic restrictions such as excluding women from land and property ownership; discriminating against women in education and jobs to assure their economic dependence on men as well as a variety of genital operations that are practiced in different forms, depending on the preferences of the men in control.

Sexual mutilations are not limited to Africa and the Middle East, as shown in this chapter. Only the forms of the practices and how they are enforced differ. The notion that women are "emotional" is shared by men all over the world. The perception by men - and thus society - is that women are possessed by sexuality, that they are unable to control. Hence the fear by men and their laws to control female sexuality - "for the good of society and the family."

As the anthropologist Ashley Montague so aptly states in **The Natural Superiority of Women:** "Never was the truth so madly inverted. The truth is that men are possessed by sex, while women possess it." [2] It is, of course, male sexuality which is dangerous and out of control and linked to violence. Rape and sexual assault by men are the universal crimes that far outstrip all other crimes in both frequency and violence all over the world.

Instead of controlling men and strictly punishing male sexual assault and sexual violence, man-made laws, rules, prescriptions and interventions are designed to restrict, persecute, mutilate and even kill women who dare to assert independence or dare to control their own bodies and lives. The world-wide anti-choice movement today, which is becoming increasingly violent, for instance, in the United States, is another manifestation of usurping the right of women to control their own bodies and fertility.

Despite the violence and danger of male sexuality that is amply documented in every country and in every area of the world, it still is claimed by men that female sexuality is dangerous and has to be controlled. This has resulted in an orgy of violent repression of female sexuality, while male sexuality is given free rein; rather, it is often claimed that women are responsible for male sexual assault. Despite the staggering rape statistics in every society, one looks in vain for any group of men working against sexual assault. Where are the male leaders who speak about the dangers of the sexuality of men and teach their own kind to control themselves?

The Country Reports on Human Rights Practices, published annually by the Department of State in the United States and sent to Congress according to law, for several years have reported on violence against women in the family, including sexual assault. [3] In all the 191 countries listed in the 1992 report, family violence against women is listed as a human rights violation. Male assault against women in their families is practiced globally.

Hard-core pornography - the depiction in magazines and films and videotapes of sexual torture of women - is a huge and very profitable male-owned industry, selling entirely to male clients. It flourishes throughout the Western World; recently its products have also been exported to developing countries and can be found on newsstands in practically all capitals. The selling of sexual violence against women in graphic form has become a multimillion dollar industry. As the enormous increase of sexual assaults shows, it certainly affects the behavior of young men. Despite the protests of women, this all-male business is growing everywhere. Prostitution and female sexual slavery also are an international business by and for men of huge proportions and is extensively documented. (See Section of Women and Violence in **WIN NEWS**.)

Though female sexuality is never violent, represssion and stringent social control of all female sexual expression are practiced by a variety of means in literally all societies, past and present. The objective of all patriarchal societies everywhere is to control women's sexuality and fertility as strictly as possible. But patriarchal leaders tolerate male sexual violence and cover up wife beating in order to "preserve the family" it is claimed. This is used as cover for patriarchal control.

The male motivation where women's sexuality and fertility are concerned is similar everywhere, regardless of race, color, country, background, age or education. Female fertility is, of course, the greatest good. Men are aware of and have internalized their own inferiority vis-a-vis women which haunts them and leads them to violence. Driven by their inferiority complex, men shrink from nothing in their quest to control women's bodies, women's fertility and women's sexuality. All this is documented in this Report.

A survey of the history of female genital mutilation in the Western World shows that though the objectives of men are the same, the methods used in controlling female sexuality and reproduction in the West are different from those practiced in African and Oriental countries. Clitoridectomy, infibulation and circumcision have been practiced by individual men on their wives throughout history and in many areas of the world: for instance, by medieval lords in Europe, by pathologically jealous husbands everywhere and by male physicians who are doing genital mutiliations all over the world for profit.

However, outside of Africa and the Middle East and in isolated cases in Asia, such physical means of sexual control have never been imposed by men on the entire female population of their ethnic group, tribe or society. Further, in the Western World, female genital mutilations (FGM) are for the most part inventions and practices used by individual men of means who could afford devices or services to restrain female sexuality and who in this way tried to assure paternity.

Historically assured paternity was all-important, especially among ruling and influential families where marriages were arranged as a means of political influence. Daughters were never consulted; indeed realistic options for young women to choose a marriage partner did not exist in most propertied families and still don't in many areas of the world today. The control of women's bodies was and is linked to property and inheritance. Therefore control of women, that is, their genital organs, was important to wealthy men of influence.

The Western form of infibulation is by mechanical means rather than the Oriental and African method of fusing the flesh of the female genitalia by scarification. One form of infibulation practiced in the West consists in pushing some rings through the labia which are then closed by wires or a padlock. This form of control has been practiced since Roman times, for instance, to control slaves, specifically to prevent conception by female slaves. "Infibulated girls fetch a higher price on the Egyptian slave markets," Carl Gosta Widstrand reports, and "it was quite general in the case of female slaves to prevent them from becoming pregnant." [4]

The idea of chastity belts is said to have been brought to Europe by the Crusaders from their voyages to the Holy Land and the Semitic East nearly a thousand years ago.

Chastity belts were used mainly by the aristocracy, the knights and lords on their wives, since they were expensive to make; skilled craftsmen fashioned them for those who could pay for such a special device.

Elizabeth Gould Davis describes the contraptions - some of which can still be seen on exhibit in medieval European castles, for instance, in Austria and Italy:

> "The device consisted of an iron or silver corset with curving between the legs, a tight-fitting metal bar perforated with a narrow opening surrounded by rows of sharp teeth. Into this instrument of torture the woman was locked, the key carried only by her husband. It was bad enough, no doubt, when the husband was at home to unlock the contraption occasionally and allow the poor woman to relieve herself and wash up, but at times when the lord and master was off to the wars and months and even years went by, the accumulated filth can hardly be imagined . . . " [5]

Gould Davis provides several other descriptions such as the device invented by the Provost of Padua "which encased the whole lower part of his wife's body." The reason for chastity belts is explained by Gould Davis:

> "This monstrous apparatus was devised by a ferocious jealousy of the husband in order to ensure the marital fidelity of his wife . . . and made her a victim of permanent and truly atrocious torture." [6]

E. J. Dingwall relates that chastity belts were imported from the Near East during the 12th century. [7] The girdles also came to France via Italy, where they were called "ceinture a la Bergamasque" or "belt of Bergamos," and were mentioned by Rabelais in **Pantagruel**: "Il boucle sa femme a la Bergamasque" (he closes up his wife in the fashion of Bergamos) is related in that story. Dingwall also mentions that "a man tried to sell some girdles of his own make in the market in St.Germain in France but was chased away by two young courtiers."

The concept of virginity in relation to property in Europe in the Middle Ages becomes quite clear if one considers the "ius prima noctis" (the "right of the first night") - also called "le droit du seigneur" ("the right of the master"). This virtually means that each noble lord and master had the right of first sexual intercourse with the bride of any of his peasant subjects before the husband could take possession of her. A woman of course had no say in any transactions regarding her body.

Other graphic descriptions of chastity belts by Gould Davis show that these devices were not as rare as one might think. An ironmonger's invention is described as "a belt and a piece which came up under and was locked in position so neatly made that once a woman was bridled, it was out of the question for her to indulge in the gentle pleasure, as there were only a few little holes for her to piss through." [8]

But, these practices did not stop with the Middle Ages.

From a publication in 1722 in Latin, published in Leipzig, Widstrand quotes a statement by Franck de Franckenau that "women . . . were castrated by means of infibulation . . . to make copulation impossible; this is accomplished by putting metal rings through their labia, as is done with horses to prevent conception." [9] Widstrand, whose account of infibulation is perhaps the most complete, assembled a great deal of information on the subject. He also relates this story which was published in 1737 in England by **The Gentlemen's Magazine and Historical Chronicle.** It states that one George Baggerly was imprisoned for two years as he

> ". . . wickedly, barbarously and inhumanly did force . . . needle and thread into the private parts of Dorothy Baggerly . . . and did then and there sew her up to the great damage of said Dorothy and against the Peace of our Sovereign Lord the King, his Crown and Dignity." [10]

It seems that Mr. Baggerly, who had to go to work fives miles from home, "was afraid to leave his wife to her inclinations." But she immediately told her mother and some neighbors what he had done to her. Mr. Baggerly pleaded guilty. "As he went to trial, the women scratched him terribly."

In 1880, as Elizabeth Gould Davis reports, a French merchandising house distributed a prospectus selling a "camisole de force," a petticoat of restraint, which is described as follows:

> "The advantages are manifold. Not only will the purity of the virgin be maintained but the fidelity of the wife exacted. The husband will leave the wife without fear that his honor will be outraged and his affections estranged. Fathers will be sure of their parenthood and will not harbor the terrible thought that their children may be the offspring of another. It will be possible for them to keep under lock and key things more precious than gold." [11]

Widstrand relates other case histories from medical files, mainly of infibulation with rings and padlocks. Such cases were reported from countries as far apart as Italy, Germany, France, Czechoslovakia and India; some were quite recently discovered by the Immigration Service of the United States. [12]

One Dr. F. Legros reported that in 1825 in his clinic at the Hotel de Dieu, a hospital in Paris, he had a woman with a hole in each labium. A Russian physician, P. Soloviev, was consulted about 1807 by a woman who complained of violent pains and was unable to walk. She was found to have three rings threaded through the labia majora, closed with a copper padlock, all heavily corroded. Her fiance had knocked her unconscious and first fastened the rings and later added the padlock. Widstrand quotes a similiar case from India, where a severely beaten woman with a broken arm was brought to the hospital by the police. When she was examined, it was found that she had silk ligatures through both her labia majora. Her husband, who used to chain her up each time he left the house, also planned to put iron wires through the silk loops and fasten the whole contraption with a lock. [13]

Gould Davis cites two cases of infibulation reported by the U.S. Immigration authorities, one in 1894 of German immigrants, and another as recently as 1906 from Eastern Europe. All immigrants coming to the U.S. had to undergo medical examinations. Thus, the infibulation of the women - by means of rings and padlocks - was discovered.

These cases of mechanical infibulation are examples of isolated practices by pathologically jealous husbands who inflicted these tortures on their wives. However, they demonstrate that the same ideas of restraining women exist in the male mind everywhere, just as rape and sexual assault are universal. No doubt there are many more astonishing stories in the files of male physicians to which women have no access.

The concepts of virginity, hymen worship and family honor, on which male control of female sexual behaviour are built, are one reason given for infibulation. The other is paternity. In the chapter on hymen worship, Elizabeth Gould Davis relates that the proof of virginity - a bloody sheet displayed after the wedding night - was a requirement in much of Europe until quite recently. It still is in most of the Middle East today and also in parts of Moslem Africa. In turn, innumerable tricks were and are invented by women to simulate virginity and produce the desired results.

In 19th-century Europe and the U.S, the male medical professionals began to take over matters of sex, advising husbands and husbands-to-be about virginity, and how to detect a "fallen woman". For instance a book by a Dr. T. Bell, published in 1821, advises young men about to be married about different methods to identify virgins. Among other signs he states "defloration alters the tone of a woman's voice" - but unfortunately he fails to state how. [14]

With the rise of the obstetrical and gynecological professions in the latter part of the 19th century, which soon became an all male domain after women were excluded from all medical education, the control over women's bodies and sexuality entered a new phase. Control over women's bodies was no longer important just to assure male paternity or as a means of enforcing male sexual superiority; but women's bodies came to be used as objects to satisfy the professional ambitions and greed of physicians by experimenting with new surgical techniques, using female genitalia. The objective was not only to reap high fees but also to gain professional acclaim and recognition for the skill of the physician and admiration from his male colleagues.

Barker-Benfield [15] reports on the invention of numerous new operations from castrations (removal of ovaries) and hysterectomies to the removal of all sex organs. Dr. E. W. Cushing of Boston, a famous surgeon, declared in 1897 that "the female sex's sexuality does not lie in the sex organs, as man's did", it was his belief that "orgasm was disease and cure was orgasm's destruction."

To satisfy the gynecologists' unlimited greed, a woman's genital organs became a gold mine especially if her husband was a man of means. The female body provided almost endless opportunities for lucrative, unnecessary surgery on the genital organs. Besides greed, the male motivation was control over female sexuality, as Barker-Benfield documents. The latter is a quite similar incentive to those that make African and Middle Eastern men subject their daughters to excision and infibulation, though in Africa and the Middle East they are reinforced by the brideprice and family honor.

Infibulation was tried out as a medical procedure by physicians in the 19th century in Europe as a remedy for prolapse of the uterus and to repair vesico-vaginal fistulae (ruptures of the vagina), which at that time were much more frequent due to inadequate birthing assistance for poor women. After repeated failures, the operation was discarded as a useless remedy. [16] No one ever reports what happened to the hapless women who were thus mutilated for the benefit of the surgeon's professional standing and prestige.

No matter how they tried, physicians could find no reason to perform infibulations as a salable operation. But clitoridectomy offered all kinds of possibilities. Surgery on women especially those of the upper classes always has been a lucrative source of income for physicians and this continues to this day. For instance, hysterectomy, as reported in a recent series of articles on medical practices and costs in **The New York Times**, is the most frequently performed, unnecessary operation in the U.S.A. with hundreds of unnecessary deaths as a result. [17] Wherever hysterectomies are included in health insurance policies, the number of these operations increases in comparison to where they are not.

Clitoridectomy was introduced first in England and then taken up in the U.S.A, quite independently of existing African practices, which were entirely unknown to the Western surgeons involved, some of whom prided themselves on having "invented" this procedure. The operation was performed as a surgical remedy against masturbation and to control female sexuality. It was used to repress sexual gratification of women, the foremost tabu in Victorian times, especially for those of the upper classes. Talk of sex was frowned on as far as the ideal of Victorian womanhood was concerned. Polite society did not recognize that women had any interest in sex whatsoever, and a lady was bound to deny that her most normal functions existed at all.

This mutilation was a very lucrative procedure for the M.D.'s involved in England. This was recognized by their professional colleagues in the United States, who promptly copied it. It was discreetly kept quiet, of course, by all involved; thus records are scarce. Well-to-do husbands brought their wives to be operated on, having been persuaded by physicians that clitoridectomy was a remedy for a large number of unspecified ailments of women under the heading of "hysteria".

Ashley Montagu, writes:

> "Hysteria for 2,000 years. . .was considered an exclusively feminine disease . . .Apart from the fact that the disease was 'limited' to women, the condition gave quite a number of 19th century medical men the opportunity to remove women's ovaries and to remove by knife or cauterization the clitoris in an attempt to 'cure' the disorder. It seems difficult to believe that such drastic operations, in spite of all rationalizations by way of 'explanation' , were altogether motivated by a desire to benefit the patient. . .Since the sexual involvement could hardly escape the attention of a perceptive 19th century physician, it is not difficult to surmise why it really was that the surgical attack upon the sexual organs was made - for 19th century ladies were not supposed to be sexual at all - men were avenging themselves upon women." [18]

And Montagu concludes there is fair evidence that men are at least as often victims of hysteria as women, and possibly more often.

The ailment of hysteria, the reason given by 19th-century physicians in Europe and the U.S.A. to perform a whole series of genital operations on women but especially clitoridectomy, has an interesting history. The name "Hysteria" goes back to ancient Greece: Hysteria is the Greek term for uterus; hence 'hysterectomy".

Already in antiquity, it was reported by men that women suffered from all sorts of unexplainable ailments such as fainting, loss of speech, breathing difficulties, convulsions, and more. In the absence of any other explanation that could be found by the physicians in 400 B.C., they blamed these disorders on the "globus hystericus". [19] It was believed, and Plato published a discourse on the subject, that the uterus was wandering about inside the body of a woman and that it was an animal desirous of conception. In fact, a woman was not considered to be human. The wandering of the uterus inside a woman, as the famous physician Galen in A.D. 150 also claimed, was the cause of all kinds of ailments, especially if the uterus was not in use, that is, if the woman was not pregnant.

These ideas were readily accepted and propagated by male physicians throughout the Middle Ages and elaborated on. All women who did not have the opportunity to "satisfy" their genitalia in ways sanctioned by society were considered sick or mad. Marriage and pregnancy were recommended as the cure. Other therapies recommended by medical men to return the wandering uterus into position were all kinds of expensive salves, and smoke baths were used to fumigate the vagina.*

Hysteria - the ailment of women - and the idea of the wandering uterus were taken up by the Catholic Church in the 16th and 17th centuries. Since the time of Augustine, the Church interpreted "the madness" of women as being possessed by the Devil. Thus, it became a concern for the Inquisition. Recurring witch-hunts instigated by the Church are documented throughout the Western World. Finally, the sexuality of women became the illness itself that had to be abolished by sword and fire.

The basic attitude of men toward femaleness seems to be the same everywhere and throughout history. The "weakness" of women was taken up in the 18th and 19th centuries as a concern by and for physicians who followed the lead of the Church. The weakness of women was interpreted as a moral weakness of her entire person; indeed, her bones are smaller, the way she is built is weak (compared to men - the measure of all things), her skin is more sensitive and her brain is smaller; her whole body is prone to disorder (that is, hysteria) - it was claimed.

It was stated by physicians that a regular bath by male sperm was necessary to keep the uterus in order. However, it was unnecessary to consider the wishes of a woman. Duden and Schatten in **The Uterus, the Hungry Animal: History of Hysteria,** quote Victor Hugo: "The man has been given by nature the key with which he can wind up his wife every 24 hours. If in the process the clockwork becomes frigid, that should not deter him." [20]

The medical men were not interested in what a woman wanted or desired, as they had discovered that conception had nothing to do with female sexual satisfaction - as had been previously believed. A woman's whole and only destiny in life was motherhood.

In the second part of the 19th century, hysteria was identified as an illness of middle- and upper-class women who were not ready to succumb to the norms imposed on them by the patriarchy and who refused and reacted against their oppression and the matrimonial requirements of self-sacrifice and continuous childbearing.

Female hysteria became an all-encompassing ailment of well-to-do women, which also happened to provide the new profession of gynecology with almost unlimited opportunities to ply this trade and make money. Clitoridectomy became one of the favorite operations. Besides hysteria, many other different disorders were given as reason for the operation, especially masturbation, which physicians claimed leads to insanity and the "most serious constitutional effects", referring to masturbation as "moral leprosy".

---

*Both in Somalia and the Sudan, smoke baths (that is, sitting over a fire with strongly smoking herbs) are used at the present time by women after delivery and as a remedy for ailments connected with childbirth.

The 19th-century American physicians' view was that the practice of masturbation was "very injurious to the health of both males and females. While men occasionally practice it, for women it is much graver". They found that masturbation was the cause of "many women's diseases, such as uterine haemorrhage, falling of the womb, cancer, functional disorders of the heart, spinal irritation, palpitation, hysteria, convulsions, haggard features - emaciation, debility, mania - many symptoms called nervous. . ." [21]

The medical remedy prescribed and carried out was clitoridectomy. The American physicians as stated above learned about this operation from Europe, where a famous surgeon, one Isaac Baker Brown (1812-1873), published his cure for "Epilepsy, Hysteria and Some Forms of Insanity". This cure consisted of clitoridectomy. In 1866, the very year Baker Brown was elected president of the Medical Society in London, as a world famous gynecologist he published his book on the **Curability of Certain Forms of Insanity, Epilepsy, Catalepsy, and Hysteria in Females.** [22] He claimed that the cause of spinal irritation, idiocy, a number of nervous afflictions, mania, epileptic fits, insanity and death as a result of the above ailments is due to "peripheral excitement of the pubic nerve" or masturbation. The cure he offered: clitoridectomy.

The story of the rise and downfall of Dr. Baker Brown, at first so greatly honored by his colleagues, is interesting. [23] It appears that the objections against him which were voiced by his peers after he had achieved professional honors and fame, were mainly directed at the methods with which Dr. Baker Brown publicized himself and his cures.

No doubt Dr. Baker Brown's method of advertising himself was as repugnant to his professional brethren as it was lucrative for him. That Dr. Baker Brown also founded a London Surgical Home no doubt aroused jealousy among his colleagues. There he performed his operations "on females of unsound mind". A controversy followed, carried on in part in the **London Times**. Finally, after a battle of letters in the **British Medical Journal** and the **Lancet,** during which time Dr. Baker Brown continued with his now famous operations on "female lunatics" in his own establishment, the Obstetrical Society called a special meeting and he was expelled.

Later, Dr. Baker Brown also was made to resign from the Medical Society. But the London Surgical Home continued to flourish for some years and Baker Brown continued his operations. One of the reasons for expelling Baker Brown was that he dared to discuss the "dirty" subject of female masturbation which was absolutely tabu, even in the medical profession. The statistics of case histories which were published as a result of this controversy are truly horrendous. It appears that the mortality from the various operations performed on women was staggering. But, no one, including physicians who criticized him, was at all concerned about the women involved. The same blindness to the horrible suffering and needless mutilations to which women are exposed by the greed of gynecologists continues to this day.

Though Dr. Baker Brown's Surgical Home was finally closed and the operations abandoned, his "ideas of the effects of masturbation on the nervous system persisted both in England and elsewhere for many years", **World Medicine** reports. [24] The warnings by the medical profession against the terrible damage done to children, both male and female, by the "solitary indulgence" continued for a long time without any basis in fact.

The worry about masturbation that spread through the middle and upper classes of Europe and the U.S. and the belief that it leads to insanity were reflected in child rearing guides. Karen Erickson Paige [25] reports that the fear of masturbation, which had been regarded as a sin since Biblical times, was widespread. She writes, "Parents looked to physicians for answers and the physicians responded with alacrity". The treatments prescribed included diet, moral exhortations, hydro-therapy, marriage, and such drastic measures as surgery and physical restraints. Circumcision was also recommended.

Masters and Johnson, in their research work on **Human Sexual Response**, also investigated masturbation in some detail. They write: "The superstition that physical or mental deterioration results from excessive masturbation is firmly entrenched in our culture. . ." [26] They also relate that persons questioned in a large sample, not only practiced masturbation themselves but described as "excessive" anything above the frequency to which they admitted - no matter how often they stated they were masturbating.

It should be added here that male cultural bias against women's sexuality is perhaps even greater than their ignorance about it. This ignorance is not only rampant throughout all male-dominated societies but also terribly damaging. As a result, everything that is written by men including physicians on female sexuality and sexual practices but especially on the subject of female genital operations is of course quite distorted by male prejudice. This prejudice is greatest on the subject of masturbation, where both cultural bias and ignorance reinforce each other.

Clitoridectomy was brought by physicians to the U.S. as a remedy against masturbation, after the operations were abandoned in England. In the U.S. the operation was recommended to cure a whole range of diseases newly "discovered" by physicians, mainly for their economic gain.

G.J. Barker-Benfield reports on the origin and development of the Orificial Surgery Society in an article on the history of women's health care. American gynecology, in its present form, was developed in the latter part of the 19th century, with the invention of a number of operations - including ovariotomies and castrations. "A third operation was invented in the late 19th century for the control of female disorders"[27] - this was female circumcision.

From about 1890 through the late 1930's, female circumcision was performed by physicians in the U.S.A.

The Orificial Surgery Society had been formed in the 1890s and published a journal which advocated that any deviation from the normal clitoris requires surgical attention. A number of operations on the clitoris were promoted. Barker-Benfield reports that the American orificialists, believing that Dr. Baker Brown had gone too far, wanted to replace clitoridectomy with female circumcision and that the same results could be achieved in the treatment of masturbation and other neuroses by "proper attention to the hood of the clitoris". Nevertheless, some of their followers continued to perform clitoridectomy.

Orificial surgery was recommended for everything from measles to melancholia, including kleptomania and promoted by the **Journal of Orificial Surgery.** Descriptions of case histories of clitoridectomies and vaginal operations abound, claiming that the operations had cured a variety of ailments including hiccups. One woman, after an extensive operation described in the journal which included circumcision, repair of the cervix, trimming and dilation of the rectum and removal of ovaries and tubes became a missionary after she recovered from her ordeal.

Dr. D.E.H. Pratt, a member of the Orificial Society, wrote in 1898: "If one were to choose the most important spot in point of influence over the entire (female) system, it would have to be the clitoris and its hood". Barker-Benfield cites Dr. Pratt:[28]

> "When it becomes. . .appreciated that the clitoris and its hood constitute the most sensitive electrical button, which can be pressed to arouse this entire sympathetic nervous system to increased activity, the importance of proper treatment of this delicate and influential anatomical spot will be more thoroughly established. . .The clitoris is a unique and accessible point from which the entire female system could be activated."[29]

A whole series of new symptoms and diseases was discovered and labeled with new names: Of course they required all kinds of new operations. Barker-Benfield describes the reasoning of the male physicians recommending such operations of the clitoris to husbands: The operation would save men from their wives' "demanding explosive sexuality" and it was sold to husbands as a means to secure sexual control over their wives - assuring women's subordination.

Female masturbation of course was a special target for the surgeons, and to curb it required the removal of the clitoris. Dr. Benjamin Dawson invented vulvoplasty, the correction of the female genitals, leading to the claim of men's control of all aspects of female sexuality. His statements were accompanied by the usual rhetoric about motherhood. This all ocurred at a time when midwives were purged from the American scene by the male-dominated professions of obstetrics and gynecology.

Finally, the orificialists also tried to sell mothers on the idea that female infants should be routinely circumcised, much as circumcision of male infants had been sold by the medical profession on pseudo-medical grounds to the American public. It is interesting to note that male circumcision today is the most frequently performed operation in the U.S. It is performed in all hospitals a few days after the baby is born.

The medical advice, until recently in the U.S. has been overwhelmingly pro male circumcision. The operations seem to be performed almost exclusively for the financial benefit of the physicians, mostly obstetricians - to the tune of 200 million dollars annually, so Karen Ericksen Paige states. Circumcision on boys is paid for by medical insurance in the U.S. At present groups of men and health professionals have begun to oppose routine male circumcision in the U.S. especially since the American Medical Association had to admit that all medical studies supporting male circumcision as beneficial to health were flawed. There is no medical indication to perform male cicumcision and in most European countries it is no longer done, except for religious reasons. [30]

The lure of doubling their income by performing circumcision on female babies as well, certainly was persuasive to the physicians. The orificialists argued that there was a need for female circumcision on grounds of equality between the sexes; and what was good for boys was good for girls as well. The operation also would free a woman and "liberate her clitoris", orificialists claimed.

The argument for female circumcision as a routine operation on babies continued through 1937, promoted by the orificialists. Fortunately, women were suspicious, though through the advocacy by Dr. Pratt - one of the leaders of the orificialists - and his campaign the operation achieved some acceptance in the medical profession. Medical journals also were receptive to Pratt's and other physicians' pleas to help educate doctors about "the need" for female circumcision.

To have the operation adopted in the end depended upon the parents and especially the mothers. Fortunately, women did not fall for any of the physicians' arguments and propaganda. The circumcisors' appeal to equality was too transparent, nor could the hygienic argument be made that was so persuasively used in the case of boys. There was also disagreement among advocates as to when the operation should be performed.

In the end, routine female circumcision on newborn girls advocated by physicians in the U.S., was rejected by women. After the 1930s the obstetricians who had done the operations, stopped recommending clitorial surgery. The fear of masturbation supported for a long time by the medical profession, which had prevailed especially in the middle class, also faded. Similarly, the recommendations for drastic treatment of masturbating children and women given in various medical textbooks were eliminated.

At present, the fear of female masturbation, first propagated by male religious leaders and then taken up by the male-dominated medical profession, has been relegated to the junk heap, as another one of the unfounded myths used to attack women for the purpose of controlling female sexuality. However, all such myths die hard. All claims by physicians that masturbtaion is damaging finally had to be discarded as completely unfounded: on the contrary, masturbation, it had to be conceded, provides needed relief from sexual tensions. Yet, the Catholic Church continues to condemn it as a mortal sin, with the Pope himself continuing to propagate this ignorant and damaging myth.

The self-serving myths of Freud, such as penis envy, on pseudo-scientific constructs which he called "research" (he was expelled from the medical association of his hometown, Vienna, for unscientific and untrustworthy research data) have damaged women ever since. Freud's theories about women have been successfully sold all over the world to the tune of millions of dollars establishing a veritable cult of followers - as lucrative for the practitioners as it is damaging to women.

The financial success of Freud's as well as the orificialists' propaganda shows that our patriarchal societies are still willing to give credit to a variety of damaging myths designed to subordinate, exploit and mutilate women. This unfortunately continues to the present, as one can watch every day on many TV talk shows featuring guests - often women - relating stories of violence, opression and sexual assault by men closet o them.

The disappearance of the orificialists in the 1930s has not stopped certain proponents of genital operations on women, who no doubt saw the operations as a potentially lucrative source of income. Recently, various genital operations have been propagated as a cure for frigidity including female circumcision.*

The Boston Women's Health Book Collective, in a letter to the editor written in 1978 to **Medical World News,** reported on the activities of one Dr. James C. Burt, a gynecologist from Dayton, Ohio. Dr. Burt "is performing a type of vaginal reconstruction operation that he claims makes the clitoris more accessible to direct penile stimulation, so that a woman can have more frequent and intense orgasms in intercourse. He says he has 'perfected' the procedure and has hired a New York public relations firm to publicize his technique. He is appearing on TV talk shows with his wife." [31]

> "Dr. James Burt. . .claims he has found a way to improve upon the female anatomy. . .Burt's 'reconstruction' consists of mutilating the major muscle between the vaginal and rectal walls. . .cutting back the clitoral hood, and tightening up the vaginal opening.
>
> Critics of the surgery note several serious side effects for women: the severing of the. . .muscle significantly increases the risk of the uterus and the rectum collapsing; infection and urinating difficulty are highly likely due to the urethra being pulled into the vagina; natural childbirth is made virtually impossible. . .
>
> All of these changes happen to a woman's body under the guise of bringing about sexual 'pleasure' for her - but a surgery that brings with it such potential pain, not to mention an entirely alien set of genitals for a woman, clearly has men's interests at heart, and men's alone . . . " [32]

Dr. James Burt, using his wife as live advertisement for his procedure, is a stunning example of the attitude of some American male gynecologists, whose main interest seems to be the manipulation of female genitalia to make money. Dr. Burt finally was forced to stop his very lucrative surgical business when some of his women patients began to sue him for malpractice, which was reported in the news. Finally, the hospital where he did his surgery was picketed by women's groups and the hospital reluctantly - as his surgery was very profitable for this institution - expelled him from the staff after he lost his medical license due to malpractice.

Another astounding example of male attitudes in the Western World towards female sexuality came to light in a Sunday newspaper supplement that is distributed (free of charge) to local community papers all over the U.S. Financed by full color ads for liquor, cars, cigarettes, etc., the **New National Black Monitor** [33] is published by a consortium of 12 male, African-American community newspaper publishers from all over the U.S. The publication prides itself on its financial success - according to statements published in the **Monitor**.

In October 1980, the **New National Black Monitor,** in its editorial, "The Monitor Microscope" (all the rest is advertising) - carried an article on "Female Circumcision". The operation is described as the removal of the clitoris and the partial but temporary closing of the vaginal entrance.

> ". . .the reasoning is that to protect the integrity of females, this extra organ (the clitoris) should be removed. There are many who would hold on realistic philosophical and social scientific grounds that this practice. . .may have some practical or social basis as well.
>
> So far as tribal Africa is concerned, female circumcision - involving in many cases a partial but temporary closing of the vaginal entrance - has practically eliminated premarital teenage sex as a major social problem. By contrast teen sex and teen parenthood in America have reached what are called 'epidemic proportions' . . .Why should not the United States and Europe be investigating the possibilities of hygienic experimentation with female circumcision as a social safeguard." [34]

---

* One of the operations that is on the list of elective operations not funded by health insurance programs in the U.S. is circumcision of the female clitoris (for frigidity). But male circumcision is paid for by most insurance programs.

The editors further suggest that too many teenagers, due to pregnancy, are prevented from getting an education and developing their potentialities: Female excision and infibulation of girls would take care of that!

The article is illustrated with drawings including one of a surgeon in a cap, mask and rubber gloves ready to perform the genital mutilations in hygienic ways.

This obscene and distorted editorial published by the **New National Black Monitor** and distributed all over the U.S. evidently was designed to encourage African-American fathers to have their daughters mutilated following the example of their African brothers - with the implication that this will protect their daughters from pregnancy and and help them become more African by adopting this tradition.

Typically, the article says nothing about protecting young African-American women from the skyrocketing incidence of rape and violence in their communities in all American cities - which is a constant menace but ignored by the male publishers.

WIN NEWS cited the above passages from the "Monitor Microscope" and also sent copies of this article to women's organizations and health groups all over the country. The **Monitor** was swamped by letters; **WIN NEWS** [35]published two pages of excerpts from these letters repudiating the outrageous claims of the **Monitor** editors. Finally, the **New National Black Monitor** had to print a public apology to women after printing the medical facts about the damage done by genital mutilation.

Tola Adenle, the editor of the Nigerian women's journal **EMOTAN**, after seeing the **Monitor** statement in **WIN NEWS**, published an open letter addresed to the **New National Black Monitor** publishers pointing out that many of the claims made by the **Monitor** about Africans were "fallacious and presumptious . . .may we suggest that there are better ways in which our lost bond can be strengthened." [36]

An investigation of the present-day situation concerning genital mutilation in Western countries shows that wherever immigrants from Africa and the Middle East settle, they bring the operations along. Many continue to impose them on their daughters, even if the children are not going to return to their country of origin. Cases of operated girls - mostly of infants - have been documented in a number of European countries, including France, U.K., Sweden, Italy and Germany, and the issue has been also discussed in Australia and Canada.

Little girls are sexually castrated according to the custom of their parents' countries of origin, even though in many cases, the immigrants have declared their intention to become citizens of their host country or have already changed their nationality. They pledge to abide by the laws and customs of the country of their choice. But, even when the parents are temporary residents, for instance guest workers from West African countries in France, they are subject to French laws, their children go to French schools and are taken care of by French health services. The same is true of all countries that accept immigrants; they must abide by and are subject to the laws of the country that has accepted them including child abuse laws.

It is clear that genital mutilation is not acceptable from the health point of view; from the legal point of view, it is severe child abuse and a criminal offense in all Western countries, according to existing legislation.

In Sweden, in Autumn 1979, a series of articles about excision began to appear in major Swedish papers including the **Aftonbladet, Dagens Nyheter** and the Sveriska **Dagbladet**, condemning the operations in the strongest terms. Women's organizations, including the Immigrant Women's Union and the All Women's House of Stockholm, spoke against the operations.

It had come to light that daughters of new immigrant families from Africa and the Middle East, had been subjected to the operations. A Swedish surgeon and professor of gynecology had performed the operation on immigrant Moslem women, one paper reported. The women had come to him, he said, asking for the operation for religious and family reasons stating that they were under great stress by the men of their families to have the operations done.

The paper of the Swedish Cooperative Movement reported that the physician claimed he did the operations because the women insisted and he claimed the operation was not different from any other cosmetic surgery. This created an uproar in Sweden, since all health services in Sweden are paid for by the government - that is from citizens' taxes. The matter was discussed in Parliament and involved the Director of Health Services as well as the Minister of Health. [37]

Sweden already has legislation on its books forbidding all forms of corporal punishment of children - genital mutilation is covered by this law on child abuse. Nevertheless, all political parties demanded specific prohibitions - to prevent Swedish physicians from performing the operations on the young daughters of immigrants.

RIFFI - the International Association of Women Immigrants in Sweden - joined by more than 60 other organizations, appealed to the government. This appeal states in part:

> "Through a law here against circumcision on females, Swedish society can give the immigrant women support in their struggle for liberation. A law against circumcision on females in Sweden is an act of solidarity. . ." [38]

A resolution was passed by the All Women's House (Alla Kvinners Hus) making these points:

> "The Women's House of Stockholm. . .looks upon female sexual mutilation, so-called circumcision, as part of a traditional way of oppressing women. . .Men and women should be equal on all levels, including sexuality. . .Female genital mutilation must be abolished. . .The sexual mutilation alters the personality of the female and interferes with her normal development.
>
> A similar operation on a male child designed to interefere with male sexuality and sexual development would be categorically condemned by all. The same standards must apply to females. . ." [39]

The resolution also states that the transfer of the operations into hospitals under the pretext to save lives, is mutilating children by modern methods, and is quite unacceptable.

Sweden was the only country that, at the Plenary Meeting of the United Nations Mid-Decade Women's Conference at Copenhagen, offered assistance to all countries that wished to prevent the ongoing mutilations. [40]

In February 1981, the Swedish newspaper **Dagens Nyheter** reported that Elisabeth Holm, the Swedish Minister of Health, proposed a law against sexual mutilation: "By introducing a new law, we could show our solidarity with women - for instance immigrant women - who belong to cultures where this is being practiced", she said. There is already legislation against maltreatment of children; this new law will be specifically for women.

NORAD, the Norwegian Agency for International Development, wrote in reply to an inquiry concerning the criminalization of sexual mutilations that "no such law is being discussed; however, the Norwegian Health Directorate has issued a circular to all public hospitals prohibiting the practice of genital mutilation on all females. . ." [41]

In France, **F Magazine** reported repeatedly that little girls, often babies, the children of immigrants or guest workers from West Africa, were being excised. Benoite Groult, the well-known French author, in the feature article of March 1979 on Sexual Mutilation, [42] reports that African immigrants living in Paris, though they are very poor, pay for excisors to come from Africa to operate on their children. The women of these African families are mostly illiterate, and accept the operation of their children as a normal event: The arrangements are, of course, made by the men who also pay for the operations and the travel costs of the operators from Africa.

In a later issue of **F Magazine,** [43] some case histories are reported of little girls from Mali, some of them born in France, who have never been to Africa but who were excised and even infibulated right in Paris.

Renee Saurel, a French writer concerned about the story of a four-year-old girl from Mali who was excised in France, began to investigate the background of this incidence, which she describes in "La Petite Oumou". This became the first of a series of articles published in **Les Temps Modernes,** which were later published in a book **L'enteree vive.** [44]

Saurel researched the historical, Islamic, philosophical and anthropological background of the mutilations in more depth than anyone else, providing a unique and brilliant analysis. The chapters on the sexual ethics of Islam and her research on pre-Islamic Arabia and the life of Mohammed make many scattered resources accessible for the first time. She also documents the lack of action both by the international agencies as well as by the responsible organizations in France.

Some of the school teachers and physicians in France know what goes on, as all school children have medical examinations. But those in charge say nothing on grounds of "cultural tradition" and because of the reaction of African men; it invariably is: "what right do you whites have to tell us what to do with our children?" Yet, whether one is white or black makes no difference: No one has the right to mutilate a child!

The mutilation of little girls from Africa living in France continued for a long time with no action taken despite the above reports, with health officials in decision-making positions refusing to take note or to act. A pediatrician, Marie-Helene Franjou, working at Mother and Child Health Clinics (PMI)* in the suburbs of Paris, started an investigation and published an article in the **Medical Daily** in March of 1981, documenting the facts from her own practice. [45] By questioning the mothers of African children who come to the clinics, she collected a number of case histories. It appears that the majority of the children of African women - including those from Senegal, Mali, Mauritania and other Francophone African countries - who come to the clinics were mutilated; their clitoris and small lips had been cut out. When asked, the mothers stated it was their tradition and the husbands insisted on it.

Dr. Franjou stated: "Whatever the problems, we must remember that under all circumstances a child must be protected. Quite aside from the terrible physical problems, the psychological trauma is just as great - especially since the little African girls are in school with white children, none of whom have been subjected to such an ordeal."

Dr. Franjou, who as pediatrician is working for the governmental health system, took up the issue in the health sector and proposed that health education is the best route for change: All immigrant families should be provided with health and reproductive information and education.

CHOISIR, in their September/October 1981 issue, published an article by Dr. Franjou stating that sexual mutilations must be dealt with from a public health point of view. A petition, drawn up by Dr. Franjou and signed by 70 French physicians all concerned with mother and child health, was sent to the heads of the Ministries of Health, Interior, Women's Rights, Justice, and Foreign Affairs; it also was sent to WHO and UNICEF, and was supported by many French Feminists. [46]

The petition, after summarizing the health facts of female sexual mutilations, asserts that this problem concerns all French physicians: We appeal to those responsible in our country, and those responsible at WHO and UNICEF:

> "To start coordinated health education programs on this subject;
>
> To support scientific research, specifically concerned with the eradication of sexual mutilations;
>
> To condemn unequivocally all practices that mutilate without justification defenseless children." [47]

At the end of July 1982, a three-month-old girl whose parents were from Mali died as the result of an excision operation. Her death made headlines all over France and was also reported by the **London Times**. [48] It appears she was operated on by an excisor brought from Mali. Her father, an employee of the local government in a suburb of Paris, had lived in France for ten years. His older daughter had also been excised in France some years previously

---

* PMI - Centre de "Promotion Maternelle et Infantile". All health care in France is paid for and controlled by the government. The health of all children born in France is followed up at these clinics including immunization, nutrition, etc.

The baby girl, Bobo Draore, a healthy child, was brought to the hospital three days after the operation: she had bled to death. Her father took her to the hospital too late. Mr. Draore was arrested and charged with criminal negligence; the Ministry of Justice, as was reported at that time, would decide what to do.

The French Ministry of Women's Rights confirms that the operation is a breach of several articles of the French penal code. The father, who was questioned for hours by the police, refused to admit that he was responsible for the death of the child - though he paid an excisor for the operation. Still, the French authorities did not send him to jail.

Another similar case came to trial: A Malian father whose child spent two weeks in the hospital in 1980 after he had excised her himself with a penknife was prosecuted. Fortunately the girl survived. The judge questioned the man why he would mutilate his own child: The father, Mr. Koukara, replied that this is always done when the girls are a few weeks old; he seemed to have no idea of the danger or damage involved, though he and his wife had lived for some years in France. He saw nothing wrong with what he had done: According to Article 312 of the French penal code, a prison sentence of 2-5 years goes with physical abuse and injury of a minor child. [49]

The formation of a Commission for the Abolishment of Sexual Mutilation and other oppressive practices against women including polygamy, forced sterilization, forced motherhood, illiteracy, etc., was announced by Awa Thiam at the United Nations Mid-Decade Conference in Copenhagen. The founding members of this private group (C.A.M.S. - Commission International Pour L'Abolition des Mutilations Sexuelles) included besides Awa Thiam and the members of a black women's movement in France and West Africa, such international women leaders as Simone de Beauvoir, Benoite Groult, Giselle Halimi, Dr. Marie-Helene Franjou and other French feminists. Their headquarters was moved to Dakar under the leadership of Awa Thiam, whose book **La Parole aux Negresses**, describing the oppression of African women, was a great success.

C.A.M.S. organized a number of conferences and meetings in Paris and Dakar as well as one at the United Nations Mid-Decade Conference in Nairobi. The most recent meeting held at UNESCO in Paris was in December 1988 under the general theme of violence against women including FGM with some participants and speakers from Africa. A long list of resolutions was formulated after this meeting including some against FGM suggesting that information and education campaigns should be organized. [50] But no programs or any other activities for women in Africa were undertaken by that group.

In Paris another organization with a similar name - G.A.M.S. (Groupe Femmes pour l'Abolition des Mutilations Sexuelles) - was organized by Dr. Marie Helene Franjou to work with the African immigrants making health their priority. [51] G.A.M.S. started its work among immigrants by first taking a survey of the number of immigrants from African countries affected by FGM and preparing an estimate of the number of girls and families "at risk". Their latest figures of 1991 show that some 20,.000 girls of African immigrant families in France may be threatened by FGM.

Other women's groups in the Paris region, where most African immigrant families live, are working together on this issue in France. But none of them are working in Francophone West Africa. Yet the Cooperation, the French government's international development program, spends a lot of money in West Africa but not for women's development or health: To date, the Cooperation has completely ignored FGM.

As stated elsewhere in this report, there is practically no medical research on FGM done by anyone from France or funded by France. Not even the prevalence or distribution or any of the basic facts that are necessary in order to develop effective programs to stop the mutilations have been researched. Yet all kinds of cultural ethnographic and anthropological investigations and sophisticated theories on the African indigenous belief structure are published and discussed - while African girls die from FGM. .

The French health and hospital system has been institutionalized all over West Africa and only French drugs and French hospital equipment exported by France are used throughout the former French colonies with huge profits for French firms. But nothing is done to stop the mutilations, not even by helping ongoing campaigns such as the one in Burkina Faso or the African groups affiliated with the IAC (Inter African Committee).

In France FGM done by immigrants finally landed in criminal courts in the 1990s, but only after three little African girls had died. They bled to death after the operations were performed at their fathers' homes, sometimes by excisors brought to France specifically for that purpose or by the father himself (see above). The proceedings in the criminal courts were continuously delayed. In the hearings all kinds of anthropological expert witnesses explained the wonderful African traditions and their importance - traditions that kill thousands of children and mutilate millions of women - but of course the male experts called don't care what happens to women and children. They are solely interested in their theories about the African belief structure and mythology. [52]

The deaths or narrowly prevented ones provided the French press with the opportunity of publishing all kinds of sensationalized stories and romanticized investigations into African traditions illustrated with spectacular photographs. But none of these stories ever give a realistic view of the misery, poverty, abuse, exploitation and terrible pain African girls and women endure by the hands of African men. Not one story ever mentions the responsibility of the French government, which never has done anything to protect the human rights of women and children in Africa in their former colonies. Yet France had the power and the obligation to intervene from a humanitarian view. Even now the French government fails to speak for the human rights of women and children, and French women's organizations are silent - yet women's taxes support the Cooperation.

Finally, in early 1993, a women from Gambia, the mother of two baby girls, was sent to jail for having her daughters excised in Paris. This was reported all over the world, including by the **New York Times.** [53] Of the five years' sentence, four were suspended but she will have to serve one year. Only once previously, an excisor working in France who was sentenced was actually sent to jail. In all previous trials - eighteen so far - even if the officials indicted the parents and even if the children died, none of the fathers who paid or otherwise procured the operations went to jail and not a single man has been punished by the patriarchal, male-dominated French courts.

It is of course typical that only women have been jailed for the mutilationof girls for which men always are responsible in France as well as anywhere else, wherever girls and women are mutilated as this Report documents and as everyone concerned knows. But the French authorities don't punish African men - evidently for political reasons. As long as they don't, the operations will continue in France and in Africa, making the French government and legal system accessories responsible for the mutilations.

In France as elsewhere, FGM is used for pornographic purposes with sadomasochistic overtones for the entertainment of certain kinds of perverted males. For instance, one can find movies showing girls being excised in Africa that are shown in certain theaters in both New York and Paris and even publicly advertised. It also appears that some enterprising Africans in Paris have taken up showing off the mutilation of little African girls, using live victims, to make money from tourists. The following anonymous letter was received at the beginning of September 1982 by **WIN NEWS**, written in English. The writer seems to have been a German tourist in Paris, judging from the words and spelling he uses. This is the letter in its entirety exactly as received:

> "Dear President of **WIN NEWS**:
>
> Yesterday, I was asked to pay FF. 1000 to see real exzision done to a young French-African girl, by a man at Platz Pigalle. I am most ashamed but I was curious so I went to see it. There were about 20 turists in the flat, each paid FF. 1000 like me.
>
> You had to pay FF. 100 for each photo if you wanted to take one.
>
> A little girl was brought, drunk or drugged, about six or seven, hands tied at the back. Her legs were by force opened and she was held on the table by three strong young men in such way that she could not move and defend her little sex. She was gagged but could be heard crying for help. A black woman, middle-aged dressed in African jewellery danced, gyrated and chanted some jumbo-mumbo, pure sham.
>
> The girl had her little cunt lips cut out very slowly by one of young black men. She was crying terribly. It took time because people were taking photos. Afterwards her klitoris or part was taken out with a scalpel.

I got an impression that she might has been through similar torture once, because there were scars already at the beginning and it looked that part of the klitoris was missing. I don't know for sure.

We returned by a minibus to Pigalle. I still hear ringing in my ears cries of this little child, cries which we paid for.

(Signed) Ashamed." [54]

After this letter appeared in **WIN NEWS**, the issue was taken up in the European Parliament, as one of the **WIN NEWS** subscribers was a woman delegate from Italy: She challenged France at a hearing , and this created a furor. The European officials requested France to investigate the issue as a human rights violation. The French Ministry of Women's Rights and Ministry of Interior were charged with conducting a thorough investigation but could find no evidence. Mme. Yvette Rudy, the Secretary of State of the Women's Rights Ministry, talked to me about this, claiming that this letter surely was a hoax. Unfortunately, based on my experience in Africa, I don't think so. What is more, who could ever make up such a story and who would profit from this?

In other European countries, wherever immigrants from Africa and the Middle East settle, the mutilations are brought along with other customs and traditions and often are continued, even if the immigrants do not plan to return to live in their country of origin. For instance many Somalians always went to Italy to work and study, as the southern part of Somalia was an Italian colony in the past; this long before the present influx of refugees. The teaching language of the University in Mogadishu was Italian, as Italy financed the institution. There is little doubt that among Somalian families in Italy, the operations were practiced, especially since the belief in traditions by Somalians is almost absolute. But the Italian government shut its eyes.

Italian feminists reported this at the United Nations Mid-Decade Women's Conference in Copenhagen in 1980. But officially no one takes any note of what is done to Somalian girls living in Italy or anywhere else. However, AIDoS (the Italian Association for Women in Development), which was organized in the early 1980's, took on the issue. They held a meeting in Rome for Italian women to inform them about FGM and the issues involved, which in Italy - much as in most of the rest of Europe - are quite unknown. AIDoS also supported and provided technical help to the national FGM eradication program in Somalia, working closely with the Somalian Women's Democratic Organization. [55] (See "Case History : Somalia")

There are every so often newspaper reports in Italy about FGM being practiced, including that the mutilations are done by health and medical personnel. But Italian officials have "other priorities." No one has done a comprehensive study to document the facts and that is essential in order to persuade governments to act.

From Australia also recurrent reports have reached **WIN NEWS** for the past few years that female children of immigrants are being genitally operated on. Australia has recently accepted immigrants from Middle Eastern and African countries and also from Asia such as Malaysia and Indonesia where the operations are practiced by devout Moslems. The Humanist Society of New South Wales, led by Marjorie Saul, investigated and took up the issue in Australia. [56] The Australian College of Pediatrics stated in a letter to the Humanist Society that it condemns any mutilating operations that are performed without medical reason. Australian doctors with any personal knowledge of such opertions were asked to advise the Humanist Society in confidence. [57]

Australia's Ethnic Affairs Council, which has the task of dealing with the many different immigrant groups, has failed to deal with this issue, the Humanist Society reports. "The host country and the immigrants need to show mutual tolerance - there are certain customs that immigrant groups should be prepared to give up if they wish to make their home here," so an article titled "A Two-Way Street" states in the **Sydney Morning Herald**, reporting on sexual mutilations. [58] Since that time this issue has been taken up by the press in Australia every few years, each time causing concern and much discussion. But to date not one case has been definitely established which can only be done by a gynecological examination. (See "Case History: Asia")

It would be strange if these mutilations could not be found in England, the goal of immigrants from all over the world, especially from Asia, but also from her former colonies in East and West Africa, including Nigeria. In July 1982, a British weekly [59] that is distributed to 30,000 hospitals and physicians printed an article that ritual genital operations on females are taught in British medical schools. The institution specifically cited in the article was the Liverpool School of Hygiene and Tropical Medicine. The report by the **Hospital Doctor** cites the Ministry of Health: "Junior Health Minister, Lord Trefgarn, admitted in a written answer that methods of performing female circumcision were being taught at certain British medical schools." [60]

That this admission by the British Ministry of Health (this was several years before the legislation to prohibit FGM in Britain was passed) represents the thinking and attitudes of a number of male professionals working in tropical medicine was confirmed by a letter I received in September 1979. A Dr. David Stevenson, senior lecturer at the Liverpool School of Hygiene and Tropical Medicine - the same institution cited by **Hospital Doctor** three years later - sent me a proposal on how to perform excisions in hygienic ways. [61] Dr. Stevenson supplied a description of how the operations are modernized, including the surgical tools to be used, and he proposed to teach this in Africa - having devised the idea following a trip to Sierra Leone. It appears that the art of mutilating little African girls quickly, efficiently, and in medically sound ways was now taught as a contribution to the modernization of Africa by Western medical professionals at British universities.

Dr. Stevenson wrote that he was concerned about the mutilations he saw in the hospitals in Sierra Leone and therefore **WIN NEWS** should publish about his great contribution to women's health in Africa and make his proposal known. He detailed the tools to be used (small surgical scissors to excise the clitoris and cut the labia minora) and how to stitch up the wound to reduce bleeding - with emphasis on hygiene. This he claimed would "respect African culture" but reduce mortality and morbidity and still be "an impressive procedure removing the girls male organ"!

It is of course known that FGM is done in hospitals all over Africa by physicians for money (see "Case History: Nigeria"). Fathers pay, as they don't want to lose the considerable amount of money for brideprice if their daughters die from FGM. But the letter of Dr. Stevenson with a proposal made evidently in all sincerity connotes a frightening perversion of values and distortion of the male mind that is difficult to comprehend for women. Yet what this man, with considerable power over women due to his profession, represents is unfortunately not unique but is responsible for endless pain and misery for women. What would this doctor think (and his numerous like-minded colleagues) if boys rather than girls were involved? Would the doctor write to men's magazines to publish his hygienic version of amputating penises of little boys - which is the equivalent of what he proposes?

In the **Hospital Doctor** article cited above, the probability of the excision being performed in private clinics in London is also mentioned. Shortly after that, the British **Observer** [62] provided proof of this allegation by printing an interview with a Harley Street surgeon who admitted doing the operations on African women from Nigeria. The physician, Dr. Sunit Ghatak, who trained in Calcutta, charged L 800-1000 for this surgery - which was quite legal at that time in the U.K. Dr. Ghatak stated that a number of such operations were done privately, but if the Royal College of Obstetricians would ask him not to do them, he would comply.

The operations he described in the article were done on adult women from Nigeria - both brought by their husbands One could not conceive and believed it was because she had not been excised. Another woman had to have a cesarean when she gave birth because, according to her husband, she had not been excised as a child - therefore he wanted her to be excised now.

In 1983 the Prohibition of Female Circumcision Act was finally passed in Britain [63] after lengthy debates, especially in the House of Lords, and several postponements due to various objections by organized physicians' groups. This stopped enterprising surgeons from doing FGM openly for wealthy African men, and it also stopped misdirected physicians and medical schools in Britain from teaching how to do FGM. But it would be naive to believe for a moment that this would put an end to the matter.

One direct positive result, however, was the organization of the Foundation for Women's Health, Research and Development (FORWARD) in London, which, under the leadership of a woman from Ghana, Stella Efua Dorkenoo, started in 1984 to develop a variety of programs, education and training activities for African immigrants to the U.K. [64] Besides publishing all kinds of educational materials on women's health and organizing meetings as well as neighborhood programs, in the summer of 1992 FORWARD organized the first European Study Conference with participants from France, the Netherlands and Italy as well as the U.S. and Canada. A declaration was formulated that categorically rejects all forms of FGM or injury of female genital organs and outlines a "unified approach for the abolition of the practice in Europe and other Western countries." [65]

The issue of the medicalization of FGM is unfortunately not about to disappear and will no doubt continue as long as patriarchal socialization continues and men profit from it because in the final analysis this is a power struggle between two very opposite views of life - which Riane Eisler has so perceptively and descriptively called the "dominator versus the partnership" view. [66]

The issue of the medicalization of FGM perhaps more than any other illustrates the depth of this division as expressed by the views of Dr. Stevenson cited above. He claims to support African culture by mutilating little girls with modern surgical instruments. What is "culture" and most of all **whose** culture are we talking about? Is it culture that prescribes the mutilation and torture of our daughters? Whose culture? It is the culture of men. Who defines culture? Men. Whose culture covers our world with war and glorifies war to boot? It is the culture of men. Whose culture uses violence and rape as an instrument of control? The culture of men. And it is the culture of men that has institutionalized FGM and the culture of men that is now trying to medicalize it for profit.

Nowhere was this so persuasively documented as in an article on "Female Circumcision" published in October 1983 in the British journal **Forum**, which lists a number of Ph.D.'s on its board including internationally known sexologists and psychotherapists. [67] The anonymous writer, who refused to give his name, but obviously is a surgeon, after discussing what he calls " female circumcision," provides a detailed description on how to perform an infibulation, including where and how to place the stitches "using a large curved needle with cutting edges." At the end the thighs are bandaged together and "after 17 days the labia will be firmly adherent."

The doctor describes the health problems that often arise from the traditional way the operations are done and then states his operation will prevent all that. To prohibit the operation was useless, he claims; people will do it anyway as the law against circumcision in the Sudan shows. This article appeared at the time when the Prohibition of Circumcision Act was discussed in the British Parliament. And he claims, "People with money should be allowed to spend it." Apparently he has made a lot of money from mutilating the little daughters of wealthy African men, and he did not want to give this practice up, as he would be compelled to do if the prohibition was enacted. This article was evidently a scheme to sell his operations. In a letter to **WIN NEWS** he claims that women should be gratified that "he made public his simple and safe procedure."

In the article the anonymous writer also claims that he talked to midwives in the Sudan (where most women are infibulated after being excised) who assured him "that sexual feelings of women are not impaired by the operation. It is quite astonishing how many men, including physicians and sexologists, make such obviously absurd statements and why. But this is another myth that male researchers propagate - after claiming they talked with African or Sudanese village women who, the men claim, talked to a male stranger about their intimate sex lives in a foreign language - a considerable feat.

Anyone who has ever been in the Sudan knows that in this very conservative Moslem society sex is not discussed under any circumstances anywhere and least of all between women and men or with "foreigners." Nevertheless, the claim continues to be made that excised or infibulated African women discuss their sex lives with Western men, stating that they experienced "normal orgasm," which is as absurd as it is obscene. Still, one can read such statements again and again in the literature or it is presented at international and African reserach conferences.

But the issue here is health. And for a physician to perform mutilating surgery with no medical indication or necessity is a fundamental offense against medical ethics and human rights. Greed certainly is a basic motif that underlies the medicalization of FGM - which acts as an incentive everywhere in the world.

This was recognized by the World Health Organization and that is evidently why WHO already in 1982, three years after the Khartoum Seminar on "Traditional Practices Affecting the Health of Women and Children," published and circulated worldwide a statement on the medicalization of FGM. At the seminar this issue was discussed in great detail and finally categorically rejected by the health department delegations of all participating African and Middle Eastern countries. But everyone knew at that time, given the attitudes and views of many of the physicians present, that this was not the end of it. (See: "World Health Organization Seminar")

The key points of the WHO statement of 1982 read:

> "WHO has consistently and unequivocally advised that female circumcision should not be practiced by any health professionals in any setting - including hospitals or other health establishments.
>
> WHO supports the recommendations of the Khartoum Seminar of 1979 on Traditional Practices Affecting the Health of Women. These were that governments should adopt clear national policies to abolish female circumcision and to intensify educational programmes to inform the public about the harmfulness of female circumcision."

Still, as this report documents again and again, the medicalization of FGM comes up in different Western countries and societies, especially now due to the growing number of refugees from civil wars in African countries where FGM is a widespread practice. More and more refugees from these conflicts come to Western countries - with their tradition. - to Europe as well as the U.S. and Canada.

Since the upheaval in Somalia, large numbers of Somalis have come to the Netherlands, a very liberal country that has served as a haven for refugees from all over the world. The Netherlands has publicly funded health services. In the clinics physicians, midwives and nurses were confronted with the problems, especially in childbirth, of the infibulated Somali women. The professionals of the health services of the Netherlands, much as in other countries when first faced with an infibulated woman giving birth or seeking help for a gynecological problem, were obviously concerned and did not know what to do.

But when Somali immigrants then came to the health clinics demanding to have their small daughters infibulated - a service that had been available in the past for instance at the general hospitals in Mogadishu (see "Case History: Somalia") - the Netherlands Ministry of Health had to deal with the issue. The usual reaction of officials is to ask an independent group to conduct an investigation of the issues involved.

The Netherland Section of Defence for Children International was charged to collect all the available data on the subject, as a doctor and nurse working with Somali refugee women had made recommendations to the publicly funded health services, "pleading for legislation of mild (so-called 'non-mutilating') forms of FGM in particular the incision known as 'sunna' (the so-called 'mildest' form of FGM), under very restricted conditions (in hospitals, by specialized doctors: gynecologists/obstetricians)." [69]

The communication by Defence for Children International, asking me for information, continues:

> "The reasons the researchers give for this recommendation are:
>
> - it will reduce the amount of severe forms of FGM
>
> - these cultural and religious reasons of these refugees should be respected.
>
> The Minister is seriously considering this recommendation. . . Research has shown that a large number of physicians re-infibulate women when they ask for it (that is after birth) and do the 'sunna' circumcision if women are asking for it. . ."

The Health Ministry seriously considered making such a recommendation to Parliament to introduce legislation to legalize the procedure so that public health services would pay for it. This means that women taxpayers in the Netherlands would be compelled to subsidize the mutilation of female children of immigrants. The ministry needed a research study to back this decision; hence Defence for Children International was asked to provide information and they finally contacted me.

For physicians to ask for legislation in order to be paid for these procedures from taxes is a betrayal of the very mandate of medicine. For a health ministry of a liberal country like the Netherlands to seriously consider such legislation defies the directives of WHO (see above) and the United Nations Human Rights Office findings condemning FGM quite aside from countering the UN Convention on Discrimination. Any attempt to legalize FGM in any form furthermore is done in opposition to the commitment against medicalization of FGM by the IAC - the Inter African Committee on Traditional Practices Affecting the Health of Women and Children.

The issue could not be concealed from the public and especially women. There were protests of all kinds including demonstrations and petitions to stop the ministries involved - both the Ministry of Health (Directory of Public Health) and the Development Cooperation Department. of the Ministry of Foreign Affairs. The Ministry of Health in a letter to **WIN NEWS** wrote:

> "The Netherlands shares the view both you and the World Health Organisation have adopted, namely that the circumcision of girls and women, in whatever form and wherever it occurs, is inadmissible and should be combated. This means that governments should also adopt strategies to eradicate female circumcision. In the Netherlands, mutilating forms of circumcision are against the law, falling within statutory provisions relating to physical abuse or the unauthorised practice of medicine.
>
> As the Netherlands has been confronted with an increasing number of Somali refugees, independent experts have conducted a study of circumcision among Somali women. They concluded their report with a number of recommendations on prevention, information and professional care. . . one of the recommendations relates to the possiblity of making a distinction between **mutilating and non-mutilating forms of female circumcision**. Those responsible for the study concluded that a small incision (such as a prick or scratch) in the foreskin of the clitoris may be regarded medically as non-mutilating and might serve to prevent more serious forms of female circumcision. Most likely the government will **not** adopt the recommendation. . ." [70]

In the end no public official could be found who was willing to take responsibility for the proposal to legalize "a non-mutilating mutilation." In correspondence with the above ministries **WIN NEWS** was assured that they were "opposed to FGM in any form." A conference of gynecologists was held to discuss the issue, which in the end became what to recommend to Parliament. But the real question is: Why was the misguided recommendation by one single physician and nurse ever taken seriously? The matter was finally only settled in February 1993 after many months of debate and controversy. The Council of Ministers agreed with the recommendation of the Minister of Health, the State Secretary of Health and the Minister of Justice "**that no form of FGM is permissible** because this tradition implies female repression". The following communication was sent to **WIN NEWS** by the Ministry of Foreign Affairs, which is summarized here:

> "**STANDPOINT**:. . . female circumcision is a practice which runs contrary to prevailing attitudes in the Netherlands on the equality of women and their place in society. It is viewed here as a form of repression, and the Dutch policy aims to combat repression of women; it opposes all forms of circumcision.
>
> This policy is in keeping with various relevant international instruments such as the UN Convention on the Elimination of all Forms of Discrimination against Women. the European Convention for the Protection of Human Rights and Fundamental Freedoms and the UN Declaration of the Rights of the Child . . . We also confirm that the Netherlands endorses the recommendation of the World Health Organization to develop strategies aimed at eliminating the practice worldwide. . . " [71].

WHAT IS THE LESSON OF THESE EVENTS? Women always must be vigilant - as apparently we are never safe from attacks on our physicial integrity, our bodies and our sexuality. After all the debate no one in the Netherlands is now willing to take responsibility for advocating the medicalization of FGM. On the contrary, the Ministry of Foreign Affairs in the above quoted seven-page report also explains the legal view that "FGM does constitute intentional or negligent assault. . . and the unlicensed practice of medicine". Measures to prevent FGM, support for women refugees and asylum seekers and giudelines for professionals are also outlined in the report; "the offer of assistance from Somali women to be involved in providing information will be utilized."

Did no one in the Netherlands know that a massive national campaign against FGM was underway in Somalia assisted by Italy when the civil war engulfed the country? The Netherland Embassy in Somalia - as well as all other missions - took part in the opening ceremony, held in the Parliament, of the International Conference in 1988 in Mogadishu on "Strategies to Bring about Change". (See "Case History: Somalia")

In the end this must be said: **What a deplorable waste of time, energy and money!** If the Health Ministry and all the other Dutch Ministries and organizations and people who spent countless hours and money on this affair would have put the same time, money and effort into teaching Somali refugees about reproductive health, they could have freed all the Somali refugees from their damaging misconceptions.

It is men who must be made to change as they are responsible for the mutilation of their daughters, since they make the family decisions and not women. Until women have equal power in all decisions, men must be held legally responsible. It is only fair to inform all male refugees when they are granted permission to stay in another country that they are responsible for following its laws and that they will be held responsible if their female children are mutilated: It is a criminal offense everywhere in the Western world to mutilate a child and if the men don't like it they can always go back to where they came from.

In the case of the Netherlands all the time and money spent on investigations and protests, etc.,, could have been spent on positive education of the refugees. Surely it is not beyond the highly educated population of the Netherlands to use their skills in positive ways to show the Somali and other African refugees who cling to such deplorable customs a better and healthier way of life. It is quite possible to teach people from all parts of the world how their bodies function, something that is useful and beneficial and will do away with damaging traditions and myths.

WIN NEWS sent, for a start a hundred **Universal Childbirth Picture Books (CBPB)** with Additions to prevent Infibulation to a new foundation - "Foundation Pharos" in Utrecht - set up on January 1, 1993, for refugee health care. [72] More will be sent later including the Somali translation of the books, which are being published in the spring of 1993[73] and will help Somali refugees understand why their traditional practices of FGM are not acceptable anywhere in the Western world.

Canada faces very similar problems as the Netherlands, since it is accepting many refugees and recently large numbers from Somalia. But Canada has, nevertheless, adopted very different policies. When the problem regarding infibulation of Somali women became evident in Canada, which, much like the Netherlands, has a publicly funded health system, clinics and doctors were compelled to deal with the health problems of infibulated Somali women, especially in childbirth. And much like in the Netherlands the issue of infibulating Somali girls born in Canada demanded an official response as fathers wanted to have their small daughters infibulated at the publicly supported clinics.

Most of the refugees from Somalia are settling in eastern Canada and predominantly in the province of Ontario, where community groups and refugee organizations were informed and alerted about the issue. FGM according to Canadian law represents "an assault causing bodily harm, or an aggravated assault involving the wounding, maiming or disfiguring of the child. A doctor performing that kind of operation on a child would likely be liable to conviction for committing assault or aggravated assault." [74]

But the critical response - setting the direction for Canada's reaction both on the governmental as well as private level - came from the College of Physicians and Surgeons of Ontario in early 1992 after studying the issue as more and more physicians were confronted with the health problems of infibulated Somali immigrant women.

A widely publicized press release by the professional medical sector states in part:

> "The Council of the College of Physicians and Surgeons of Ontario announced today that the performance by an Ontario physician of female circumcision, excision or infibulation will be banned. As well as forbidding these procedures, the College notes that during the course of a vaginal delivery of a woman who has been previously subjected to this practice, a physician may find it necessary to surgically disrupt the scar tissue resulting from the earlier procedure. In this circumstance, the physician, at the conclusion of the delivery, must not endeavour to reconstruct the infibulation but should confine activities to repairing the surgically incised area.
>
> Over the past few months, the College has received inquiries from concerned physicians being asked to perform this procedure . . . Legislation prohibiting female circumcision, excision or infibulation already exists in several countries including Sweden and Great Britain where performance of the procedures carries a penalty of imprisonment. The College will be bringing its new policy to the attention of the Federal government and asking the government to develop similar legislation in Canada.
>
> To help physicians provide effective, sensitive care to women who have undergone these procedures, the College has asked its Education Committee to study educational initiatives to assist physicians in treating these patients. . . The College wishes to emphasize that physicians should treat patients who have had this procedure with sensitivity and compassion.
>
> A physician who is requested to perform this procedure must decline and also refuse to refer the matter to any other person. In the event that a physician learns of a person performing female circumcision, excision or infibulation, the matter should immediately be brought to the attention of the College." [75.]

Regarding national legislation to prohibit FGM in response to an inquiry of **WIN NEWS** the Canadian College of Physicians and Surgeons stated in a later reply that the federal government had responded that prohibition of FGM was already covered by existing legislation on child abuse. Health and community groups in Canada as well as women's organizations and immigrant and refugee centers are taking on the issue in the context of health, working with immigrant families. But the leadership from the medical and health sector certainly is all-important and provides an example.

Such leadership is entirely missing in the U.S. Despite repeated letters to the AMA - the all powerful American Medical Association - which speaks for the opinions of physicians as well as letters to the federal public health authorities and the surgeon general and the Department of Health and Human Services, the issue has been entirely ignored. The only response received was from the National Institute of Health, stating that they would look into working with other federal agencies such as the Immigration and Naturalization Service. I had suggested in my letters to them in 1992, pointing to the Canadian initiatives, that immigrants to the USA should be warned that FGM represents gross child abuse according to social workers consulted. But despite follow-ups, both the AMA as well as government officials concerned with health remains mute.

In the meantime, rumors are circulating widely that immigrants from Africa and the Middle East have for years practiced the mutilations and that immigrant physicians from the Middle Eastern and African countries do the mutilations for a fee. Due to the privacy protection laws between physician and patient there is no way to bring the issue out in the open as no public moneys are involved (as in Canada and the Netherlands, indeed, most of Europe).

In April 1990 the **American Medical News**, a newspaper for physicians published by the AMA, ran an article "US doctors seeing 'circumcised' female immigrants". [76] The article states the fact that physicians occasionally see women from African and Middle Eastern countries who are mutilated and that the practice continues among some immigrant communities. But the article, which explains FGM in very general terms, provides no facts and no numbers as to how many immigrant children might be at risk. And that needs to be established first as was done in France, as well as making contact with immigrant groups and communities.

To date not a single case of a child subjected to FGM in the U.S. has been documented and certainly no deaths related to FGM have been recorded as happened in France - which greatly shocked the French public and could not be covered up by the French authorities who had concealed the facts for years. But in France it took the deaths of three little African girls and dozens of court cases before the French government was compelled to act. The only official action to date has been to send one excisor and one mother to jail. The men who are responsible for FGM in France as well as everywhere else are free.

In the U.S. physicians who do the mutilations know how to protect themselves and since health care is entirely based on private enterprise there is no way to get at the facts unless women in immigrant communities speak up for their children which is quite unlikely.

A proposal I developed to teach immigrant women from Africa - for instance from Ethiopia - using the **Childbirth Picture Books** at a local African community center in the Washington area was ignored by the Ethiopian man who runs the center. The local chapter of the National Organization for Women, who first was interested in volunteering to teach African women immigrants, backed out. In fact women's organizations in the U.S. have done nothing to even help establish the basic facts of how many children are at risk to be subjected to FGM in the U.S. which could be easily done by any national group.

Too many African-American women in the U.S. not only refuse to face the issue but accuse anyone dealing with FGM of racism, and their strident accusations have prevented so far all action by women in the U.S. The leadership should come from the health sector as in Canada, but there is no one interested or concerned. On the contrary physicians no doubt make money from the mutilations of helpless little girls as they do in Africa and elsewhere protected by secrecy.

The realistic view for refugees is - and I speak from personal experience - to learn from the new environment and its people, to seek out the best of what is new but most of all to find opportunities to contribute in building a new and different future. To cling to tradition and the past can only harm you, but most of all it will harm your children. It is the future of the children that is irreparably damaged by burdening them with a past that has nothing to do with their present life nor does it provide support for inevitable change.

Mutilating the genitalia of a child is not only a dangerous physical operation but it irrevocably damages all her future life and health: most of all it alters her personality. All this creates terrible physical and psychological burdens that none of her contemporaries face and that may well destroy her ability to create a productive life. It is essential that all refugees and especially men be confronted with these facts and be made to face the reality that in all the Western world they will be held responsible for the damage they do to their children and to women no matter what their traditons of the past. And the very future of their whole society depends on women, not on men.

What is recorded in this report, shows that the real cause of FGM is the attitude of men which is the same all over the world: the ruthless male desire to dominate and control the sexuality of women. But accusations of racism are invariably made every time the subject of FGM is discussed. In response to this it must be said that the ultimate in racism is to claim that, because a girl is brown or black, she should be subjected to a torturous mutilation which would be absolutely rejected for a white child. Yet accusations of racism are used again and again especially by men to stop all action against FGM.

Finally, this plea in a letter from a Sudanese woman in Germany, re-printed in its entirety:

> "Dear Frau Hosken:
>
> I heard of your WIN-organization from a friend. I am a Sudanese graduate in education from Munchen. I don't think you can help me, but you may help other Sudanese women, who, like me, have been through the hell of pharao operation. This operation is done to make you feel nothing but pain when you make love, so you do not ask the husband for sex but he tells you when.
>
> I was closed after being cut when I was ten. My mother was Egyptian and she was not closed, only cut. She herself, did not like me to be closed by pharao operation but she went back to Egypt to visit her relations and I was cut the next day. The daya who did it was an old woman and closed me very tight. I stayed in bed for three weeks. Women say that the tighter is the bride, the more the husband will love her.

When you are closed, it is like you are in prison in yourself.

I have been sent abroad and from German girls heard of pleasures of love. I never could do as much as touch myself. There is no feeling left and the gate is closed. In this way, it is made sure that the girl is a virgin when she is married.

I have been married for three years and have a daughter. My aunts want her to be cut and closed like they are. My husband says that the Turkish doctors, here in Germany, would do it without pain and without complications. It costs 1000-DM and it is said that when done before two years, the child will not remember a thing later. My husband says that it's either now or later, when it is more painful. Otherwise, nobody will marry her.

Why we women cannot be left with our bodies as when we are born? In a few weeks my girl, who is now two, will go to a doctor to be cut and closed. I prefer this than the torture I have been through. There is no way we can live back in Darfur if the girl is not operated. Please write to other women about our suffering. You have pleasure when loving your husband. We have nothing, there are no feelings left. The knife takes all away.

I don't give my name because you cannot help me. What was cut off will not grow again. My husband would not like what I have written. He is very proud that I was closed so tight and that he had me without help.

Let merciful God be with you and guide you. . ."[76]

In June of this year a World Conference on Human Rights will be held in Vienna by the United Nations: All over the world women are organizing, signing petitions and demanding to be heard. It seems strange but so far women have been almost entirely omitted from the international human rights agenda which seems to be solely concerned with civil and political rights of men, often forgetting that women exist.

But women's human rights are beginning to be recognized. For more than five years FGM has been included in the "Country Reports on Human Rights Practices" by the U.S. Department of State. [77] A section on women - specifically on discrimination and violence against women in the family as well as FGM - is included in each report. From every African and Middle Eastern country where FGM is practiced not only these facts are cited but the latest information is included providing a remarkably comprehensive view.

For many years I have lobbied Congress and the Department of State for the inclusion of women and specifically FGM in the Country Reports. The fact that FGM is now included and cited in every country where it is practiced makes FGM an officially recognized human rights violation all over the world. And that is a considerable change.

When I first began to report the facts about FGM in **WIN NEWS** in 1975, no publication or journal or news service anywhere in the world was willing to print this information: all international organizations and agencies participated in this conspiracy of silence refusing to acknowledge the very existence of FGM, including WHO and UNICEF.

To bring the issue to world attention and especially to the attention of international organizations and United Nations agencies, **WIN NEWS** began in 1976 to collect signatures from women worldwide under a human rights statement condemning FGM as a Human Rights violation and urging the UN Secretary General and the Division of Human Rights to work for its abolishment. Many thousands of signatures were received by **WIN NEWS** from all over the world and sent on to the the UN Secretary General, the Director of the Human Rights Division in Geneva as well as the Secretary General for Social Development and Humanitarian Affairs. The final statement of the one page letter summarizing the health facts on FGM, with the signatures attached, is as valid today as when it was written:

"The mutilation of the genital organs of the female body for any reason whatsoever is a fundamental offense against the human rights of all women in general and specifically against the female children and women who are mutilated.

THE RIGHT TO HEALTH IS A BASIC HUMAN RIGHT THAT CANNOT BE ABRIDGED."

FOOTNOTES

1. **Convention on the Elimination of All Forms of Discrimination Against Women:** Contact Centre for Social Development and Humanitarian Affairs, Division for the Advancement of Women, Vienna International Centre, P.O. Box 500, A-1400, Vienna, Austria
2. Montagu, Ashley. **The Natural Superiority of Women**. Collier Books, a Division of MacMillan Publishing Co., (New York) 1952, p. 50.
3. Country Reports on Human Rights Practices for 1992, prepared annually by the Department of State for the U.S. Congress. Available from Superintendent of Documents, Washington, DC 20402.
4. Widstrand, Carl Gosta. "Female Infibulation", **Studia Ethnographica Upsaliensa**, Vol. XX, 1964, p. 102.
5. Gould-Davis, Elizabeth. **The First Sex**. Penguin Books, 1972, pp. 154-55.
6. Ibid.
7. Dingwall, Eric John. **The Girdle of Chastity**. Routledge (London), 1931 (as quoted by Widstrand and Gould-Davis).
8. Gould-Davis, op. cit., p. 167.
9. Widstrand, op. cit., p. 199.
10. Ibid.
11. Gould-Davis. op. cit., p. 167.
12. Widstrand. op. cit., p. 113.
13. Ibid.
14. Bell, T. M.D. **Kalogynomia**, London: Stockdale, 1821 (as quoted by Gould-Davis).
15. Barker-Benfield, C. J. **The Horrors of the Half Known Life: Male Attitudes Towards Women and Sexuality in the 19th Century America**. Harper/ Colophon Books, 1977.
16. Widstrand, op. cit. p. 114.
17. **New York Times**,, January 26, 27, 28, 29, 1976 (Page One: Special Feature).
18. Montagu, Ashley. op. cit., p. 118.
19. Duden, Barbara, and Isabelle Schatten. "Die Gebarmutter das Hungrige Tier" ("The Uterus, the Hungry Animal: History of Hysteria"), **Courage**, March 3, 1978, p. 20.
20. Ibid, p. 20.
21. Duffy, John. "Masturbation and Clitoridectomy: A 19th Century View", **Journal of the American Medical Association**, Vol. 186, October 19, 1963, pp. 245-248.
22. Ibid.
23. Fleming, J.G. "Clitoridectomy: The Disastrous Downfall of Isaac Baker Brown, F.R.C.S. (867)", **Journal of Gynaecology of the British Empire**, Vol. 67 (6), 1960, pp. 1017-1034.
24. Nichol, Guy. "The Clitoris Martyr", **World Medicine**, Vol. 4, No. 16, May 6, 1969, pp. 59, 63, 65.
25. Paige, Karen Ericksen. "The Ritual of Circumcision", **Human Nature**, May 1978, pp. 40-48.
26. Masters and Johnson. **Human Sexual Response**. Little, Brown & Co. (Boston), 1966, p. 201.
27. Barker-Benfield, C. J. "A Historical Perspective on Women's Health Care - Female Circumcision", **Women and Health: Issues on Women's Health Care**. Jan./Feb. 1976, Vol. 1, #1, pp. 13-15, 18-20.
28. Ibid., p. 15.
29. Ibid.
30. National Organization of Circumcision Information Resource Centers, P.O. Box 2512 San Anselmo, CA 94979-2512: Newsletter available.

FOOTNOTES (continued)

31. Letter from Boston Women's Health Book Collective written to **Medical World News,** 1978.
32. **Letter to Science for the People** (Nov./Dec. 1978) written by The Boston Feminists Working Against Violence Against Women.
33. **New National Black Monitor**, October 1980. Editorial Offices: 410 Central Park West, Penthouse C, New York, NY 10025.
34. Ibid. See also **WIN NEWS,** Vol. 7, No. 2, Spring 1980, p. 39.
35. **WIN NEWS**, Vol. 7, No. 4, Autumn 1981, pp. 39-40.
36. **EMOTAN** (Autumn 1981 issue), PMB 70, UIPO, Ibadan, Nigeria. Tola Adenle, Publisher / Editor See also **WIN NEWS,** Vol. 8, No. 1, Winter 1982, pp. 25-26.
37. Letter from Alla Kvinnors Hus (All Women's House), Sva Svartensgat. 20, Stockholm, Sweden. See **WIN NEWS**, Vol. 6, No. 1, Winter 1980, Insert.
38. International Association of Women Immigrants (RIFFI), Vanadisvagen 7, 3tr., 113 46 Stockholm, Sweden. See also **WIN NEWS**, Vol. 7, No. 3, Summer 1980, p. 36.
39. Alla Kvinnors Hus., op. cit., resolution dated September 12, 1979.
40. **WIN NEWS**, Vol. 6, No. 3, Summer 1980, p. 36.
41. **Dagens Nyheter**, Febr. 14, 1981. See **WIN NEWS**, Vol. 7, No. 2, Spring 1981, p. 37.
42. **F. Magazine,** #14, March 1979, p. 56.
43. **F. Magazine**, October 1980, pp. 74-75. See also **WIN NEWS**, Vol. 7, No. 4, Autumn 1980, p. 47.
44. Saurel, Renee. "La Petite Oumou", a series of articles in **Les Temps Modernes** (1979-1980), Paris. Also **L'Enteree Vive**, Editions Slatkine, 1981, (Paris).
45. **Medical Daily,** March 12, 1981 (in French). See also **WIN NEWS**, Vol. 7, No. 2, Spring 1981, p. 35.
46. Franjou, Marie-Helene, Dr. **Choisir**, Sept./Oct. 1981, (Paris). For a summary translation see **WIN NEWS**, Vol. 8, No. 1, Winter 1982, pp. 26-27.
47. **WIN NEWS**, Vol. 8, No. 1, Winter 1982, p. 27.
48. **London Times**, July 24, 1982. See also "A Sexual Rite on Trial", **Newsweek**, November 1, 1982. See also **WIN NEWS**, Vol. 8, No. 4, Autumn 1982, for a summary of French press reports on the same subject.
49. **Le Monde**, October 7, 1982. See also **WIN NEWS**, Vol. 8, No. 4, pp. 37-38.
50. See **WIN NEWS**, Vol. 15, No. 1, Winter 1989, p. 28 and **WIN NEWS**, Vol. 15, No. 2, Spring 1989, p. 41. C.A.M.S., Commission Internationale Pour L'Abolition des Mutilations Sexuelle (International Commission to Abolish Sexual Mutilation), the P.O. Box maintained by Awa Thiam and this organization no longer replies (after 1991). **La Parole aux Negresses,** Awa Thiam. Denoel/Gonthier, Paris, 1978.
51. G.A.M.S., Groupe Femmes pour L'Abolition des Mutilations Sexuelles (Women's Group to Abolish Sexual Mutilations), Maison des Femmes, 9 Cite Prost 75011, Paris, France. See **WIN NEWS**, Vol. 15, No. 2, Spring 1989, p. 40. See **WIN NEWS**, Vol. 10, No. 1, Winter 1984, p. 31. This survey established that 77 percent of the African girls coming to French health clinics are at risk of a total of about 36,000 African children (girls and boys). The latest figures of G.A.M.S. are more than 20,000 girls at risk. See **WIN NEWS**, Vol. 17, No. 4, Autumn 1991, p. 36.
52. See reports "Deaths of Baby Girls of African Immigrants", French Trials and Parents/ Excisors" etc. See **WIN NEWS**, Vol. 10, No. 3, Summer 1989, p. 40. **Le Matin** , June 6, 1989. See **WIN NEWS**, Vol. 8, No. 4, Autumn 1982, pp. 36-38. **Nouvel Observateur**, July 21, p. 41. **Le Monde,** Oct. 7, 1982. **NY Times**, Jan. 11, 1993, See **WIN NEWS**, Vol. 19, No. 2, Spring 1993, section on FGM.
53. **The New York Times,** Jan 11, 1993. See **WIN NEWS**, Vol. 19, No, 2, Spring 1993.
54. Letter in author's file (Sept. 9, 1982). See **WIN NEWS**, Vol. 8, No. 4, Autumn 1982, p. 38

FOOTNOTES (continued)

55. AIDoS (Italian Association of Women in Development), via del Giubbonari, 30 int. 6, 00186 Rome, Italy. Contact: Daniela Colombo. A newsletter is available.
56. **WIN NEWS**, Vol. 5, No. 1, Winter 1989, insert.
57. **WIN NEWS**, Vol. 6, No. 4, Autumn 1989, p. 45.
58. **Sydney Morning Herald**. See also **WIN NEWS**, Vol. 6, No. 4, Autumn 1980, p. 45.
59. **Hospital Doctor**, Vol. C2, #27, July 8, l982, (Guildford, U.K.).
60. Ibid. See also **WIN NEWS**, Vol. 8, No. 3, Summer 1982, p. 51.
61. Letter in author's file. See also **WIN NEWS**, Vol. 6, No. 2, Spring 1980, p. 34.
62. **The Observer**, Oct. 10, 1982. See **WIN NEWS**, Vol. 8, No. 4, Autumn 1982, p. 39.
63. The Prohibition of Female Circumcision Act 1983, which declares an offense not only for doing the operation but also for anyone who takes part including procurement or facilitating the act. See **WIN NEWS**, Vol. 10, No. 1, Winter 1984, p. 37.
64. Foundation for Women's Health Research and Development (FORWARD), Africa Centre, 38 King St., Covent Garden, London, WC2 8JT, England, Stella Efua Darkenoo, director.
65. First Study Conference on FGM in Europe, organized by FORWARD (see footnote 64). See also **WIN NEWS**, Vol. 18, No. 4, Autumn 1992, p. 37. Conference report available from FORWARD.
66. Eisler, Riane. **The Chalice and the Blade: Our History, Our Future.** Harper & Row, Publishers, Hagerstown, Md., 1990.
67. **FORUM** magazine, October 1983, published by FORUM Press Litd., 2 Bramber Road, London W14 9PB, U.K. Roger Baker, editor. Article on "Female Circumcision," by an "anonymous" surgeon. See **WIN NEWS**, Vol. 10, No. 1, Winter 1984, pp. 38 and 39.
68. World Health Organization: Female Circumcision Statement on WHO Position and Activities, June 1982. Submitted to the UN. Sub-Commission on Prevention of Discrimination and Protection of Minorities. Geneva 27, Switzerland.
69. Defense for Children International (DCI), P.O. Box 75297, 1070 AG Amsterdam, The Netherlands. Stan Meuwese, director. See **WIN NEWS**, Vol. 18, No. 4, Autumn 1992, pp. 30-32, ; Vol. 19, No. 1, Winter 1993, p. 34-36,
70. Letter in author's file dated August 26, 1992, from Ministry "Welzijn Volksgezondheid en Cultuur" (Health Ministry), Directoraat Generaal van de Volksgezondheid, Postbus 3008, 2280 MK Rijswijk, The Netherlands.
71. Ministry of Foreign Affairs, The Hague. Netherlands Policies on Female Genital Mutilation. March 2, 1993. Signed by Head of the Legal and Social Affairs Division.
72. Foundation Pharos, Herenstraat 35. P.O. Box 13318, 3507 LH Utrecht, Netherlands.
73. Hosken, Fran P. **The Childbirth Picture Book**/Program - "A picture story of reproduction from a woman's view", pictures by Marcia L. Williams. Published by **WIN NEWS**, 187 Grant St., Lexington, MA 02420, USA. Books, flipcharts, color slides in English, French, Spanish, Arabic. Additions to prevent excision and infibulation. In the Somali translation a section to prevent infibulation is included in the book.
74. **The Ottawa Citizen**, Jan. 4, 1992. See **WIN NEWS**, Vol. 18, No. 2, Spring 1992, p. 45.
75. Press Release of January 27, 1992, of the Canadian College of Physicians and Surgeons of Ontario, 80 College St., Toronto M5G 2E2, Canada. See also **WIN NEWS**, Vol. 18, No. 2, Spring 1992, p. 46.
76. **American Medical News**, April 27, 1990, "U.S. doctors seeing 'circumcised' female immigrants". Published by American Medical Association, 535 North Dearborn, Chicago, IL 60610.
77. Letter in author's file. See also **WIN NEWS**, Vol. 6, No. 2, Spring 1980, p. 34.
78. Country Reports on Human Rights Practices. published annually in February by the Departmentt of State. See every Spring issue of **WIN NEWS**. Available from: U.S. Government Printing Office, Superintendent of Documents, Washington, DC 20402.

THE POLITICS OF FEMALE GENITAL MUTILATION: A CONSPIRACY OF SILENCE

The politics of genital mutilation are first of all the patriarchal politics of controlling production and reproduction of the wholly-owned female labor force - the primary resources of male power and wealth. They are the sexual politics designed to affirm the power of males over female sexuality and reproduction. The patriarchal family structure - a worldwide institution maintained and enforced by all man-made governments and organized religions - serves that goal.

The male-headed family hierarchy is replicated on a larger scale by the male-headed hierarchical governments - which exclude most women from participation and decision-making. This system is in turn repeated in international arrangements between countries and states where women are almost totally eliminated from making decisions such as on peace and war that directly affect life and death. Yet, the myth about democracy is propagated by men, whose power in all political systems is based on the exclusion and exploitation of women - or the majority of each society. Control over women's bodies and sexuality serves as the underpinning of this system: Female genital mutilation (FGM) directly serves patriarchal control.

The Conspiracy of Silence concerning women's rights, women's contributions and needs and women's sexuality is all-pervasive, starting in each family and reaching to the top of the male hierarchy of international decisions and affairs. Women are excluded from speaking on their own behalf and from all meaningful participation in decision making unless they are willing to support patriarchal goals.

Here, we are first of all concerned with the Conspiracy of Silence in international politics that directly affects the lives and health of tens of millions of girls and women. This conspiracy has made it possible for female genital mutilations to spread all over Africa the Middle East and even into parts of Asia. The operations on female children are now being introduced into modern health care as sexual castrations and exported all over the world: Yet the silence of the patriarchal establishment is only rarely broken and almost never with positive results for women.

For instance, UNICEF - the agency that claims to work for children and mothers under the leadership of a man, Mr. James Grant - must be held responsible for a large part of the increase in Female Genital Mutilation (FGM) over the last 12 years or since the World Health Organization Seminar in Khartoum in 1979, where specific recommendations were made on how to stop the practice. UNICEF has failed to effectively support the eradication of FGM. Worse - Mr. Grant has failed to give leadership by developing effective policies for UNICEF offices in African and Middle Eastern countries. UNICEF has also failed to support local efforts to stop FGM in many African countries where such efforts have been started (see UNICEF below).

The politics of female genital mutilation (FGM) are positively linked to the politics of ignorance - of witholding from women and the young the vital information about how their bodies and reproduction function: These sexual power politics are truly international. For instance we see today the political battles over the distribution of condoms as protection from AIDS. The same politics form the background for development decisions at the United Nations and especially those concerned with women's health.

It is, of course, a fact that if there was a will to stop FGM it could be accomplished in most urban areas in about 20 years. But this would require male leadership both international and national and broad-based male support. Without these I don't believe it could succeed at the present time. This must be kept in mind at all times when reading this report: it is men who collectively and individually are responsible for continuing the practice of FGM. The sexual politics that form the underpinning of FGM in each family, ethnic group, and country as well as the reasons given and the myths propagated by men, are documented in the Country Case Histories that form the bulk of this report.

THE PARAMETERS

The politics of genital mutilation changed with the World Health Organization (WHO) Seminar of February 1979 in Khartoum (see: "WHO Seminar"). The implementation of the international recommendations formulated at the Seminar must be seen as a tangible goal and priority. International assistance for implementation is usually available and readily organized for health concerns, for instance the eradication of smallpox, as well as regional health problems such as malaria or river blindness.

The Seminar Report[1] was published by the WHO Regional Office in Alexandria, Egypt, which sponsored the seminar, and the recommendations were widely disseminated. The recommendations were also confirmed in an article by Dr. Taba, the WHO Regional Director, which was published by the official WHO magazine. It was further publicly announced in the statement by UNICEF that was widely distributed at the UN Mid-Decade Conference for women in Copenhagen in July 1980.

These recommendations were designed to serve as guidelines for action throughout Africa and the Middle East. The first step was to make them widely known, both in Africa and internationally, to gain support for implementation. FGM, which had been hidden for hundreds of years, had to be made known before any recommendations could be implemented: The patriarchal conspiracy of silence, that prevailed around the world and especially at the United Nations, had to be broken.

The formation of the Inter African Committee on Traditional Practices Affecting the Health of Women and Children in 1984 at a meeting of international non-governmental organizations in Dakar, Senegal, which followed up on the Khartoum Seminar - was a major step forward in implementing the recommendations of Khartoum.[2] For five years - between 1979 and 1984 - these recommendations were ignored by all African countries and by all WHO and UNICEF country offices. In the Dakar Seminar with the participation of non-governmental and women's organizations from all over Africa, these recommendations were elaborated and the groundwork was laid for action by national committees. At present - in end of spring 1993 - there are more than twenty-two such committees active in different African countries (see "Case History: Senegal" and "Women and Health").

The actions in each country to implement the recommendations can be readily adapted according to local needs. But, given the economic constraints of most African countries, international financial and technical assistance is essential. For instance, family planning (FP) was introduced, with a great deal of international financial and technical support, to assist governments in developing countries to start FP programs. Great efforts are being made, supported by vast sums of money, to introduce FP in Africa; but population growth rates are still increasing.

Though FGM eradication programs could be coordinated with FP programs, as they complement each other and would greatly benefit women's and children's health, it is amazing to see that internationally supported FP programs have entirely ignored the very existence of FGM. International FP organizations, including IPPF - International Planned Parenthood Federation [3] - have done nothing to prevent FGM and have failed to even talk about it - though they obviously can no longer claim that they dont know about it.

The men who plan and design family planning programs that are internationally funded for African and Middle Eastern countries are not concerned with women's health but with "population control" or they could not ignore FGM. And that is one reason why the programs are failing in Africa despite all the money spent. It is ironic that international family planners are motivated by the same patriarchal incentives "to control women's fertility and reproduction" as the African men who are intent to father ever more children. Though they seek opposite results, the basic issues and motivations of both are the same: control over women's bodies, sexuality and fertility which is shared by men everywhere.

In both cases, women and children are the violated victims, deprived of their rights and often made to pay with their lives. When family planning experts begin to work for what is needed by African women - education and resources - so they are independent of men, they will successfully deal with their own fertility - as women have done everywhere else in the world. But that means that the experts would lose their jobs and men would lose their patriarchal sexual domination - and that is the real and very political issue in eradicating FGM as well as successful control of fertility.

Unfortunately what family planning programs have failed to accomplish in Africa may be done by AIDS. WHO statistics on AIDS in Africa have worsened with every report over the past years: They are by far the highest in the world. Sub Saharan Africa also is the region where as many women as men were infected from the start - and, as a result, also infants. This the experts found hard to explain, as everywhere else the majority of the infected were men and they never looked at women. But now women are catching up.

Already in 1986 in a letter to the **New York Times** following a series of medical reports on AIDS in Africa, I pointed out that

> "As a result of FGM, as well as other sexual practices by men that involve lacerations and the flow of blood in the female genital area, AIDS has many opportunities to reach women - who are infected during sexual intercourse. Due to genital mutilation, especially infibulation, sexual intercourse must be preceded by cutting the introitus of the artificially closed bride. Excision, or clitoridectomy, also often involves formation of hard scar tissue (especially in dark-skinned people, due to keloid formation), frequently resulting in lacerations during intercourse.
>
> In many areas of Africa, girls are married at a very young age to much older men, who can afford to pay the steep bride-price. The genitalia of the often very small girl brides are torn by the much larger males during intercourse. This is confirmed by hospital records in maternities and by midwives and nurses working there. Many young rape victims can also be found in hospital maternities.
>
> The heterosexual transmission of AIDS in Africa is clearly explained by the violent sexual practices of men: including the requirement by all Moslems (as well as some other societies) that blood must flow on the wedding night to confirm the bride's virginity; clitoridectomy and genital mutilation; child marriage; widespread sexual violence, and rape all contribute to the heterosexual transmission of AIDS." [4]

FGM continues all over Africa and the Middle East on a huge scale - but none of the internationally sponsored development programs, including those directly concerned with health and family planning, pay any attention to this. Even when deaths as a result of FGM are reported by the press, as often happens in Kenya, the highly paid international development experts - almost all of them men - still manage to ignore this. "It is the custom" they say; anthropologists hired as program advisers assert that "all traditions must be preserved". Yet tradition supports the status quo, undermining all development - because development means change.

FGM is much like wife abuse. It goes on everywhere. It is quite normal that women should be violated, beaten and horribly injured by their own husbands. For centuries. no one said anything about it; social institutions, hospitals, physicians, the police, judges and churches all protected the male abusers with their silent complicity and often they still do. Missionaries and church groups of all denominations still uphold this Conspiracy of Silence about FGM today that prevents effective intervention and eradication.But, the numbers of mutilated girls and women increase every year due to population growth: **More than 110 million is the latest tabulation**. (See: Women and Health)

THE INTERNATIONAL POLITICS OF FEMALE GENITAL MUTILATION

Most African and Middle Eastern countries where FGM is practiced have been governed by male dictatorships or authoritarian regimes of one kind or another, some of them military and all of them without any viable representation of women or women's interests. Even though it is claimed that recently a process of democratization has begun mostly due to international political pressure, such movements where they exist do not reflect the interests of women in viable ways, specifically where health or education is concerned.

The gap between literacy of men and women is still increasing everywhere in Africa, so UNESCO statistics show, but this international agency, though ostensibly concerned with education, has in recent years done literally nothing to develop any effective plans or initiative to deal with this growing gap which their experts, sitting in the comfort of their offices in Paris, keep reporting.

The United Nations Development Program (UNDP) as well as WHO and UNICEF all have offices and representatives in every African country and are busy with supporting all kinds of government programs. But the astonishing fact is that although women and children are the majority in every country and although these agencies since the beginning of the UN Decade for Women in 1975 claim to support women's development, the reality is that everywhere women are left out, ignored, sidelined and ever farther behind. Urbanization, called the engine of modernization, affects mostly men in Africa who are leaving the rural areas and subsistence farming in droves while women and children are left behind in rural areas to do all the heavy work alone. Men contribute next to nothing to their families except fathering ever more children, but the male dominated governments in Africa do not require men to support their offspring (see "Case History : Kenya").

In all towns in Africa, one can see idle men and boys hanging around with nothing to do - often drunk and a menace to everyone - while women in the rural areas are overburdened with trying to grow enough food to feed their many children, who are ignored by their fathers. All this is, of course, known to the United Nations Agencies as well as all other development programs sponsored by different Western countries who say nothing and ignore the situation of women and children.

The Convention on the Elimination of All Forms of Discrimination Against Women [5] which has quite specific clauses covering women's rights has been ratified by most African countries. It is interesting to read the reports on the status of women they are required to produce every few years which provide a vivid account of the discrimination, the indignities and injustices to which women are subjected under the jurisdiction of male dominated African governments.

Where the breach of the clauses of the convention is too blatant and the prevailing practices too obviously against the agreements signed by the governments, the male decision makers simply declare this area of the law to be "exempt", or set aside. Such exemptions usually are concerned with family law - for instance, Egypt declared all family law to be outside the scrutiny of the convention. This now has become the means by which patriarchal governments keep glaring injustices and male privileges in place.

But the United Nations and its agencies who are supposed to back up international agreements and support their implementation are similarly in the hands of men intent on protecting their own male privileges, and so they do nothing. Only 3.4 percent of decision-making jobs at the UN and its agencies are held by women according to the reports of the UN Statistical Office of the New York UN Secretariat.

The UN and its agencies do not have equal employment laws, though all the governments that financially support the UN agencies have long since implemented such legislation for women, because their women voters have demanded it. But the male dominated governments have taken care to omit such rules for the UN. Consequently the UN and all its agencies, including all those working in Africa are bastions of male privilege and grossly discriminate against women working in their offices. Many of the men are citizens of developing countries. They obviously never speak for women's rights as this would undermine their own privileges at home where "their" women are still under absolute male control. All these international civil servants are supporting FGM by their silence in solidarity with the African and Middle Eastern men.

Sexual harassment is rampant among UN staff, this brotherhood of shared privilege. Due to the absence of equal employment laws and especially the absence of an independent authority to hear and adjudicate complaints, women have no recourse as was recently again reported by the **New York Times** in an article on sexual harassment. [6] The **Times** summed up the situation at the UN and its agencies quite succinctly a few years ago - and nothing has changed where women are concerned:

> "The United Nations international staff, conceived in the organization's days of heady idealism as a high-caliber civil service organization, insulated from national politics, finds . . . its image tarnished. Winning one of the professional positions no longer depends on merit but politics, favoritism and 'knowing someone." [7]

"Sex discrimination deeply entrenched at the UN" was another front page article headline of the **Times**. The UN and its agencies are rife with discrimination against women in recruitment, hiring, placement and promotion, the article documents. [8] Such discrimination in the very agencies that should speak for women's health and development obviously has a devastating influence when it comes to issues like FGM. All UN agencies have strenuously resisted having anything to do with this issue (see below WHO / UNICEF) and to this day the silence is rarely broken.

Yet despite everything, African and Middle Eastern women have succeeded in making some gains in education and employment after International Women's Year (1975). In Africa, more women have begun to move to urban areas where they are able to make at least some contact with contemporary life and get some work and independent income. In the rural areas, their isolation is still almost complete.

But the women's economic and political toehold has been short-lived due to the World Bank/International Monetary Fund (WB/IMF) austerity programs to "restructure" the debts incurred by governments. Drastic cuts in all services, especially health care and education that affect women and children most of all, have been made as well as in all other government jobs. In African countries, what jobs exist are mainly in the public domain. Private enterprise is very limited due to the lack of capital. Women have borne most of the cutbacks in jobs - as always they are the last hired and first fired.

The economies of most African countries have not improved due to the forced WB/IMF policies. Rather these policies have proved to be a disaster for most Sub-Saharan countries with women and children suffering most of all; and there seems no end in sight. All this was reported and analyzed in the British Commonwealth Report **Engendering Adjustment for the 1990s** [9], which points out that the measures enforced by the WB/IMF for countries to pay back loans made by the men of past governments (in which women had no say and made no decisions) need not have damaged women. But the men who run the WB/IMF obviously never consider women and children at all.

The WB/IMF is not held responsible for the failures of its forced economic policies which are by now highly visible due to growing poverty all over Africa. That the chief victims are women and children even UNICEF had to admit: There is a marked increase of infant mortality in African countries where the WB/IMF policies have been in place.

Recently human rights, has received more attention in Africa, where some human rights groups have been formed. Women have been almost entirely excluded from the international human rights agenda that is only concerned with political and civil rights. For instance Amnesty International ignores women's rights except as political prisoners.

However, since the 1980s, the **Country Reports on Human Rights Practices** [10] which are published every year by the U.S. Department of State, have included women and are now reporting on FGM in every country where it is practiced, as well as on family violence against women. This is a very important step as it confirms FGM as an international human rights violation (see "The Western World"). Due to my extensive lobbying with the U.S. Congress and the State Department, the issue of violation of women and FGM is now officially recognized as a human rights violation. It is no longer possible to claim that FGM is a traditional practice and therefore beyond scrutiny. Human rights are now internationally and politically recognized to be absolute and not subject to limitations by gender or culture or tradition.

THE STATUS OF WOMEN IN AFRICA AND THE MIDDLE EAST

> **"Women are fifty percent of the world's adult population and one third of the official labor force, they perform nearly two-thirds of the actual working hours, for which they receive one-tenth of the world's income but they own less than one percent of the world's property".**

This statement released by the United Nations Mid-Decade Conference in Copenhagen has been cited all over the world, as it succinctly characterizes the status of women.

Development programs by the United Nations, by Western governments and by the hundreds of private voluntary groups including all kinds of church and charitable organizations working in developing countries have accomplished little positive change for women. Rather, development has increased the huge gap between the status of women and men. Since women and children are the majority around the world, it is now evident that the billions spent on development have not accomplished the goals set at the end of the second World War when the United Nations and its agencies were founded.

This report explains some of the reasons why. As long as development is based on a hierarchical structure of gender discrimination and damaging traditions are supported under the label of "culture", development will continue to fail with devastating economic results. The very term "development" means change. By incorporating "tradition" into development programs, change is obstructed and development fails. Nowhere is this more clear than in continental Africa, where gender plays such an important role in the division of labor. Ester Boserup in **Woman's Role in Economic Development** [11] pointed this out. But her advice was ignored by the men who make the decisions, especially in the World Bank, which finances the largest development programs

Food production everywhere in the developing world and especially in Africa is critical. Access to food and adequate nutrition is a prerequisite for the hard work of agricultural production and development. The distribution of food in each family - grown and prepared by women - is a matter of status. Studies in Africa by the UN Protein-Calorie Advisory Group (PAG) state:

> ". . .the head of the household always gets the first portions, receiving a serving from each wife -- even if food is short. . . the worst off are women , victims of tabus and male priorities. . .in many areas women and children eat after the father and all other males have satisfied their appetite . . .young women and children, especially girls, those whom we would regard as most in need of optimal health for the task of childbearing, tend to receive the dregs of meals and bear the brunt of traditional food tabus - - describing the general picture in East Africa." [12]

An analysis of the status of women in the societies that mutilate their female children is essential to form an understanding of this problem which is largely political. FGM does not exist in isolation. It can only be understood in the context of women's lives and against the background of how women are regarded by their male dominated societies. In Africa, two distinct kinds of societies are involved in FGM: First the Arab-African societies influenced by the Middle East and known for their activities as traders including many nomads; the others are the sub-Saharan feudal and tribal village societies engaged in subsistence agriculture or cattle raising.

Sub-Saharan black Africa might be characterized as a rural hierarchical, polygamous tribal society, ruled by male elders or chiefs. Most sub-Saharan women live on the land and are occupied with subsistence farming; that is, they are responsible for growing the food for their large families including all men. They also raise and support their many children while men in the past were occupied with warfare and hunting. Recently men have migrated to the towns in ever larger numbers where they try to make a living in the modern sector; but there are few jobs, given their limited education and skills.

In Arab-African societies, segregation of the sexes is the aspiration of all patriarchal families, though it cannot be achieved in rural areas: women's labor is needed in the fields or where migratory populations follow their herds. However, the seclusion of women, and their exclusion from the public and economic spheres is the norm for Moslem families. Moslemization of the traditonal Animist sub-Saharan village societies is progressing especially in West Africa, moving southward from Moslem North Africa.

When economic conditions of the rural families improve or they move into town, a woman's life in Moslem society becomes confined to her husband's or father's house, for example in the Sudan. A selected few, privileged women of elite families are highly educated and allowed to take part in political and professional life. These are the women who are permitted to hold some positions in government and who go to international meetings. But the family is every woman's first responsibility, no matter what her profession. Islam's ideal is that a woman should not work but should devote herself to motherhood and the home. Therefore, a woman's education and mobility are restricted.

In Sub-Saharan as well as Arab-African and Middle Eastern societies, females are the property of males. Upon reaching puberty, a woman is traded from her father's family to her husband's family in return for a bride-price paid to the father. All marriages are arranged between the male family heads and represent an alliance between families rather than individuals. A woman's chief purpose is to produce and raise sons, to render sexual services to her husband as well as to take care of his food and house.

In village societies and rural areas, the task of women to prepare the daily food. includes carrying water and wood for fuel, often for miles. A woman also must grow and prepare what her children eat as well as feeding all the men of her husbands family. The laborious traditional ways of subsistence farming and food preparation in Africa today, including the grinding or pounding of corn and other food grains or roots, have not changed for centuries and take hours of hard work every day. Attempts to introduce labor-saving devices and tools have at best temporarily succeeded in some places, but since such innovations have no support from men, they are often abandoned when the sponsoring international groups relinquish support in the belief that they are accepted.

It is part of the male political agenda in Africa that women must work hard and be pregnant continuously, as this keeps them under male control, therefore men oppose education and labor-saving devices for women. Alternatively men take over all new tools provided by development programs and demand payments from women for running them. But women have no cash income and cannot pay for services. In that way, many attempts to improve women's lives have failed because men hold all the power and all the resources and tools and they do not want to give up their control of women as a wholly owned labor force. In turn, women farmers are still excluded from most services of government farming agents - mostly men - to improve farming methods. The agents have no incentive to assist women as often their husbands would not approve.

Modernization and education or what is recognized by everyone as a better life is available only to a small elite in urban areas, most of whom work for their respective governments. With few exceptions, these are men. Women are excluded in Africa, as everywhere else in the world, from most of the public decision-making jobs. But women are also excluded from most of the critical family decisions that affect their personal lives such as whom to marry or when. Their lives continue to be restricted by traditional tabus and patriarchal rules that vest all rights, all economic assets and all property in men.

In Africa and the Middle East today, the reproductive function of women continues to be regarded as the only justification for their existence besides rendering personal services to men. For a woman not to marry is still today unthinkable in Africa and the Middle East. At the same time, reproduction is used as the means for women's exclusion from education and jobs, that is, economic independence. But independent women are not available for exploitation by men. This patriarchal view is not limited to Africa and the Middle East.

The classic analysis of Evelyn Sullerot [13] provides a valid analysis of the restrictions on women that even now are still largely in place. With the rise of fundamentalism in the Middle East and Moslem Africa the patriarchal control over women's behavior subjecting them to absolute servitude of men is being continuously reinforced. Sullerot claims that unless a link in the patriarchal chain that imprisons women is broken, women have no chance to escape on their own. The Case Histories in this Report quite confirm this view.

Sullerot provides a plausible framework for the ongoing mutilations of female children and the brutal sexual assaults and constant raping to which a very large part of the women in African and Middle Eastern societies are subjected by men in their own families under the label of tradition and custom.

Sullerot defines the chief elements that govern women's lives: First **Fertility and Adultery.** Before all else, a wife is considerd a breeding machine to perpetuate the male line. Therefore, the punishment for female adultery is extreme, as it is seen as a threat to the whole male-centered structure. **Domestic Confinement,** still practiced in most Moslem societies, is a direct result of the above views. The objective is to confine women in the home to restrict their activities in order to keep them under male control. **Property Rights** are the third link in the chain. Women are excluded from owning and disposing of property. A female passes from the tutelage of her father to that of her husband and finally that of her own son. The absence of property or land rights for women is also true for most African societies that are not Moslem. Land is the chief resource in agricultural societies, therefore it is controlled only by men. **Civil and Political Rights** are the fourth link in this chain. Women have no civic role and are excluded from the public sphere.*

Fertility, Adultery and Domestic Confinement:

Not everywhere in Middle Eastern/African patriarchal societies are all four elements to restrict women present. For instance, in sub-Saharan, tribal Africa, domestic confinement does not exist in the traditional social structure, as women have to do most of the subsistence farming and work in the fields. There are few restrictions on their movements, and they also engage in all kinds of market activities, especially in West Africa.

Most rural women must work in the fields, carry water, and do the hardest labor in Moslem and Arab Africa. What a woman produces, including children, belongs to her husband. But families who live in towns and who can afford it relegate women to the home, especially during their childbearing years. This is to show that the head of the household is sufficiently affluent to keep his women from working outside - it is a matter of male prestige, for instance in the Sudan. When women do go out in strict Moslem areas, they must be "covered" by a cloak or the equivalent (tobe in the Sudan).

All four factors are present where infibulation is the rule. Since strict seclusion often is impossible to practice where a woman's labor is needed, she is infibulated instead, for instance in the nomadic population groups that follow their herds including in Mali, Somalia and Sudan. Instead of secluding her whole person, her vagina is closed by infibulation. Her vital generative parts, which the male patriarchy seeks to control, are artificially closed by scarification only to be opened and used by her legitimate male owner after he pays the bride-price.

The prohibitions against adultery are most severe in Moslem areas - traditionally, death by stoning; now such murder is committed in more modern ways. Excision and infibulation seek to accomplish absolute control over female sexuality by the male guardian (or owner) of each woman - her father, her husband, and finally her son or nearest male relative, who is responsible for her maintenance. Thus, economic responsibility is used to control access to her genitalia. For instance in the Sudan, men going on long journeys frequently had their wives re-infibulated. Recently it has been reported that re-infibulation is again widely practiced. (See: "Case History : Sudan.")

The requirement that the bride must be a virgin is absolute in Moslem and Arab Africa and the Middle East. Paternity must be assured for inheritance, according to the rules that govern the patriarchal system; hence infibulation. This system, with all its economic reinforcements, is very much intact today, for instance in the Sudan.

In some societies in sub-Saharan Africa, by contrast, girls have considerable freedom before marriage, including sexual freedom. Children are welcome, even before marriage. Fertility is highly prized and of the greatest importance to women everywhere in Africa and the Middle East. It is, indeed, the chief means to legitimize a woman's existence.

---

* In antiquity, in Greece and Rome, women had no more public rights than slaves. In the USA, more than 1,700 years later, women were excluded from the document that declared "all **men** are created equal"; and women continue to be excluded to the present time. In the country that claims to be the largest democracy, more than 51% of the population (= all women) are formally and constitutionally excluded from equal rights. Ratification of the Equal Rights Amendment to the U.S. Constitution failed again in Summer 1982.

To produce sons is the road to what little power is available to a female. To produce no sons is reason for divorce, though it is the seed of the male that determines the sex of the child. But men in Africa and the Middle East refuse to acknowledge this biological fact.

To enhance fertility, rituals of all kinds are practiced - different fetishes, special amulets, potions and special herbs are sold in the markets or by special medicine men; dances and rites of all kinds are performed including dangerous mutilations. (See: "Case History: Nigeria") The belief in evil spirits, in the evil eye, in all kinds of jinns and supernatural powers is part of daily life all over Africa and the Middle East, with sorcerers and special healers plying their magic as a lucrative trade often in marketplaces. Remedies for infertility are high on their list because of the overwhelming importance of fertility for the status of a woman. A woman will try anything in case of infertility, which is the greatest disaster that can befall an African woman. Excision is among the prescribed cures for infertility, sometimes with fatal results, as hospital case histories show.

Polygamy is legal and practiced everywhere in the Middle East and in Africa. Though Cote d'Ivoire is said to have legislation forbidding multiple wives, there is no evidence that it is enforced. While Moslems are limited to taking four wives (at one time), the powerful men of tribal societies can have an unlimited number of wives.

Polygamy is a means to have many more children by the dominant males, who buy girls sometimes 30 or more years younger for wives. In rural Africa, for instance in Sierra Leone and other traditional areas, there is no limit to the number of wives a man can own. Since what "his" women produce belongs to him he can afford to buy more and more wives thus multiplying his fortune as the children, as soon as they are able, become part of the agricultural labor force and work "his" land.

Traditionally the village chief alots land to each man according to the number of wives he owns. Polygamy is a sure system of economic success for each man, as Ester Boserup already pointed out in her classic book **Woman's Role in Economic Development** [14], where she also discusses the economics of polygamy in traditional rural Africa. Moslem men of influence, for instance in West Africa, often have a dozen or more wives, though only four at one time. The obsession with fertility is shared by African and Middle Eastern men.

Property Rights:

In the past, land was a communal good in Africa, and it still is in some African rural areas. In the traditional tribal system, land is distributed by each chief to each male head of the family for his wives to till. The colonial system introduced private property and private landholding patterns, with ownership limited to men.

Women were excluded from ownership under both systems and continue to be excluded since independence and up to the present time in most African countries. Even where the law has been changed, there is no way for women to enforce their rights in the face of male control. Even if they know their rights - which in most rural areas women don't (up to 90% are still illiterate) - the male village chiefs supported by the male elders obviously will obstruct all attempts of women to assert any rights.

As the bride-price payments in cash or in kind confirm, women are regarded as property. Often a very young girl, as soon as she menstruates, is given by her father to the highest bidder to use her body for continuing his line. The bride is rarely allowed to even see the purchaser. Marriage is a financial deal between men and an alliance between families.

In the modern sector in cities of much of Africa today, women still cannot get bank credit, as they have no collateral. This is slowly changing in a few countries, at least on paper. But in rural areas, most women are overburdened with children and farm labor. Illiteracy prevents them from contact with any laws designed to help them. All laws are administered by men who are interested only in keeping women ignorant of their rights.

A Moslem woman can legally inherit only half the share of her brothers, including at times land; but in practice, such ownership is often impossible to enforce. She is usually compelled to cede her property to a male relation for "protection". Most of the time, she does not know her legal rights, and even if she does, how can an illiterate woman go to court against her own family?

Equal rights clauses are included in many African constitutions - according to statements made by African and Middle Eastern government delegates at the United Nations. Nevertheless, internationally financed agricultural and urban development programs usually exclude women from land and property ownership. Land and buildings with few exceptions are always registered in the name of a man. Thus women farmers are excluded from obtaining credit for seeds and tools, which drastically reduces their ability to produce food and especially cash crops.

Land and property rights are a basic economic and political issue. Since independence, foreigners have not been allowed to own or buy land in most African countries. But why are African women treated like foreigners and excluded from owning land and real property in their own names. Are they not considered citizens? Why are African women excluded from owning the land they till? Is that not slavery?

Civic and Political Rights:

Where Moslem law is strictly observed, women are excluded from the public sphere. They cannot even go into the street alone and must be covered from head to toe with a cloak. Saudi Arabia provides the much admired model for African men, due to its oil wealth and due to its orthodox religious practices. Their restriction of women is the model for African Moslems, whose goal is to participate in the annual pilgrimage to Mecca.

Though women's formal exclusion from the public sphere is not a rule in tribal and black Africa, there are no female chiefs except among a few ethnic groups in Ghana and in Sierra Leone. Traditionally all the village elders and chiefs who make decisions, including when and on whom excision is to be performed, are men.

In the modern sector, one can find a few exceptional women serving their governments in decision-making positions. That means that the talents of nearly half the population are wasted in countries that can ill-afford to waste anything. The "brain drain" is frequently internationally deplored: Or that many educated men leave their developing nation to work in the industrialized world. But the brain drain due to discrimination - excluding some of the best minds from education for decision-making jobs because they come with a female body is nowhere mentioned. It is also ignored by advisors on international development, who apparently are afraid to upset their African brothers' patriarchal rule.

While Islam uses religious grounds to exclude women from the public sphere, discrimination in education, especially in higher education and in scholarships for study abroad, is the means to exclude women from participation in public life in black Africa. Going back to colonial times, neither Britain nor France nor any other colonial power provided scholarships for women, let alone invited women to study at a university abroad.

Illiteracy is, of course, a massive barrier for political participation of women everywhere in the world; it is especially formidable in Africa, where in many countries, up to 90 percent of rural women are illiterate, and little or no headway is being made. The educational gap between women and men is increasing everywhere in Africa and is the highest in the world in Moslem Francophone West Africa. As Sullerout states:

> "To educate the masses of illiterate women is not philanthropy undertaken in a spirit of egalitarian idealism or as a democratic crusade. It is a vital need in the modern world, a question of life or death for many, and for all a choice between stagnation and progress. Without female education, progress can be transmitted to each generation either not at all or very slowly, since it cannot be passed on in the home." [15]

THE SEXUAL POLITICS OF AFRICAN AND MIDDLE EASTERN MEN

Women's only legitimate purpose in life - according to African men - is to serve men and bear their children. Yet women are mutilated in such a way as to make childbearing a harrowing ordeal of exhausting, prolonged suffering which often costs them their lives. This, so men can prove their sexual superiority. But apparently, even this is not enough. Man-made traditions give African and Middle Eastern men the right to use physical violence against women to impose their will; and they claim the right to divorce which means to throw out a wife without any resources or any means of support - after taking away her children in a display of unmitigated cruelty.

Divorce is very frequent, especially in Moslem Africa, where men often discard their older wives to replace them with young and fertile ones, whose labor and childbearing will increase their male owners' wealth.

The economics of FGM are quite sophisticated in how they work for the benefit of men. The bride-price, which is collected by the father, can only be assured in many societies by selling a daughter who is excised. If it is a Moslem ethnic group, infibulation may be required; it guarantees virginity. No father would risk losing such a considerable sum in cash or in kind as the bride-price, by failing to have his child mutilated; the earlier, the better because if he waits, she might make a fuss. If it is done at an early age and the girl dies, not much is lost; he can always make another. It is no effort for him.

In turn, the male family head will not accept a daughter-in-law unless she is mutilated. He often has to pay the bride-price to buy wives for his young sons so he decides with whom to deal and refuses to buy brides who are not operated. This, in turn, makes it "necessary" to have his own daughters "done" so they are not rejected. And so the rules are made by the male head of each family, who then claims FGM is a "women's affair".

To claim - as many African men do (as well as male, Western anthropologists) - that women are the ones who perpetuate the operations in societies where women have never had any choice about anything, least of all their bodies, is ludicrous. Clearly, it is a matter of male sexual politics. As soon as men stop demanding FGM as price for marriage and stop paying for having their daughters mutilated, the operations will stop.

If one speaks to African representatives at the United Nations or African diplomats, they frequently pretend that FGM is a women's affair that they know nothing about; an absurd claim considering that they have sexual relations with excised women and frequently have several wives, besides paying to have their daughters "done".

Men in Africa, whether illiterate or intellectuals, know very well that they derive power from mutilating women's genitalia and sexuality. It is a matter of political control. The fear of female sexuality is after all shared by men around the world; just as male attempts to castrate females' sexuality goes on everywhere (see "The Western World").

Though women took an active part in the struggle for independence all over Africa, the male heads of the newly independent African countries ignored all women's rights, though they loudly proclaimed their own rights. Excision and infibulation continued without a word. Jomo Kenyatta, the leader who became president of Kenya, after the fight for independence - which relied on the collaboration of women - stated that no real Kikuyu male would marry a woman who is not excised (see "Case History: Kenya").

Modernization has been welcomed by African leaders who surround themselves with imported technology, Western tools and Western luxuries of every kind; but they have their daughters "done", that is excised - preferably in a modern hospital equipped by a Western donor using antibiotics donated by Western health programs with the mutilations performed by a Western trained African physician.

The sexual politics by which African men pursue power and sexual control over women through mutilation and violence are now collapsing with the onslaught of AIDS. And AIDS is spreading like wildfire all over Africa, faster and farther than on any other continent, as men are unwilling to control their sexuality. But once more the majority of victims are women and girls who have no protection from the violent and bloody sexual assaults by men, that are regularly reported by the press, for instance in Kenya.

The objective of male sexual politics in Africa and the Middle East are the same as those of men all over the world: to assure female dependence and subservience by any and all means. First through economic control, by denying women education, modern tools, equal pay and jobs, making economic independence impossible and marriage or dependence on a man compulsory. Next through segregation, by excluding women from the public sphere and all decisions that affect their lives. Overburdening women with continuous childbearing so they are unable to take on public responsibilities accomplishes the same results. Finally through physical control - violence, rape, physical and sexual assaults, child marriage, bride burning, excision and infibulation. Some or all of these "measures" are pesent in all patriarchal societies.

The sexual politics in Africa and the Middle East are quite explicit. By mutilating girls especially if done at an early age, women are made into pliable posessions of men. Their psychological resistance is broken by the ordeal of the operation and their will power reigned in or destroyed. The mutilations deprive women of one of the mainsprings of life. Their sex drive is permanently associated with pain; sexual pleasure and satisfaction, a principal source of happiness and relaxation, are forever out of their reach.

Women are made into sexual tools for the satisfaction of men without any possibility of participation. They become sexual objects owned by men and must suffer intercourse which is forced on them. Instead of being pleasurable, it often is a painful ordeal they cannot avoid. But to have children - which is the only way to gain status - they must submit.

The sexual politics of African and Middle Eastern men have as an objective to keep women dependent on men. The purpose of a woman is to serve her husband and master, to provide him with food, comfort and sexual services and to bear and rear **his** children. If she does not please him, she can be instantly divorced. FGM assures the superiority of men. In turn, to assure that the practice continues, an astonishing proliferation of myths, irrational beliefs, stories and justifications of why FGM is necessary are circulated.

THE REASONS GIVEN

The stories to promote, defend and propagate FGM may sound to us quaint and sometimes absurd or ridiculous justifications for practices that are unacceptable from our view. According to our way of thinking no one would take seriously such advice, let alone follow it. But in rural areas, women, who are illiterate with no contact with the rest of the world or with any rational explanations, of how their bodies function, have no way to evaluate what they are often told over and over by men of influence in their communities.

In the absence of any education on reproduction and sexuality or about the biological facts of life, what in the West is referred to as "myths" is the reality for too many people in Africa and the Middle East. Sex education is not taught in the schools and missionaries who introduced school education initially certainly excluded this subject and to this day it continues to be omitted. But in societies that so greatly prize fertility, it is of primary importance. Instead dangerous fertility rituals, fetishes and witchcraft are practiced.

In the traditional environment, communities are convinced of the necessity of the operations; many women believe that FGM is practiced everywhere; hence there is no alternative. It is the tradition; it has always been done. To question customs in a traditional village society simply does not occur. Decisions are made by the chief and the elders, all of them men, for the **group** and never by an individual, least of all by a woman.

To anyone without any acquaintance with science or biology, the process described, for instance, explaining reproduction, may be more mysterious and strange than any of the stories told in Africa. What proof can we show that a cell divides the way it does unless we have a microscope? Or how can we demonstrate that there is such a thing as an egg or sperm? How do we explain that bacteria are responsible for infections and not the evil eye of a neighbor or an evil spirit that needs to be appeased?

The most persuasive reason why FGM is "necessary" is that without it women cannot have children and that it enhances fertility. The status of African and Middle Eastern women in large part depends on the number of children they produce - especially sons. Lack of fertility is cause for divorce or for taking another wife in case the first one cannot produce enough children fast enough to satisfy her husband.

For instance, in the rural areas of Kenya, it was universally believed by women until the 1920s that excision was necessary to have children; consequently every woman was eager to undergo the operation. In West Africa, the most often cited reason is that excision is required by the ancestors and no one will run the risk of offending the all-important ancestors. This belief is often translated as simply "it is the custom".

Everywhere in Africa, custom seems to be reinforced by fear. Over and over, the notion is expressed that "a terrible fate is in store for those who defy custom or the wishes of the ancestors." Thus, responsibility is evaded. Even if a girl dies from the operation, this is fate or is caused by an evil spirit or the evil eye or even the girl herself; no doubt she has done something wrong (such as having sexual relations before excision). Neither the operations nor the operators are ever blamed in case of death.

"Waywardness of girls" is the reason most frquently given all over Africa for FGM. Girls will run wild unless they are excised. There is no way to control a girl who is not operated on. This reason is given in East and West Africa and among very different ethnic groups, expressing the notion that a female is unable to control her sexuality. In the Sudan and other Moslem countries, a girl is told that she is incapable of resisting men; and thus, she is bound to dishonor her family. It is on her virginity that the honor of the family rests. Thus, the only remedy is to excise and infibulate her (see "Case History: Sudan").

The need to "control girls" is related in many different countries and societies. The Sierra Leone Muslim Men and Women's Association Kankaylay responded that no specific reason has been advanced for circumcision of either boys or girls in this country, but custom has it that a girl who fails to be initiated in the Secret Society - which means she is excised - will become a liability in society (see "Case History: Sierra Leone").

In turn, what is said in Nigeria, for instance in Cross River State, is very similar. It is believed that circumcision is the first step to control waywardness in girls and uncircumcised girls are considerd abnormal, since, according to the belief, they have both male and female organs. These girls "are regarded as unclean and are always subject to ridicule and abuse. The members of their families are also subjected to ridicule".

Time and again and in almost every society, waywardness in girls, promiscuity, lack of sexual control of females and the need to preserve the family are reiterated as reasons for excision and infibulation, both by animist sub-Saharan black African population groups, as well as by Moslems in Egypt, Somalia and the Sudan.

"Girls who are not excised cannot be controlled and are promiscuous" is the reason given for the operation also in Ethiopia where genital operations are practiced throughout the country. The Amhara, the dominant population group of Addis Ababa, who are Ethiopian Christians, excise their girls shortly after birth, "so the girls are gentle and easy to control".

Similar sayings are "girls who are not excised play rough", "a girl has to be operated to become a faithful wife". One school teacher stated his opinion in the letter column of a West African magazine: "Since polygamy is the custom of our society, excision is essential as a man could not satisfy all his wives. It would ruin his health."

In Mali, in turn, as Assitan Diallo points out (see "Case History: Mali"), it is widely believed that boys and girls are born with both male and female sexual attributes, the foreskin and the clitoris respectively. Both have to be eliminated to establish the sex of the adult without question. Excision is considered essential for a girl to become a woman and to enter adult society. This belief is cited throughout West Africa by many ethnic groups. A woman cannot be accepted as a serious and responsible adult unless she is operated.

In turn, all kinds of magic beliefs are tied to the operation, for instance by the Bambara in Mali. Since many girls die from excision, the danger of the operation is tied to an evil spirit called "Wanzo" who inhabits both girls and boys and must be removed before they can enter adult society. The Mossi in Burkina Faso believe that the clitoris is a dangerous organ that will kill the baby during birth, so the clitoris must be removed before having children. This belief circulates all over West Africa with different variations.

One of the variations is that the clitoris is dangerous for a man who should not have intercourse with a woman who has a clitoris as this will make him impotent. Another version is that the clitoris may kill him during intercourse. The story about the dangerous clitoris also surfaces in the East African literature with a different twist. It is claimed that women in Ethiopia suffer from "hypertrophy" (= an unusual enlargement) of the clitoris; therefore it has to be cut off. This was the reason given when the Catholic Church approved the mutilations among their converts - and it has been used ever since all over Africa (see: "History"). But a gynecologist working for many years all over Ethiopia never found such an enlargement among the thousands of women he examined.

If anything goes wrong during a group excision and a girl bleeds to death, this mishap is never blamed on the operator. The ritual was not correctly performed according to the rules or the girl must have done something very bad so she is being punished. It never occurs to anyone to question such a drastic punishment. On the other hand, the necessity for the operation is not questioned either; it simply is "the custom".

The French sexologist Gerald Zwang in a recent article sums up some of the reasons given by African and Middle Eastern men for promoting FGM:

> "In many Moslem countries, the clitoris is regarded as a vile attribute that allows women to enjoy themselves, with another man besides the one who owns her or also by herself without any man at all. This means disgrace for the husband and danger for society. Excision of the clitoris means health and tranquility. The tranquility husbands enjoy knowing they will never be cuckolded. It is a healthy outlook for women who feel at peace with their bodies and who therefore are ready to do all the work men expect them to do and which they are created to do. It is the clitoris that gives to the Western woman that freedom of action, of dress, of manner, which is scandalous in the view of the Islamic believers and the animists of Africa." [16]

Many of the Moslem sheiks and marabouts still teach that exicision is a requirement for the truly faithful Moslems (see "Case History: Senegal" and "Case History: Sudan") and of course the religious argument is a most persuasive reason to mutilate a daughter. This quite recently was shown in Paris, where an illiterate Moslem woman from Gambia had her two infant daughters mutilated because she claimed it is a religious requirement as well as an essential custom. Nevertheless the French judicial system is sending her to jail (see "The Western World"). "It is the custom" always is the ultimate explanation.

"Beauty" is another reason sometimes stated, for instance in Egypt or Sudan, why excision is necessary. The normal genitalia of a woman are ugly and disgusting and must be removed as well as all body hair to make a bride "clean" and ready for the husband. "Tahara", the word used for FGM in Sudan means cleansing and purification in Arabic and this is the reason given in southern Egypt and Moslem Sudan for the removal of all female external genitalia. A woman must be clean to pray. The "Sunna" operation is widely promoted by Islam as an "embellishment" though what is mostly practiced under this name is the removal of the clitoris.

It is interesting to note that the various Christian denominations active in Africa did not prohibit the mutilations except for the Scottish Missionary Society in Kenya (see "Case History: Kenya"). The Catholics quite openly tolerated it and still do today with official support from Rome (see "History"). And the Catholic Church has much influence especially in West Africa. In Cote d'Ivoire, the largest Catholic cathedral anywhere was built by the country's Catholic president. This cathedral was recently visited by the current Pope, who gave it his blessing. In the shadow of this church thousands of helpless little girls continue to be horribly tortured and mutilated with the full knowledge of the Catholic priests who have never lifted a finger to protect them from these terrible mutilations.

These are the politics of African and Middle Eastern men, often supported by men from other parts of the world. The stories cited above are but some of the many reasons given and promoted by men in order to continue to mutilate their own daughters to assure patriarchal rule. Women in these societies, deprived of education and with limited contacts outside their own communities, have no way to resist or stop what men demand. **No man will marry a woman who is not mutilated.** This is why these appalling tortures continue to the present time and why women are compelled to submit their own daughters.

No matter from what ethnic group, men know that FGM is the best way to establish male power and control over women. The myths, the rituals, the stories, the embellishments, and all the reasons given all serve to disguise the facts and make them easier to sell. The real reason is to preserve patriarchal power - no price seems to be too high, especially since most of it is paid by women

There are many highly educated powerful African and Middle Eastern men: None of them have ever spoken up, let alone started any actions to stop the continuing mutilations of many thousands of helpless children every year. The Secretary General of the United Nations - Boutros Boutros Ghali - is an Egyptian: of course he knows that in his country millions of girls and women are horribly mutilated and that these operations continue to be practiced all over Egypt - including infibulation. But he has done nothing and he has ignored the letters he was sent asking for his support to eradicate FGM.

"The Reasons Given" show how little control women have over their bodies and lives.

But the silence in the rest of the world is a testimony that the patriarchal system of female oppression is quite international. reaching all over the world: It is a shame that men and especially those working in international health have so far utterly failed to take this issue seriously by challenging the men who are directly responsible for the horrible crime of mutilating their own children.

The Economics of FGM.

Excision and infibulation are very profitable for the operators, including trained health personnel and physicians in the cities; the mutilations are also performed in many hospitals. In more and more countries, wealthy men pay surgeons for the operations performed on their daughters, frequently as infants so they dont remember later. But the physical and psychological damage is permanent. It is often a shock for an educated young woman to find out what was done to her as a child by her family.

The Sudanese physicians at the Khartoum Seminar advocated strongly that the language of the recommendations should be ambiguous to make it possible to perform the operations under hospital conditions, that is for a fee. They argued it would save lives. But in the end this was rejected (see: "WHO Seminar"). Economic gain reinforces the continuation of genital mutilation. In many countries, the price paid to the operators is considerable. There is no competition in rural areas as this is often an "inherited" trade.

It is frequently reported that a certain caste, such as the blacksmith caste in West Africa, or the Midgen caste in Somalia, are the operators. The practice is retained by certain families. Barbers perform the operations in some towns on the male and female children. For instance in Egypt or in Northern Nigeria among the Hausa, barbers traditionally function as surgeons.

In Kenya, circumcisors are particular people who are known in each community to be specialists in this practice. The job usually runs in the families, so the young women learn the trade from their grandmothers or mothers or where men do the operations, from their grandfathers or fathers. The circumcisors are considered to provide an important and respected service to the community. The money is paid in appreciation for the service rendered. During the circumcision period, circumcisors can perform the operation on 40 or more girls a day, earning more money than they could make any other way.

In West Africa , including Mali, each village has a resident circumcisor who also travel from village to village during the season of circumcision, which provides a good income for the practitioners. In the Sudan, the traditional midwives or birth attendants follow this profitable trade. Each village and community has such a practitioner and the operator is well paid. The money in each case is provided by men as women have no cash income. Therefore the claim that men have nothing to do with the mutilations is entirely untrue.

In Egypt, the dayas or traditional midwives similarly derive much of their income from these operations; there are also male circumcisors who sell their services from booths in the streets, including Cairo. Local clinics, physicians and trained health personnel are similarly involved In Egypt today: At least half the female children continue to be excised. In most African countries, both trained and traditional health workers perform the operations for a fee; sometimes they are done in the hospitals. (See: "Case History Mali")

In the Letter Column of the **DRUM**, a magazine distributed throughout Nigeria, a circumcisor, Alhaji Jimoh Ala-Bede, wrote about his trade:

> "Circumcision is the profession of my family. I have built two houses with the proceeds from circumcision and I have several children in different schools. I circumcise both males and females, and inscribe tribal marks on people who want them. I have dealt with almost all ethnic groups in Nigeria on the question of circumcision for female children. Our forefathers believed in it, and there must always be tradition. What damage does it do to the female organ? As far as I am concerned, it does no harm. Even the Quran supports circumcision for both males and females." (See "Case History: Nigeria"). [17.]

To stop the operations the excisors must be persuaded to stop their trade: their income has to be replaced with other equally lucrative and respected means of support. One of the programs of the Inter African Committee addresses this problem.

THE WORLD HEALTH ORGANIZATION // THE CASE OF UNICEF

The World Health Organization (WHO) and UNICEF are the two largest international institutions concerned with health and, in the case of UNICEF specifically, with children's health. But both the mandates and the activities of these organizations are very different.

WHO is an international organization of health ministries, and virtually all governmental health departments all over the world are members. They meet every year in early spring in Geneva at the WHO headquarters where health ministers set the agenda and make decisions for future activities. These activities are devided among its regional offices; in addition there are WHO offices in every member country. WHO also has research departments covering major professional health concerns and publishes large numbers of research and conference reports of seminars and professional conferences sponsored by WHO all over the world. The WHO Seminar in Khartoum on "Traditional Practices Affecting the Health of Women and Children" was such a technical regional seminar to which health ministries of all African and Middle Eastern countries were invited to send delegations (see: "The WHO Seminar").

Another essential responsibility of WHO is international health regulations. For instance, WHO develops the requirements for what kind of immunizations are mandatory to travel to specific countries or regions of the world; governmental health departments then enforce these regulations. WHO also is responsible for the international regulation and administration of health through health ministries as well as dealing with major international health threats, such as AIDS and other infectious diseases, or health problems that affect large areas of the world, such as malaria.

UNICEF by comparison is an organization that works on the local level, assisting and helping to organize local programs for children or mothers with small children, including immunizations and initiatives against childhood diseases, child feeding programs, all kinds of child care education, nutrition programs, and much more. UNICEF raises money mainly from the private sector by a variety of initiatives - for instance, by organizing fund-raising programs of all kinds such as their greeting card division.

There are UNICEF support groups in all Western countries - with many women volunteers who raise money for UNICEF. Therefore the agency must listen to the wishes of these organizations as well as work with private groups of all kinds in the child health field. Their public image is of great importance, as UNICEF depends on wide public support. But UNICEF also gets large annual contributions from governments - to which women as taxpayers contribute as well.

Both WHO and UNICEF have offices in every country with their own staff and headed by international administrators who usually rotate every few years to different countries and assignments. These administrators are in charge of the country programs and in the case of UNICEF work with local private groups as well as governmental departments and with the national health ministries in the case of WHO. That is, these country officers and their staff are of course well informed on the health needs, programs, and priorities of the country where they work and are in constant contact with the health problems, health needs and diseases of the population; many local people are directly employed by them. They are also required to follow policies decided by their respective headquarters

Given these general parameters, one must ask: How is it possible that these two large, influential and prestigious organizations that are recognized and supported all over the world have so utterly failed to address Female Genital Mutilation (FGM), which affects the lives and health of more than 110 million girls and women in a huge region of the world. By any definition, FGM must be be classified as a major regional public health problem, affecting many tens of millions of families.

How is it possible that both these powerful international agencies, charged with health around the world, refused for many years to acknowledge FGM or deal with the health problems resulting from these damaging mutilations. What is more, how could these agencies, supported by public funds and voluntary contributions in order to serve people around the world - especially children for UNICEF - intentionally conceal the mutilation of little girls, including the terrible health results, for such a long time?

By now, the secrecy is broken and the information about FGM cannot be hidden any longer because African women have taken up the issue and are organizing in most African and Middle Eastern countries where FGM is practiced to stop this violent interference in the normal reproductive health of women. Both agencies certainly are experienced in organizing all kinds of health information campaigns with positive results - the small pox eradication campaign by WHO and the child-immunization campaigns of UNICEF are excellent and successful examples. Why have these agencies failed to take some of the most urgent and necessary actions to help initiate information and education campaigns against FGM or support those that exist ?

Both UNICEF and WHO have organized national, regional and international campaigns on many other issues, including ongoing breast-feeding campaigns, the recent grass roots campaigns against de-hydration and child-malnutrition, aside from the ones listed above and many other local and regional problems. Over the years **WIN NEWS** has reported on dozens of important health campaigns by WHO and UNICEF, both global and regional, that have succeeded in mobilizimg extensive resources and involving many different groups. What then has prevented both these agencies to deal with FGM and inspire the kind of initiatives they have successfully conducted in many other areas.

The Khartoum Seminar Recommendations of 1979 (see: "World Health Organization") certainly provide useful guidelines, and the organization of the Inter African Committee (IAC) on Traditional Practices Affecting the Health of Women and Children in 1984 provides an institutional framework. But the kind of long-term, continuous support that is necessary to effectively sustain the far flung activities of the IAC and its affiliates has never materialized. Both WHO and UNICEF are highly qualified to provide this support in all the countries where FGM is practiced, as the leadership all over Africa by now has publicly rejected the mutilations.

Neither the national campaign in Somalia in 1985-88 nor the ongoing government supported current campaign in Burkina Fasso to eradicate FGM has had the kind of institutional support that agencies like WHO or UNICEF are able to provide.

And this lack of international support must be challenged because each year more and more girls are mutilated. Children are now subjected to FGM at an ever younger age - which has been the main change - so that more and more women will suffer for the next 60 or more years not only pain but also all kinds of debilitating health damage. This is not only a personal problem for the women and their families but has very costly results for the national health care budget of each country (see: "Health Facts and Overview").

Already in 1960 in a United Nations seminar "On the Participation of Women in Public Life", held in Addis Ababa, the African participants asked the World Health Organization to undertake a study of the medical aspects of "operations based on customs, to which many women were still being subjected all over Africa".

The participants expressed that "The World Health Organization could show that this mutilation has no medical justification and that rather it is harmful to health and should be abolished forever." [18] Even before that, the Commission on the Status of Women and the Economic and Social Council [19] had invited the World Health Organization to undertake a study "of the persistence of customs which subject girls to ritual operations and on the measures adopted or planned to put an end to these practices."

WHO at that time took the position that the operations in question were based on "social and cultural backgrounds", and therefore, were outside its competence.[20] That WHO physicians and officers were well-informed on the terrible health problems resulting from the operations is documented in their own published literture. For instance, WHO published in 1975 a technical report on the Epidemiology of Infertility [21] which details the terrible permanent health damage resulting from FGM as well as problems in childbirth and the harmful effects of FGM on fertility.

In 1976, WHO published a study by Dr. R. Cook on the "Damage to Physical Health from Pharaonic Circumcision: A Review of the Literature". In the Summary, Dr. Cook writes: "The sum total of suffering and disability consequent upon pharaonic circumcision is, therefore, considerable." [22]

WHO continued to claim for years that the organization could do nothing without specific requests by the governments of the countries involved. But WHO has taken an active part in many other preventive campaigns, such as smallpox eradication, measles shots, and other preventive innoculations. Governments are regularly persuaded to follow WHO's advice in implementing all kinds of health measures, including preventive ones.

At the present time, many of the African leaders who formerly supported or even propagated FGM - for instance, President Kenyatta in Kenya - are gone. Many political leaders have spoken against FGM. For instance President arap Moi of Kenya prohibited FGM in public speeches and directives at least twice since 1982: Why did neither WHO nor UNICEF offer to organize and/or support an education campaign against FGM that could have become a model for other countries in Africa. (See: "Case History: Kenya")

That WHO could initiate such a campaign given the great success of the 1979 WHO Seminar in Khartoum is evident from the objectives of its own constitution. These statements of special importance to women are included in this document:

> ". . .to provide information, counsel and assistance in the field of health. . .
>
> . . .to assist in developing an informed public opinion among all peoples on matters of health.
>
> . . .to promote maternal and child health and welfare. . ." [23]

WHO refused not only to deal with FGM but refused to acknowledge that FGM was a major regional public health problem until the 1979 WHO Seminar, which was scheduled only after my article on the Epidemiology of Female Genital Mutilation appeared in summer 1978 in the **Tropical Doctor,** [24] the most influential international journal on tropical medicine. The article documented that FGM was not an isolated practice, as had been claimed by both WHO and UNICEF, but that many millions of women and girls were mutilated in a broad region of Africa - from the Red Sea to the Atlantic coast. Interviews with gynecologists in hospitals in East and West Africa were included in the article, confirming that the operations were also being practiced in the cities and that far from dying out, the mutilations represented a major and growing public health problem.

The 1979 WHO Seminar for the first time provided African health professionals and health department delegates the opportunity to speak on this tabu issue at a professional meeting: the Recommendations to abolish the practice resulted from those discussions. The Seminar also legitimized discussion of the subject internationally, and the health delegations from Africa and the Middle East to the Seminar expressed interest in international collaboration.

After decades of delay, WHO led the way and also actively supported the organization of the IAC, though it took from 1979 to 1984 to accomplish this. Unfortunately, since then, the support by WHO has been very limited. The political reality is that the health ministries around the world that set the agenda of WHO have "other priorities" - a statement that is made over and over by institutions of all kinds about women's concerns. But it is a fact that WHO offices in Africa have not taken any visible action that could be noted here. Even though **WIN NEWS** has repeatedly offered free copies of our **Childbirth Picture Books (CBPB)** with the Additions to Prevent Excision and Infibulation to all African WHO representatives for distribution, there has been hardly any response. The response by UNICEF offices in Africa to the same offer has been much more productive - with the help of UNICEF offices thousands of books continue to be distributed.

THE CASE OF UNICEF.

It took UNICEF a very long time to even acknowledge the existence of FGM. When I contacted UNICEF first in 1973 after returning from Africa and went to their headquarters in New York to get some information on FGM, my inquiries were met with complete lack of interest. I was sent from office to office at their headquarters in New York and finally to the Director of Information. "We have no information about female circumcision" was the standard reply. "But UNICEF has representatives all over Africa. Don't they know what is being done to girl children in the countries they serve?", I asked the Information Director. "We know nothing about this; we have other priorities", was the sum of the evasive replies.

UNICEF maintained this posture of knowing nothing and doing nothing until nearly a year after the WHO Seminar in Khartoum in 1979. The information director at UNICEF headquarters in New York, Mr. Alistair Matherson, who in 1973 claimed to know nothing about genital mutilation of African girls, published an article on the subject in the **London Observer** [25] in September 1979 after his retirement from UNICEF, half a year after the WHO Seminar. He praised UNICEF's policy of doing nothing "out of respect on the part of the Agency for cultural traditions." It seems to be of no concern to UNICEF, who gets large contributions from women to take care of children's health, that thousands of little girls die or are tortured and permanently maimed due to traditions UNICEF upholds!

At first, I could not believe that a huge organization ostensibly devoted to the welfare and health of children in the developing world simply took the posture that the mutilation of millions of helpless girls is not their concern. I tried again and again to find someone in this extensive bureaucracy who cared enough to take an interest. As editor of **WIN NEWS**, I repeatedly wrote to Mr. Henry Labouisse, the executive director at UNICEF headquarters in New York at that time, and kept up communication after Mr. James Grant took over the leadership in 1980.

Why a man should be in charge of an agency serving children has never been explained. What is more, Mr. Grant had no discernible qualifications or experience regarding children's needs. He had run a private research firm in Washington publishing political policy papers on international development after working for US AID. His own business openly discriminated against women - not a single woman professional worked on his staff. At present, almost all of the UNICEF offices in Africa are headed by men. Yet, especially in Moslem countries, all activities concerned with children and childbirth are in the hands of women - some of them secluded - who are not allowed to have contact with men, least of all foreigners.

On my many visits to Africa, I made it a point to visit not only maternities but also UNICEF offices as well as WHO representatives. I found that some of these international civil servants had never visited a maternity or talked to midwives in the countries they served.

For instance, the first time I visited Somalia in 1979, I learned from the UNICEF representative there, a Mr. Kennedy from New Zealand, that he did not discover that infibulation was practiced on all girls and women until he had been in the country for one and a half years. He told me he made this discovery quite by accident. The antibiotics given to midwives in the midwifery boxes and kits, distributed by UNICEF in many developing countries, kept needing replenishment. But antibiotics are only needed when surgery is required and not for normal births. Kennedy finally asked why so many more antibiotics were required in Somalia than anywhere else. A midwife then told him that every woman was infibulated and had to be cut open to give birth. Mr. Kennedy shared with me his "discovery" - which was indeed quite amazing to a man from New Zealand who obviously knew nothing at all about the people he was supposed to serve.

However, it is not only his ignorance that is appalling but also that UNICEF sends people all over the world to administer multimillion dollar programs to assist children and mothers without giving them any information or training about the social and health conditions of the people whom they are supposed to serve, for which they are well paid

It is also totally counterproductive to have UNICEF represented almost everywhere by men who in many countries are not permitted to communicate with the women and who therefore are not able to learn what children really need. It appears that the agenda of this agency, instead of being based on children's needs, is set by men based on male political priorities. Very few women are in decision-making positions at UNICEF, much like throughout the UN system, which still has not implemented equal employment rules.

UNICEF in hindsight claimed to have participated in the WHO Seminar in Khartoum, where representatives from most UN bodies concerned with women's health sent delegates. But the Sudanese UNICEF representative never bothered to come. UNICEF headquarters in New York ignored the meeting as well as the Recommendations and none of its African representatives were informed on the Seminar until nine months later. UNICEF continued to "respect FGM as a cultural practice" - as the information director of UNICEF wrote in his internationaly distributed article (see above).

In October 1979, UNICEF headquarters changed its politics after I was invited to give a presentation to the New York staff, where I also showed a movie on female excision in western Sudan. Many male staff members in the audience were visibly upset. The next day UNICEF sent to **WIN NEWS** a statement on "UNICEF Position on Female Circumcision" that they published worldwide. The opening paragraph reads:

> "The health hazards and psychological risks, long-term as well as immediate, to young girls as a result of the practice of female circumcision in its varied forms, are a serious source of concern to the United Nations Children's Fund . . . "[26]

The statement reiterated the Recommendations made in Khartoum and then went on to outline four UNICEF activities, all limited to meetings and research in Egypt. UNICEF also claimed that "field offices are being briefed on the subject and recommendations of the WHO Seminar, and are being requested to convey the Fund's readiness to cooperate with the concerned governments in all possible ways."

At the United Nations Mid-Decade Conference for Women in July 1980 in Copenhagen, UNICEF, together with WHO, published a press release on a "Joint Action Program" by the two agencies, the result of an inter-agency consultation that took place at the end of March1980 in Alexandria Egypt at the regional WHO Office. The press release stated that the agencies were ready to support national efforts, collaborate in research, and participate in health training as well as respond to community-initiated activities. [27] But all these policy statements, consultations and press releases cost a lot of money, use lots of paper but have no positive results in Africa, as UNICEF field offices were and are almost exclusively run by men who don't want to hear about FGM, let alone talk about it..

At the UN Mid-Decade Women'sConference, UNICEF issued another special press release on "Female Excision: UNICEF's Position" (#IN/80/8 - 7 July 1980), where again the same statements were reiterated and the recommendations of the Khartoum Seminar were cited, though UNICEF never participated. This widely circulated press release also proposed strong advocacy efforts and was worded in such a way, citing specific cases, to create the impression that the agency was activating its far-flung network to finally get something positive done to prevent FGM, which even now is entirely untrue.

UNICEF sent a large delegation to the Mid-Decade Conference Forum to gain the support of women. The agency members participated in a number of meetings, including some on FGM organized by **WIN NEWS** to show the prototype of the **Childbirth Picture Book** for comments to potential users. Women from all over the world who attended these meetings and who were concerned with the issue believed the agency's sincerity.

But when I visited the UNICEF office in Cairo in October 1980, I met with Mr. Ulf H. Kreuger, its director.The purpose of my visit was to discuss the implementation of the Khartoum Seminar Recommendations, in which Egypt had participated, and to learn in in practice about the assistance offered by UNICEF at the Mid-Decade Conference (see above). Egypt has long-standing legislation to prohibit the operations; nevertheless, FGM is practiced all over Egypt including Cairo (see "Case History: Egypt").

Mr. Kreuger, when asked if any programs were being planned or supported to stop FGM, stated that he had received a proposal from the Coptic Church of Egypt to combat female circumcision, [28] but he had turned it down. "The issue is too controversial," he stated. This in spite of the fact that his office had participated in the joint WHO-UNICEF consultation in Alexandria less than a year earlier to specifically deal with FGM - which UNICEF had also cited at the 1980 Mid-Decade Conference. Evidently all the UNICEF press releases were designed to mislead women, as UNICEF depends on women to raise funds for their male-dominated bureaucracy.

The proposal, developed by the Department of Education of the Coptic Church, which is affiliated with the Middle Eastern Council of Churches, represents a coordinated effort to eradicate FGM over a period of years. It gives special attention to the creation of awareness about the operations on the part of the church leadership. The program is based on training sessions for all community and religious leaders and represents a comprehensive effort to reach all members of the Coptic Church and its many millions of followers in Egypt, including activities at community centers. Booklets, movies and other training materials, both audio and visual, were going to be prepared.

The Coptic Church program was not only a first but addressed the entire Coptic community. It could have been an important contribution by UNICEF and could have set an example. But UNICEF refused to provide assistance, and UNICEF has failed up to the present time to make the kind of contributions that a children's agency of such international standing and means should be morally obligated to do.

It was by pure chance that I discovered this program in the UNICEF files. There may be many more such requests for UNICEF assistance in UNICEF offices all over Africa and the Middle East that were turned down or ignored. It appears that the agency is unwilling to see that their publicly announced policies are implemented. The male representatives in Africa - there are almost no women - evidently refuse to work for the eradication of FGM regardless of what headquarters direct. As my experience in Somalia shows, UNICEF representatives do not even care enough to find out what the real problems of children and mothers are in the countries where they have offices.

This shows that the promises made by UNICEF at the 1980 Mid-Decade Conference for women were nothing but a political move by UNICEF to silence women who, in growing numbers, had written from all parts of the world demanding that the agency do its job and free girls from these terrible mutilations. After information from the WHO Seminar and with it information on FGM began to be published especially in European women's magazines, many women wrote to UNICEF to challenge this failure to act. Until then the media had been entirely silent. At international meetings, the subject was never mentioned. Whenever anyone dared to say anything, he or she was instantly accused of racism by African men. UNICEF, WHO and all other international agencies employ many African men - including many polygamists who make sure that the subject of women's rights or FGM is never discussed or taken seriously.

UNICEF is supported by direct fund-raising actvities in all Western countries. UNICEF greeting cards are well-known everywhere. This is a multimillion dollar industry. UNICEF's fund-raising National Committees in many countries - for instance, the U.S. Committee for UNICEF in New York - continuously organize fund-raising campaigns.

Women are urged to contribute and women work as volunteers to help raise money for UNICEF. We must make it known around the world that we require UNICEF to live up to the UN Charter, to serve women and children according to their needs and not according to political pressures by governments or according to their own sexual politics. Article 100 of the UN Charter states:

> "In the performance of their duties, the United Nations staff shall not seek or receive instructions from any government or from any other authority external to the Organization. They shall refrain from any action which might reflect on theirposition as international officials responsible only to the Organization . . . " [29]

UNICEF has betrayed this mandate even more than other UN agencies as it was set up to serve children who cannot speak for themselves. Despite this commitment for independence, UNICEF representatives continuously claim when challenged why they fail to support programs to stop FGM that now exist in many countries that they cannot act without governmental instructions. But UNICEF even fails to support government campaigns against FGM, for instance the ongoing campaign in Burkina Faso.

By claiming to work for children, UNICEF has built a male-dominated bureaucracy that serves itself and has forgotten its purpose while squandering enormous amounts of money on unnecessary luxuries, fleets of cars, lavish offices and services for their male administrators overseas. All this goes on in the poorest developing countries. Not only is this a gross abuse of its mandate and misuse of funds, but it sets a terrible example. There is no reason whatever why a children's agency should be run by men - it is high time that women take over UNICEF, send its director packing and clean up. There are many qualified women who can run and staff this agency and who can put UNICEF back on a track of service and humanitarian goals which were the original objectives.

The politics of UNICEF will not change until women protest around the world. UNICEF cannot function without public support. The case history of UNICEF's failure to support African girls and free them and their countries of these horrendous mutilations which is documented here is a shameful record of international male sexual politics.

Up to the present time, summer 1993, 14 years after the Khartoum Seminar, which opened the issue of FGM to international discussion and the eradication of FGM to international leadership, the male-dominated international leadership has remained silent. Indeed the issue of FGM continues to be quite deliberately ignored by international health activities and development, though it directly affects the lives and health of more than 110 million women and girls and their families. The conspiracy of silence continues, as well as the politics of claiming ignorance. But this has become increasingly difficult due to the thousands of African refugees, who, due to the growing number of civil wars in African countries and greater mobility, are spreading FGM all over the world: Health ministries in Europe and Canada have had to deal with the issue. (See "The Western World.")

WHO after their annual meeting this spring published another press release on "Female Genital Mutilation" calling "for the elimination of harmful traditional practices." But no actions are even proposed, though the usual clause is added that WHO is ready to support national efforts. WHO was evidently persuaded to break the long silence - ever since the 1979 Seminar in Khartoum - because several US senators, led by Senator Kennedy, recently sent WHO a letter inquiring what had been accomplished regarding prevention of FGM. This press release was not prompted by any concerns for women's health but by politics, that is senators have influence on US contributions to WHO. [30]

THE CONSPIRACY OF SILENCE

Why have African women in rural areas who are most affected by FGM not spoken more forcecefully to break the silence is often asked. Benoite Groult points out the reasons:

> "Each one is isolated in her cell, isolated in the family in the service of a man and master, in the love of her children. The term 'cell' describes it all. Even if we add up all the isolated women's lives, they don't make a movement that could demand justice. Women today remain the largest enslaved group because each one is separately exploited." [31]

In addition, woman is pitted against woman where polygamy is the rule, as in Africa and the Middle East. To keep silent and to keep women in "their place" by supporting tradition have been the gist of the politics of international agencies as well as charitable organizations, missionaries, church groups and even family planning programs who presumably are concerned with change. The UN agencies, quite aside from the patriarchal African governments, all follow the same line. As long as they observe the same rules, nothing will disturb the silence. The male-headed bureaucracies and international agencies share an interest in preserving the patriarchal system and power structure. Therefore, they discourage all investigations into and publications on FGM.

Women were never sent overseas by the US Agency for International Development (US AID) to work as development or health professionals until about 1980. On my first visit all over Africa in 1973, there were only men running all development programs including at all UN agencies except for a few secretaries. Development was an all-male enterprise much as the diplomatic staff at the embassies. Men held all decision-making positions and communicated with the male government officials - women were never heard or asked to speak and were entirely ignored. Even now most of the development experts and consultants who continuously tour the globe are men. They do not ask questions about women or talk to women as the male government officials might object.

Though at present some women are sent overseas by US AID and by European governments which support international programs, most decisions are made by men in every area, especially in the critical program plans. Besides that, the government ministries that administer the programs are entirely male dominated.

For instance in Kenya the "circumcision controversy" was widely discussed in colonial times and the debate reached London; this completely stopped with independence. The fight for independence was cleverly linked by Kenyatta to the institutionalization of FGM as an essential tradition. The silence in Kenya was not broken until after the death of President Kenyatta in 1978, when the Kenyan press once more found its voice to report on FGM. Though the prohibition of FGM by president Moi in 1982 was widely reported, there was no follow-up information or education and silence once more descended, until this year. (See: "Case History: Kenya.")

In Francophone West Africa, discussion of genital mutilation never existed. Few medical articles were published and hardly any research has been conducted, let alone any clinical studies such as those in the Sudan and East Africa. Silence on the subject is almost total. Even now, the terrible truth is quite safe from the wealthy French and European tourists who visit the resort hotels around Dakar for winter holidays. They would never guess that many of the attractive young women who perform African dances in the luxury hotels may be sexually mutilated according to medieval African rituals.

In Kenya also, the steady stream of tourists flocking to Nairobi, and from there to the game parks, would never believe the truth - which is entirely concealed. Any questions from tourists are answered - as mine were - with: "These practices no longer exist." Or, circumcision is explained as a colorful, traditional coming-of-age ritual with all kinds of celebrations, dances and feasts by African villagers. And until now, all Kenyan women's organizations have also been silent, on political grounds, as the dominant ethnic group, the Kikuyu following their revered leader Kenyatta, support FGM.

It is, however, astounding that no charitable organization or church group working in health in Africa - and many of them set up their own clinics and hospitals - never even published the most basic information about the damage done by FGM. Except for the Scottish Church Missionary Society in Kenya (see "Case History: Kenya"), there was literally nothing published when I began to send out questionnaires in the 1970s to internationally listed missionary and church groups and organizations working in Africa.

I had to piece together information from many different medical articles and miscellaneous health publications, from the questionnaires I sent all over Africa - in English and French - as well as from the ethnographic literature. No one had ever put the facts together about FGM or coordinated the scattered reports to at least make an estimate of the magnitude of the problem. Silence, myths, false rumors and tradition protected the spread of the mutilations. And silence today protects the practice in the cities where FGM is also done in clinics and hospitals without discussion. Why? Because FGM continues to be a marriage requirement made by men. Everyone knows it but no one says a word, and all mention of the facts, particularly the terrible damage and suffering of girls and women, is immediately squashed. This is much like wife abuse, which goes on everywhere in Africa and around the world, but until quite recently no one said a word.

Besides the politics of WHO and UNICEF, which are outlined above, the politics of other UN agencies should be examined. First of all, the Center of Social Development and Humanitarian Affairs: under its auspices, all UN activities for women are organized, including the Decade for Women and its conferences as well as the one planned for 1995.

Early in the campaign to make the facts about genital mutilations known, I contacted Secretary Helvi Sipila, who headed the International Women's Year Conference and was director of the Center of Social Development and Humanitarian Affairs until she retired in 1981. Since 1976, thousands of signatures of concerned women and men from all over the world were sent by **WIN NEWS** to UN Secretary Kurt Waldheim, to Secretary Sipila, and to the UN Human Rights Division, stating that genital operations are a violation of the human rights of all women. The human right to health must be protected as assured by the Human Rights Declaration of the UN. But this initiative was entirely ignored.

Recently the Country Reports on Human Rights Practices published by the US Department of State have become one official document that recognizes FGM as a human rights violation. (See Introduction.)

The official UN activities related to the Decade for Women all but denied the existence of FGM, which was never discussed at any of the three governmental Women's Conferences held in Mexico in 1975, in Copenhagen in 1980, and in Nairobi in 1985. WHO did provide an extensive report on the WHO Seminar at the 1980 Conference.

But at the Forum, the non-governmental week-long meeting that is held with every UN conference, the issue could not be suppressed. At the 1980 Copenhagen Forum, the first presentation on the subject was by Renee Saurel, who had recently published a series of articles on genital mutilation in France. [32] The meeting attracted a capacity audience; most of the women from all over the world who attended her presentation had never heard of genital mutilation and were totally shocked by what she said.

To provide factual information on FGM for those to whom this subject was quite unknown, I organized some workshops at the Forum summarizing the information that I had presented at the WHO Seminar a year earlier and the second edition of the **Hosken Report** which was published by then. I also organized some meetings to show and discuss the new **Childbirth Picture Book** (CBPB)/**Prototype** [33] with the additions to prevent excision and infibulation, with African women and health professionals from all over the world, to get their comments and ideas. The program and book are designed as a positive means to teach reproductive health from a woman's view and to prevent the mutilations. They have been published in English, French, Arabic and this year in Somali with the Additions. More than 50,000 copies have been distributed in Africa and the Middle East.

At the 1980 UN Conference Forum, African women were finally persuaded to organize a panel discussion on "Female Circumcision", chaired by Eddah Gachukia, the leader of the Kenyan delegation and a member of Parliament, with presentations by Awatif Osman from Sudan, Edna Adan Ismail from Somalia, and Mary B. Assaad from Egypt. (See "Case History: Kenya.") The meeting was announced in the Forum newspaper under a different title to disguise the subject, following the wishes of the Kenyan women. [34]

Eddah Gachukia, backed by Wangari Maathai, the president of the National Council of Women of Kenya (NCWK), claimed that no research existed on the extent of the practice in Kenya and due to lack of information they could not say anything. Offers to assist doing such research were immediately turned down by all Kenyans.

Edna Adan Ismail, who is by training a midwife and was for many years in charge of women's health training and midwifery in the Ministry of Health of Somalia, described the health problems encountered by girls and women in her country due to FGM and so did her counterpart from Sudan, Awatif Osman. The spread of sexual mutilations in Egypt was described by Mary Assaad, a sociologist, whose research shows that even in Cairo the operations are far more widespread than anybody was willing to admit.

The discussion, during which a number of African women in the audience spoke, centered on what to do. Very little of a tangible nature was proposed by the panelists or other speakers. The women in the audience from Denmark and Europe and other Western countries were eager to support any proposal made by the African/Middle Eastern women panelists who were unable to suggest any actions as they had no support in their own countries or communities where the subject was still tabu and no discussion allowed.

But this was the first time ever that the issue of FGM was discussed by African women at an international open meeting where everyone could participate. In many ways this was a breakthrough. Regrettably no action resulted, though the WHO Seminar recommendations were distributed and UNICEF passed out a press release that they were willing to assist, a promise that never materialized. (See below The Media and the Message.)

The Inter African Committee (IAC) organized 4 years later in 1984 has greatly contributed to opening up viable discussion and cannot be silenced or ignored as most other women's groups were in the past. Since their start, they have formed affiliates in more than 22 African countries and have held two regional conferences. They organized a series of meetings and discussions at the 1985 Nairobi UN Conference Forum and their president Berhane Ras-Work has spoken at many other international meetings: The message is loud and clear. But by comparison to long-established international organizations that are financed to the tune of millions of dollars annually with many years of experience and a large following, the IAC is still struggling for financing and backing. Therefore, it is important for all international organizations to join in the commitment for change and incorporate preventive action in all programs in Africa (see "Women and Health").

The silence maintained by almost all Christian denominations and missionaries has not changed with internationalization of the issue by the WHO Seminar. For instance a survey of genital operations was made for **WIN NEWS** at a Catholic missionary girls' school in the area east of Mount Kenya: All the girls, the daughters of converts going to the school, were excized, the survey showed. The director of the school to whom I sent a package of **CBPBs** for the school, claimed that there was no time in their busy curriculum to teach the girls about reproductive health, yet most of them will probably bear eight or more children. (See "Case History: Kenya.")

When I first began to systematically collect information on FGM I sent questionnaires to large numbers of charitable organizations and church groups working in health care in Africa and to their international headquarters. After I was asked to present a world review of FGM at the WHO Seminar I broadened this research. I contacted health ministries and well-known international organizations such as CARE, OXFAM, Save the Children, IPPF and others in the population field, also the World Council of Churches and many other church groups.

The responses to the questionnaires received from Africa showed that the mutilations were very wide-spread and that large numbers of female children were mutilated. Many of the international organizations replied that they knew nothing about FGM or that these were cultural practices and not their concern but up to African women. Even now very little has changed, though the Inter-African Committee and their affiliates have organized action groups in most African countries where FGM is practiced (see "Case History: Senegal" and " Women and Health").

An exchange of letters with the Christian Medical Commission of the World Council of Churches is typical of the attitude of many church sponsored health and hospital programs in Africa. When I asked for their help in gathering information on FGM, the reply from Marit Kromberg, M.D., the Director of the Commission, stated that she did not consider it wise to do such research and consequently, they would not help. Even today, this and most other Christian groups go by the prescription that ignorance is bliss. The commission, so Dr. Kromberg explained, serves as an "enabling organization and has developed a network of contacts. . . At no time has the subject of female circumcision come up in our discussions. . . The Commission is deeply involved in the development and promotion of health care in Africa and many other countries." [35]

It is difficult to understand how any organization can be involved in health care in Africa, where many women have more than eight children, without noticing the terrible problems in childbirth due to FGM. When I visited maternity hospitals in Africa, every midwife and physician I asked talked about the problems they encounter in deliveries including obstructed labor due to FGM. Surely it is an obligation of health professionals to prevent deliberately inflicted health damage. More than a year later Ms. Nita Barrow took over as the head of the Christian Medical Commission: She later headed the Forum at the UN Decade Conference in Nairobi. Though Barrow is a nurse by training and had great influence as leader of this Commission, one of the most powerful international charitable organizations, she was no more willing to talk about FGM, let alone extend any help to prevent the mutilation of African girls whose health and lives often depend on programs of organizations like the one Barrow headed.

The policy of seeing nothing, hearing nothing and doing nothing by church groups and their hospitals continued after the WHO Seminar opened the issue for international discussion and action: It goes on to this day. Unfortunately, it is a fact that the children of Christian converts of all denominations are excised and mutilated as frequently as followers of all other religions, with the full knowledge of the Christian leadership who guide their flocks.

But what is quite incredible is the continuing silence on FGM maintained by all the initiatives to promote "Safe Motherhood" with millions spent on high-level meetings, conferences and research conducted by physicians sitting in their plush offices at WHO in Genva or at US universities, without ever mentioning FGM. Obstructed labor was identified from the beginning as one of the six major causes of death in childbirth; and it is cited especially in Africa. But the fact that obstructed labor is frequently caused by FGM has not been mentioned at all though the highest per capita death rates in childbirth are recorded in sub-Saharan Africa in the regions where FGM is practiced.

The Safe Motherhood activities started in 1987 with a World Bank sponsored "Safe Motherhood" Conference, co-sponsored by WHO and UNFPA, which was held in Nairobi in the early part of February. [36] The objective was to draw attention to the unnecessary deaths in childbirth in developing countries that could be prevented by applying health measures that are well-known and readily available: 500,000 deaths in childbirth - so WHO reports - take place annually, almost all in the developing world.

This silence is maintained by all organizations and programs on "Safe Motherhood" active in Africa today. It must be greatly applauded that this terrible annual death toll of women in childbirth - most of them in developing countries - has finally attracted world attention and concern. But it is outrageous that the organizations and agencies dealing with the problem continue to suppress all information that FGM is one of the major causes of childbirth mortality in sub-Saharan Africa: the highest childbirth mortality is documented in sub-Saharan countries where FGM prevails. Also very damaging are the many dangerous traditional cultural practices that still surround childbirth and pregnancy in most of the developing world and especially in Africa. But these are not discussed.

A large number of delegates from health ministries from all over the world and especially from Africa attended this high-level World Bank sponsored "Safe Motherhood" conference - including international health experts - but not one word was said during the entire meeting about FGM. Since the meeting was held in Nairobi, all that delegates, many of them physicians, would have had to do was to visit a maternity hospital in Nairobi and they could have observed that a large number of women delivering there are mutilated and the problems that result. Instead the conference participants - most of them men - spent a week in Nairobi's luxury hotels on this midwinter safari without any mention that more than 110 million girls and women are mutilated in continental Africa with terribly damaging results for childbirth, causing thousands of unnecessary deaths every year.

This conference and the resulting "Safe Motherhood Initiative" were organized by Family Care International of New York, [37] which continues to hold high level regional conferences all over the world involving a great deal of expensive travelling as well as printing thousands of glossy publications; but most women dying in childbirth cannot read. By now the World Bank department on Women and Development, headed by Barbara Herz, which was assigned to deal with Safe Motherhood activities, has been reorganized and completely changed. But it is nowhere mentioned that the World Bank/IMF economic restructuring programs, imposed especially on African countries, have caused drastic cutbacks of the already underfunded health ministries: This is responsible for thousands of unnecessary deaths of women in childbirth for lack of basic services and medicines.

In all the voluminous papers produced under the heading of Safe Motherhood by the World Bank and by Family Care International, one looks in vain for any hint that FGM is one of the major causes of death in childbirth in Africa - complete silence is maintained up to the present time - summer 1993. But it is doubtful that the health department officials, mostly men, who go to these high-level "Safe Motherhood" conferences have taken any initiatives to save women's lives - maternity services in developing countries are the most neglected part of each health budget. What is more, in many countries, especially in Africa but also in much of Asia, for instance India, most women deliver at home.

A recent report by Family Care International states that though the overall death rate from childbirth has fallen by 5 percent in the past 5 years, the number of women giving birth has grown: Therefore the overall number of women dying in childbirth has continued to increase. One can but wonder if the methods used to organize conferences attended by officials and health experts can ever have the desired results: What is needed is a grass-roots approach to reach traditional birth attendants and midwives and childbearing women everywhere. Such a grass roots initiative has been successfully introduced with spreading the message on "Oral Rehydration" for children by WHO and UNICEF and many others. At the very least the high-level conferences - which are needed - must be backed up and conducted simultaneously with grass roots community mobilization and childbirth education for the whole family. (See: "Women and Health".)

The World Health Organization, which cosponsored the original conference publishes a newsletter, **Safe Motherhood**, [38] three times a year by their Division of Family Health. It is available free in English and French and includes lists of resources and contacts. But one looks in vain for any mention or discussion of FGM. US AID has also funded an activity called MotherCare, which is run by John Snow - a large for-profit contractor - who has organized many other multimillion dollar development programs for US AID. Large amounts of literature is published, also a newsletter, **MotherCare Matters**, [39]: But not one word on FGM is included and complete silence on the subject continues.

It is difficult to understand the motivations of health-care professionals who, as the above record shows, deliberately ignore major health problems that affect women, such as FGM, which damage the lives and health of millions of women and their families as well as the economies of many African countries: this quite aside from the terrible suffering and pain inflicted on innocent victims who are denied both the information and care they need by these professionals.

Why do these men - and international health is still an entirely male affair with very few exceptions - keep these problems silent? How is it possible for a responsible human being and health professional who knows the consequences of his silence to act in this way? These people have enormous resources available and have access to communication which enables them to introduce and support change. Instead, they keep the issue silent and hide from their responsibilities.

When I first began to learn about FGM and the unwillingness of the international health officials to speak the truth, I did my best to mobilize communication and to publish the facts. At that point - twenty years ago - most people in the Western world and especially women were quite unwilling to believe these facts. When I accused WHO of doing nothing, they reacted by cutting off all communication with me and directed all their personnel to send me no information and answer no inquries.

After some time, especially when my research was beginning to be published by well-known medical journals, they had to act: The WHO Seminar in 1979 in Khartoum was the result. But unfortunately WHO has done nothing since except publish press releases - they have not even done any more research, let alone initiate any education programs as they have done and are doing on other problems. And though the Inter African Committee was organized with their help, WHO has failed to provide the necessary in-country support in Africa that is so urgently needed by their affiliates.

What is the reason, at this stage, when the dimensions of the problem of FGM are known to anyone working in health in Africa, to keep up this conspiracy of silence which still is the rule among international health professionals? How can one keep silent about this terrible, preventable torture and suffering that the international health community has within its power to change? Are these international health officials afraid of African men, or what is the reason for this continuing silence and denial?

The interest of African men who have their daughters mutilated is quite clear - it is control over women, a higher bride-price and their approval by other men in their communities.

The interest of those who earn a living from doing the mutilations in traditional communities is also quite clear as well as the motivations of those in the health sector in Africa - both men and women - who do the operations in clinics and hospitals for money. Indeed there are some so misguided as to claim that it is better to do the operations the medical way.

It is also clear that most women in the traditional environment have no choice as all decisions are made by men. They will be unable to find husbands for their daughters, since men require the mutilations for marriage. What is more, the vast majority of women in rural areas is illiterate and therefore cut off from all modern information - including on health. UNESCO and others charged with teaching literacy have utterly failed to reach women. And health professionals have failed to teach about reproduction in ways that all people can understand: That is the most devastating result of the conspiracy of silence.

But how can the many population organizations and international family planning programs that work in Africa claim that they introduce contraception to save women's lives and then turn around and refuse to acknowledge that FGM exists and deny women and families the education about FGM they so urgently need?

And finally how can health professionals working in Africa for WHO or UNICEF or for the many private or religious organizations involved in mother and child health continue to try to conceal FGM? It is their failure to speak that stops effective preventive action. These people have nothing to gain from their silence. Why then keep it up, as the many examples cited above show? This is impossible for me to understand: as human beings we all share the same pain. How can such persons face themselves?

DISCRIMINATION IN DEVELOPMENT

First some background and an overview. Development as an organized, internationally funded activity by governments started after World World II after the founding of the United Nations, some 45 years ago. The UN agencies have been engaged in development activities ever since in the South, that is the developing countries, while the industrialized North has funded these activities, cooperating with different countries and governments. Development first of all is concerned with economic activities of all kinds including building the necessary infrastructure for transportation (harbors, roads, airports, etc), communication including electricity networks, telephone, TV, etc., as well as buildings and plants of all kinds - everything necessary to run a modern productive economy. Agricultural development makes it all possible. But development is also concerned with organizing modern health care, education and schools as well as training to use modern tools and much more. This is the first time in history that economically established countries have undertaken in a systematic way to assist new emerging nations, providing support for their economies with the stated objective of benefitting their people as well as gaining new trading partners.

The vast majority of development programs sponsored by UN agencies, the US and European governments, as well as Canada, Japan, Australia and other industrialized countries are planned and organized by **men** in cooperation with the government ministries of developing countries headed by **men** to organize programs that teach, train and assist **men** in developing countries to implement and finally take over the projects. Women always have been entirely ignored. The sponsoring countries use these programs to introduce their products with the expectation that at the end of the program they will continue to be bought. That is, most development programs have also commercial objectives which may create problems, as documented in the development literature.

In sub-Saharan Africa development activities started after independence - mostly during the 1960s and differed with each country. The former colonial powers in most cases also became the major sponsors of develpment programs undertaken by request from and in cooperation with the respective ministries or government bodies of each country. There is also a large number of private or nongovernmental organizations, charitable and church groups active in international development all over Africa. All development activities and programs must first be approved by each government; they can proceed only with government approval which can be revoked anytime.

How are women's lives in Africa and the Middle East affected by development, the collective term for policies of modernization pursued by their countries and their political leadership? Development, associated with visions of a better life, is measured most often in terms of economic growth. Specific economic goals are set by national development plans, usually made for three or five years, which include everything from road building to health training, improvement of the technical infrastructure and social services most of which did not exist in the past in traditional societies: All countries in Africa and most of the developing world have such development plans.

To carry out development plans successfully and to improve the standard of living or well-being of the people are, of course, the stated objectives of each government and the UN agencies designated to assist specific efforts with financing and technical advice. Besides the multilateral development programs of the UN and the European Community, there are many bilateral assistance programs of individual countries sponsoring cooperative development projects many of them carried out by private groups. All this takes place in a policital setting: In sub-Saharan Africa development activities have been repeatedly disrupted by civil wars, devastating large regions and destroying all productive activities.

International development activities started with high hopes and great idealism. By now, several decades later, much of the enthusiasm has given way to disillusionment, as few of the development goals have been achieved. Politicization of agencies and plans has skewed priorities, and the male-dominated bureaucracies are once more failing the poor. Everywhere most of the poor and the poorest of the poor are women. In the search for reasons for these failures, it seems strange that few development planners have discovered that women - or half of each nation - have been quite left out by most development plans everywhere in the developing world.

Among the positive actions in the US was an amendment to the Foreign Assistance Act passed in 1973, the Percy Amendment, named after the chairman of the senate committee, which requires that special attention must be given to women's needs in development programs assisted by the US - "thus improving their (women's) status and assisting the total development effort." - A second amendment passed in 1974 directed to the UN agencies, of which the US is a contributing member, broadened the "integration of women" to include all UN development activities. [40]

The United Nations Decade for Women - Equality Development Peace - 1975-1985, sponsored three world conferences and specific development plans: its continuing objective is the support women's development around the world, drawing attention to the needs of women which are entirely neglected in all international development programs. This internationally supported global initiative represents the first internationally organized government effort on behalf of women. The objective was and is to mobilize women in developing countries, providing them with the opportunity to speak for themselves with international support, as well as to mobilize women in the industrialized countries to join these efforts and raise support and resources for women in developing countries. Another UN World Conference for Women is planned for 1995 to be held in Beijing. [41]

But in each recent evaluation - required by the UN Decade for Women Plan - of the progress of women in developing countries, it was found that the situation of women had not only not improved but had measurably deteriorated in comparison with men. For the first time systematic research efforts carried on by women documented and published many of the dismal facts and economic statistics regarding women especially in education, training, health, nutrition, maternal mortality and the many damaging traditional practices to which women were subjected on gender grounds. These include bride burning in India, widespread food tabus in Asia and Africa and genital mutilation in sub-Saharan Africa, quite aside from seclusion and polygamy in large regions of Asia and Africa. Fortunately such practices as footbinding in China have stopped.

It would seem, given these traditions, that development and what it promised - to improve social and economic living conditions - would first of all be addressed to women, who clearly were in urgent need for change. Instead, the research documents just the opposite: Women were almost entirely excluded from development programs.

In turn, countries that sponsored development programs and especially the UN agencies all but excluded women from decision making and professional positions in that new and promising field. As a result women in developing countries had no one to speak for them.

Barbara Rogers, who did fieldwork and research in Africa and all over the developing world, shows in her book, **The Domestication of Women,** how male development planners transfer their own prejudices and preconceived notions about women's place to the programs they design. Rogers writes:

> ". . . A combination of law and policy [is] directing the flow of cash to and from each household through its 'head'. . . 'land reform' involves land being allocated to heads of households as outright owners; all other claims, especially women's, are suppressed . . . Measures to 'protect,' segregate and/or domesticate women often [are] built on, or reinforce, local gender segregation and the division of labor. . .
>
> Excluded from education by missionary prejudice, women and girls [are] excluded from paid employment by entrepreneurs. . . The ideology of their domestic destiny is strongly advocated, through the teaching of Western-type domestic skills and moral teachings about their place being in the home. . ." [42]

The discriminatory effect of "development" on women is by now recorded in numerous studies made by women: The research documents the disenfranchisement of women in developing countries by denying them the tools and training they need. But even now the male development experts - for instance the many hundreds of economists who work for the World Bank - take no interest in such research. It is astonishing that the male-dominated development bureaucracy does not acknowledge the role of women. Where women are traditionally the farmers, as in much of Africa, the traditional food supply is often jeopardized as a result. The domestication of women - that is the subjection of women under male control - is the gist of "development."

Though women are now organizing all over the developing world, it is very difficult to make up for 40 years of systematic disenfranchisement and exclusion. The failure of development strategies, especially in the huge rural areas of Africa, is by now entirely obvious to anyone who wishes to really see.

UN debates have for years been dominated with acrimony between "South" and "North" - the developing and industrialized countries, respectively. The frustration over the visible lack of success of "development" has been expressed in the demands for a "New International Economic Order" (NIEO), in the belief that this will address the imbalance between the rich North and the poor South and promote social and economic justice. But the imbalance between women and men is far greater and has an enormous impact on the well-being of each country and its majority - women and children - which was never recognized at all by the NIEO, which was formulated by men.

Most development plans stop at the household level, treating the family as an economic unit without ever examining who does what within each family. In much of Africa, women are the productive members of the family. Men, for example, in Kenya, form the bulk of the unemployed in the urban areas; Nairobi and other African cities are swollen with idle, jobless, alienated men. They spend on drink what little they occasionally earn. Women of these families, left behind in the villages, are overburdened with household work, subsistence farming and child rearing of the ever larger families fathered by men who spend their time away from home claiming to look for work which does not exist and who fail to assist their families. Yet, it is the male head of the family who is singled out for all development assistance and in whose name all land is now registered, land that he does not work. Martha F. Loutfi from ILO (International Labor Organization) explains:

> "Since it is individuals who work, . . . analysis and policies cannot stop at the household level. This is made more imperative by recent evidence that the income and status of females, relative to male household members, have often been adversely affected by changes thought of as beneficial for development . . . "[43]

It finally had to be recognized that male household heads do not share their income and development benefits with women and children. But if women are the beneficiaries of development programs, the well-being and nutritional status of the children improves.

Experience shows that the trickle-down theory does not work, not on the international level, not on the national level, and least of all on the community and household level, especially where male privilege and male domination are traditional or where the needs of women and children are traditionally put last, as in most of Africa and the Middle East.

In turn, the failure of international assistance to reach those for whom it is intended has been documented, for instance, in the case of refugees especially in Africa. Most of the refugees are women and children who are abandoned by the men of their own families. The supplies intended for the refugee camps are often diverted by men and can be found on the local markets. The most recent example is Somalia, where the women and children were left to starve by their gun-toting men and boys - their own fathers, husbands and brothers - who prevented all food assistance from reaching them.

To the customary restraints on women in Africa and the Middle East, which include such traditions as genital mutilation, the bride-price, polygamy and child marriage, the discriminatory practices of what is termed "development" are added. Yet the only way that women can escape from the damaging practices and traditions, which have kept women in their place as the property of men, is through change, that is, "development."

And this is the dilemma. While "development" quite blatantly discriminates against women as documented throughout the development literature written by women, it is the only hope for change. International development programs can be influenced where they originate - at the international level - by women whose governments are involved in planning, financing and, most of all, technical assistance. Technicians and advisers in the past have been almost exclusively male: this is slowly beginning to alter now. **WIN NEWS** is devoted to the proposition to change all that, by providing information, tools, access to resources and networking. Legislation such as the Percy Amendments to the Foreign Assistance Act in the US (see above) need enforcement: Stronger legislation is needed now and in many more countries that sponsor development programs.

International development is based on economic partnership between nations, between the sponsoring and developing countries and societies: a partnership among all nations for mutual economic success, productiveness and the improvement of living conditions of all members of each society. Economic development starts at home, in each society, community and family.

Economic development cannot be accomplished by policies that eliminate women from economic participation and productiveness - to make them "dependents" of men in order to enhance male power. Economic development must be based on partnership within each family - the basic social building block - and then within the family of nations. It is within the family that a child learns and is socialized: Inequality, with all its destructive consequences, is first learned at home and in each family.

Violence between nations and between ethnic groups within countries and states and the exploitation of whole populations are the result of power relationships based on inequality - which are quite similar to those between families as well as between individual women and men in each family. Inequality destroys the dignity of nations as well as the dignity of individuals as members of a family.

Power corrupts the family of nations, much as it corrupts the relationships in each family. Until and unless we recognize these facts and work for change in the relationships between women and men, development will continue to remain an unfulfilled promise. Yet it is within the grasp of each of us to affect that change.

Sub-Saharan Africa is still the least urbanized region of the world today. In most African countries, especially those with which we are primarily concerned here, where girls are subjected to genital mutilation, the vast majority of the population lives a rural life. Egypt is the exception, where more than a third of the population lives in urban areas. From Somalia and the East African coast to Senegal's Atlantic Coast and the Gulf of Guinea, 80 to 90 percent of the people lead a rural way of life. The vast majority is dependent on subsistence farming and traditional activities. Nigeria is the exception in West Africa: It is the most densely populated country with many urban settlements, and due to its large oil revenues, it is also the wealthiest and most rapidly changing and urbanizing area.

African capitals show the highest urban growth rates in the world: Many cities are increasing their population through immigration from rural areas - added to the natural growth - by more than 10 percent a year. This means a doubling of their inhabitants in less than 10 years.

Many African towns were founded by Arab traders or by colonists or had been small settlements in the past. They are not equipped to handle this influx of people; they have neither reliable water supplies nor sewer systems, electricity or other services. Most of the immigrants are unskilled, without any means of support and are strangers to an urban way of life.

Urbanization has been called the engine for development and change. It means a new way of life, contact with the rest of the world, with many different people and new ideas. Despite the squalor of the shantytowns of immigrants and what outsiders regard as terrible living conditions, most urban immigrants prefer these to going back and living in the rural areas they came from.

What does this migration to cities do to the lives of women? Urban life means a complete change from traditional rural living conditions and attitudes. It means a break with tradition, with the past, with village life, where everyone knows everyone else's business. In the village, the individual is subordinate to the hierarchical group. The head of the patriarchal family makes all the important decisions, and the wishes of an individual, especially if female, are not considered at all.

In the city, the opposite is true. The initiative of the individual is all-important; each person must speak for herself / himself and compete. And each individual is responsible for her/ his own decisions. The restraints of the feudal village life are gone; there is no one who tells you what you must do. You have to make your own decisions according to your choices. Even if they are limited, these choices offer many more options than village life. But the support of the group in the village also is gone - you are alone and on your own.

Most African cities today have a large surplus of men; men have been leaving the villages in large numbers to seek paid work and an easier life in the towns, but cities offer few jobs. Many men leave their wives and children behind in the villages to fend for themselves and only come home once or twice a year to rest and to father another child. Some men have a wife in the village and another one in town, though they cannot support either one by their meager earnings; employment is uncertain at best.

In the cities, men have access to new ideas, education, modern technology and tools, and they have contact with the rest of the world - all of which can be summed up as "change." But the rural areas remain in the past, where things are done according to tradition rather than by rational examination. In the village, the orders of the chief and the male head of the family are carried out without question, and the ancestors' wishes are strictly observed. The gap beween men and women is growing. It is the gap between present and past, and often it is the gap beween an urban and a rural way of life.

Recently, however, women are beginning to follow men into towns in many areas. Young women especially, who want to escape the crushing burdens of village life, are beginning to flock into the cities looking for a better life, attracted by the bright lights and a promise of change. Most of them lack the basic education and skills to get a job.

Literacy is of crucial importance for finding work in the modern sector. All kinds of new skills are needed that girls and women coming from the villages simply do not have. What is more, men have arrived in the African towns long before the women; they already hold jobs and have acquired new skills. Men do not want women's competition, and they do not want women taking "their" jobs. Therefore, though there are no traditions that can be cited as reasons for excluding women from occupations that did not exist in the past, African men everywhere are declaring "as unsuitable for women" a long list of the best paid, modern jobs, often referring to Western-inspired prejudices, many from a generation or more ago.

The men who run development programs often reinforce the African men in their efforts to exlude women from education and training for new occupations and jobs, claiming that women have no time to attend the training and meetings because they have to look after their children and their homes.

The struggle to preserve male privilege and male authority can be witnessed in towns all over Africa. For this purpose, the media are also enlisted including TV, first of all admonishing women to uphold all African traditions which make women submit to male authority. In addition, every Victorian and colonial prejudice against women continues to be trotted out by the male-dominated African press to convince women of their inferiority and to keep them in line - that is, subservient to and dependent on men.

It was astonishing to hear President arap Moi of Kenya invoke tradition when he was confronted by the Green Belt Movement, led by a woman, Professor Wangari Maathai. He tried to build a huge high-rise building in Uhuru Park, the largest open green space of Nairobi. When faced with his opposition, he stated it was against African tradition for a woman to speak up publicly: "A woman has no right to criticize" he claimed. That very public controversy took place quite recently - in November 1989. [44]

Throughout Africa men still ridicule "Western women's lib" and claim it has no place in Africa, though they obviously do not know what they are talking about. However, their constant assertion that women's rights are irrelevant in Africa shows their fear, and this fear is also the motivating force in the continuing male support of FGM: To preserve the morality of women is the reason most often given by men, most of whom are polygamists.

Prostitution is very widely practiced in all African towns, in all Moslem areas and also where excision and infibulation are the rule, including in the Sudan. The reason why women turn to prostitution is because this is the only way they can support themselves.

It is ironic that the men who prevent their daughters from getting an education in order to keep them under male control in fact support prostitution. Many young women who now run away from their villages, the hard labor and limitations of rural life and go to town have no way to support themselves except by prostitution. This also immeasurably contributes to the rapid spread of AIDS throughout sub-Saharan Africa.

Kenneth Little, in **African Women in Towns,**[45] discusses prostitution with examples mostly from West Africa, though , of course, it goes on in all African and Middle Eastern towns everywhere. What he reports from the 1970s is still true today. Women who live alone, that is, not with their families, are automatically regarded as prostitutes almost everywhere in Africa and the Middle East, especially in Moslem societies.

Little shows that prostitution was traditionally tolerated by many ethnic groups, contrary to the claims made that it was introduced with colonization. For instance, it is the custom, as also described by Kenyatta, [46] for a chief or other influential man to offer his guests the choice of any of his wives for the night, as a gesture of hospitality. In urban areas, women who are divorced take up prostitution as a source of income, as they have no other way to earn a living. Many women practice this trade with the consent and support of their families as it pays well. If children are born as a result, they are sent back to the village where they are welcomed as additions to the labor force.

In most African towns, prostitutes work in the marketplaces or bars, but in Moslem communities, they are secluded and work out of their homes. Since there is a shortage of young women in towns as men leave their wives in the rural areas and polygamy is widespread (mainly older men marrying young women for the second, third or fourth wives), young men turn to prostitutes. Far from preventing prostitution, polygamy encourages it and so does the institution of the bride-price.The question of how to define prostitution must be raised here. Is not a girl made into a prostitute by her father who trades her in return for a bride-price? In fact, the fathers sell their daughters' sexual services and fertility to the highest bidders, without asking the daughters who are forced to accept the men to whom they are sold.

Venereal disease including AIDS is rampant in African towns as WHO statistics document. It is spread by men to the rural areas when they go home to visit their families.

Perhaps the most important difference between rural and urban life is that in towns and cities, women see something new and they are also able to get together and organize. In the rural areas, families often live too dispersed for the women to meet. Family groups often change location, moving to new land. Large numbers of people follow their herds and live a nomadic way of life, for instance in the Sudan, Somalia and in many countries of West Africa. Women under such conditions have little opportunity to form supportive relationships with other women, to talk about themselves or to compare their conditions. They have even less opportunity to learn.

Polygamy pits woman against woman, and segregation often prevents women from different families to meet. In the Middle East and Egypt, it is the custom to marry between cousins, which further limits outside contacts. In rural areas, women are burdened by a constant round of daily chores, with little time to think about their future, or their lives - let alone change or what is called development.

To become conscious of one's situation first of all requires a basis for comparison and an alternative or some choice. But women who have never lived away from their families lack both. To ask such women what they want - as development advisers suggest - makes no sense, as women do not know what is available. But urban life offers quite new opportunities for women that simply do not exist in traditional rural life, including education, change and development. Urban life means not only social and economic change, but it offers women the chance to achieve some independence, to learn something different and new and to see another way of life. Most of all it provides women the opportunity to become conscious of their own condition. Urbanization and modernization are closely linked, offering essential ingredients for development and change.

Urbanization is dramatically changing African traditions which support, unchallenged, male authority and control over every part of women's lives. The injustice of the condition of women's lives and the exploitation by men become glaringly obvious in the setting of a modern urban environment. More and more women perform the same jobs as men, often better. Everywhere the traditional claim of male superiority is exposed as nothing but a hoax. Male privilege is shown up to be based on self-serving oppression by men which is quite incompatible with the development goals proclaimed by all African governments and politicians.

Urbanization is the yeast that is essential for raising the consciousness of African women to organize and work for change and most of all to develop their own talents and abilities. Urbanization has only just started to affect women who are moving into the cities and are learning that there are choices; they are beginning to realize the power that they really hold. This is only the beginning of a social revolution that is long overdue: It will change for the better every part of African life.

Women always have been the productive force of Africa: To ignore their talents and abilities instead of providing women with the opportunities to develop themselves and modernize their activities has resulted in economic disaster for much of Africa, as the record shows. The present economic crisis must be put at the doorstep of the male development advisors and UN bureaucracy but most of all of African men.

Many development programs are funded by various kinds of loans: as a result of the very enthusiastic development activities in the early 1980s and before many poor countries, now that the loans have come due, are unable to pay the money back. Many of the projects have failed to pay a return and the governments find themselves unable to pay back the loans. This, in a greatly simplified way, is what is happening now as not only interest but capital repayments become due. This is also why the World Bank/IMF is able to impose economic restructuring on so many countries especially in Africa in return for new loans that many African governments can't do without.

Women in developing countries have been left out of development programs, but they are most affected by the economic austerity, as like women everywhere else, they are the first to lose their jobs. Since they take care of their children, they are directly affected by price increases and lack of consumer goods. In Africa, where most women still live in rural areas, they have been entirely ignored by development, but the steep price increases of basic consumer goods due to the economic problems of the government greatly affect their and their children's lives.

These economic problems and their terrible impact on women in developing countries were discussed in a series of teaching kits and publications sponsored by NGOs (Non Governmental Organizations) for Women and Development at the United Nations in Geneva. [47] These materials explain the development problems from women's views. As DAWN (Development Alternatives with Women for a New Era), a women's group from developing countries, led by Peggy Antrobus, summarizes the problem:

> "The almost uniform conclusion of the Decade's research is that with a few exceptions, women's relative access to economic resources, incomes and employment has worsened, their burden of work has increased, and their relative and even absolute health, nutritional and educational status has declined." [48]

Development programs that in each country are designed and implemented in cooperation with the government introduce men to new technologies and tools and teach men new skills and ideas. Women, it is claimed by male development experts supported by anthropologists, should stay within their "traditions" no matter how laborious the work or how damaging the traditions, for instance FGM.

Men are taught to use tractors and ride them through the fields. Women one can see in the fields all over Africa working bent over with hoes and traditional tools. This backbreaking agricultural labor could be made much easier if women were taught to use modern tools. But that is called "interference" and immediately discouraged by men, claiming it disrupts family tradition. And the development advisors - almost all men - side with the African men. Women are still excluded from owning any of the land they till though most of the men in Africa have left the rural areas presumably to get work in towns and cities. Women are the majority of the subsistence farmers on land owned by men: They are excluded by tradition from ownership, and they are not paid for their work. There is a term that defines such a relationship: It is called slavery.

Women and children are left behind in rural areas to do all the subsistence farming alone, ignored by the international development planners and the agricultural agents of their own countries who are only interested in export crops. The women are not only physically left behind, illiterate and isolated in the rural areas, but they are left out of modernization and education with no access to information or new ideas while overburdened with work.

Ester Boserup, an agricultural expert who was the first to look at what was happening with women in developing countries, summarized the situation:

> "Economic and social development unavoidably entails the disintegration of the division of labour among the two sexes traditionally established in the village. With modernization of agriculture and with migration to the towns, a new sex pattern of productive work must emerge, for better or worse. The obvious danger is, however, that in the course of this transition, women will be deprived of their productive functions, and the whole process of growth will thereby be retarded. . ." [49]

Boserup's book documented what she encountered all over the world - how women's exclusion from modern economic development and discrimination against women are literally built into all development projects. She predicted that this exclusion will result in more and more economic failures of not only projects but the failure of countries and regions to improve the standard of living of their people. And she was proved right. It should be obvious that if you exclude half the productive population - that is women - from modernization and do not educate them or provide them with training and new tools, economic development will suffer and so will the entire population of each country and region. But this was not accepted for instance by the World Bank or UNDP, the largest funding agencies of development, who must be finally held responsible because they are the leaders in economic development quite aside from US AID, which has one of the largest development budgets of any country.

Boserup's analysis and warnings were ignored by the planners - all of them men. Today more than 20 years later and billions of dollars wasted, there is more poverty, and successful development programs especially in Africa are hard to find. More women are illiterate than ever while the literacy gap between women and men is constantly growing, so UNESCO statistics confirm. And illiteracy is highest in sub-Saharan Africa: But UNESCO, the UN agency charged with education, seemingly is ignoring the education of women. One result of failing to educate women is population growth, which in Africa despite billions spent, is still out of control. One reason obviously is the exclusion of women from development and education.

In 1991, in recognition of Boserup's ground-breaking work which is still ignored by the international development institutions, another book **Persistent Inequalities: Women and World Development** [50] edited by Irene Tinker, was published. In this book Tinker candidly evaluates the situation today paying tribute to the original analysis by Boserup, who also contributed a chapter. Tinker also expounds on the faith most of us shared - naively - she states. We believed, that once the problems Boserup explained were fully exposed such as the biases against women's education, the lack of economic support and training of women would be corrected, because it is in the interest of economic development.

I remember that at the 1975 UN International Women's Year Conference in Mexico, women were told by the many development experts and program representatives, for instance from US AID, that what they needed was research as very little information on women in developing countries was available. To include women effectively in economic development programs, it was necessary to learn more about women's activities. The need for information was accepted by women everywhere. But as Tinker shows and the title of her book pinpoints, though hundreds of books and research reports of all kinds, including conference reports and long lists of recommendations have been published since then by women from all over the world, inequalities continue and discrimination against women is pervasive in all development programs. Though more women are employed for instance by US AID, few of the critical decisions are made by women.

There are so many books and research studies published today that it is hard to keep track of them. But the research and publications by women have not changed development programs nor how they are implemented. Despite the Decade for Women declared by the UN, all UN agencies discriminate in hiring. With only 3.4 percent women in decision-making positions according to the UN statistical office, it is clear why women are neither heard nor seen in development programs, as all decision makers are men. This scandalous situation replete with sexual harassment continues as is regularly reported in **WIN NEWS** in the sections on Women and the UN/ and Development. [51]

There are still hardly any women overseas for instance in the offices of UNICEF, UNDP and WHO: I repeatedly visit or contact their offices in Africa, and almost all decision-making positions are occupied by men.

Development as a profession is still a prime stronghold of patriarchy with terrible results for women in developing countries. And this patriarchal domination of development results in great damage to women as well as the failure of development programs. For instance many of the multimillion dollar health programs in Africa by US AID in the 1980s have failed. Some had to be closed down by request of the respective governments and others simply had no positive results. But the situation at the World Bank is the worst one for women as the World Bank/IMF structural adjustment policies especially in Africa have greatly damaged millions of women economically.

The Commonwealth Report, **Engendering Adjustment for the 1990s,** [52] documents that these damaging policies are the result of the failure of World Bank planners to examine the impact of their plans on women: The report documents that the bank's planners could have avoided the economic damage they continue to cause women without impairing the projected results. But for the World Bank what happens to women is irrelevant.

While the World Bank now has agreed to make environmental impact examinations of their program plans, they continue to disregard the impact of their programs on women. Environmentalists have demonstrated in Washington in front of the bank headquarters repeatedly to demand changes in policies until the president of the bank agreed. There were full-page ads in **The New York Times** about the horrendous devastation of the environment by programs designed and financed by the bank, for instance in Brazil.

But no one has ever demonstrated for justice for women, either in front of the bank or at the UN in New York, though the bank and the UN - especially UNDP - have over the years inflicted devastating damage on women by excluding them from development and re-inforcing patriarchal exploitation. Development programs also have done terrible damage to women's and girl's lives and health by failing to prevent FGM for instance in all health and family planning programs, as the section on population control documents and as **WIN NEWS** has continuously reported since 1975.

Ignorance about women, despite the extensive research and publications now available, as well as disparagement and contempt for women pervades the entire development community. Instead of telling African men that women cannot be treated as chattel and property in any internationally sponsored programs, culture and tradition are invoked regularly to exclude women and discriminate, even if this risks the success of the program: because the male development planners are afraid to risk offending the men. So development programs modernize and fortify traditional exploitation of women and continue to tolerate such practices as FGM and many other traditions that damage women and girls as I have pointed out in my Congressional testimonies (see below). But even where women in African countries are speaking up - for instance in Burkina Faso or in Nigeria and other countries where IAC (Inter African Committee) affiliates are working to prevent FGM - US AID family planning and health programs have ignored them and provided no support despite promises made.

Now that women in the US, Canada and in all European and other Western countries are major participants in the labor force and are increasingly economically independent of men, the developing world, especially Africa and parts of South Asia are the major strongholds of male domination and patriarchy. That is not about to be changed as long as men are in control of development. Women must finally recognize that development is designed and planned to reinforce male control and to keep women subservient because in this way the men who finance development keep themselves in control.

Keeping women backward, uneducated and dependent makes sure that the developing countries will not get ahead: because it is impossible for a country to achieve economic success as long as the majority of the population is illiterate and unable to function in the modern world. What is more, women transmit their knowledge to children: How can women teach the younger generation something they do not know? Therefore, each generation starts with an enormous handicap which will continue as long as women are excluded from education, training and development.

Who profits from this situation? Those in control in every country - men. And in turn the men in the industrialized world can exercise control over developing countries through their international institutions, for instance the World Bank/IMF, UNDP and other international bodies. Women are the unpaid labor force that makes it all possible. In Africa women do the essential subsistence farming which keeps the entire population fed, for which they are not paid at all; they are only a small fraction of the paid labor force.

Nowhere in the world are women paid for housework, including hundreds of family related jobs without which the entire economy of every country would stop. Now that women are a major force in the labor market, they are demanding ever louder to have their household related work monetized: This will finally force men not only to pay women equal wages but to take on their share of housework.

And it also is becoming increasingly clear that what goes on in Africa and other developing regions is slavery of women. In Kenya more and more women who are educated are refusing to marry. In the US the recent census found that more and more successful women have children without husbands because why should a self-supporting woman go home to serve a man? The statistics on violence by husbands or partners certainly makes this a sound decision.

What I describe and analyze here provides the political background why the male dominated Western development community has never objected to the wholesale mutilations of female children in Africa and the Middle East even after they cannot claim any longer that they "did not know"! What is, however, astonishing is the uniformity with which the development agencies and organizations reacted when I began first to contact them regarding FGM. Unfortunately today very little has changed.

From the start of my investigation into female genital mutilation, I contacted US AID. The agency has sponsored for years programs all over Africa, some of them in health. I asked the physicians of the AID Health Unit about mother and child health (MCH) programs in Africa and what was being done to prevent genital mutilation. At a meeting in 1976 at the AID offices in Washington, DC, it turned out that the physicians present, even those who had worked in Africa, did not know what I was talking about, and I had to explain the basic facts about genital mutilation to them. I don't think they believed me, and the matter was ignored.

I also contacted the international development assistance programs of Britain, Sweden, Germany, Denmark, Canada, Australia, Austria, France, the Netherlands, the EEC, Norway and more. What responses I got were more or less the same and can be summarized by: "We know nothing. This is a cultural matter and not our concern. We only respond to requests made by governments."

Women in development programs which began about the time of the International Women's Year in 1975 initially consisted mainly of all kinds of small handicraft projects which later became "income-generating projects". These projects were promoted by women NGO groups especially and were funded for instance by US AID to be able to claim that they were doing something for women's development. One useful program was the development of a worldwide Directory of Women's Organizations: the first one ever put together. I was asked to take on this project because I had traveled all over the world as an international journalist and planner and had many contacts in developing countries as well as knowledge of several languages.

This directory was supposed to be US AID's contribution to the International Women's Year and was to be sent free to all developing countries. But first it sat for two years at AID - after my work was completed and delivered - due to internal squabbles and politics. It was 1977 when it was finally printed. In the meantime some addresses had changed. Despite my urgent advice to computerize it and/or print it in such a way that it could be updated regularly - since it is an invaluable resource for women - this was refused. Later, with the permisison of US AID, I tried to get the directory updated and published in the private market and sent a proposal to all well-known directory publishers. They all refused: there was no money to be made with it, they all claimed. Recently, however, a major global women's directories has been published, to which I contributed. [53]

In the early 1970s, women's development was a new idea: Women in developing countries had been largely ignored, but due to the widely publicized UN International Women's Year, most countries that sponsored and funded development programs started "Women in Development" departments. I wrote to most of them asking about their programs for women's development and health, to write about in **WIN NEWS**. After the 1979 WHO Seminar I also inquired about FGM, sending literature and offering them copies of **the Childbirth Picture Books** with the Additions to prevent excision/infibulation. I got some replies including this typical response from the Administrator of the Women's Development Program of Canada: "We only react to requests. We assist governments with technical help and financing for programs they ask for. We do not initiate and we can do nothing about genital mutilation unless we are asked to help." It was the same policy everywhere.

However, it is an amazing fact that family planning, which was not only unheard of but actively resisted by a majority of developing countries in all parts of the world, in a few years - or since the UN Population Conference in 1974 in Bucharest - has become "accepted", indeed a priority for most developing countries in all parts of the world. Practically all foreign assistance agencies of Western governments sponsor population programs now. While family planning was rejected throughout the developing world up to the 1974 conference, there are now family planning programs everywhere.

Though I sent information to all international development agencies about genital mutilation including the WHO Seminar recommendations, only the research offices of Sweden and Britain even acknowledged this, despite the fact that the literature documents the mounting health costs as a result of mutilating a large part of the female population. But no interest was shown and no action was taken anywhere.

The European Community also has financed programs in many African countries under the Lome Conventions, a broadly-based trade and aid agreement between European and African as well as Caribbean countries. I wrote to the Commissioner for Development of the EEC who at that time was Claude Cheysson, who later became Foreign Minister of France, and asked him to make the facts on FGM known through their publications and sent along information on FGM. The editor of the **Courir**, the official development magazine of the EEC, which continues to publish, invited me to submit an article on the health facts regarding FGM. After the article was sent, which was a factual report on the health situation of women and an overview of the spread of the operations in Africa and the Middle East, there was a long silence. After many inquiries to follow up, the **Courir** refused to publish the article claiming that the subject was "too sensitive" though by then my article on the Epidemiology of FGM was published in London in **The Tropical Doctor,** a journal that is distributed and read all over the world.

Aside from individual governments sponsoring development, the EEC and UN gencies especially UNDP, there are very large numbers of non-governmental organizations working in Africa and sponsoring all kinds of programs, quite aside from numerous church and missionary groups. The latter were the first ones to set up schools and organized education programs for children in Africa that never existed in the traditional African or Middle Eastern communities, starting with teaching literacy.

Church groups also concentrated on setting up health services and hospitals wherever they went to spread their religions in Africa. Though schools were nationalized after independence in all African countries, the influence of the missionaries continued, including their teaching. Reproductive health and the biological facts of childbearing as well as sexuality continue to be largely excluded. The very information needed most by all young people in Africa and especially girls and women, whose lives and health are on the line due to the demand by all African men for more and more children, is not taught anywhere even now.

Neither schools nor the missionary health services teach girls and women the facts about their own bodies and health despite the widespread damaging traditional practices that the hospitals need to deal with, such as terrible injuries and hemorrhage due to FGM and many problems including obstructed labor in childbirth. But silence on these matters continues even today in most education and development programs.

It was, however, revealing that when President arap Moi publicly prohibited FGM in Kenya in 1982 the chief medical officer of the government released an order addressed to all hospitals and health facilities - those of the government and all others run by missionary and church groups - that henceforth all excision operations were prohibited. This confirms what had been rumored that missionary hospitals were performing the mutilations (see "Case History: Kenya"). It is a fact that not only in Kenya - where it is now prohibited - but everywhere in African cities FGM is now done in hospitals.

Congressional Testimonies

From the start of the investigation into FGM, I contacted the Washington headquarters of US AID to get information on their programs all over Africa, many of them in health. During the 1980s several multimillion dollar health programs were developed and implemented - for instance in Sudan, Somalia and Mali, which I visited in each of these countries. I testified in Congress several times including before the Appropriations Committee-Subcommittee on Foreign Operations, since Congress votes the funds for all large development programs, quite aside from funding the agency according to their budget. My objective was to draw attention to the neglect by AID of the needs of women in most countries and especially in Africa where AID had major programs in health.

I regularly contacted AID over many years to check on their health and family planning programs in Africa and to send them information about FGM to circulate to their program development teams. This had some positive results for instance in Somalia (see "Case History: Somalia") as the US health team finally began to ask questions of their counterparts in the health ministry about FGM. It came out that the Somalians had already started to work on developing programs to prevent infibulation, but neither side had been willing to discuss it. The Somalians of course assumed that FGM was not known in the US, so they did not talk about it and it was excluded from the AID health survey.

But women and women's health continued to be ignored. AID also entirely ignored the Recommendations of the Khartoum WHO Seminar, though I gave a special presentation to the Africa department of AID when I returned from Khartoum and my extensive visit to East and West Africa in 1979 and flooded them with literature. In my testimonies before the Subcommittee on Foreign Operations of the Appropriations Committee, which control AID program funding, I cited specifically that FGM was entirely ignored in three multi-million dollar health programs in Sudan, Somalia and Mali, though almost all women are drastically mutilated in those countries. *

Infibulation is the rule throughout Somalia and Moslem Sudan and also widely practiced in Mali. I asked that women's health needs must be considered in all health programs by AID and that prevention of FGM, which affects almost the entire female population in the three countries, must be made a priority. For instance, in my testimony in 1980 before Senator Inouye, who chaired this powerful Committee for many years I stated:

> "My research shows that genital mutilations are increasingly performed in the modern sector in Africa, including in hospitals, often on newborn babies, as sexual castration of females, stripped of all traditional rites. This is a gross abuse of modern medicine and we must advise this Committee that increasingly health equipment and training contributed to the countries where these operations are practiced, are used to mutilate female children. Speaking for American women and taxpayers, I strenuously object to the use of U.S. moneys and contributions to carry out clitoridectomies and infibulations on non-consenting children in Africa and the Middle East, with U.S. contributed equipment and tools." [54]

Senator Inouye was visibly shaken by those revelations and questioned me. I told him that AID was not actively involved in the "modernization" of the mutilations but their failure to take preventive measures allowed this to happen. The Senator then requested AID to review the situation and to give him a report, and he added that whether by commission or by ommission, AID must be held responsible.

---

* $ 8 million - Sudan: Primary Health Program
$14 million - Somalia: Rural Health Delivery Program
$ 4 million - Mali: Rural Health Project

In the reply to the senator, the AID health administrator whitewashed their lack of attention to women's health needs and failed to answer the questions I had raised in my testimony. As Senator Inouye so aptly stated, whether by commission or by ommission, the results are the same: The failure to take preventive measures results in the modernization of the operations and their introduction into the modern health sector.

The failure not only by US AID but by charitable and church groups to introduce preventive actions and to teach against FGM while teaching about health and family planning is the reason why FGM is now increasingly practiced in the modern sector by western-trained health care professionals. The ommission of preventive actions by development programs is also the reason why FGM is being spread by immigrants all over Europe - indeed worldwide (see "The Western World").

I testified on many other occasions and before different committees on women's development and health urging greater support for women's development and asking that prevention of FGM should be included in all family planning and population programs in Africa and especially Egypt. I was confronted mostly by all male committees who are well briefed that culture must be respected, especially when it comes to Africa, or they may be accused of racism.

In June 1993 just after a new AID administrator took over, I again submitted testimony to the Foreign Operations Subcommittee of the Appropriations Committee, Senator Patrick Leahy of Vermont, Chair. [55] My testimony was concerned with the widespread discrimination against women in all UN agencies, including rampant sexual harassment, and also at the UN Secretariat. The UN still has no effective equal employment policies, as there is no independent judicial authority to adjudicate complaints. UNDP recently developed what they call equal employment policies. [56] But without an independent body to decide on complaints, the policy is not worth the paper it is printed on.

While all governments that fund the UN have implemented equal employment laws in their own countries, no such requirements have ever been made of the vast UN bureaucracies and its agencies. Women will never be included as equal partners in development and health programs until women hold decision-making power equal to that of men in the institutions and agencies that formulate and implement the programs. In the summary of my testimony I stated:

> "We urge this Committee to attach binding requirements for Equal Employment of Women and protection from sexual harassment - including an independent board to adjudicate disputes and complaints - to all funds contributed/donated to United Nations bodies and international institutions, including and especially the World Bank/IMF, the UN Secretariat, WHO, UNICEF, FAO, etc. They should be required to develop affirmative action plans, much like institutions have to in the US." [57]

Most of my testimony dealt with the persistence of FGM and the failure of US AID and its contractors and international agencies to which the US contributes including UNICEF, WHO, UNFPA, IPPF and others, to address the problem and to incorporate preventive education in all health and population programs in countries affected by FGM and especially in their large family planning programs all over Africa.

> "We urge that US AID and their contractors be required to integrate FGM prevention in all their Family Planning and Health Plans and Programs in affected countries in Africa and the Middle East, and that every possible support shall be provided to local groups in Africa and the Middle East working for the eradication of FGM. We also request that all private organizations working for US AID do likewise and be required to provide surveys of their actions and document results of their teaching."
>
> "Similarly, all funding of family planning organizations, and especially UNFPA (United Nations Population Fund) and IPPF(International Planned Parenthood Federation) should be made subject to a requirement to include teaching the prevention of FGM in all family planning programs in all affected countries. IPPF, UNFPA and other family planning organizations to which the US contributes money must be held accountable and show proof of results of their teaching. We also strongly suggest that all immigrants to the US from FGM affected countries should be informed that these mutilations are unacceptable and a criminal offense." [58]

THE POLITICS OF POPULATION CONTROL

Great efforts are being made, supported by vast sums of money, to make population control effective in Africa, the only continent where population growth rates are still increasing. That is, the annual percentage of growth is increasing almost everywhere in sub-Saharan Africa. Even in the poorest countries and in the areas where infant mortality is the highest in the world - in Francophone West Africa - the population growth rate is steadily inching up. Kenya until quite recently held the record for population growth, with more than 4.5 percent annual growth rate, or about eight children for every woman in the country. Population growth is pushed by the pronatalist and macho attitudes shared by most African men seeking self-aggrandizement in the form of children. The demand by African men for ever more children is expressed in their national and personal politics.

While Islam requires men to support their children at least theoretically, there are no such requirements in African traditional societies. In the rural areas each woman has to grow the food for her family. Each wife must feed all her children from the food she grows - and the husband as well when it is her turn to sleep with him. Each wife is assigned a piece of land by the family head and husband - as Kenyatta explained in his book **Facing Mt. Kenya,** where he described African traditions (see: "Case History : Kenya").

Therefore, polygamy is among other things a very profitable enterprise for men as women and children are each man's wholly owned agricultural labor force. The more women and children, the more land can be tilled and the greater his wealth: the proceeds of what is sold in the market grown by his wives belongs to each man. Therefore, the more wives and children a man posesses, the greater his wealth and power.

Urbanization and modernization, which go hand in hand, quite reverse this situation. Children in a modern urban economy are very expensive. But it takes time for this to be understood and even longer to be translated into action: that is, to limit the number of children. African politicians, expressing the feelings of their fellow men, at first called the introduction of population control an imperialist genocidal plot by the North.

The pill was cited by Kenyan parliamentarians as a danger to women's health, asking that it should be outlawed. But the fact that large numbers of women die from the strains of continuous childbearing has never disturbed any African man! Death rates due to childbearing are, predictably, the highest in the world in Africa's pronatalist countries where genital mutilation is practiced.

Though by now more African politicians have recognized that birth control is necessary if their economies are to develop, it is still a very controversial issue and not accepted in rural areas. But it is amazing that even now most international population programs are designed to address women though it is known that all family decisions, especially where children are concerned, are made by men. When I asked the midwives in the city hospitals in West Africa where family planning had been finally officially introduced, they said that they are authorized to give out free contraceptives to women after childbirth. But they also told me of husbands who divorce a wife when they discover that she uses contraceptives.

International family planning organizations and programs belatedly recognized that especially in Africa it was necessary to work with men if any positive results are to be achieved. It is difficult, however, to find men willing to listen. Especially in rural areas it is hard to provide convincing arguments why polygamists should reduce the number of children they make since they are not held responsible for child support and their status in the community and among men depends on the size of their families.

To be sure family planning has been introduced only quite recently in some African countries. For instance in West Africa the countries formerly under French colonial rule adopted all French legislation upon independence which included prohibitions to distribute contraceptives. While this was changed long ago in France, this legislation in West Africa was only revoked recently. It is doubtful, however, that contraceptives reach many rural areas or are used by women in rural areas most of whom are illiterate.

It is unfortunate that what family planning seemingly is unable to achieve in Africa because of the unwillingness of men to use contraceptives AIDS will accomplish.

Sub-Saharan Africa has already the highest AIDS infection rate in the world. The latest figures by WHO are eight million; no doubt in reality the number is much higher. [59] The infections are spreading rapidly due to sexual practices by men and so are all other sexually transmitted diseases (STD). For years WHO has warned about a gonorrhea epidemic in Africa. But population programs pretend this is not their concern. Yet the cause of the spread of AIDS, other STD, the failure of family planning and the increase of FGM is the same: the sexual behavior of men.

The history of population control as an international movement and activity is very short. It officially began only after the UN World Population Conference in 1974 in Bucharest, where a world plan was made by all governments except by the Vatican, which still opposes all effective birth control. Almost all governments of developing countries agreed that the systematic control of population growth was essential to achieve economic development and that too rapid population growth would result in more poverty and deprivation and eventually political unrest.

The discussions at that population conference where the non-governmental organizations held a series of separate meetings with speakers from all over the world, covered a wide range of topics from demographics to health. Everything was discussed except women: The viewpoint of the female half of the world was entirely ignored; women were excluded from all governmental and non-governmental discussions.

It was an amazing performance: Here was a world meeting discussing the control of reproduction without ever mentioning women, who were treated throughout as objects to be controlled by men. A small group of women activists at the conference whom I joined, only through intensive lobbying, finally achieved the inclusion of a short amendment on women in the World Action Plan. [60]

The UN Fund for Population Activities (UNFPA) [61] was created following the population conference in 1974. It is involved in planning and funding all kinds of population programs from demographic record keeping to fertility surveys as well as working with governments on a variety of family planning education programs. UNFPA, much like other UN agencies, has representatives all over the world who are engaged in field activities and work with pertinent government departments and help with setting up programs. UNFPA is the only UN agency headed by a woman, and she has been working in the administration of the agency from its beginning.

UNFPA publishes annual reports that survey their activities as well as a newsletter and all kinds of statistics, information and literature. It should be added here that UNFPA has given at least some support for prevention of FGM, working with IAC (Inter African Committee) affiliates in West Africa. They are the only organization in the international population field that has provided any tangible help.

Besides UNFPA, most governments that fund development programs also support population programs throughout the developing world, assisting governments to introduce these often very new and nontraditional activities. US AID (Agency for International Development) has developed and supported the most extensive population programs for many years and the US Congress has provided more money for population activities, about $150 to $200 million annually, than for any other AID programs. The US also contributes funds regularly to UNFPA and IPPF (International Planned Parenthood Federation), [62] a private family planning organization, as well as funding many other population activities and programs.

However it is astonishing that women were not only ignored at the initial population conference in 1974, which was conducted by men as if women did not exist; but ever since women as persons with the right to make their own decisions and women's health have been ignored. Population planners, most of them men, have dominated this new and often highly paid field; they treat women's bodies as objects to control in order to achieve their plans. While family planning is essential for women all over the world to control their fertility and preserve their health, the objective of the population planners is to achieve measurable demographic goals.

Besides IPPF there are large numbers of private US based organizations in the international population field, many of them also get government grants.

Family planning has been introduced and promoted in Africa and the Middle East in the countries where FGM is practiced without paying any attention to women's health - pretending FGM does not exist. Even now family planning programs in FGM- affected countries entirely ignore the ongoing mutilations even in their program areas. It is hard to understand how this is possible especially when introducing IUDs. A few years ago a US AID sponsored population program planned to set up clinics in Khartoum to distribute contraceptives, especially IUDs. The physicians - all men - who designed the program "overlooked" that almost all women in Khartoum are infibulated!

But it is outrageous that the men who design and plan population programs in Africa refuse to deal with FGM as a health issue and have never included any preventive teaching to stop FGM in family planning education nor in the training of health and family planning workers.

For instance, a survey on excision which was made in some of Cairo's family planning clinics found that most of the women coming to the clinics for services were mutilated and they had or were planning to have their young daughters operated. When the family planning clinic staff was surveyed it turned out that the women, trained to provide family planning services and education, were planning to have their daughters mutilated, besides being excised themselves. It appears that the training programs for the clinic staff never taught that FGM is a dangerous practice that inflicts permanent damage, or the facts about reproductive health. Every hospital in Cairo gets many cases of severely bleeding little girls, the victims of excision (see: "Case History Egypt").

The Cairo Family Planning Association, [63] a private organization that predates the governmental program, started teaching prevention of FGM under the leadership of Aziza Hussein, its director, in the early 1980s, several years before the IAC (Inter African Committee) was organized. By now the Cairo Family Planning Assocation, which sponsors a special coordinator of all FGM-prevention activities, has more experience than any other group. They have organized numerous conferences with press coverage as well as public information campaigns, broadcasts and special training programs for medical and nursing schools, hospitals and much more. The many different activities they developed can serve as education for other groups who can learn from their experience - as regularly reported in **WIN NEWS.**

Unfortunately the Cairo Family Planning Association is still the exception in Africa. In the international arena Population Action International (PAI - formerly Population Crisis Committee) [64] is the only private organization that for many years has had a "Special Projects Fund" that has assisted different African groups and programs concerned with the eradication of FGM. PAI has shown what can be done by thoughtful well-organized support and is presently involved in a major program in Kenya. But it is obvious that one single organization, no matter how committed or successful, cannot alone deal with these dangerous practices all over sub-Saharan Africa. (See: "Women and Health")

Women's groups in the developing world are by now loudly criticizing the damaging disregard for women's health by population program planners (see below). But for population planners to deliberately ignore genital mutilation going on in their own program areas makes them accessories to the fact. It would be an easy matter to integrate prevention of FGM into all family planning education programs in Africa. Both women and men should be taught about reproductive health by all family planning programs: The dangerous damage done to women by FGM should be shown also to men, including the problems the operations cause in childbirth, as the **Childbirth Picture Book** does.

US AID is not alone in failing to include preventive education in their multimillion dollar population programs in Africa. IPPF, which gets contributions of many millions every year from the US quite aside from many other sources, has affiliates all over Africa in countries where FGM is the rule. But they have not even tried to develop any effective ways to include preventive education in their programs or assist their African affiliates to do so. IPPF at first ignored the WHO Seminar but finally included a short report in their worldwide publication, **People.** The WHO recommendation were shortened so they could be read to mean that the operations should be done by trained personnel. When I demanded a correction, it took a year to print it. I still suspect that this distortion was quite intentional, since many African physicians who work with IPPF also do these mutilations.

IPPF has all along resisted publishing the truth about FGM. They have shown their lack of concern for women's health by failing to advocate prevention of FGM, and they have said nothing for years on the subject, though **WIN NEWS** has kept them informed. To date, there is no policy to prevent FGM. Though IPPF has educational materials of all kinds, there is nothing available to discourage the many damaging traditional practices related to childbirth and pregnancy especially in Africa and for the prevention of FGM.

When IPPF belatedly printed a small flyer on FGM only two years ago, they reiterated what had been published long ago stating the health facts. But there was no positive proposal included to encourage eradication let alone any help or tangible support for education in prevention of FGM. IPPF used to lead in developing family planning education and in introducing contraceptives. But now they suddenly have lost their voice - why? So much for the leadership of IPPF. Yet the easiest way to raise consciousness about FGM is when introducing family planning.

Patriarchal attitudes toward women are not unique to IPPF. Unfortunately IPPF dominates the entire population movement even now. Yet it must be clear even to the IPPF management, quite aside from all others in the population control field, that their best allies are women. Even in Africa, despite the enormous pronatalist pressure exercized by men, women do not want a child every year.

In response to my request for information, IPPF sent a statement by their International Medical Advisory Panel dated November 1991 on FGM [65] (more than 11 years after the WHO Seminar which opened the issue for international action). This statement reiterates the health damage done by FGM and then suggests that Family Planning Associations (FPA) "should inform themselves on the prevalence and characteristics of FGM in their own countries." Finally the statement suggests that the FPAs "should join efforts with other governmental and nongovernmental organizations already working on this issue". And finally the advisory suggests "discussions on the subject and actions for eradication should be introduced into broader programmes aimed at improving the reproductive health of women. . ."

One can but wonder, where is the leadership of IPPF? Instead of being in the forefront as they were when introducing family planning, the advisory talks about joining existing efforts. But there is no indication that any action was taken or that this statement was even forwarded to any affiliates - there are no incentives offered to act or to prepare a program nor any suggestions on how to obtain financial support. It is just another piece of paper with words. It is quite ironic to suggest inclusion of information on FGM in health education by family planning programs in view of the "Women's Declaration on Population Policies" made in preparation for the 1994 World Conference on Population. (See below) Women from all over the world are protesting the lack of concern for women's health by population programs and demanding fundamental changes in population policies - giving women an equal voice. Where are the "broader programmes for reproductive health" into which the advisory panel suggests FGM prevention should be included? They evidently do not exist, according to women who prepared the "Declaration" (see below).

But there are many other international organizations concerned with population control besides IPPF, though IPPF is the largest long established group that in the past was a leader. Now it has become another unresponsive international patriarchal bureaucracy.

Pathfinder Fund [66] which saw themselves as pioneers as their name indicates, was entirely privately financed for many years and independent of government dictated policies. But as many others in this field, they began to accept US AID funding and as a result became more conservative. They work all over the world including in Africa with a regional office in Kenya. Over the years **WIN NEWS** has kept them informed on FGM and I have repeatedly met with their management to persuade them to initiate some preventive actions in their programs in Africa: They have done nothing at all and even refused the **Childbirth Picture Books** I offered. One of their African representatives some years ago sent me a report on excision and infibulation in East Africa from his field experience - so they have been well-informed all along. But evidently no one cares that the families they serve with contraceptives mutilate their own children.

There are many other organizations that have lucrative contracts from US AID to organize and run population and health education programs all over the world including in Africa; some of them maintain overseas offices, especially in Nairobi as it is a very pleasant place to live - all of it paid by US taxpayers. But to date all the money spent on population programs has achieved few positive results in Africa. And the programs have done little for women because of their damaging patriarchal approach, supporting culture and traditions: As long as the traditional social, sexual and economic subordination of women in Africa continues, population control will not succeed.

None of this has been recognized by the men who develop the population programs - since their own male egos are involved. They are not about to relinquish control. For instance Dr. R. T. Ravenholt, who for years was the chief of the Population Program at US AID, developed the first population policies for the agency which set the direction for the future. He was determined to implement strict population control all over the developing world by any and all means. He characterized FGM as "nothing but a traditional way of regulating population growth" and proposed to me that I should write an article expounding this idea in the **Population Report**, a US AID funded journal that is distributed worldwide. [67] When I refused, he demanded my research and said he was going to have someone else write it. I refused again.

US AID has maintained health and population officers in their missions worldwide, including in Africa, which I have often visited and where I sent many hundreds of **Childbirth Picture Books** for distribution especially to midwifery schools. But though the AID officers often are in each country for years and know by now about FGM, not the slightest effort has been made in any of the family planning and health programs to include preventive measures, though this could be easily done at no extra cost.

During the 1980s I testified in Congress repeatedly to demand that preventive measures should be taken, especially since US AID-imported training and tools are used to "modernize" - that is medicalize - the mutilations, stating that US AID had a responsibility to safeguard the health of girls at least in their own program areas.(See Development.) For instance in Burkina Faso the government started a national program to eradicate FGM with a special office devoted to this activity. Yet the US AID sponsored family planning program in Burkina Faso has done nothing to cooperate with this effort.

In the summer of 1988 Berhane Ras Work, the president of the IAC, was in Washington and visited US AID to talk to the program coordinator in population and health for Africa. She explained the objectives of her organization to Dr. Gary Merritt who sent a cable to all health and population officers describing the work of the IAC. The cable suggested that the mission officers in each country should support the activities of the local IAC affiliates and work with them. [68] The cable also made specific suggestions for action, for instance "including information on harmful traditional practices in all MCH (mother and child health) and family planning service delivery and education projects". This certainly sounds like a great success. But this communication, though sent by official route and the proposed actions needed no funding, was completely ignored by all US AID Missions.

During the Reagan and Bush administrations due to political pressure by the Christian Right and the anti abortionists all population programs were cut down and all kinds of restrictions were imposed. Despite this, US AID has introduced and expanded population programs in Francophone West Africa, as well as in Nigeria, quite aside from the large ongoing programs in Kenya and Egypt. But to date nothing has been said, let alone done, to prevent FGM. This despite the fact that FGM has been cited as a human rights violation in all African countries for the past five years in the **Country Reports on Human Rights Practices** [69] which are prepared every year by the State Department for Congress, as required by law. Congress has the power to cut all funding for AID programs and curtail trade agreements with countries that show persistent human rights violations.

US AID is an agency of the Department of State. Therefore all human rights violations first of all affect US AID programs. But now we have the amazing situation that while the State Department condemns FGM as a human rights violation, US AID by their failure to stop the ongoing mutilations in their program areas is supporting FGM. That means US AID is an accessory or contributor to human rights violations cited by the Department of State, which is technically the head of US AID.

In my Congressional testimony this past June I said again that preventive education must be included in all population and health programs in Africa that are funded by US AID or to which the US contributes. Everyone knows by now what is going on: There are no more excuses. While the IAC's work is pioneering and groundbreaking and shows the way, only a budget as large as the one US AID spends on population programs can make real progress in eradicating FGM. In my testimony I summed up:

> "There is no reason why Family Planning Programs should not discourage FGM and speak about the terrible damage done by FGM which is graphically shown in our **Childbirth Picture Books**. All family planning workers trained by US AID in African countries where FGM is practiced must be taught about the damage done by FGM, urged to stop the mutilations and encouraged to teach against them. . . The silence about FGM on the part of US AID sponsored family planning programs - now that African leaders have opposed FGM - is totally irresponsible because this **silence supports the continuation of FGM**. . .
>
> We urge that US AID and their contractors be required **to integrate FGM prevention in all their Family Planning and Health Plans and Programs in affected countries** in Africa and the Middle East, and that every possible support be provided to local groups in Africa and the Middle East working for the eradication of FGM. We also request that all private organizations working for US AID do likewise and be required to provide surveys of their actions and document results of the effectiveness of their teaching. This requires no special programs and no special staff. All AID health programs and contractors, especially those concerned with family planning, should be required to teach prevention of FGM as part of their contracts and should include comprehension tests about FGM as they do about family planning. . .
>
> All funding of family planning organizations, and especially UNFPA (United Nations Population Fund) and IPPF (International Planned Parenthood Federation), should be made subject to a requirement to include teaching the prevention of FGM in all family planning programs in all countries where these mutilations are practiced. IPPF, UNFPA and other family planning organizations to which the US contributes money must be held accountable and show proof of the results of their teaching. . ." [70]

The Women's Declaration on Population Policies [71] prepared for the 1994 International Conference on Population and Development is an important statement of goals by women and for women reacting to the fact that "women's fertility has been the primary object of both pronatalist and antinatalist population policies". In the preamble the Declaration states: "We call for a fundamental revision in the design, structure and implementation of population policies, to foster the empowerment and well-being of all women. . ."

First, the "Fundamental Ethical Principles" are set out which define women's rights including "whether, how and when to have children and how many". The responsibility of men for their sexual behavior is cited next and that sexual and social relationships between women and men must be governed by principles of equity, non-coercion and mutual respect and responsibility". FGM is specifically included in this statement:

> "Violence against girls and women, their subjugation or exploitation, and other harmful practices, such as genital mutilation or unnecessary medical procedures, violate basic human rights. Such practices also impede effective health - and rights-oriented population programs. . ."

And finally it is emphasized that the "fundamental sexual and reproductive rights of women cannot be subordinated". A section on "Minimum Program Requirements" defines how population policies and programs should be designed and implemented "to eliminate pervasive inequalities". In the end the "Necessary Conditions" are spelled out which include that "using participatory processes at least 50 percent of decision-making positions in all relevant agencies shall be filled with women who agree with the principles described. . ." This declaration was drafted, reviewed, modified and agreed on by large numbers of women and women's organizations all over the globe, and more are joining all the time. We have come a very long way from the UN Population Conference in 1974 where women were neither seen nor heard: but there is much more ahead!

THE MODERNIZATION OF FEMALE GENITAL MUTILATION

The introduction of female genital mutilation (FGM) into modern health care services takes place in two ways: by omission and by commission. The most frequent way is by omission that is by failing to oppose FGM for instance on the part of providers of health care or other related services such as family planning. The other way is by commission, by doing the operations like other kinds of surgery or by training others in the procedure.

Somalia is the only country where a medical report is available on how infibulation was performed in a hospital in Mogadishu by specially trained male nurses (see "Case History: Somalia"). In Egypt, Sudan and Nigeria, and no doubt in most urban areas of Africa, surgeons are paid by the male family heads to do the operations on their daughters - as this "modern way" is quicker and more efficient. In Kenya FGM was practiced in most hospitals, which became public knowledge when President arap Moi prohibited FGM in 1982 and had all hospitals notified, including the missionary ones.

The excision of a three-year-old girl in a Nigerian university hospital was reported by a physician who described it as "medically uneventful," and, the physician continued, "judging from the skill and speed with which the surgeon performed the simple intervention, he must have done it lots of times before" [72] (see "Case History: Nigeria").

The Egyptian statutes against the operations are written in such a way as to give physicians a monopoly; that is, unqualified personnel (which means mainly dayas or traditional midwives) are forbidden to practice such surgery but physicians are not.

Under the excuse "to prevent worse harm," physicians in the Sudan do the operations when families (= fathers) insist - which was discussed at the Fifth Obstetrical/Gynaecological Congress in Khartoum in 1977 as well as at the 1979 WHO Seminar. But to have the mutilations done by trained surgeons costs the father more money. Only families living in large towns or the capital have access to any modern medical services. Most of the time the operations are done by the traditional excisors who have always made a living from this activity and have learned it as apprentices from experienced practitioners.

There can be little doubt that the operations are now done by trained health personnel for a fee, almost everywhere where the operations are "the tradition." Indeed, some physicians believe that they are providing a good service by sexually castrating little girls in sanitary ways because this saves them from infections. Fathers in turn are willing to pay physicians because this way they are sure the girl will not die, otherwise the father risks losing the considerable bride-price, and he can sell her as soon as she is done.

It is interesting to note that Dr. Bannerman, the WHO representative in charge of the traditional health programs, who was sent to Khartoum to participate in the 1979 Seminar, argued that Africans cannot be deprived of this important tradition and that, therefore, the operations should be done in the hospitals (see: "WHO Seminar"). Dr. Bannerman is a physician from Ghana, and there are plenty of other physicians who share his views. One can but wonder how Dr Bannerman and people of his ilk propose to satisfy this need for observing African tradition: Would they invite excisors and their helpers into hospitals to carry on group excisions with their traditional tools, or does he propose to build special clinics in the bush for his purpose to mutilate little girls in an authentic environment?

The most detailed medical description of an infibulation operation was provided in 1982 in a British sexology journal called **Forum**, which on its masthead prints a list of consultants that include some of the best-known sexologists, psychotherapists, physicians and Ph.D.s in the UK and US and provides this information: "**Forum** Magazine is the International Journal of Human Relations published in six countries." The **Forum** deals with sexuality and sexual problems according to its own description. [73]

The article was written by a physican/surgeon who did not give his name - the heading was "anonymous." The six-page feature, which was published at the time when the law against circumcision was debated in the British Parliament, claims to deal with "the facts of the matter." The anonymous writer then explains the damaging physical health problems resulting from the traditional way the operations are done and then proposes "that people with money should be allowed to spend it as they wish" adding there is an "obvious advantage . . . to have this type of operation performed under modern conditions with anaesthesia and a proper surgical technique."

The article then claims that to pass legislation to prohibit the operation - referring to the bill in Parliament - is quite useless, citing the prohibition in the Sudan from the 1940s. But this was written in 1983, and London is not Khartoum.

Then, the anonymous writer provides a detailed medical description of the operation- including what surgical tools to use to do an infibulation in an operating room. The description includes where and how to place the stitches "burying the clitoris completely and as effectively as excision," using "a large curved needle with cuting edges" and placing "a deep suture through the labia 5 mm. below their origin." More stitches "are placed similarly at 7 mm. intervals... The thighs are bandaged together for several days . . . after 17 or so days, the lips of the labia will be found to be firmly adherent . . . " [74]

This promotion of FGM operations in a widely distributed magazine as surgical procedures done for a fee on girl children who have no way to protect themselves is really quite amazing, considering that this journal has some internationally known physicians and sexologists listed as "consultants," including Dr. Malcolm Potts of Family Health International in North Carolina and Dr. John Money of Johns Hopkins University.

The editor of **Forum**, Mr. Roger Baker, replied to my letter which first questioned why a reputable author would publish in a reputable magazine "anonymously," stating that physicians and surgeons in the UK are not allowed to publish under their own names. This is entirely untrue as every British medical journal shows. And the anonymous author/ surgeon replied that "Ms. Hosken ought to be highly gratified that we have made public a simple and safe procedure . . ." Obviously the surgeon took pride in his "invention" which he describes as a "kind and humane method, safe and simple, causing no mutilation, no risk and minimal discomfort." And the author ends his article with the claim that midwives in the Sudan had assured him that "the sexual feelings of the women were unimpaired by the operations."

There is no doubt that surgeons in London, quite aside from Africa, do the mutilations for money on the daughters of the well-to-do. Unfortunately, the author is quite correct in stating that laws will not stop the surgery - apparently he knows his professional brothers very well - that is, they will do anything for money.

But there are also physicians who are motivated by other concerns. In September 1979 I received a letter from a Dr. David Stevenson, senior lecturer in international community health at the Liverpool School of Tropical Medicine, [75] who contacted me for information about the Khartoum WHO Seminar.

Dr. Stevenson, a specialist in tropical medicine, had participated in a medical congress in Sierra Leone in November 1978. At this congress, Dr. Stevenson evidently learned about genital mutilation, wich is practiced in often drastic form on most girls of that country (see "Case History: Sierra Leone"). Therefore, he prepared a proposal - which he sent me asking to have it published in **WIN NEWS** - on how to do the mutilations in the hospital or in hygienic, modern ways.

Dr. Stevenson outlined the medical procedures on how to cut the genitalia of the little African girls with Western tools and Western gynecological efficiency, to preserve the "African" traditions. He proposes "the use of modern, small surgical scissors" - to remove the clitoris and labia minora - and "perhaps stitching to stop the bleeding, possibly with fine catgut or another absorbable suture, with emphasis on hygiene . . . to reduce morbidity and mortality." And he also suggests that perhaps "the operations could be reduced to removal of the clitoris only - with possibly a ligature tied around its base . . bleeding and scarring would be greatly reduced but there would still be an "impressive procedure," and the "girl would still lose her male organ."

Like other physicians, Dr. Stevenson claims that he would prefer to see genital mutilation done away with - and adds this may happen more quickly by showing respect for the culture of the society. That his method, as experience shows, results in the opposite, never occurs to the doctor. Introducing the operations into modern health services practically guarantees that they will never be eradicated as long as physicians can make money from them. But as with some other surgeons, not money but fame evidently was his objective - perhaps the operation could be named for him, he thought.

It is quite difficult sometimes for women to discover just what goes on in the minds of men where sexuality is concerned. The doctor thought that his surgical invention was so important that women would flock to him to thank him; **WIN NEWS** as an international journal could be instrumental in making his contribution known to women everywhere!

Dr. Stevenson no doubt is teaching his African students in tropical medicine at the University of Liverpool just how best to mutilate the female children in their countries - preserving the "impressive" procedure of sexual mutilation but reducing the risk of killing the girl because, after all, this means that the father would lose a considerable sum for the bride-price. So, the doctor suggests that "sympathetic modern practitioners" might gain the "confidence of the elders" by "discussing what actually happens and its meaning and importance to the community."

It is astonishing that this physician - and he is not alone - sees no conflict between "an African tradition" and the use of modern, Western medical tools. One can but wonder about the ethics of a physician, indeed a teacher of medicine, who uses his professional skills to teach how to sexually castrate and mutilate helpless female children because they are black or brown, under the excuse of "culture." This man, as all other physicians, has sworn to use his skills and knowledge to heal.

Nowhere in Stevenson's proposal is anything said about the teaching of reproduction, human biology and sexuality to the elders and to the women, men, girls and boys, to prevent these mutilations. Prevention is never mentioned at all.

In an article recently published in **Hospital Doctor**, a professional medical newspaper distributed to hospitals in the UK, it is claimed that medical students are now taught how to do genital mutilations and the Liverpool School of Hygiene and Tropical Medicine is named (see "Women and Health").

These examples of commission no doubt can be multiplied. But the issue of omission is a far more widespread and insidious one.

The conspiracy of silence, which is outlined above, not only assures the continuation of the operations but by not opposing the practices and not teaching against FGM, the spread into modern health services is assured. By saying nothing to discourage the operation, it can be easily assumed, for instance by those being trained in health such as traditional birth attendants, that it is quite all right to use their newly acquired skills, tools and antibiotics to mutilate children. When a traditional practice is not discouraged for whatever reasons, it is certain to be continued in a new form. This is precisely what is happening with FGM, which is modernized using newly introduced techniques.

For instance, in the Sudan, though in the midwifery schools the students are taught that they must never do the operations, it is a fact that everywhere trained midwives do infibulations; indeed, much of their income is derived from FGM. Until and unless other means of economic support for the operators can be found, it is likely that these operations will be continued for economic reasons by the very people who should teach against them. Though this is widely known in the health sector of many African countries, none of the internationally financed health programs have addressed this fact. Yet, training of midwives, which is supported internationally, continues without any attempt to enlist their cooperation by finding and substituting other sources of income for them; for instance, the distribution of contraceptives and family planning information.

The omission of prevention is especially glaring in internationally financed and supported health and family programs in Africa and the Middle East, developed with the assistance of Western health experts. US AID over the years has sponsored a large number of health programs in Africa, quite aside from supporting many multi-million dollar family planning programs, for instance, in Egypt, Kenya and, most recently, in Nigeria.

Though in the Sudan US AID funded an $8 million Primary Health Care program in the early 1980s that also dealt with training of health workers, nothing in that program ever mentioned FGM - despite the fact that just about every woman in the program area is infibulated, causing more health problems than any disease. And although originally the program proposal included a mother and child health section, this was deferred for later - so Dr. Osman Modawi, the chief of the department of gynecology, told me.

But later never came - so women's needs were again left out. However, 2,000 copies of our **Childbirth Picture Book (CBPBs)** were sent to the Sudan by US AID, as soon as they were translated into Arabic, by request of the primary health department of the ministry for this program. Unfortunately, though the **CBPB**'s have Additions to Prevent Excision and Infibulation which we make available free, they were not included.

In Somalia, a $14 million Rural Health Delivery Project started implementation in the early 1980s - it included all kinds of training programs also for women. But the fact that infibulation is a major health hazard for all Somali women was never stated, though all other health problems were enumerated, affecting only a few percent of the people.

This very ambitious program, planned for more than two years, was beset by logistical and many other problems and finally had to be withdrawn before implementation. But this time I sent the pertinent office at US AID information on FGM and specifically information on infibulation in Somalia, resulting in discussion of the issue with the Somalis who had already started their own program to prevent FGM. Despite this, nothing on infibulation was included in the AID program. Nor was anything said about FGM in the US AID Family Planning Program, the first one ever in Somalia.

In Mali, a Rural Health Program, designed with US AID assistance and financing, tried to initiate a new rural health delivery system. This project never even got started - most of the money was wasted.

These are but a few examples from the field of the failed activities of USAID in the area of health, which is so very important for African women. But women were never involved in any of these initiatives. For instance, in Somalia when I urged representatives of the official women's organization, the SWDO (Somalian Women's Democratic Organization), to make their needs known to the program directors at the time I visited Somalia in 1983, it turned out that the women did not even know that such a program existed. Yet the SWDO was a governmental body, and health care was one of the priorities.

Though all the health programs cited above were organized some time after the Khartoum Seminar, the Recommendations of the seminar were entirely ignored by USAID and they continue to be ignored to this day. After the failures of the multimillion-dollar health programs in Africa, US AID did not sponsor any more.

But it is the same with the population programs of US AID: all family planning activities, though they are for women, do not even recognize the existence of FGM nor do they include preventive teaching (see above: "The Politics of Population Control").

As a direct result of ignoring FGM, the operations are modernized, that is, the training, tools, drugs and equipment imported to implement health and family planning programs are used to mutilate children because nothing is done to stop this. Since the mutilations are ignored by the program sponsors, the obvious assumption by the local participants and health workers trained by US AID is that the modernization of the operations is an improvement, especially since some money can be made by doing them.

After returning from Africa, I arranged to give a presentation to the Africa bureau of US AID in Washington, to report on the Khartoum Seminar and to discuss the Recommendations - with the objective to influence policies. A year later, after nothing changed and the Recommendations continued to be ignored, I decided to testify before the congressional committee that is concerned with appropriations for US AID. Attacking the money sources is always effective when pursuing changes in policies.

In the spring of 1980, I testified as editor of **WIN NEWS** before Senator Daniel Inouye, who then was the chairman of the Subcommittee on Foreign Operations of the Appropriations Committee, which approves all US AID budgets. I presented the facts about the Khartoum Seminar and that the Recommendations were made to stimulate also international action. I also cited the failure of US AID and UN agencies, including UNICEF, to implement the Recommendations. An analysis of major ongoing health programs of US AID was included (see Development), showing that these multimillion-dollar programs still ignored the needs of women and pretended that genital mutilation did not exist. At the end of my testimony I stated:

> "My research shows that genital mutilations are increasingly performed in the modern sector in Africa, including in hospitals, often on newborn babies, as sexual castration of females, stripped of all traditional rites. This is a gross abuse of modern medicine and we must advise this committee that, increasingly, health equipment and training contributed to the countries where these operations are practiced, are used to mutilate female children. Speaking for American women and taxpayers, I strenuously object to the use of US monies and contributions to carry out clitoridectomies and infibulations on non-consenting children in Africa and the Middle East, with US-contributed equipment and tools." [76]

Senator Inouye was visibly shaken by those revelations and questioned me. I told him that though US AID was not actively involved in the "modernization" of the mutilations, the failure to take preventive measures allowed this to happen. The senator then requested AID to review the situation and to give him a report, and he added that whether by commission or by omission, US AID must be held responsible.

US AID, in its reply to the senator through Dr. Stephen Joseph, deputy assistant administrator for Human Resources Development, whitewashed their lack of attention to women's health needs and did not answer the critical questions I had raised in my testimony about the modernization of FGM.

As Senator Inouye so aptly stated after my testimony, whether by commission or by omission, the results are the same: The failure to take preventive action results in the medicalization of genital operations and their introduction into the modern health sector all over Africa and the Middle East, and that is going on now.

During the following years I repeatedly testified before the Appropriations Committee, Subcommittee on Foreign Operations and also the Foreign Relations and Foreign Affairs committees on FGM and on women's development.

FGM is not only modernized in Africa, but immigrants from Africa bring it with them wherever they go: if it is ignored and no preventive actions are taken, the practices continue, as they have for many years, for instance, in France. There the fathers of African immigrant families pool their meager resources to bring traditional excisors to Paris, for instance, from Mali, to have their daughters mutilated - as many African men don't trust Western physicians to do a thorough job.

Though these facts were published in the **Medical Daily** [77], a professional newspaper for physicians, in March 1981 by several women pediatricians who had discovered mutilated African girls in French schools in the Paris region, the French health authorities typically ignored the issue and refused to even acknowledge it. Then, in July 1982 a three-month-old girl died as a result of the operation - she bled to death. [78] The father carried his baby daughter (an otherwise healthy girl) to the hospital, but it was too late. Her death finally made headlines all over France, and the facts could no longer be denied by the French authorities responsible for health, as all health serives are publicly financed.

The parents of the dead girl had lived in France for 10 years; the father - according to newspapers - spoke French well and worked for the government. The family also had an older daughter who was similarly excised but did not die. Therefore the father claimed he could not understand why the baby died and would not accept the fact that the operation killed his child. Though he was questioned extensively by the police, he did not acknowledge that he had done anything wrong.

As a French woman who is familiar with the situation stated to **WIN NEWS**, "We only hope that the little girl has not died in vain." But the father was never punished. Though these operations continue to be practiced by Africans in the Paris region, nothing was done until this year.

The French courts finally had to take notice after three more girls died. The issue now has reached the criminal courts. Only suspended sentences were given to several fathers and couples who paid for the mutilations or, in one case, a father cut up his own child with a penknife. But finally this year a jail sentence was imposed on an illiterate woman from Gambia, who had both her daughters mutilated by an excisor.[79]

But no man has ever been sent to jail up to the present time - though the mutilations in France, or wherever they are done, are always paid for by the fathers. But now that it is known that FGM will be prosecuted in the criminal courts and that there is no longer any hesitation about imposing jail terms, many little African girls are sent back to Africa to have the mutilations done there by their extended families.

The French government never took any actions to stop FGM, neither in colonial times nor after independence, in West Africa where France is still heavily invested, nor in France itself where thousands of African immigrants come to find work. After the deaths of several children, GAMS - Women's Group for Abolishment of Sexual Mutilations (Groupe Femmes pour L'Abolition des Mutilations Sexuelles) was organized, by French and African women, led by a pediatrician, Dr. Marie Helene Franjou. [80] Health care in France is free and paid for by the French government, and all are required to bring their children for checkups. This brings African women together at the clinics which makes it possible to teach them about health and about the damage done by the mutilations. GAMS used some of the Childbirth Picture Books in French by **WIN NEWS** for their teaching programs and finally also printed their own adaptions.

CAMS - the International Commission to Abolish Sexual Mutilations [81] - organized by Awa Thiam in 1980 held several conferences in Paris and Dakar in the 1980s. The most recent one was held in December 1989 in Paris. The discussions, besides dealing with FGM, covered violence against women, rape, polygamy, contraception, abortion and more with a long list of resolutions formulated by the participants from Africa and France. These conferences under the leadership of Awa Thiam certainly created much attention among the intellectual leadership in Paris, but no programs or actions were developed to reach and teach African immigrants or to start any actions in Africa.

At the end of 1984 a booklet was published by the Ministry of Women's Rights under the leadership of Yvette Roudy on **Sexual Mutilations in France of Today** [82] providing a survey and count of how many African women immigrants are actually in France and how many female children therefore are "at risk". The facts and background were provided by GAMS; other parts of the report were written by different contributors including, unfortunately, the usual statements by anthropologists praising "customs and traditions". Especially in France it is impossible to get away from such influences that still have a strong hold on policies in Francophone West Africa, which has always tolerated horrible abuse of women and children and the worst human rights violations in the name of "African culture".

A long list of recommendations is included in this publication sponsored by the government but no money was provided by the Ministry of Women's Rights to implement any of them (see: "The Western World"). No medical research or fact finding on FGM has been sponsored or supported by France. FGM was never mentioned officially, let alone any campaigns to stop FGM such as the one in Kenya or Sudan organized by the British. Therefore FGM not only flourishes but is done in hospitals for instance in the Gabriel Toure Hospital, the largest city hospital in Bamako, Mali.

A roundtable discussion on sexual mutilations was also held by the Secretariat for Women's Rights of the French Socialists in November 1984 at the National Assembly. [83] Mme. Yvette Roudy, the minister for women's rights at that time, led one of the discussions. More than 200 women and men including many from Africa participated as well as representatives of many different groups. But neither from this nor from any other meeting held in France on FGM did any action plan result despite another long list of recommendations. Mme. Roudy was both active and outspoken against FGM; but soon after the 1985 Decade Conference on Women in Nairobi, where she led the French delegation, she left as minister due to political changes in the French government. Indeed there is no more Ministry of Women's Rights in France.

Most of the activities described here and many more, including television programs and discussions, continued among the French intellectual elite but had no influence on African immigrants who continue to mutilate their female infants as reported by the press. And there are no prevention programs except the one by GAMS, which has little official support and can only teach a few women (see above). Nor is there any support for the prevention or eradication of FGM in Francophone Africa (see "Women and Health").

In 1985 Renee Saurel a well-known writer and feminist who had shocked the women at the 1980 UN Women's Conference in Copenhagen with her outspoken talk on FGM, published a most critical book, **Bouches Cousues (Mouths Sewn Closed)**. [84] This well researched book is a scathing evaluation of the French medical establishment and bureaucracy, which controls all health care, and their utter failure to protect immigrant girls from being mutilated.

In sharp sarcastic language she describes what is being done to little African girls whose parents came to live in France mostly in and around Paris and who go to school with French children. Yet they are being mutilated the traditional way right in Paris with horrible consequences for their health and lives and their ability to adjust to their classmates and schools - the world around them. Yet, so Saurel charges, nothing is done by the convoluted French bureaucracy, neither the governmental education system nor the governmental health system protects the children from this kind of "modernization" of FGM. The mutilations continue in the suburbs of Paris while those in the French bureaucracy keep their mouths shut (see "The Western World").

But the criminal court cases continue as serious injuries and deaths of children, often small infants, cannot be hidden even by the bureaucracy which up to now is taking no effective preventive measures. What did create a furor and investigation in France a few years ago was the letter which I received from a tourist who had visited Paris. I published this anonymous letter in **WIN NEWS** in autumn 1982. It subsequently was discussed in the European Parliament, as one of the women MPs from Italy who was a subscriber read it at a Parliamentary meeting and demanded an official explanation from France.

In the letter the tourist to Paris describes how he and other visitors were taken one evening in a mini bus from Place Pigalle for a high fee to a suburb of Paris to watch a live exhibition of an excision operation on a small African girl. All this was arranged by a group of Africans who charged the visitors extra for each flash picture they were allowed to take while a young black man cut out the clitoris of a partially drugged, moaning small girl on top of a table. (see "The Western World").

The letter sent to **WIN NEWS** from Germany [85] describes the facts without comment. I published it because it seemed impossible to imagine how anyone could make this up: What would the writer gain from sending it? But the fact that it was brought to the attention of the European Parliament not only shows that it was taken at face value but it forced France to investigate. The European Parliament can require any member state to investigate any internal problems that are cited in Parliamentary discussion.

The issue landed on Mme. Roudy's desk in the Ministry of Women's Rights as well as the Ministry of Interior. But, as expected, the French government claimed that they could find no evidence whatever to verify this incident. Unfortunately even this did not result in any actions by the French government to deal with the issue of FGM in a constructive way that is to start preventive education of African immigrant families especially those who have children. But with Mme Roudy no longer in power and with a conservative government in France, it is unlikely that anything will be done in the near future.

In France up to now the government has not organized any FGM prevention programs for African immigrants within their extensive health and education system to teach African immigrants in a systematic way why FGM is damaging and why it is prohibited in France, indeed all over Europe and the rest of the Western World. Instead the lawsuits continue hauling immigrants into court after the fact, that is after their children have been mutilated. These lawsuits often drag on for years and accomplish nothing. The French government similarly did nothing to discourage FGM in West Africa during colonial times and even now the French pay no attention to FGM, though they enjoy considerable influence.

For years **WIN NEWS** campaigned against the modernization of FGM, collecting signatures and writing letters to WHO and especially the WHO African regional offices. In Autumn 1981 **WIN NEWS** began to circulate a press release on the "Introduction of Female Genital Mutilation into Health Care Practices and Institutions". This Press Release was addressed to the World Health Organization in Switzerland and to the two regional offices in Africa and the Middle East and was sent to them with hundreds of signatures of women and men from all over the world.

The press release states:

> "Genital operations are performed on non-consenting female children by health professionals (physicians, surgeons, trained midwives, trained nurses and trained health workers), often using equipment, tools, and pharmaceuticals contributed by international assistance programs in hospitals/clinics/and other health care settings in Africa, the Middle East, and parts of Asia. The operations are also now being performed in many other parts of the world on children of African/Middle Eastern immigrants including in France, Germany, Italy, Sweden, Australia and more and are being spread all over the world. . ." (* See "Appendix").

But there was no response. Therefore in the early 1980s **WIN NEWS** began to distribute the **Childbirth Picture Books** with the Additions to Prevent Excision and Infibulation in Africa and to African refugees and started to organize actions to prevent the spread of the mutilations that was taking place all over the world and especially the modernization of the operations, as described above. This comprehensive campaign has these objectives which are as valid today as when first published in 1982: [86]

- to abolish all forms of female genital mutilation anywhere in the world, specifically exicision and infibulation;
- to promote the health and integrity of female children, both physical and mental;
- to criminalize female genital mutilations in modern health care systems and to expel from their professions, health practitioners who perform female genital operations on healthy girls and women;
- to show that genital operations, performed on healthy girls and women, are unethical, immoral, contrary to national development objectives, and a violation of human rights.

The campaign especially urged that health peer groups should be organized by professional health workers to support each other in developing preventive actions. One way of doing this is by "twinning", that is cooperation between specific African and Western community organizations to promote women's health on the local level and prevent FGM by health education using the **Childbirth Picture Books** (see "Appendix").

There are other possibilities of organizing mutual support, sponsorships and cooperation between health professionals especially those working on the community level both formally and informally. Forming sister health groups of women health activists and professionals for mutual support between communities or between countries and exchanging information and resources are other ways to support women's health. That is starting on the grass roots level and working up for support rather than down from the top which is used by all governmental programs and activities. But experience shows there often is little or no trickle down. There are many avenues for working together especially in health care, which affects everyone.

In June of 1982 WHO released a "Statement of WHO Position and Activities" which reconfirms the 1979 Khartoum Seminar Recommendations stating that WHO has assured governments of its readiness to support national efforts against FGM, adding that:

> "WHO has consistently and unequivocally advised that female circumcision should not be practiced by any health professionals in any setting - including hospitals or other health establishments." (see "Appendix")

Unfortunately this important advisory by WHO did not get the exposure it should have had and that WHO has available through its own communication system, but the statement was buried among many other documents.

While in France FGM is prohibited by the existing penal code under child abuse, in Britain it was claimed that a law to formally ban FGM had to be enacted. After long debates in Parliament which continued over several years, this finaly took place in 1985 (see "The Western World"). It finally happened because the papers uncovered some cases where Harley Street surgeons performed the mutilations for a high fee. For instance, **The Observer** ran an article in October 1982 citing a physician who openly admitted he had done the operations on Nigerian women brought to him by their husbands, and no doubt other cases could be found.

The article reports:

> "Dr. Ghatak, who trained in Calcutta, explained why he had performed the operation on two of his patients, both Nigerian women. One was brought by her husband because they could not conceive and believed it was because she had not had a clitorectomy. 'Another lady had had a baby by caesarian section. Both she and her husband thought it was because she hadn't had the necessary operations as a child', he said." [87]

According to British law there was no offense involved and a surgeon could do genital operations without any penalty. Therefore new legislation was passed.

But as a result of the British bill "The Prohobition of Female Circumcision Act of 1985", which outlaws FGM and especially the modernization of the mutilations, financial support could be provided by the government for preventive and educational activities. FORWARD - The Foundation for Women's Health, Research and Development [88] - was organized in London and housed in the Africa Center and has been active ever since. FORWARD has sponsored a number of conferences quite aside from continuing educational activities, teaching programs on health and training of government health and community workers and teachers and even staging plays and more. These preventive activities seemingly have been successful as not a single case of FGM has been found and certainly no deaths have been recorded such as in France. But unfortunately it cannot be prevented that such activities go underground. FORWARD in July 1992 held a conference for all organizations in Europe working on the prevention of FGM.

But it is necessary to always be vigilant. That some men have some very twisted ideas about women was recently shown by a national newspaper supplement the **New National Black Monitor** published in New York and distributed as a Sunday supplement to local black community papers. An article, the only one of the supplement which is made up of colorful ads, advocates the introduction of excision and infibulation in black communities in the US as a means to control teenage pregnancy claiming that this is the best way to keep girls in school. The **male Monitor** editors are so concerned about the education of girls that they advocate to mutilate them! (See "The Western World").

Unfortunately, this proposal to mutilate, indeed infibulate, black teenage girls for their own good is not an obscene joke, but describes - full of admiration - what is done in Africa suggesting that black communities in the US should learn from this. This particularly perverse mind set of the black editors is built on a quite common perception of many if not most men that women's bodies are owned by men to control, use, abuse and cut up and change in whatever way a man desires.

All over Europe practically all countries by now have circulated to their health systems prohibitions to practice any form of FGM since all European countries have government funded health care. Or they have passed some form of official directive against FGM and at least on this level, it seemed, the issue was settled. That is until summer 1992 when I received a seven-page fax from a children's organization in the Netherlands, "Defence for Children International" [89]

The organization asked for information on FGM, specifically what legislation exists in Africa. This was needed for a research report requested by the Dutch Health Ministry in preparation for proposing legislation. The facts in this amazing affair were that the Netherlands, a very hospitable country, accepted a large number of Somalian refugees and was confronted with their custom of infibulation which was entirely new for the government clinics and hospitals. Quite aside from the health problems the medical facilities had to treat, the families asked the clinics to infibulate their daughters as many evidently were accustomed to do in Somalia.

It appears that one physician and one nurse who had worked with the Somali refugees proposed that the mutilations should be medicalized or as the health ministry subsequently claimed do "a non-mutilating" operation. I wrote to the health ministry and sent them the WHO advisory against the introduction of FGM in any form into health care. But instead of rejecting such a preposterous idea - paying gynecologists and hospitals for what the health ministry called a "non-mutilating" mutilation - the bureaucratic wheels evidently could not be stopped. For more than a year this outrageous affair continued, with hundreds of newspaper articles, demonstrations by women and much more

It is impossible to explain why the government proceeded on a nonformal suggestion by two people who evidently had no experience with Africans. One line in a report started this appalling wasteful and useless debate that in the end had only losers. For the Somali refugees, already traumatized by fleeing the horrible situation in their country, it drew attention to their worst customs. For the government it meant time and money wasted in useless debates and being attacked by all kinds of citizens' groups quite aside from all women. The Ministry of Justice, the Ministry of Foreign Affairs and many others in the government became involved, taking time and money away from constructive pursuits.

For women in the Netherlands it meant spending time and money - which most of them could ill afford - on organizing and protesting and trying to stop the government. In the end no one in the government was willing to take **responsibility** for this affair and every department involved claimed it had been opposed to FGM in typical bureaucratic evasion of responsibility. In **WIN NEWS** this affair is described in great detail in three issues as it unfolded (Autumn 1992, Winter and Spring 1993) because it is an important lesson that women always have to be vigilant to protect their bodies. Therefore, it is important to draw some lessons from these unfortunate events.

In the end this must be said: **What a deplorable waste of time, energy and money!** If the Health Ministry and all the other Dutch ministries, organizations and people who spent countless hours and money on this affair would have made the same effort to teach Somali refugees about reproduction, they could have freed them from their damaging misconceptions. Especially the men, who make all the decisions, need to be convinced that these mutilations are a serious threat to health of both mother and child, therefore they are prohibited in most of the world. With the help of graphic teaching aids such as the **Childbirth Picture Books** - they could have persuaded **all** the Somali refugees in less time than it took for this affair. What is more it is only fair to inform all refugees that these mutilations are a criminal offense and they must obey the laws of the country where they want to live.

All the time and money spent on investigations on protests and meetings could have been spent on positive education of the refugees. Surely it is not beyond the highly educated population of the Netherlands to use their skills in positive ways to show the Somali and other African refugees who cling to such deplorable customs a better and healthier way of life. It is quite possible to teach people from all parts of the world how their bodies function, something that is needed by everyone: But evidently that was not done.

The Ministry of Foreign Affairs finally in February 1993 sent a long statement about their decision which is summarized here:

> "It is important to stress again, at the outset, that female circumcision is a practice which runs contrary to prevailing attitudes in the Netherlands on the equality of women and their place in society. . . We would also confirm that the Netherlands endorses the recommendation of the World Health Organisation to develop strategies aimed at eliminating the practice worldwide. . .
>
> Although female circumcision as such is not punishable under the Criminal Code, it does constitute intentional or negligent assault (article 436 of the Criminal Code) and the unlicensed practice of medicine (articles 300-309 of the Criminal Code). . .
>
> The Dutch Association of Obstetricians and Gynaecologists has recommended that the Ministry of Welfare, Health and Cultural Affairs set up a support committee. Doctors and gynaecologists are to refuse to perform any form of female circumcision. . . [90]

The Dutch government set up the "Foundation Pharos" [91] January 1993 to work with refugees, taking over the activities of the Refugee Health Care Center and others to develop an information and consultation center on FGM, with the purpose to prevent girls being mutilated and to improve assistance to refugees and asylum seekers who are already operated. The project serves professionals in the field as well as refugees. The emphasis will be on Somali women - this according to a communication from the Ministry. Perhaps, after all, some lessons have been learned from and about women.

THE MEDIA AND THE MESSAGE.

The media play an important and often double-sided role where controversial issues are concerned and especially on everything that affects women. Female Genital Mutilation (FGM) certainly is such an issue. Keeping silent - in support of patriarchal domination and ignoring whatever women do or say, disregarding women's needs - is one side of the media treatment. The other side is to distort the facts to make women appear ridiculous or to create controversy between women.

The objective always is to keep male power firmly in control of what is published by whom and how. Of course, recently women's publications, women's papers and magazines are proliferating all over the world and have broken the stranglehold of absolute male control of what is published and by whom.

WIN NEWS has published a section on **Women and Media** for many years, printing information on women's serial publications worldwide, which are increasing everywhere, establishing communication and networking independent of male media control. Research by women on discrimination by male controlled media and TV has been distributed and the media are being monitored. In the US most major newspapers and TV networks had to be sued for discrimination before opening all positions to women equally. Discrimination practiced by the global media makes independent networks like **WIN NEWS** essential for communication by, for and about women and to provide information that is not biased, sexist or abusive of the female majority.

The issue of genital mutilation is a good example of how those who run the media silence and distort reality exploiting women's desperate plight and needs. First, all information on FGM was silenced and ignored. When that was no longer possible, a few of the Western-educated African women working for their male-dominated governments or the equally patriarchal UN agencies were persuaded to lend their names to media attacks on Western women speaking against FGM.

Publishing the terrible facts of traditional ritual mutilations and abuse was regularly called interference or cultural imperialism by the press and at the UN, and women who dared to say the truth were attacked as racists and strident feminists who did not understand African culture and traditions.

All of this supports control by men. For instance many of the men from Africa and the Middle East who hold decision-making positions at the UN agencies, have their own daughters mutilated. They can be relied on to oppose all information or discussion of FGM. In turn they can count on the solidarity of their male counterparts. For instance the media director at UNICEF, until after the Khartoum Seminar in 1979, denied that FGM was a problem and then published an article in an international magazine attacking "Western Feminists" for their lack of respect for African culture (see above).

Recently a columnist for **The New York Times**, Mr. A. M. Rosenthal, suddenly discovered FGM, complaining that no one was paying any attention to this "torture". He presented his version of FGM though he clearly knows nothing about it. [92] In typical male chauvinist fashion he ignored all women who have worked for years to make the issue known against enormous obstacles such as the male-dominated press represented by **The New York Times**. For Rosenthal FGM is of course a ready-made issue to shore up his lagging readership - which he evidently discovered as he wrote twice on the subject.

Instead of giving women credit he cited a British male controlled publication, **the Minority Rights Report** which almost never publishes on women. A few years ago they asked some women editors to put together a short pamphlet of previously published information, including information from **WIN NEWS**. This booklet landed on Mr. Rosenthal's desk, so he stated. This is another typical example of how male journalists and the media put women down while exploiting them. The abuse of women by the press and TV is done so routinely that it has become the accepted media style all over the world.

With a few exceptions the male dominated media have kept almost total silence on FGM, joining the conspiracy of the UN agencies and all other male institutions that over so many years have perpetuated the practice and supported its spread to ever larger regions by failing to report any of the facts.

Until quite recently, it was astonishing how all the media from academic journals to newspapers absolutely refused to publish anything at all on FGM. Though my articles on other subjects were regularly printed by well-known newspapers such as the **Boston Globe** or the the **Christian Science Monitor** as well as many international and professional publications, it was impossible to persuade anyone to print one word on FGM though I submitted dozens of articles from my trips to Africa in the 1970s and 1980s.

In 1976 for the first time a small publication concerned with African rèsearch, the **Munger Africana Library Notes** by the California Institute of Technology, published my article **"Genital Mutilation of Women in Africa"**. [93] This was the first time the subject was discussed in a comprehensive way in a non-medical publication. Shortly after that a more extensive research article I wrote **"Female Circumcision and Fertility in Africa"** [94] came out in **Women and Health** published by the Biological Sciences Program of the State University of New York in Westbury. This article was subsequently translated and appeared in France, Germany and Italy in women's journals.

Although this was a breakthrough, dozens of other articles and reports were rejected continuously: "We cannot deal with this topic" and "Sorry this subject is unacceptable" were the usual responses. By now I have published dozens of articles on FGM in many different publications and languages, but there is, nevertheless, still a great reluctance by the media to present the truth. The facts about FGM are frequently disguised by all kinds of cultural embellishments or surrounded by descriptions of colorful festivals and clothes. This kind of misguided praise of cultural traditions, published by anthropologists, continues to this day .

Shortly after my article appeared in **Women and Health**, I was asked by the editor of **Tropical Doctor** published in London, the most prestigious international medical journal, to submit a report on FGM based on my experiences visiting African maternities: **The Epidemiology of Female Genital Mutilation,** [95] was published in July 1978, which included the first comprehensive map of Africa showing the spread of FGM. Unfortunately the number of mutilated women cited at that time had to be increased several times since, nearly tripling the number of girls/women initially estimated to be affected. The editor of the **Tropical Doctor**, Prof. Bruce Chwatt, had written on FGM in Kenya and knew that my report was groundbreaking in establishing the facts of the spread of FGM.

A month after the article appeared, I was invited to present these facts at the seminar which was planned by WHO for Khartoum the next year and give a presentation on my research as well as be a member of the WHO Conference Secretariat and temporary advisor on FGM. But even though the WHO Seminar in February 1979 finally broke down the international barriers of silence that had prevailed ever since the United Nations and its agencies were organized, perhaps an even greater barrier still exists: ignorance and discrimination against women.

Traditional and patriarchal attitudes especially by African men who constantly charge interference and racism often stop all information. Women too often do not want to hear about these horrible brutalities as it is too upsetting. But it is essential to make the facts known in order to initiate change and to eradicate FGM.

People working internationally for the many organizations involved in development and especially in family planning cannot be allowed to continue to evade their responsibilities and make excuses such as "these are cultural traditions" and "it is racist to interfere". They must be confronted with the reality: should a girl because she is brown or black be subjected to the torture and lifelong health damage of FGM, a practice that everyone categorically rejects for a white child? That is the real racism and must be absolutely stopped. Yet at every one of my lectures someone in the audience always claims: but we must preserve traditions! And the issue of tradition is continuously raised in the press.

Pictures, films and videos are a powerful method to communicate, especially in Africa where literacy is very low (among women in rural areas often less than 10%) and visual communication - TV and movies - are limited to major cities. Electricity has not yet reached many of the vast rural areas of sub-Saharan Africa. But if you bring along your own powersource visual presentations can make an enormous impression and pictures of all kinds can be effectively used for education.

A number of films/videotapes have been made* for information and consciousness-raising in Africa and abroad. For instance one film made in Burkina Faso with the support of the national government and distributed by a French filmmaker is used throughout the country for local meetings. Aptly named "My Daughter Will Not Be Excised", the film provides a strong message to local decision makers, chiefs and fathers, dramatizing the situation of young village girls and the conflicts between tradition and change. This movie is used all over the country in the government campaign against excision and was made locally for that purpose. It is also distributed internationally to draw attention to and gain support for this campaign (see "Case History: Burkina Faso").

The IAC (Inter Africa Committee) is distributing a videotape, made about their work in Africa by a Swedish filmmaker. The problems of FGM are shown and discussed from the view of African women from different countries and to seek support for the activities of the IAC. Made in large part in Nigeria it provides a realistic view of the magnitude of the problem of FGM as well as the many other damaging traditional practices that are still ignored by all development programs.

There are other films and videotapes available that have been made in different countries of this huge continent, which show local conditions, recently some have also been made by women. Some are shocking to viewers showing the unmitigated brutality of these mutilations, but too often colorful clothes and dancing are used to disguise reality.

The BBC (British Broadcasting Corporation) made a documentary on FGM filmed in the Sudan and directed by Louise Panton in the early 1980s which was finally shown for the first time in March 1983. It is ironic that Panton spent two years in the Sudan making this remarkable document with the cooperation of many medical professionals who in that country have been actively opposed to the mutilations and campaigned against them for decades. But in the end the male management of the BBC opposed showing the film and finally was only persuaded to compromise by cutting out some of the critical footage that showed the operation. [96]

At the present time it would be impossible to make such a film in Sudan where the Moslem fundamentalist government has been increasingly restricting women and cutting off all outside communication except with Iran. But the impact of this TV program was quite temporary despite the fact that the whole controversy surrounding its showing was repeatedly discussed in all the papers. It seems that, like with so many other media events, there is always something new and more exciting that comes along to claim the attention of the public and what was shown a week ago is forgotten.

In France also, for a time in the 1980s, all kinds of TV programs on FGM were shown, meetings and discussions were held and many articles were published. But though all of this no doubt raised the consciousness of some sophisticated people in France and elsewhere in Europe, it had practically no effect on the lives of women and girls in Africa: due to population growth and because the operations are done to ever younger children, more and more girls are mutilated every year.

These mutilations also go on in areas where family planning and health programs are introduced, financed by European countries or the US. But the decision makers and program planners quite aside from the men who run the UN agencies concerned with health and development do nothing: they pretend to see and know nothing; therefore there is no reason to protect the girl children at risk, which would upset their fathers.

A translation of the **Hosken Report "Les Mutilations Sexuelles Feminines"** [97] was published in France by Denoel in November 1983, and I went to Paris for media promotions. I was interviewed by various radio and TV programs and talked to the press. But though a major article of mine - a report on my 1983 research trip to sub-Saharan East and West Africa - appeared at the same time in **Marie Claire,** one of the most widely distributed women's magazines of France, the publishers failed to advertise the book, and it was largely ignored. [98] The French are not ready to face what is really going on in West Africa in their former colonial empire where French economic and intellectual influence is still very strong; nor is it really acknowledged that FGM is practiced in Paris.

---

*See list of Films/Videotapes in Bibliography

The mutilations were and are discussed quite candidly in the abstract by the media in Paris, accompanied with sophisticated philosophical theories and psychosexual analysis by anthropologists. These intellectual adventures seem to have no relation to reality or any impact on decisions by the Cooperation (the development ministry of the French government). The discussions in the media in Paris on FGM are entirely unrelated to the stark realities of the mutilations practiced in Africa.

With an ever larger population of immigrants in Europe including more and more from African countries, the attitudes now are changing toward dealing with the problems at hand due to immigration and away from what goes on in Africa. The media report from Africa about seemingly endless and ever more brutal civil wars, about repeated droughts and famines and growing poverty as well as the pandemic of AIDS that is beginning to engulf most of sub-Saharan Africa, making all other problems pale by comparison. But they do not report that the reasons for many of these disasters may have something to do with customs, behaviour and traditions: that no one has dared to even hint about.

At the 1980 Mid-Decade Conference in Copenhagen the international press and media from all over the world were present as at all UN conferences. Awa Thiam from Senegal spoke candidly and forcefully against FGM: She had recently published her first book **La Parole aux Negresses** [99] an outspoken feminist statement for the rights of black women in Africa and internationally and against the African traditions that exploit and damage African women including FGM.

Her message - women must work together globally and join hands against all forms of oppression - was well received. She announced the formation of a Commission for the Abolishment of FGM (CAGM). [100] This organization which sponsored two conferences - one in Dakar and one at UNESCO in Paris - has not been heard from recently though it rallied considerable support for several years during the 1980s.

In 1985, CAGM together with women from West Africa and France organised a meeting at the UN End of Decade Conference FORUM in Nairobi. Unfortunately most of the English-speaking East African women were unable to participate as the meeting was held in French. Awa Thiam, after completing her studies in Paris, returned to Dakar in the late 1980s where the international headquarters of CAMS was located; but there has been no evidence of any activity for several years.

But the issue of FGM also offers all kinds of opportunities to gain attention to some who have learned to use the media for personal advancement especially at UN conferences. At the Copenhagen Conference for Women, another African group of women did not share the commitment of Awa Thiam for women to work together. AFARD/AAWORD (Association of African Women for Research and Development) [101], led by Marie Angelique Savane, loudly protested all discussion of genital mutilation at the FORUM and she with others by shouting tried to disrupt some of the meetings on FGM. At a meeting of their own, AWORD refused to let white women participate and declared that all white women were excluded on racial grounds from their research organization in Dakar.

Savane even attacked UNICEF for offering help to African community organizations who wanted to work against FGM and gave interviews on her opposition: her accusations were printed on the title page of the conference newspaper and picked up by the international press, giving her instant attention. That as well as her attacks on all women speaking against FGM earned her a lot of international coverage which evidently was her objective. She was cited all over the world by the press for her attacks on Western women, complaining they were dominating the conference and third world women.

Savane not only attacked all attempts to make the facts about FGM known but she condemned all international campaigns against FGM, and charged that FGM was the result of "underdevelopment" and therefore the North was responsible. All these statements were eagerly used by the international press to claim that women from developing countries and European/Western women were fighting and that feminism was rejected by women from the third world as irrelevant. Savane's attacks have been used by the media ever since when the Copenhagen Conference is discussed. Though Awa Thiam, also from Dakar, did not agree, her call for unity and collaboration between all women everywhere was ignored by the press.

Savane, in the **International Child Welfare Review**, in 1979, [102] had published an article defending female genital mutilation with these words: "what can be offered in exchange to the little girls who look forward. . . to that important moment of their lives?" And this publication is distributed worldwide speaking for children! **ISIS**, an international women's magazine published by Jane Cottingham and Marilee Karl in Geneva, provided Savane with another opportunity to publish, claiming that "excision has an essential function", where she attacked all international actions to prevent FGM as "cultural imperialism". As a result, citing Savane's statement in **ISIS**, the Swedish International Development Authority (SIDA), refused to provide previously promised funding to programs to stop FGM - no doubt other organizations were similarly discouraged from offering help.

As expected, this media campaign of Savane's, making clever use of the international press to promote herself among the most conservative power brokers at the United Nations, was rewarded. After being invited to conferences all over the world (women from developing countries are always paid when invited to participate by international and UN meetings and get research grants for their papers and work), she got several well-paid UN assignments. Recently she has been rewarded with a permanent high-placed administrative job at the UN in Geneva, no doubt for her activities supporting patriarchal rule. African men especially enjoy much influence at the UN and are delighted to support a woman speaking for FGM and "their" traditions to keep women under control.

These kinds of politics, publicized by the media, which play a key role in all controversial matters, make the UN and its agencies what it is today, a morass of personal and venal politics of the lowest kind that have left their mark on everything touched by this corrupted system. [103] And all this could not exist without the manipulation of the media who are key players, as the press is able to arouse the public over an issue that might otherwise be ignored, especially when feminism can be attacked and women made the losers.

For obvious reasons, every UN agency has an extensive press department which publishes huge amounts of literature, press releases, glossy multicolored expensive booklets praising their great "accomplishments", whatever the issue. If the money wasted on this useless redundant literature of self-aggrandizement would be instead given to women's groups to further their own activities and for local development, it would really accomplish much positive change and local development.

For instance if the money wasted by UNICEF and UNDP, quite aside from the FAO, UNESCO and UNFPA on glossy full-color expensive and wasteful publications, would be used to train midwives and traditional birth attendants, the maternal mortality related to childbirth could be substantially reduced. Or if the money would be used to pay TBAs in Africa to stop excisions and instead distribute contraceptives in rural areas, this could result in measurable change. Instead, all the so-called Safe Motherhood programs publish more and more expensive literature in the US; but this sophisticated publicity does not help communities who need basic educational materials in simple usable form.

The publicity published by the information offices at all UN agencies is competing for attention, creating pollution and drowning everyone in paper. It is increasingly difficult to distinguish between fact and media hype, and in the process the importance of the real message is diluted. And the message that all media should focus on is:

Female Genital Mutilation must be stopped here and now.

It is an intolerable, violent attack on girls' health and a human rights violation.

FGM has been perpetuated and spread locally and regionally for 2,000 years to ever more people and areas by myths and traditions, mostly by word of mouth. The media for many decades have supported these mutilations by their failure to report the truth and have deliberately suppressed all factual information - as stated above. Even now the message still does not come through loud or clear: It is a basic responsibility of the media, I believe, to finally make the truth about FGM known all over the world. The mutilations are being spread worldwide due to much greater mobility of the people directly involved. The other essential media task is to educate the affected societies in Africa and the Middle East by communicating the basic health information on reproduction - as the **Childbirth Picture Book/Program** tries to do. There are many different effective ways today for the media to reach people with the essential message about their own bodies and health.

In the past several years, more and more articles have been published in the US, in Canada and in Europe due to the fact that FGM is being imported now all over the world by African refugees (see "The Western World"). It is unfortunately inevitable that enterprising writers and publishers of all kinds use this subject which can be easily sensationalized and used for pornographic purposes to sell more publications. Recently FGM has been publicized with yet another twist: Alice Walker fictionalized and embellished the issue making it the centerpiece of her new novel **Possessing the Secret of Joy**. The book grossly distorts all the health facts of FGM and presents an Americanized view with all kinds of psychiatric overtones that have nothing to do with the reality in Africa The subject - FGM - though it is not really discussed at all, with the help of clever promoters has landed the book on the best-seller list: Walker, a black woman, cashed in on FGM.

In our media-dominated culture where violence of all kinds is exploited and torture of women sells, it is unfortunately only a question of time until some TV or movie entrepreneur will find a way to make money from even more sensational presentations of FGM. In fact, in some New York and Paris movie houses films on excision made in Africa can be found in theaters where pornography is featured.

Though - as stated many times - the first step is to break the conspiracy of silence, it is important to stress the objective constantly: to protect girl children from these mutilations and free the women of African and Middle Eastern societies from the damaging cultural traditions and practices that have no place in the world today. And that cannot be done by talking or publishing articles or making movies and videos or holding conferences and meetings in the rest of the world.

In the final analysis, this can only be done in Africa by a coordinated long-term and continuing effort to educate the people involved and to teach them on their own terms about health, about their own bodies and how reproduction functions: And then they will decide for themselves that these mutilations must stop. It is a long, hard and laborious process of education that is needed now, which is neither glamorous nor financially rewarding, but I am afraid this is necessary and has to be done if we are serious about the goal - to eradicate female genital mutilation permanently so it will never and nowhere be practiced again.

There is no one in Africa and for that matter anywhere else who is not interested in reproduction - how our bodies function. How children are made is and has been a prime concern for people and especially women always and everywhere. This precisely is the topic of the **Childbirth Picture Books,** which teach with pictures as the title states and can be understood by people everywhere as our experience in many countries and translations into a dozen or more languages shows. And more teaching materials with these objectives are needed.

Not only in Africa but all over the world the most damaging silence for girls and women is the silence surrounding the essential life-giving biological process of our bodies - how reproduction functions. This silence is dictated by the elderly men in power who run every society - the politicians and military rulers together with the religious leaders of every denomination. In the introduction of all the **Childbirth Picture Books**, I state:

> "The failure to learn about the natural biological process of giving life, or how a baby is made, continues to be the cause of great suffering, pain and tragedy; quite needlessly. Yet, millions of women and girls continue to live in fear and ignorance of their own bodies and life-giving functions. In many areas of the world, more women still die of childbirth than of any disease; yet this is entirely and easily preventable. The biological facts of reproduction continue to be the best kept secrets in many parts of the world, often distorted by damaging myths, taboos, and fears that threaten and debase the lives and dignity of women.
>
> We hope that this book and program will be helpful by making the vital information on reproductive health accessible and available to women and men, and especially the young, all over the world: it is designed for those who, so far, have not been reached with this vital information." [104]

FOOTNOTES

PARAMETERS

1. World Health Organization Seminar Report on "Traditional Practices Affecting the Health of Women and Children," February 10-15, 1979, Khartoum, Sudan. Available from: WHO Regional Office, P.O. Box 1517, Alexandria, Egypt.
2. Inter-African Committee (IAC), 174, rue de Lausanne, CH-1202 Geneva, Switzerland; and c/o Economic Commission for Africa, ATRCW, P.O. Box 3001, Addis Ababa, Ethiopia.
3. International Planned Parenthood Federation, P.O. Box 759, Inner Circle, Regent's Park, London NW1 4LQ, England.
4. **The New York Times**, December 15, 1986. Author's letter to the editor, "Why AIDS Pattern Is Different in Africa."

THE INTERNATIONAL POLITICS OF FEMALE GENITAL MUTILATION

5. Convention on the Elimination of Discrimination Against Women, Division for the Advancement of Women, DC-2, 12th Floor, United Nations, New York, NY 10017; also contact: International Women's Rights Action Watch, Humphrey Institute, 301, 19th Avenue South, Minneapolis, MN 55455.
6. **The New York Times**, December 20, 1992, "Sexual Harassment at the UN." See **also WIN NEWS,** Vol. 19, No. 1, Winter 1993, p. 9.
7. **The New York Times**, July 22, 1979, p. 1.
8. **The New York Times,** October 18, 1981. See also **WIN NEWS,** Vol. 8, No. 1, Winter 1982, pp. 7-8.
9. **Engendering Adjustment for the 1990s**, Report of a Commonwealth Expert Group on Women and Structural Adjustment, Commonwealth Secretariat, Marlborough House, Pall Mall, London SW1Y 5BX, England. See **also WIN NEWS**, Vol. 16, No. 4, Autumn 1990, pp. 9-12.
10. Country Reports on Human Rights Practices, prepared annually by US Department of State for US Congress Committee on Foreign Relations and Committee on Foreign Affairs and is available from the US Government Printing Office, Superintendent of Documents, Washington, D.C. 20402.

THE STATUS OF WOMEN IN AFRICA AND THE MIDDLE EAST

11. Boserup, Ester. **Woman's Role in Economic Development.** St. Martin's Press, Inc., NewYork, 1970, pp. 54-55.
12. "Women in Food Production, Food Handling and Nutrition with Special Emphasis on Africa." Study by the Protein-Calorie Advisory Group (PAG) of the United Nations. **PAG Bulletin**, Vol. 3, Nos. 3/4, September/December 1977, p. 45. See also **WIN NEWS**, Vol. 4, No. 1, Winter 1978, pp. 20-23.
13. Sullerot, Evelyne. **Woman Society and Change**. World University Library, McGraw Hill Book Co., New York. 1973, pp. 20-26.
14. Boserup, op. cit.
15. Sullerot, op. cit., p. 173.

THE SEXUAL POLITICS OF AFRICAN AND MIDDLE EASTERN MEN

THE REASONS GIVEN

16. Zwang, Gerald. **Le Nouvel Observateur**, November 14, 1977 (summarized and translated from the French). See also **WIN NEWS**, Vol. 4, No. 1, Winter 1977, p. 52.
17. **The Drum**, the national magazine of Nigeria, 1977-78, Letters column. See **also WIN NEWS**, Vol. 5, No. 2, Spring 1979, pp. 57-58.

THE WORLD HEALTH ORGANIZATION

18. Document ST/TAO/HR/9 from United Nations Seminar "On the Participation of Women in Public Life." Addis Ababa, Ethiopia 1960, paragraphs 60, 61 and 62.
19. United Nations **ECOSOC Resolution 680 BII (XXVI)** and Document #E/3592.
20. Ibid.

FOOTNOTES (continued)

21. World Health Organization Report on "Epidemiology of Infertility", 1975. Technical Report No. 582.

22. Cook, Dr. R. "Damage to Physical Health from Pharaonic Circumcision (Infibulation) of Females: A Review of the Medical Literature," 1976. Dr. Cook was Regional MCH/ NUT Advisor to the WHO Regional Office of the Eastern Mediterranean, P.O. Box 1517, Alexandria, Egypt, when this was written.

23. Constitution of theWorld Health Organization, signed July 22, 1946. For copies write to the WHO representative in your country or to the Department of Information, WHO, 1211 Geneva 27, Switzerland.

24. Hosken, Fran P. "The Epidemiology of Female Genital Mutilation". Published in **Tropical Doctor,** July 1978. Documentation of spread of genital operations in Africa.

25. Matherson, Alistair. "Unkindest Cut of All", **The Observer** (London), Sunday, September 19, 1979.

26. "UNICEF Position on Female Circumcision." UNICEF, 3 United Nations Plaza, New York, NY 10017. See also **WIN NEWS**, Vol. 5, No. 4, Autumn 1979, pp. 26-27.

27. World Health Organization Press Release #WHO/11 (1 April 1980), "Female Circumcision: UN Agencies Decide on Joint Action Programme." WHO, Division of Public Information, 1211 Geneva 27, Switzerland.

28. Project on Combating Female Circumcision by the Coptic Church of Egypt. See **WIN NEWS,** Vol. 7, No. 1, Winter 1981, pp. 37-38.

29. United Nations Charter, available from every UN office around the world.

30. World Health Organization Press Release #WHA/10 (12 May 1993), "Female Genital Mutilation: World Health Assembly Calls for the Elimination of Harmful Traditional Practices." See also **WIN NEWS** Vol. 19, No. 3, Summer 1993, p. 46.

THE CONSPIRACY OF SILENCE

31. Groult, Benoite. **Ainsi Soit-elle**. Editions Grosset and Fasquelle (France), 1975, p. 109.

32. Saurel, Renee. "L'Enterree Vive," **Les Temps Modernes** (26 rue de Conde, Paris 6, France). Editor: Jean Paul Sartre. A series of nine articles published in 1979/80. Subsequently published in book form: **L'Enterree Vive (The Buried Live: An Essay About Female Sexual Mutilation).** Preface by Simone de Beauvoir, Editions Slatkine, Paris, 1981 (in French). See also **WIN NEWS**, Vol. 6, No. 4, Autumn 1980, p. 47, and Vol. 8, No. 2, Spring 1982, p. 31.

33. Hosken, Fran P. **The Childbirth Picture Book/Prototype** was circulated for two years throughout developing countries for comments from women's and health community groups and international health and family planning organizations.

34. Mid-Decade Conference Forum 1980, Copenhagen, Panel Discussion: "Sex Education/Female Circumcision." See **WIN NEWS** Vol. 6, No. 4, Autumn 1980, pp. 42-43.

35. World Council of Churches, Christian Medical Commission, 150 rue de Fernay, 1211 Geneva, Switzerland. Letters of March 3, 1976, and February 17, 1976, signed by Stuart J. Kingma, M.D., and Marit Kromberg, M.D.

36. Safe Motherhood Conference, Nairobi 10-13 February 1987. Contact: The World Bank, Public Information Dept., 1818 H St., N.W., Washington, DC 20433. See also **WIN NEWS**,Vol. 13, No. 2, Spring 1987, pp. 23-26.

37. Safe Motherhood Initiative/Conference organized by Family Care International, 588 Broadway, Suite 510, New York, NY 10012; Tel: (212) 941-5300.

38. **Safe Motherhood** - a newsletter published by WHO three times a year, in French and English by the Maternal Health and Safe Motherhood Programme, Division of Family Health, World Health Organization, 1211 Geneva 27, Switzerland.

39. **MotherCare Matters** - published by John Snow, Inc. (a contractor of US AID - US Agency for International Development), 1616 N. Fort Myer Drive, 11th Floor, Arlington, VA 22209.

FOOTNOTES (continued)

DISCRIMINATION IN DEVELOPMENT

40. Percy Amendment to the Foreign Assistance Act of 1961 (named after Senator Percy, who chaired the Foreign Relations Committee and proposed the amendment).

    The amendment directed the Agency for International Development to administer the US foreign aid effort in such a way as to promote the integration of women into the national economies of recipient countries, thus improving the status of women and assisting the total development effort. The Percy Amendment on the Integration of Women, Sec. 33. Chapter 3 of part III of the Foreign Assistance Act of 1961 is amended by adding at the end thereof the following new section:

    "Sec. 305. Integration of Women. - The President is requested to instruct each representative of the United States to each international organization of which the United States is a member (including but not limited to the international Bank for Reconstruction and Development, the Asian Development Bank, the Inter-American Development Bank, the International Monetary Funds, the United Nations, and the Organization for Economic Cooperation and Development) to carry out their duties with respect to such organizations in such a manner as to encourage and promote the integration of women into the national economies of member and recipient countries and into professional and policy-making positions within such organizations, thereby improving the status of women." (Proposed by Fran P.Hosken)

    See Congressional Record, 93rd Congress, Second Session, Dec. 4, 1974, No. 168.

41. United Nations Division for the Advancement of Women, DC-2, 12th Floor, United Nations, New York, NY 10017; Secretary General: Gertrude Mongella (Tanzania), Chair of the 4th World Conference on Women - 1995.
42. Rogers, Barbara. **The Domestication of Women: Discrimination in Developing Societies**. Kogan Page Ltd., London, 1980, pp. 39-40.
43. Loutfi, Martha F. **A New International Order Begins at Home - Rural Women: Unequal Partners in Development**, an International Labour Office publication, Geneva, 1980, pp. 25-26.
44. **Sunday Standard** (Kenya), November 12, 1989. See also **WIN NEWS,** Vol.16, No. 1, Winter 1990, p. 52.
45. Little, Kenneth. **African Women in Towns: An Aspect of Africa's Social Revolution**. Cambridge University Press, 1973.
46. Kenyatta, Jomo. **Facing Mount Kenya**. Vintage Books, Division of Random House, New York, October 1965 (originally printed in 1930).
47. **WOMEN AND THE WORLD ECONOMIC CRISIS - KIT NO. 6.** The JUNIC/NGO Programme Group on Women and Development, The United Nations Non-Governmental Liaison Service, Palais des Nations, CH-1211, Geneva 10, Switzerland. This kit on the economic development and others of the series were published in 1991/92 in book form, one book on each topic, by Zed Books: UK - A A Distribution, Ltd., Dunhams Lane, Letchworth, Herts SG6 1LF; USA - Humanities Press International, Inc., 171 First Ave., Atlantic Highlands, N J 07716. See also **WIN NEWS** Vol.16, No. 4, Autumn 1990, p. 7.
48. **DAWN** - Development Alternatives with Women for a New Era. University of West Indies, School of Continuing Studies, Pinelands, St. Michael, Barbados, West Indies. See also **WIN NEWS,** Vol. 18, No. 3, Summer 1992, p. 11.
49. Boserup, Ester. **Woman's Role in Economic Development**. St. Martin's Press, Inc., New York, 1970, Preface, p. 5.
50. Tinker, Irene. **Persistent Inequalities - Women and World Development**. Published by Oxford University Press, Inc., New York. See also **WIN NEWS,** Vol. 17, No. 1, Winter 1991, pp. 12-15.
51. **Women and Development** is a regular section in every issue of **WIN NEWS**, published quarterly since 1975.

FOOTNOTES (continued)

52. **Engendering Adjustment for the 1990s**, Report of a Commonwealth Expert Group on Women and Structural Adjustment, Commonwealth Secretariat, Marlborough House, Pall Mall, London SW1Y 5HX, England. See also **WIN NEWS** Vol. 16, No. 4, Autumn 1990, pp. 9-12.
53. **WOMEN'S MOVEMENTS OF THE WORLD - An International Directory and Reference Guide**. Edited by: Sally Shreir. Published by: Longman Group UK Limited, Longman House, Burnt Mill, Harlow, Essex CM20 2JE, United Kingdom. Distributed in the US, and Canada by The Oryx Press, 2214 North Central Ave. at Encanto, Phoenix, Arizona 85004.
54. Hosken Fran P. **Testimony - Subcommittee on Foreign Operations of Appropriations Committee**, US Senate, Senator Daniel Inouye, Chair, April 1, 1980. See also **WIN NEWS**, Vol. 6, No. 2, Spring 1980, pp. 32-33.
55. Hosken Fran P. **Testimony - Subcommittee on Foreign Operations of Appropriations Committee,** US Senate, Senator Patrick Leahy, Chair, Washington, DC 20510-6025. Public Witness Hearings, June 15, 1993. See also **WIN NEWS,** Vol. 19, No. 3, Summer 1993, Editorial (Summary).
56. See **WIN NEWS** column on **Women and the United Nations** (every issue) on sexual harassment at the UN. See **WIN NEWS,** Vol. 19, No. 1, Winter 1993, Section on **Women and Development**, pp. 7-9 and Editorial; UNDP Sexual Harassment Policy, see **WIN NEWS** Vol. 19, No. 3, Summer 1993, p. 7.
57. Hosken, Fran P. **Testimony - Foreign Operations Subcommittee, Committee on Appropriations**, US Senate, Senator Patrick Leahy, Chair, June 15, 1993, page 8.
58. Ibid.

THE POLITICS OF POPULATION CONTROL

59. WHO statistics on AIDS in sub-Saharan Africa. World Health Organization, Div. on AIDS, Information Dept., 1211 Geneva 27, Switzerland. See also **WIN NEWS,** Vol. 19, No. 3, Summer 1993, p. 29.
60. Report of the Population Conference 1974 in Bucharest. **See WIN NEWS** Vol. 1, No. 1, Winter 1975, pp. 19-21.
61. United Nations Population Fund (UNFPA), 220 East 42nd St., 18th Floor, New York, NY 10017; Dr. Nafis Sadik, Executive Director.
62. International Planned Parenthood Federation (IPPF). P.O. Box 759, Inner Circle, Regent's Park, London NW1 4LQ England.
63. Cairo Family Planning Association. 50 Goumhouria St., Cairo Egypt; Aziza Hussein, Director. Annual Reports available. FGM Coordinator Ms. Aziza Kamel Mahmoud.
64. Population Action International (PAI), formerly Population Crisis Committee (PCC). 1120 19th St., NW., Suite 550, Washington, DC 20036-3605; Special Projects Fund, Dr. Gordon Wallace, Director.
65. International Planned Parenthood Federation (IPPF) (see Footnote 4). Statement on Female Genital Mutilation by the International Medical Advisory Panel, Nov. 1991.
66. Pathfinder International, Nine Galen St., Suite 217, Watertown, MA 02172-4501.
67. **Population Report**, published by the Population Information Program, Center for Communication Programs, The Johns Hopkins School of Hygiene and Public Health, 527 St. Paul Place, Baltimore, MD 21202 See also **WIN NEWS** Vol. 5, No. 1, Winter 1979, p. 33).
68. Cable sent to all US AID African Missions; From: Dr. Gary Merritt, Chief HPN Div./Office of Technical Resources Africa Bureau AID, Washington, DC 20523. See **WIN NEWS,** Vol. 14, No. 4, Autumn 1988, pp. 21-22.
69. Country Reports on Human Rights Practices, US State Department, see footnote 10.
70. Hosken, Fran P. **Testimony Submitted to the Foreign Operations Subcommittee, Committee on Appropriations,** Senator Patrick Leahy, Chair, June 15, 1993.
71. **Women's Declaration on Population Policies**. Contact: International Women's Health Coalition, 24 East 21st St., New York, NY 10010.

FOOTNOTES (continued)

THE MODERNIZATION OF FEMALE GENITAL MUTILATION

72. Personal communication in author's files.
73. Response to October 1983 issue of **Forum,** anonymous article on FGM surgery. **Forum** is a journal published by FORUM PRESS LTD., 2 Bramber Road, London W14 9PB United Kingdom. Editor: Roger Baker. See **WIN NEWS,** Vol. 10, No. 1, Winter 1984, pp. 38-39.
74. Ibid.
75. Letter in the author's files. See also **WIN NEWS**, Vol. 6, No. 2, Spring 1980, p. 34.
76. Hosken, Fran P. **Testimony Subcommittee on Foreign Operations of Appropriations Committee,** US Senate, Senator Daniel Inouye, Chair, April 1, 1980. See also **WIN NEWS**, Vol. 6, No. 2, Spring 1980, pp. 32-33.

    Other Testimonies by Fran P. Hosken:

    Foreign Affairs Committee, US House of Representatives, Representative Clement J. Zablocki, Chair, March 13, 1981.

    Foreign Relations Committee, US Senate, Senator Charles Percy, Chair, April 22, 1981.

    Subcommittee on Foreign Operations of Appropriations Committee, US Senate, Senator Robert W. Kasten, Jr., Chair, May 14, 1981. See also **WIN NEWS,** Vol. 7, No. 3, Summer 1981, pp. 34-38.

    Subcommittee on Foreign Operations of Appropriations Committee, US Senate, Senator Robert W. Kasten, Jr., Chair, June 8, 1982.
77. **Medical Daily,** a professional newspaper for physicians. March 12, 1981. See also **WIN NEWS,** Vol. 7, No. 2, Spring 1981, p. 35.
78. **Le Monde,** July 22 and 23, 1982. **Le Matin,** July 21, 1982. See also **WIN NEWS** Vol. 8, No. 4, Autumn 1982, pp. 36-38.
79. **The New York Times,** January 11, 1993. See also **WIN NEWS** Vol. 19, No. 2, Spring 1993, p. 50.
80. G.A.M.S. (Groupe Femmes pour L'Abolition des Mutilations Sexuelles), 8, cite Prost, 75011 Paris, France.
81. C.A.M.S. (Commission Internationale pur l'Abolition des Mutilations Sexuelles), B.P. 1969, Dakar, Senegal, Awa Thiam, President. Editor's Note: This latest address in Senegal does not respond. See **WIN NEWS,** Vol. 15, No. 1, Winter 1989, p. 28.
82. **Les Mutilations du Sexe des Femmes Aujourd'hui en France (Sexual Mutilations in France of Today).** Published by Editions Tierce, 1 rue des Fosses St. Jacques 75005, Paris, France. Sponsored by the Ministry of Women's Rights, Mme. Yvette Roudy, Minister, 53, avenue d'lena, 75017 Paris, France.1984. (Ministry no longer exists)
83. Les Mutilations Sexuelles Feminines en France (Female Sexual Mutilations in France - Roundtable Discussion). Organized by the National Secretariat Fighting for Women's Rights of the Socialist Party, November 10, 1984 at the National Assembly. See **WIN NEWS,** Vol. 11, No. 1, Winter 1985, p. 35.
84. Saurel, Renee. **Bouches Cousues: Les Mutilations Sexuelles Feminines et Le Milieu Medical (Mouths Sewn Up: Female Sexual Mutilations and the Medical Establishment).** Published by Editions Tierce, 1, rue des Fosses, Saint-Jacques, 75005 Paris, France. See also **WIN NEWS** Vol. 12, No. 1, Winter 1986, P. 42.
85. Anonymous letter addressed to **WIN NEWS**. See **WIN NEWS,** Vol. 8, No. 4, Autumn 1982, p. 38.
86. Campaign of **WIN NEWS** to eradicate FGM. See **WIN NEWS,** Vol. 8, No. 4, Autumn 1982, p. 40. Campaign regularly reported since then in **WIN NEWS** (once a year).
87. From: **THE OBSERVER** (UK),October 10, 1982. See also **WIN NEWS,** Vol. 8, No. 4, Autumn 1982, p. 39.

FOOTNOTES (continued)

88. FORWARD (the Foundation for Women's Health, Research and Development), 38 King St., London WCZE 8JT, England. Director: Stella Efua Dorkenoo. The purpose and activities of FORWARD have been repeatedly written up since 1986 in **WIN NEWS,** including many FORWARD publications; a newsletter is available.
89. Defence for Children International, P.O. Box 75279, 1070 AG Amsterdam, The Netherlands. See **WIN NEWS**, "The Medicalization of FGM in the Netherlands", Vol. 18, No. 4, Autumn 1992, pp. 30-32; **WIN NEWS,** Vol. 19, No. 1, Winter 1993, pp. 34-36; **WIN NEWS,** Vol. 19, No. 2, Spring 1993, p. 45.
90. See **WIN NEWS**, Vol. 19, No. 2, Spring 1993, p. 45, "NETHERLANDS: ALL FORMS OF FEMALE GENITAL MUTILATION OFFICIALLY REJECTED", Ministry of Foreign Affairs, the Netherlands, Contact: P.P. van Wulfften Palthe, Head of the Legal and Social Affairs Division; also Ministry "WELZIJN VOLKSGEZONDHEID EN CULTUUR" (Health Ministry), Directoraat Generaal van de Volksgezondheid, Postbus 3008, 2280 MK Rijswijk, The Netherlands.
91. Foundation Pharos, Herrenstraat 35, Utrecht, The Netherlands; Mr. Evert Hartog, Director. See **WIN NEWS**, Vol. 19, No. 2, Spring 1993, p. 45.

THE MEDIA AND THE MESSAGE

92. Rosenthal, A.M. Editorial Column, **The New York Times**, December 29, 1992, and July 26, 1993.
93. Hosken, Fran P. "Genital Mutilation of Women in Africa", **Munger Africana Library Notes**. Published by Munger Africana Library, California Institute of Technology, Pasadena, CA 91125. Issue #36, October 1976.
94. Hosken, Fran P. "Female Circumcision and Fertility in Africa", **Women and Health**. Published by Biological Sciences Program, State University of New York, College at Old Westbury, Old Westbury, NY 11568. Vol. 1, #6, Nov./Dec. 1976, pp. 3-11.
95. Hosken, Fran P. "The Epidemiology of Female Genital Mutilation". Published in **Tropical Doctor**, July 1978. Documentation of spread of genital operations in Africa.
96. **BBC Forty Minutes: Female Circumcision,** a film produced by Louise Panton. Also available as video tape. See also **WIN NEWS**, Vol. 9, No. 2, Spring 1983, pp. 62/66.
97. Hosken, Fran P. LES MUTILATIONS SEXUELLES FEMININES, Editions Denoel, 19, rue de l'Universite, 75007 Paris, France, 1983.
98. **Marie Claire Album**, 11 Bis, Rue Boissy, D'Anglas, F 75008 Paris, France. Nov. '83.
99. Thiam, Awa. **La Parole Aux Negresses**. Denoel/Gonthier, 19 rue de l'Universite, 75007 Paris, France, 1978.
100. Commission for the Abolishment of Genital Mutilation (CAGM). Latest known address: Siege Social de la Commission pour l'Abolition des Mutilations Sexuelles, B.P. 1969, Dakar, Senegal.
101. Association of African Women for Research and Development (AAWORD), B.P. 11007, C.D. Annex, Dakar, Senegal. Some of the founding members: Marie Angelique Savane, sociologist from Dakar; Fatima Mernissi, sociologist from Morocco; Dr. Nawal el Sadaawi, M.D. from Egypt, Malica Vajrathon from Thailand.
102. Savane, Marie Angelique. "Why We Are Against the International Campaign", **International Child Welfare Review**, #40, 1979, published by the International Union for Child Welfare, Rue de Varembe 1, 1211 Geneva 20, Switzerland, pp. 37-39.
103. **Sunday Times** (UK), August 15, 1993, **FOCUS** Section, "Talk Poor by Day; Live Rich by Night", cover page and pages 10-11.
104. Hosken, Fran P. **The Universal Childbirth Picture Book**, English Edition, from the Introduction.

WOMEN AND HEALTH: ACTIONS FOR CHANGE

BACKGROUND AND CONTEXT

The purpose of this final chapter is to provide an overview of positive initiatives in Africa to eradicate female genital mutilation (FGM) and to describe the actions in different countries, including local as well as international support. But first some background information on the prevailing health conditions and beliefs that are widely shared in Africa is needed. And since the issue is health, the question must be raised why, after nearly 15 years since the WHO seminar recommended international action, FGM has been steadily increasing in continental Africa from an estimate of 84 million in the early 1980s to more than 110 million estimated now. After nearly 20 years of intensive investigation, field work and constant advocacy, the experiences reported here should provide a basis for what needs to be done. But what is described here is a moving target: There are new initatives being started all the time. The objective is to learn from the experience of those who are working in the field and to exchange information.

The Recommendations of the WHO Seminar in Khartoum were made nearly 15 years ago at a time when the dimensions of FGM and the problems involved were only beginning to be defined. When I began to collect and put together the facts, documentation was scattered throughout the medical and ethnographic literature in four languages and had to be coordinated. It was necessary to travel all over Africa to visit maternity hospitals and talk to midwives and physicians about their experiences. At first it was not at all clear what approach to take. FGM had been so politicized in Africa in the past 50 years, and so well hidden for centuries, that the facts were very difficult to establish.

Through fieldwork and personal contacts as well as through thousands of questionnaires sent all over Africa, I was able at the time of the WHO Seminar to provide an overview of what was practiced and where. Yet my estimates of the numbers of people involved were still far too low. Still it was clear even then that FGM was a public health problem of huge dimensions that had been deliberately neglected and ignored by WHO, UNICEF and all others concerned with health in Africa.

Though in 1979 the very existence of FGM as a health problem was still denied for instance by UNICEF and most other international health programs in Africa and many still try to today, it became clear that the only hope to deal with the issue was going the health route. There are, of course, political, economic, psychological, and sexual problems directly involved, quite aside from ethnic and cultural ones; and the power of "tradition" often is overwhelming, given the absence of formal and especially scientific education in most of Africa, besides the fact that the vast majority of women are illiterate.

In many African countries tradition is further supported by a strong belief structure in magic and supernatural influences, which are quite inaccessible to what we call rational arguments. It is quite futile to argue about beliefs with people convinced of the power of whatever spirits they claim to worship or whatever gods they feel control their lives.

But there is one area that affects everyone's life and where actions can be correlated with tangible results and that is health. Even that approach is often difficult as traditional medicine men and healers as well as traditional birth attendants still have much influence and promote FGM as well as dangerous fertility rites and childbirth practices. But ever since the Khartoum Seminar it has been clear that promoting health is the best avenue for change. This has also been the priority from its start in 1984 by the Inter African Committee and all their affiliates. Health was the center of the first government-supported national program against FGM in Somalia and health is the basis for the oldest and most comprehensive program by the Cairo Family Planning Association.

Health has been a priority in all African development activities to which family planning has been added in the past 15 years in East Africa and recently also in West Africa.

As pointed out in the chapter on Politics, it is astonishing to see that Western health care is introduced and promoted in Africa quite selectively. There has never been any reluctance to propagate new ideas about nutrition or to introduce antibiotics, family planning, malaria campaigns, vaccinations, modern hospitals and surgery and much more - none of which existed in Africa and that some traditionalists opposed. Despite local resistance the smallpox campaign by WHO was a success. In fact, now the problem is that essential drugs and medicines, health equipment and tools, which have to be imported, are very scarce and the most urgent needs cannot be met due to the World Bank/IMF imposed austerity, which puts enormous restrictions on imports.

The point is that by now Western health care is accepted and in great demand especially in urban areas of all African countries, which can be seen by the long queues of people lined up daily in front of every hospital and clinic waiting for services.

It is ironic that the World Bank started the Safe Motherhood Conference and Campaign in 1984, but the World Bank austerity is responsible for the drastic shortages of the most necessary drugs and equipment in maternities all over Africa, causing many unnecessary deaths in childbirth, as I saw for myself when visiting maternities again in 1988 in East and West Africa. If some of the money wasted on glossy publications and "research" by male medical experts would be used to buy urgently needed medicines for women or pay for desperately needed trained midwives, many women and babies could be saved.

Maternities everywhere in Africa are overcrowded, with women two to a bed, and others on the floor: I have never seen sheets in any African maternity -- but no one looks or cares. The Safe Motherhood campaign organizers jet around the world to high-level health ministry conferences in luxury hotels to listen to male "experts". But I don't think they have ever visited an African maternity and seen what I have regularly seen from East to West Africa where even the city hospitals have nothing left to provide maternity services, as their budgets have been cut to pay back the World Bank: So women continue to die.

But this question must finally be asked: Why does the Western health system based on a scientific approach deal with health problems in such selective ways? How is it possible that this system works for the prevention of measles, diphtheria and other childhood diseases and ignores the man-made injuries of thousands of children due to genital mutilation? Why does it deal with malaria but ignores childbirth, though childbirth causes more injuries and deaths than malaria? Why does the Western health care system, which is supposed to serve all people according to need, serve some and not others - especially if they are female? Why are the special needs of women and children so glaringly short-changed, and in the case of genital mutilation, entirely ignored?

Does a little girl suffer any less from an intentionally inflicted mutilation than from a mutilation resulting from a disease such as polio or from being run over by a truck? Why do Western health care systems, supposedly concerned with the prevention of disease, refuse to prevent deliberately inflicted injuries because of "tradition"? Why do we try to prevent assaults and personal attacks and punish those who cause them but allow people who are ignorant about the health facts to mutilate and assault their own children with impunity? Those are the questions that must be asked.

It is always said that it is up to the people involved to make their own decisions: quite true; but they can only do so if and when they have the information they need to make a viable choice in the interest of themselves and their children. At present, as the chapter on Politics shows, such access to information has been denied, especially to women. What is more, the children directly affected are quite unable to speak for themselves. To do nothing to protect girls from the mutilations, saying they and their families should decide, is a cynical evasion of responsibility. The primary victims are mostly too young to even know what is being done to them; yet they will have to live with the consequences of the mutilations for their entire lives. The tragedy is that where women bear a dozen children or more no one has bothered to teach these people the basic biological facts about their own bodies in a form which they can understand.

Yet both WHO and UNICEF proved a few years ago with the global Oral Re-Hydration program that illiterate women on the grass roots-level can be taught new ways to take care of their children - even if it is against tradition - and save them from certain death.

Traditional Practices and Health Education

All the research in Africa and the Middle East, as reported in the country case histories, makes it clear that none of the people involved in traditional practices have a realistic knowledge about their own bodies or about the biological facts: They lack the most basic concepts of health despite many years and millions spent on "development". Mass communication has never been used in the service of health or in an organized way to teach the people in Africa how their bodies function. The same is true in most other developing countries. Family planning has reached most areas, but one looks in vain for any health education program, though radio reaches most rural areas in Africa.

The first need is health education and information before real choices can be made. Only when the biological facts of reproduction, based on scientific and factual grounds, are available to all families, can they knowingly and responsibly decide if they wish to have their children operated - after they weigh the health and social facts. For instance, every delegate who spoke at the WHO Khartoum Seminar in 1979 emphasized the same overwhelming need for health information and health education for all the people, not just the few involved in the delivery of health care.

Since then, everyone in Africa with whom I talked about FGM emphasized the need for basic health and sex education; but unfortunately in many countries the missionaries got there first and started schools. Sex education was excluded from the start, and though governments took over the schools long ago, the curriculum has been influenced by the missionaries and they were the ones who taught the present teachers. But it is not necessary to look to Africa for the failure to teach young people what they need to know; the battle against sex education has been going on in schools all over the US for years.

As a result, most of the health problems that women face due to genital operations are not attributed to their cause. Though it is known that the operations are dangerous, the health problems and the fatalities that result are almost never blamed on the mutilations. Rather it is believed that they were caused by all kinds of evil spirits or because the rituals had not been properly observed or because the victim was bewitched or had done something wrong. Cause and effect are not related.

In the absence of any education on reproduction and sexuality or about the biological facts of life, the stories and traditional myths are the reality for most people in Africa and the Middle East who practice genital mutilation. In the traditional environment, people are convinced of the necessity for the operations; and most women believe that they are done everywhere else in the world - hence there is no alternative. To question customs in a collective village society simply does not occur. Decisions are made by the chief and the elders for the group and never by an individual.

To someone who has no acquaintance with science or biology, the process described - for instance in a scientific explanation of reproduction - may be entirely mysterious and strange. What proof can we show that a cell divides the way it does unless we have a microscope? How do we explain that bacteria are responsible for infections and not the evil eye of a neighbor or an evil spirit that needs to be appeased?

Therefore it is important to provide information in ways that are understood which is the reason why the **Childbirth Picture Books (CBPB)** teach with pictures: they have separate sections on excision and infibulation. But to understand the damage done by the mutilations, it is necessary to first understand how normal reproduction functions. To make sure that the **CBPB**s are understood, they were first sent in loose-leaf form for comments to midwives and health educators all over the world. (See Appendix.)

But where most people are illiterate, tradition wins. Despite the mandate of UNESCO, which is charged with education and literacy training, more then 45 years after the Agency was established, there are more illiterate women than ever and the literacy gap between women and men is constantly growing. Without being able to read, education remains a closed door and custom is the only way information is transmitted from one generation to the next. While many customs may be useful, evolved to solve everyday problems in often harsh rural environments, the traditional practices in health or the absence of any scientific approach, results in early death, as the life expectancy statistics confirm - which are still the lowest in the world in Africa.

In the search for answers to problems, tradition is regularly invoked. "It is the custom" is usually the most persuasive justification for almost any practice - especially where health measures are involved. Everywhere, custom is reinforced by fear. Over and over the notion is expressed that a terrible fate is in store for those who dare to defy custom. What we call myths is the reality for people who have no access to the biological facts of life. (See: The Politics of FGM: The Reasons Given)

In turn, the information about reproduction and sexuality that comes from the West instead of being freely available and openly taught is similarly mystified and concealed, especially from the young, who need this information most of all. Our bodies and normal physical functions are treated as being shameful and surrounded by patriarchal tabus - much in the same way as many of the traditional beliefs.

How is a young person growing up with so many conflicting ideas and tabus about reproduction and sexuality to know the truth? How can a girl or young woman, who often pays with her health and even her life for her ignorance, learn what she most urgently needs to know? She is indoctrinated from early childhood into believing the traditions. Even if she is going to school, no one teaches about reproduction or human biology, least of all, about sex. Formal education and schools were introduced in most of Africa by Christian missionaries; they also introduced the idea that sex is sin and reproduction a subject that cannot be discussed, let alone taught in the schools. Though millions are spent on family planning, factual information about reproduction is still mostly unknown.

"Why should anyone trust the medicine from abroad when so many people die when they go to the hospital?"; "Why ask the man at the clinic who hands out some pills when the potion of the local medicine man has cured your friend?"; "Why use some new medicine instead of doing what your grandmother told you to do?"; "It has always been done this way; it is the wish of the ancestors and they know best."

All over Africa, it is still widely believed that uncircumcised women have difficulties in childbirth, though exactly the opposite is true. In some ethnic groups, cuts into the vagina are made in addition to excision, for instance in Kenya and Sierra Leone, "to make childbirth easier". The result, on the contrary, may be fatal.

The idea of excessive growth of the clitoris - or hypertrophy - seems to be propagated in the most diverse regions, for instance in Ethiopia as well as Nigeria and Burkina Faso. Hypertrophy of the clitoris appears in the historical medical literature going back to Roman times (see "History"). It is interesting that one can find the notion that hypertrophy of the clitoris afflicts African women also in some medical articles (all written by men), and of course, it has been propagated by the anthropologists, quite aside from Catholic missionaries (see Case History: Ethiopia). Thus, the clitoris has to be amputated for reasons of health. But why a large clitoris is "unhealthy," while a large penis is not, none of the men, including physicians, have ever been able to say.

In West Africa, men claim that the clitoris is "dangerous"; that it is injurious to a man to have intercourse with a woman who has a clitoris and impairs his potency. It is also claimed that it damages the baby during birth and is a dangerous organ that obstructs intercourse and must be removed. (See :he Politics of FGM: The Reasons Given.)

Given this sample of health beliefs, which are still very widespread, it would seem especially important that the biological facts be openly discussed and made widely known to protect the younger generation. Radio by now reaches most of the villages; cassette tapes can be played most everywhere and also in privacy, even where there is no electricity; to listen, you don't need to be able to read. Communication technology is inexpensive and ubiquitous. Rock music and its stars are known everywhere, including in African villages, because their tapes go everywhere. The same technology could be used to teach about health - it costs much less to prevent problems than to build hospitals.

The question of who should teach the young about reproduction and sexuality has not been solved: In Africa and the Middle East, the problem is acute because the majority of the people and therefore also all teachers have been brought up with the same misconceptions about human biology. Contrary to what one might believe the internationally designed family planning programs have failed to transmit even the most basic facts about reproductive health, especially to women.

Health is a big business in Africa. Traditional remedies of all kinds, including protective necklaces, bracelets, amulets, are sold in most local markets, ranging from snakeskins to fertility dolls, dried animal parts and organs, as well as secret herbal potions , roots, powders and pastes to be ingested or smeared on the body. Traditional healers sell their wares and their skills in all markets. Their secret remedies including various kinds of surgery are surrounded by magic. The procedures include all kinds of cuts and tribal markings, most of them dangerous, especially those related to childbirth. They advocate their remedies with all kinds of propaganda and attract unsuspecting customers, promising instant cures in the absence of factual health education.

Schoolteachers in Africa and the Middle East have little access to basic health publications and even less information about reproduction - they certainly are not equipped to teach about health practices let alone about reproduction. A few years ago I talked to the minister in charge of primary education in Kenya - which is far ahead of many other African countries where schools are concerned, though even Kenya cannot meet the demand. Ms Julia Ojambo told me, when I suggested sending the schools copies of the **Childbirth Picture Books,** that there were no teachers who could introduce such a subject. And she quickly added they had no money to train them.

Education about reproduction should be the responsibility of the health departments and taught from a health point of view, especially since fertility is so important in African and Middle Eastern life. But health departments, despite their name, are mostly concerned with illness and curative care, following the imported Western model of institutionalized medicine. What is called health education in Africa and the Middle East is almost exclusively concerned with training of a professional sector; that is, those who make a living from health care rather than educating the general public in what all people most urgently need to know. Thus, health education for the people and especially information about reproduction and sexuality, in countries where women's entire adult lives are spent on childbearing and childrearing, are not available and never in a form that is accessible regardless of language or literacy. Therefore the damaging traditions continue.

To compound the problem, it is estimated by WHO that probably only a small percentage of the population in the rural areas of most African countries has any contact with modern health care during their entire lives. Therefore, health education by audio and visual means is especially important: it also costs far less and can reach many more people than curative care. But the education of the average woman and mother in the fundamentals of keeping healthy is entirely ignored by all health departments because it is not considered a professional concern.

Among the many damaging traditional practices that were first discussed at the WHO Seminar in Khartoum is the practice of cauterization, that is, burning the skin with red hot irons or needles, which is very widespread as treatment for many ailments in the Sudan, the Middle East and also Nigeria. For instance, a baby's stomach is burned with a hot iron as treatment against diarrhea or stomach ache. Most of the time the wound becomes infected; if the children die from the remedy, the death is blamed on evil spirits rather than on the treatment.

Another treatment is cutting the uvula out of the throats of babies, which is practiced in Ethiopia, Nigeria and other areas as well. Many of the babies die as a result. "It is necessary," the people say, but no one can explain why it is done. Cutting or filing of teeth is another of the many health traditions that have so far been mostly ignored claiming that "culture and tradition must be preserved". Attempts to assist victims for instance of FGM are frequently accompanied by charges of "interference" by traditionalists supported by anthropologists - especially where damage to women and children is involved.

Many of the beliefs propagated today in Africa and the Middle East about women's bodies, reproduction and sexuality (see Country Reports) can be found in historical accounts of medieval Europe. Indeed, many of these beliefs existed all over the world up to and including Victorian times (see The Western World). It is also interesting to note that though some Protestant missionaries, for instance in Kenya, opposed female genital mutilation, especially medical missionaries, they never taught women or men about reproduction and health, nor do the missionaries today.

The Implication of Religion in Health

Cleanliness is a reason frequently cited all over Africa when advocating FGM, implying purity is an important virtue of women, with religious overtones. Though it is stated that FGM is not a religious command either by Moslems or Animists nor that it is promoted by any other religion, the facts given here speak for themselves.

In Sudan it is said that a woman is unclean unless she is operated, and this belief - that excision is necessary for cleanliness, health and purity as becomes a moslem woman - is very widespread also in Egypt. The Arabic name for the operation, "Tahara", means purification, with religious implications. The notion that a woman's sexual organs are a source of pollution and that all her normal sexual functions, such as menstruation, are dirty and shameful, is widespread not only in the Middle East and in Arab and Moslem countries, but the very same ideas are also found in Christianity and continue to be propagated via the Bible around the world.

In many African and Middle Eastern countries, especially those under Moslem influence, the idea is propagated that women's sexuality is dangerous; that girls who are not operated "run wild" and are promiscuous and prostitutes, damaging the honor and religious standing of their families. The operations, it is said, must be done because women cannot control their sexuality. This is, of course, an exact description of male sexuality - which is aggressive and promiscuous - transferred onto women by those who seek to control women's sexuality and lives: men. As elsewhere in the world, female sexuality is defined by men and religion is used to uphold and enforce male power and control.

Christianity, Islam and Judaism all originated from the same Middle Eastern area and background; they all share to a remarkable degree their attitudes toward women's bodies, sexuality and health, as well as ideas about chastity and reproduction. The inferiority that is bestowed on women and the contempt expressed for women's normal, healthy, biological functions by the male leadership is shared by these three man-made Middle Eastern religious systems and has been upheld over the centuries by their male hierarchies. They also support food tabus, which especially damage pregnant women.

This claimed inferiority of women, decreed by these religious systems, is based on total ignorance of the normal and healthy biological functions of women's bodies. Therefore, the religious hierarchies preserve ignorance and mystify or withhold the biological facts. Women's reproductive functions are called dirty and despised because they are different from those of men, and thus not "normal", since "man is the measure of all things". But, since men depend on women for children and for sexual pleasure, this dependence is the reason for attacks on women's bodies, sexuality, and biological functions because nothing is so difficult for men to bear than dependence - which connotes inferiority.

It is, of course, maddening for a man to realize that he totally depends on a woman to reproduce himself to have an heir and perpetuate his line. This has been sufficient reason throughout history for the bloodiest orgy against women's bodies and health - which goes on to the present time under various disguises, not the least of which is our modern, technologized, male-dominated medical system.

Historically, the ignorance and fear of women's natural, biological functions and sexuality are documented in countless traditional rituals, for instance those related to menstruation, about which women have published much recently. Most of these rituals are damaging to women's health and self-respect. For instance, girls and women who menstruate are locked up in separate huts, are not allowed to eat with the family and are isolated from everyone. Such punishing customs are not limited to Africa, but are also traditional in parts of Asia, and so are many food tabus for women.

The ignorance about women's bodies is, of course, maintained and exploited by all religious systems organized by men, to establish their own superiority and maintain "on moral grounds" the inferiority of women. The objective is control of women's bodies and sexuality, by declaring the biological superiority of women "dirty, polluted and inferior". Ignorance about the biological truth has to be maintained at any price; hence, even now, sex education is banned from most schools by the ruling patriarchal system in all parts of the world.

Religious systems, especially Christian and Islamic, as well as the various African Animist beliefs that are prevalent in the areas discussed here, where female genital mutilation is practiced (often under the label of health), all have a vested interest to keep women ignorant about their own bodies and biological potentialities - thus under male control.

Christianity, historically and to the present time, has controlled female sexuality, claiming female sexuality is sinful. For instance, even now, the Pope decrees that masturbation is a mortal sin - it is said to be damaging to health, though this is entirely untrue and contrary to biological fact.

Health is often the reason given for all the different methods used by men to control and destroy women's bodies and natural biological functions: Organized religion, no matter what the system, has everywhere in the world (not only limited to Africa and the Middle East) been the ready tool to subjugate women by strictly regulating female sexuality and by mystifying the natural processes of reproduction, which are then distorted to fit religious rules: Priests and medicine men are often the same.

In medieval European history - which was so strongly dominated by the Catholic Church - one can learn about practices brutalizing and abusing women's bodies and health and exploiting women's biological functions similar to what goes on in some areas in Africa today including beliefs in witchcraft and supernatural powers which then serve as excuses to persecute women. But African men have succeeded beyond the wildest dreams of men anywhere else in the world: They have persuaded women to mutilate their own female children knowing the horrible pain and permanent damage this causes.

A child psychologist, who works with abused children, once explained this to me: You can gain the allegiance of a child by inflicting some terrible torture or punishment. This child will then do whatever you want and become dependent on the abuser once the torture has broken his or her will. I had asked this question in seeking an answer to why a mother would torture her child much as she was tortured herself. After being exposed to this terrible subject for so many years, as a mother I find this impossible to understand.

If you know that generation after generation girls are mutilated in this terrible torturous way which makes childbirth a horrendous ordeal that African men force on women year after year, it seems that there must be something missing, women's resiliance is gone, they become dependent victims of men who use them and abuse them at will. After centuries of such abuse apparently the very possiblility of revolt no longer exists, there is no psychological resistance left and women become malleable victims with seemingly no will of their own and unable to oppose FGM.

In the past, traditional practices that often greatly damage women's bodies and health could be attributed to ignorance about the biological facts (see The Western World). This is no longer true today. However, organized religion, whatever the faith or name, is, as the record shows, a constant danger to women's health and sexuality.

In most of Africa, the Middle East, parts of Asia and also in some countries in Latin America, girls often are married very young without their consent; that is they have no viable choice. A married woman - and this is sanctified by all organized, male-headed religions - cannot refuse sex or to bear children, even if it means her death.

In most societies today, religious institutions backed by the patriarchal system are in the forefront of denying women access to biological facts and in propagating damaging myths about women's sexuality under the label of "morality".

The myths about female genital mutilation persist to this day - yet no one, not governmental health departments or family planning organizations or development advisors or least of all educated Africans in their own countries, do anything to teach the truth about women's health and the facts about reproduction. Rather, religion continues to be readily available to be used as an excuse to mutilate female children under the label that this is the way to keep "order" in society and enforce morality.

It is interesting to note that many African men after getting an education at a European or an American university go home, marry several wives and have all their daughters mutilated. I interviewed some UN officials from African countries who readily admitted that they had all their daughters done because "this is our tradition".

INITIATIVES TO ERADICATE FEMALE GENITAL MUTILATION

IAC - THE INTER AFRICAN COMMITTEE ON TRADITIONAL PRACTICES AFFECTING THE HEALTH OF WOMEN AND CHILDREN

The Inter African Committee was organized in 1984 at the Seminar on Traditional Practices Affecting the Health of Women and Children in Dakar five years after the WHO Seminar in Khartoum of the same name was held for government health departments. Already in 1979 in Khartoum it was proposed to hold another seminar in West Africa, because few Westafrican countries were able to send delegations due to travel problems at that time. (See: WHO Seminar and Case History: Senegal.) [1]

The Dakar Seminar was organized by the Working Group on Female Circumcision/ Sub-Committee on the Status of Women, a Non-Governmental Organization accredited to the United Nations in Geneva, which was headed by Berhane Ras-Work from Ethiopia and was hosted by Senegal with WHO and UNICEF providing technical and financial support. The Recommendations of the Khartoum Seminar in 1979 on Traditional Practices Affecting the Health of Women and Children were unanimously accepted and confirmed at that meeting and were detailed and expanded, providing the basis for an action plan adopted by all IAC affiliates. The IAC has been headed since its organization by Berhane Ras-Work and has offices in Addis Ababa at the ECA (Economic Commission of Africa) regional center and in Geneva.

From the beginning the IAC has endeavored to set up local groups in all African countries where FGM is practiced in order to start and carry on education and information programs about the dangers and damage done by FGM. These local committees carry on workshops and training programs; they distribute educational materials and bring the issue of FGM to the attention of policymakers. The IAC and their local groups have succeeded to inform especially the leadership as well as a large part of the population in each country about the dangers of FGM and other damaging traditions, such as child marriage, food tabus and damaging childbirth practices.

At the Forum of the 1985 UN Women's Decade Conference in Nairobi, Kenya, in July 1985, the IAC organized a number of workshops and panel discussions to overflow audiences. These meetings were coordinated by Berhane Ras-Work with women from many different African countries discussing the situation regarding FGM in their countries and outlining plans on what to do. Several physicians, including Dr. Koso-Thomas from Sierra Leone, first explained the medical facts to the women from all over the world in the audience, many of whom had never heard about FGM. [2] Reports from Sudan, Gambia, Togo, Senegal, Mali, Benin, Gambia, Ghana, Nigeria, Liberia, Sierra Leone and Egypt were included. A representative from the Health Ministry of Kenya explained the prohibition of FGM by President Moi, but Kenya had not organized a committee affiliated with the IAC. There were also a number of other meetings on FGM: This was quite a contrast to the previous United Nations Women's Conference in 1980 in Copenhagen where a group of African women organized by Marie Angelique Savane from Dakar disrupted meetings on FGM and attacked those who tried to speak for the victims of FGM - which attracted a lot of press attention. (See The Politics of FGM.)

The IAC is committed to holding regional seminars every few years in order to bring together all the affiliates, set priorities and adopt an action plan. The most recent meeting was held in Addis Ababa in November 1990, and another one is proposed for February 1994. The week-long meeting in 1990 [3] was held at Africa Hall of the ECA the regional UN agency. Among the opening speeches was one by the UN Under Secretary and Executive Director of the ECA, the Minister of Health of the Ethiopian Government (which since then has changed) and other influential national and international leaders.

THE INTER AFRICAN COMMITTEE (continued)

Delegations from IAC affiliates from more than 20 countries participated and spoke at the 1990 Conference. Due to the political problems and civil wars that continue all over Africa, some of the IAC affiliates had to be reorganized since, as in many African countries, all organizations are part of the government. When a government changes, all organizations lose support. Therefore, the number of IAC affiliates changes, but recently there have been between 22 and 26.

A regional network such as the IAC has developed is all-important in the battle against FGM as otherwise each group from each country would compete for scarce financial support against all others. Especially initially, support from like-minded groups and financing is needed. What is more, educational and training materials can be shared as well as the experience gained from one country or area that can be most useful elsewhere. In a recent IAC president's report, the many different activities are outlined which are summarized as follows:

- Special Training and Information Campaigns;
- Training or Orientation of Traditional Birth Attendants and Other Practitioners;
- Setting up of National IAC Committees and Supporting Zonal Meetings;
- Preparation and Distribution of Reports on Seminars and Workshops, as well as of Educational and Information Matertials;
- Support of Research Activities; Evaluations; Advocacy; Fundraising. [4]

A number of Resolutions and Recommendations were made at the 1990 Conference, which are printed in their entirety in the Conference Report, which was published a year after the Conference and is one of the most comprehensive documents on the subject of FGM. A specific resolution regarding the definition of the practice was passed at that meeting and has made a worldwide impact:

> "Considering that the term 'female circumcision' could be misleading and may not fully describe the extent of the practices, the delegates of this conference recommend that this term be replaced with 'Female Genital Mutilations' (FGM)".

Included among the international recommendations were that regular meetings should be held between the countries concerned to exchange information and that follow-up and supervisory visits should be made regularly. Immigrant populations from Africa in Europe, America, etc., should be supported and the religious leaders of all denominations should be invited to publicly denounce FGM.

In the closing speech Berhane Ras-Work encouraged everyone "to appeal to your respective governments to consider seriously the resolutions. . . and instruct the relevant institutions to implement them. . . to free women from practices that diminish them mentally and physically. . ."

A film about the work of the IAC - now made into a videotape - was shown for the first time at the 1990 Conference- made by Swedish filmmakers. It covers some of the activities of IAC affiliates, for instance in Nigeria: In rural areas and marketplaces male excisors still operate quite openly on dozens of little girls - many only a few years old. Interviews with a number of African women from different countries are included who reject the operations and describe their terrible ordeals. In the introduction of the film African women leaders including Berhane Ras-Work and the head of the Nigerian IAC Committee Dr. Irene Thomas speak about the objectives of the IAC and its activities. This videotape is now distributed by the IAC office in Geneva.

In a 1993 activity report of the IAC some of the programs by affiliates in different countries are summarized which include training and information campaigns, training of trainers' programs and sensitization activities. Workshops are conducted for different groups for instance, of women's leaders and community health workers. The experience gained in one area or country can be usefully applied in others. For instance, the teaching materials and training of trainers'-programs developed by AIDoS - the Italian Association for Women in Development initially for Somalia have been adapted for use by the IAC and adopted for training by different countries. (See Case History: Somalia.)

THE INTER AFRICAN COMMITTEE (continued)

Another IAC program is concerned with providing former excisors with training for other ways to earn their living as the economic incentive is considerable. At the 1990 IAC Conference in Addis Ababa a group of local women, former excisors, organized a fair for conference participants, showing and selling their craft products from handwoven traditional women's scarfs to a variety of household products. It is essential to develop some other income-generating activities for excisors in order to persuade them to stop doing the operations which provide them with a good income as well as respect in their communities. FGM practitioners will continue to do the operations underground even where it is prohibited unless some other way is found to enable them to earn their living.

The activities of the IAC provide an important framework of mutual support, exchange of information and financial support, which is invaluable. Most of allthe IAC brings those who are working to stop FGM together and out of their isolation of being associated with activities that many in their own communities do not approve of. Quite aside from the important financial support, the IAC is able to provide by fundraising all over the world on behalf of the many local groups. Mutual support, recognition of their work and encouragement are essential. The Africa-wide IAC Conferences, as well as regional meetings, serve also as educational experiences for affiliates and for personal contact.

Exchange of information and especially exchange of technical skills - how to develop and structure programs as well as training - are invaluable support services by the IAC. Since FGM is spread over so many countries with many different local practices and ethnic groups involved, speaking different national and local languages, it is essential to have regional leadership and coordination which the IAC is providing. The attitudes toward FGM vary greatly with different countries, regions and ethnic groups. Therefore it is important to set priorities and to focus on what has been successful and this the IAC, as a network, can supply. One objective, is to continue to build national organizations.

For years international agencies, for instance UNICEF and WHO, had been able to claim that "Female circumcision is a local custom by a few isolated groups that is dying out" and therefore it did not merit any attention. The IAC has forcefully been able to assert the fact that FGM is a major public health problem that requires international attention.

The IAC as an African organization speaks for African women both in Africa and around the world. At the recent OAU (Organization of African Unity) Conference on Assistance to African Children in November 1992 in Dakar Senegal, Berhane Ras-Work spoke on the subject of girl children in Africa. Her statement was included in the final conference report where she stressed the necessity to "protect the female child from all forms of harmful traditional practices and in particular to the elimination of such practices as female genital mutilation. . ." [5]

The IAC participated in the UN Human Rights Conference in Vienna in June 1993 and called on delegates to adopt legislation to prevent the performance of FGM and other harmful practices. A workshop on FGM was also organized at the Fôrum, the parallel Conference organized at every UN Conference by the Non-Governmental Organizations. The IAC recently has been granted consultative status by the Economic and Social Council of the UN. which greatly strengthens its status and ability to gain support from governments as well as United Nations bodies - especially WHO and UNICEF.

Another IAC Conference is planned for February 1994 in Conakry, Guinea, in West Africa. This meeting had been originally scheduled for Sudan but had to be postponed and moved to West Africa due to political conditions. This will also be the 10th Anniversary of the founding of the IAC, which should be credited with changing the attitudes of governments and most of all of people all over the world.

In Africa today the IAC has become an important influence and is accepted as speaking for women's health concerns. This is a remarkable achievement, since until ten years ago no African woman dared to speak about FGM in Africa and no African government would tolerate any discussion of what was then called "female circumcision". That the IAC is speaking for African women's health also all over the world should be continuously emphasized especially now when in Europe and the US FGM is starting to be exploited by some and used as a media event. But the real concerns and needs of African women, representd by the IAC, need much more effective support to implement change.

THE INTER AFRICAN COMMITTEE OF NIGERIA

The Nigerian IAC [6] is headed by Dr. Irene Thomas ,the first woman physician of Nigeria, and is the most active IAC affiliate. In Nigeria, the most populous African country, a majority of the population practices FGM, and many other damaging traditional practices are widespread (see Case History: Nigeria). Ms. E.M. Alabi, a midwife and health educator, is the coordinator of the extensive activities of the Committee which are outlined below. A newsletter **My Task** is published biannually, which reports on the national and international activities of the Nigerian IAC and is summarized here:

> **Training and Information Campaigns (TIC)** to sensitize and mobilize communities are organized to think, talk and act against all harmful traditional practices. It is a three tier program - on the Federal, State and Local level. At the Federal level, a workshop was held for officials of the Health Ministry and international organizations such as WHO and UNFPA and representatives from various Ministries and different States of the Federation. The participants went home well-equipped for the campaign against these practices. Six states of the Federation also held workshops with a total of about 700 participants in attendance. The objective is for participants to mobilize and sensitize the communities on the grass-roots level - creating awareness for positive action. The third phase is taking place at the community level where people from all walks of life assemble for mobilization. It is envisaged that the communities continue the crusade using churches, mosques, women's and other groups as well as house to house campaiging to sensitize and mobilize people.
>
> **Training of Traditional Birth Attendants** (TBA) and traditional healers who are the core of health care providers at the grass-roots level. These groups of health care providers complement the services of health personnel; it is essential to educate them in order to update their skills, knowledge and practices as well as to sensitize them about harmful traditional practices. Training programs have been conducted in many locations with hundreds of TBAs trained and health workers retrained.
>
> **Training of Trainers**: They will train and retrain TBAs in their communities. Regular meetings should be held with TBAs where experiences are shared and problems solved. With education and sensitization of TBAs and other health workers, enlightenment of communities toward eradication of harmful practices is accomplished: Once trained, they become members of IAC. They are expected to join the campaign against FGM and other harmful traditional practices, to hold regular meetings and organize fund-raising activities. Follow-up visits are made regularly.

A Plan of Action is prepared once a year, the Executive Council meets and a general assembly of the Nigerian Committee is held in Lagos. Talks are organized for professional groups, for influential and religious leaders, for decision makers and for NGOs; also radio and TV talks and campaigns on harmful traditional practices in churches, mosques and youth clubs. Other actions planned are to lecture in the schools on FGM. A task force on the eradication of fistulae and on child marriage has been organized. Other actions include:

- Three-day programs on Training and Information Campaigns (TIC) in ten state capitals and a one-day program in fifteen local government areas;
- Training of Trainers (TOT) to continue with the further training programs and supervision of TBAs within their states of origin;
- Seven research grants to study and document the prevalence and influence of certain harmful traditional practices.

Membership throughout the Federation is increasing as more Nigerians including school children join in the crusade against harmful traditional practices and hold discussions in rural and urban settings to raise awareness.

In a research paper on "Traditional Methods of Childbirth in Africa - The Nigerian Experience" Ms. Alabi, the IAC coordinator for Nigeria, discusses not only the traditional methods of delivery but also dietary restrictions and prenatal care as well as postpartum treatments that are threatening women's health - making the activities of the IAC especially important as women's health needs have been quite ignored.

The traditional childbirth practices to which Nigerian women are subjected even now result in some of the highest childbirth mortality figures anywhere in Africa. Despite the oil wealth of the country, women's health needs have been very much neglected. Yet all men demand large families and fertility is considered all-important. One of the most damaging traditional practices discussed by Ms. Alabi are the "Gishiri" cuts made in the vagina by traditional operators to widen the birth canal. (See Case History : Nigeria). Ms. Alabi outlines some of the health care problems of women in Nigeria:

> "Nigeria, which has a large population . . . , is faced with serious limitations such as inadequate health facilities and trained personnel. As a result, 70 percent of childbearing women depend on traditional birth attendants, traditional healers and herbalists for their health care who are usually illiterates without any formal training in delivery procedures and with strong beliefs in supernatural powers . . . " [7]

The IAC Nigerian National Committee, Ms. Alabi states, has worked since the end of 1989 " to ameliorate health and to create awareness in various communities on existing harmful traditional childbirth practices." As outlined above, the committee works on sensitizing the public by using all available media, teaching in marketplaces, schools, mosques and churches, they contact policymakers, village and district heads and community leaders.

THE NATIONAL ASSOCIATION OF NIGERIA NURSES/NURSE MIDWIVES (NANNM)

In 1985-86, NANNM [8] conducted a survey of FGM practices in all 19 states which revealed that it was practiced in 13 states, and in 5 states an estimated 90 percent of women underwent some type of FGM. From 1988-1990 the members of this professional association carried out a nationwide eradication of harmful traditional practices campaign that included FGM, child marriage and nutritional tabus with financial support from Population Action International (formerly the Population Crisis Committee) and technical assistance from PATH (Program in Appropriate Technology for Health).

NANNM conducted a program that started with a national workshop in Lagos. At the workshop, the head of the Nursing and Midwifery Council of Nigeria, Mrs. R.O. Sofenwa, said that the traditional reasons given for FGM were no longer tenable in this present age because many of the female children were permanently damaged for life through the operation. Following this, 11 state workshops were held in states chosen for their high rate of harmful traditional practices. Communication strategies were designed after NANNM members had conducted focus group discussions and learned reasons for and attitudes about the practices.

The first phase focused on training of trainers who in turn conducted training and educational activities at state and community levels. Drama, market promotions and community mobilization and educational campaigns carried the message of the harmful effects of female circumcision. The nurses also used the print and electronic media to disseminate their message. The Project Director took part in a national television talk show, and other local NANNM leaders appeared on radio broadcasts. Articles about FGM were published in national newspapers. The project stimulated open discussion about the topic; an evaluation was scheduled to be conducted in 1993 to determine what behavioral changes have taken place. Anecdotal evidence from circumcisors in Southern Nigeria suggests that their business has fallen off as reported by the **London Observer.**

WOMEN'S HEALTH ISSUES IN NIGERIA, [9] is the title of a recently published collection of research studies on women's health issues in book form, written by Nigerian women. It is edited by Mere N. Kisekka, a professor and coordinator of the Women in Development Unit of Ahmadu Bello University, and is the first detailed study on women's health problems by Nigerian women. The book includes a chapter on "Female Circumcision and Other Dangerous Practices" as well as discussions of maternal mortality and reproductive rights, sociocultural factors causing maternal mortality and morbidity, also a chapter on "Women's Organized Health·Struggles", linking the local initiatives with international ones. This book provides detailed documentation of the health problems faced by Nigerian women, showing that there is a long and difficult struggle ahead - especially against traditional practices - that has only just begun.

EGYPT: THE CAIRO FAMILY PLANNING ASSOCIATION PROJECT [10]

This program - the first one organized anywhere to stop FGM - called **"Project on the Physical Violation of young Females"** was initiated by a seminar in October 1979 in which many leaders in the health field participated and which received much publicity. The seminar studied the problem from several aspects: The health, social and religious implications were discussed as well as the official stand by the Egyptian health authorities.

A plan of action based on recommendations for educating the Egyptian public was outlined, with the aim of working toward the promulgation of a firm law. The Cairo Family Planning Association (CFPA) accepted the responsibility for implementation of these recommendations, beginning this work in October 1981. First the Coordinator made a study of 500 women aged 20 to 30. The results showed that 80 percent of them were excized; the reason given was custom. This plan was made three years before the IAC was organized and was a ground-breaking event. (See Case History: Egypt.) Recently the program was formally affiliated with the IAC as the Egyptian National Committee.

This initiative is the most comprehensive program working under conditions quite different than most others. Egypt is much more urbanized than other African countries where FGM is practiced and has a highly developed health system compared with sub-Saharan Africa, as well as one of the largest government sponsored family planning programs. The CFPA, which is privately sponsored, has always functioned as innovator and leader. The very large Egyptian Population Program, supported by the US Agency for International Development (USAID), has ignored FGM. **The Childbirth Picture Books (CBPB)** by **WIN NEWS** translated into Arabic have been widely used in Egypt by both programs since 1984; but only the CFPA is using the **CBPB** Additions to prevent FGM.

Each project by the Cairo Family Planning Association first undertakes research on the basis of which the programs are formulated. The activities of the committee are concerned with education and information, seeking "the integration of measures against harmful traditional practices in all sectors of health, education, economic and social development programs and policies. . ." After working on this problem for more than 12 years, a great deal of valuable experience has been gained.

Egypt has an extensive health and hospital system especially in metropolitan Cairo, which is a huge urbanized region, and there are many other cities and towns including Alexandria. Therefore, the work and programs to eradicate FGM in Egypt are different from the activities in most other African countries that have a mostly rural population. The project has developed many channels for reaching and educating the public including through nursing schools, women's associations and especially the mass media. Some examples of these activities are cited in their reports:

- Production and distribution of booklets and printed materials in English and Arabic;
- Personal contacts, distribution of information in childhealth and family planning centers and intensifying face-to-face campaigns with people at different meeting places, utilizing audiovisual methods;
- Using mobile units headed by social workers to reach different communities and groups as well as homes;
- Identifying and enlisting trained and professional groups and organizations such as social workers, physicians, midwives, nurses, teachers and women's groups.

In the most recent annual report, the CFPA states that it has succeeded in having information on the hazards of FGM included in family life education as well as in school curricula and medical as well as nursing training programs. Such inclusion of information especially in all family planning and other ongoing health programs is certainly the most cost-effective and the most efficient and comprehensive method to deal with FGM which could be introduced everywhere else in Africa where national family planning programs have been set up. The media campaign against FGM carried on by the Cairo Family Planning Association sets an example by involving community leaders and especially physicians, nurses and others in the health system in this broad-based campaign.

EGYPT: THE CAIRO FAMILY PLANNING ASSOCIATION PROJECT (continued)

In Egypt media development, the press, radio and TV as well as filmmaking are highly developed. This offers many opportunities for communication. Highly respected leaders in their professions are speaking out in the media against the operations. This is especially important because as reported in the Case History on Egypt, every Egyptian hospital continues to get cases of bleeding girls due to the operations, many of whom are severely injured. Yet this is hushed up and parents are seldom punishèd, though the legal means to do so exist. With the spread of AIDS especially in densely populated urban areas, any operation on the genitalia of a child - particularly since FGM is often done with unsterilized instruments - can be fatal.

Many seminars have also been held by and for physicians who work with the CFPA to spread awareness among other doctors and to prevent them from doing the operations. While the operations are prohibited, physicians are exempted and it is left to their judgment whether or not they will do the operation in specific cases. [11]

The current Annual Report announces plans to "cover massive educational, training and information campaigns in Upper and Lower Egypt". Until now most of the activities have taken place in metropolitan Cairo and its many institutions. The report summarizes:

> "Closer cooperation has been established with other organizations including the Red Cross, the Ministry of Health and Social Affairs, Ministry of Education, UNICEF, WHO, etc. . . . A pilot project was set up in the form of training for TV program designers, producers and telecasters in 3 channels. . . . Programs were telecast . . . followed by workshops for evaluation attended by TV and broadcasting personnel. . . The FGM message was integrated into selected TV programs. . . A large number of educational materials and research reports have and are being published along with posters, pamphlets and visual materials."

From the start the Egyptian program has worked closely with the medical and professional health leadership in Egypt, organizing a number of conferences and meetings that have had wide press coverage and resulted in extensive discussions of the issue in the news. With the wide experience of the Cairo Family Planning Association as basis the project is well situated to influence the health training and health education field which is far more extensive and developed in Egypt than in other parts of Africa. The Egyptian program, due to its long experience, can provide leadership and helpful examples for organizing initiatives and programs.

The United Nation's Conference on Population and Development is scheduled to take place in Cairo in September 1994; this will provide an opportunity to share the experience gained by this innovative program with many more, especially those who work in family planning in Africa who need to integrate teaching for women's health and the prevention of FGM into all family planning programs.

THE GAMBIA: BAFROW - FOUNDATION FOR RESEARCH ON WOMEN'S HEALTH, PRODUCTIVITY AND THE ENVIRONMENT, BANJUL [12]

BAFROW is a registered organization established to carry out action-oriented research, surveys and pilot projects on issues related to women's health, women's productivity and the environment. Its ultimate objective is to support institutions and agencies and in particular indigenous grass-roots women's groups in developing and implementing research, training and developmental pilot projects relating to women's health, their productivity and their environment.

A core support grant to BAFROW from Population Action International in 1993 supports a program to develop a strategy for eradication of FGM in the Gambia. Mrs. Safiatou Singateh, Coordinator of BAFROW, has been active locally and internationally for some time in efforts to eradicate FGM. She conducted a major research study in 1985 on "FGM, the Gambian Experience", on the social, economic and health implications for the Gambian Women's Bureau, which she headed for many years. This core support grant will facilitate the establishment of BAFROW to carry out innovative pilot projects in the private sector and later involve the public sector with the help of Mrs. Singateh's contacts.

SOMALIA: STRATEGIES TO BRING ABOUT CHANGE [13]

Somalia as a functioning country and society no longer exists. As this report goes to press indiscriminate killing and aimless violence are continuing: Apparently these will not stop as long as Somalian men have any weapons left. The effort, described below, to rid the country of the family customs that traditionally socialize all boys for a life of violence came too late. The mutilation and infibulation of female children in every family brutalize all males. The results can now be seen displayed before the world on TV, yet the real cause of this violence is never discussed. With the huge amounts of weapons imported and given to men who are bred for violence and respect only force, the results are predictably lethal. But the programs so thoughtfully designed and developed by women, with much international commitment and support, need to be recorded: They are positive initiatives that set an example and could be used in other countries.

In June of 1988 the SWDO - the Somalian Democratic Women's Organization with the collaboration of AIDoS - the Italian Association for Women in Development - organized an international conference under the above heading to gain support for the national campaign to eradicate FGM. Infibulation - the most drastic and damaging form of FGM - has been practiced by all ethnic Somalis, a traditionally nomadic illiterate Moslem population, for as long as anyone can remember. (See Case History: Somalia.)

It is to the great credit of the now deposed and repudiated government of Siad Barre that the SWDO was given full support to organize this national campaign against infibulation, an initiative unprecedented in Africa. The SWDO gained the financial and technical support of the Italian Government - the former colonial power that ruled the southern part of Somalia. AIDoS, funded by the Italian Government and supported by women and women's organizations all over Italy, provided not only technical and financial support but AIDoS staff members also worked in Mogadishu for several years. [14]

An office shared by Somali and Italian women at the SWDO headquarters in Mogadishu was organized as operational and training base for implementing jointly made plans and for developing education and information initiatives. A program was developed to introduce new ideas, to inform and educate - with health the priority - and to reach the people on the family level where the decisions regarding children are made.

The objective was to convince both men and women that the mutilation of their daughters is not "necessary" as they had been taught all their lives to believe, following tradition. The political and religious leaders had to be reached on their own level and convinced to change, as they have great influence on the families who follow them.

The SWDO together with AIDoS developed plans with the support of the government and all its ministries to reach each section of society on their own level with structured educational initiatives. For instance, different programs, supported by visual and educational materials, were designed for the Ministry of Health, Ministry of Education, Interior, Agriculture, etc. Each education program to stop infibulation was to be integrated with all other activities and programs of each ministry and adapted to the needs of the people with whom they worked in the field. That is, the basic programs developed jointly by the SWDO and AIDoS were adapted for each target group to be reached.

This very carefully designed and comprehensive campaign, though it was stopped by the civil war, can provide a model for other countries or areas. The same structure can be adapted for different African countries; therefore an outline of the plan is given here: [15]

> "The **objectives** of the campaign are to provide information on the health aspects of infibulation in order to influence change . . . The **focus** of the approach is to present the subject of infibulation primarily as a health issue in an effort to remove the discussion from its religious and cultural connotations."

The campaign was organized around specific **target groups** using information packets as tools which in each case are adapted to the needs of the group.

> "The choice of **target groups** has two main objectives: to reach certain social groups whose attitudes toward infibulation create an obstacle to change and to reach influential people within a given community who could influence a widespread modification of the practice of infibulation . . . "

SOMALIA: STRATEGIES TO BRING ABOUT CHANGE (continued)

The project was designed to work with the following social groups:

- women and mothers who are accepted and/or influential within their community;
- secondary school pupils; religious leaders;
- medical and paramedical personnel.

The campaign was designed to focus on increasing awareness especially on the part of doctors, religious and community leaders concerning the severe damage which is done to a woman's health from a practice which has no value nor is a religious demand. Support from these two groups can lead in future to more concern for women's health. Because the campaign addressed very different social groups, there was a need for as many "information packages" as there were social divisions. For example, the packet for medical and paramedical personnel was far more technical than the information prepared for other groups. Each packet consisted of the following:

- pamphlets, informative handouts and other publications;
- a written discussion of the information to be presented by the instructor;
- a checklist to help the instructor lead a discussion;
- a manual explaining the use of audiovisual and other equipment;
- programs for slide-show presentations and materials for overhead projectors;
- a packet for medical and paramedical personnel focusing on the negative consequences of infibulation to women's health.

The subject matter of each information packet was determined by the target group; for instance, health, education (schools), religion, law, social welfare, etc. The time allotted to the development of the packets was six months and required the collaboration of groups active in this field who were going to teach with the help of these educational materials. The campaign itself was planned to last for a year. Implementation was open-ended, though intensive action was planned for the beginning. The campaign also included strengthening the capabilities of the SWDO by training in organization and management. A Documentation and Printing Center was established at SWDO headquarters including computers and copiers and other equipment to enable the SWDO to continue to develop and print educational materials as needed.

The International Training Center in Turin, Italy, of the ILO - the International Labor Office - worked on the development of multimedia teaching materials, including videotapes, which can be adapted for different audiences and shown anywhere as part of a teaching program or as a separate presentation to initiate discussion.

In March of 1988 a national conference was held in Mogadishu, organized by the SWDO, on **The Health Hazards of Infibulation and Its Eradication** with the objective to formulate a definite national policy for eradication of FGM. A series of recommendations was made by the participants from representative bodies and organizations of Somalia , who were directly involved in the effort to eradicate FGM.

The national conference assured broad-based support for the SWDO campaign and for the international seminar which followed in June 1988. This international meeting was held in the Parliament with the participation of the diplomatic corps and all international organizations. Impressive opening and closing ceremonies were held in the main hall of the Parliament, which had a huge frescoe of a Somali woman with upraised arms covering the entire podium wall, showing hundreds of people with their faces lifted toward her. The setting and ceremonies raised the consciousness of all participants and gained support for their cause, strengthening the resolve for change which it expressed.

During the three days of workshops and discussions, invited representatives from different African countries spoke and explained their efforts to eradicate FGM, including the Sudan, Gambia and Egypt. An Indonesian physician explained that among the Moslems in his country, the practice has become today mostly a symbolic rite. Daniela Colombo, the vice president of AIDoS, spoke first, outlining the efforts in developing the program in cooperation with the SWDO. Next I reported on actions all over the world to eradicate FGM. Berhane Ras-Work spoke on the many activities of the I AC.

SOMALIA: STRATEGIES FOR CHANGE (continued)

There were working groups on health, including physicians from the Benadir Hospital for Women and Children, a working group on law, on training and information, and on religion. The meetings all took place in different halls of the Parliament, and involved many decision makers of the government.

Conference reports were continuously broadcast in order to involve as many people as possible of the local population. There certainly was no doubt left in anyone's mind that the women of Somalia wanted change and were determined to do away with these terribly damaging traditions. It had been recognized by the Siad Barre Government that in order to succeed economically and to take its place internationally, practices like infibulation would have to stop: There certainly was high level governmental support for the SWDO - AIDoS program and this conference. The formal closing proceedings left everyone convinced that this was a comprehensive, carefully planned effort that had full backing by the government as well as international support. But at the time of the Conference the civil war had already started in the North. (See Case History: Somalia)

By now Mogadishu, including the project headquarters and all its equipment is destroyed, the project staff have fled. The pictures shown on TV of mutilated bodies of soldiers dragged through the streets who were sent to Somalia so starving women and children could be fed by protecting them from the violence of Somali men have aroused the world against such vicious brutality. But it is unconscionable that once more the whole issue of FGM and the violence against girls and women, which infibulation represents, is completely ignored. In all the political negotiations Somali women are missing - which is the fault of the United Nations, whose leadership has utterly failed. The international press and TV, broadcasting from Somalia, have completely ignored Somalian women except as famine victims rather than victims of the men who dominate this society and who continue to have their own daughters infibulated. But women, half the population of the world, will no longer be ignored: We shall be heard!

The SWDO/AIDoS program sets an example of international cooperation between women: It is hoped that this may become a guide. Since 1989 AIDoS in collaboration with the IAC and with the technical support of the ILO Training Center in Turin has developed information campaigns and programs, though on a much smaller scale, using a similar approach and similar methods. They have been introduced in Ethiopia, the Sudan, Nigeria and Gambia, supported by UNFPA. [16] The ILO Training Center has, based on the experience in Somalia, developed prototype multimedia module training packages, adaptable for different African countries, as well as programs for trainers on how to use and adapt the multimedia modular training packages.

BURKINA FASO: CAMPAIGN AGAINST THE PRACTICE OF EXCISION [18]

At the present time Burkina Faso is the only African country where a governmental national campaign to stop excision is being implemented. This campaign was started in 1988 with a national conference in Ouagadougou, the capital, held in the spring of that year. (See Case History: Burkina Faso).

The **Action Program for 1992-95,** under the leadership of Miriam Lamizana, includes a budget outlining ongoing and proposed actions. This program is based on the initial meeting held in 1988, where a national committee was formed which became operational in October 1990. Some of the activities (which can be copied in other countries) are:

- Organization of an information center // Radio and TV porgrams
- Development of a videocassette on excision as a documentary with testimonies by physicians, midwives, nurses, religious leader, including comments from mothers, young girls, and excisors. The committee uses the showing of the video tape to different audiences as a way to collect opinions on the effectiveness of the message.
- Showings of the film "My Daughter Shall Not Be Excised", which was made in 1990 in a local village, to different groups all over the country to stimulate discussion.
- Organization of trips by the committee through ten provinces with meetings held and information distributed with the objective to start local groups.

BURKINA FASO CAMPAIGN (continued)

This eradication campaign takes place against a background of very limited health services as stated in the Action Program. Improvements in maternity services are very much needed as well as immunization programs for children under five and for pregnant women. Maternal mortality is very high, there is a great lack of physicians and more trained midwives are very much needed.

The campaign is short of funds, as the above cited report states. Some meetings in the provinces had to be canceled due to lack of transportation and money. Despite the fact that this is a government organized and nationally supported action, no major donors have come forward (such as the support by Italy through AIDoS in Somalia). Though this campaign started in 1988, the Action Program states that up to now the greatest problem has been that it lacks all continuing funding or any other regular source of income. Nevertheless, the report states, the committee organized 22 discussions between July and November 1992, as well as 30 visits and campaigned in 7 counties and 17 villages all over the country besides holding 4 TV Programs.

It is clear from this summary that this national campaign, the only one in Africa today fully supported by the government of this very poor country badly needs international sponsors and financial as well as technical support. Italy, which formerly administered the southern part of Somalia including Mogadishu, provided both financial support as well as extensive technical help for the SWDO campaign (see above). But France, the former colonial power which administered Burkina Faso (then called Upper Volta), has provided no help. While AIDoS - the Italian Women's Organization - worked with the SWDO, there is no French women's group working with and providing technical assistance to the women in Burkina Faso or to the National Committee against excision. Much more could be accomplished, as the government backs this initiative, if the necessary support could be found.

The campaign is based first of all on consciousness raising using the film "My Daughter Will Not Be Excised", [19] which was taken in Burkina Faso and shows a real-life situation. A physician comes back to his village with his small daughter whom he is trying to protect from being excised against the wishes of his own father and his family. The topic is used as basis for discussion and to raise questions among the audience, often for the first time, why excision is performed, explaining the health damage that results. Most of all, the film is used to raise doubts in the minds of the very traditional viewers about the usefulness or necessity of this practice - questions that in the rural environment of this country have never been raised, let alone discussed.

This consciousness raising approach - quite different from what was done in Somalia - may be useful in many other rural areas as the film raises personal questions. The viewers, most of whom have little exposure to films, see themselves represented in this story. But this is only a beginning in this very conservative society. Much more is needed to introduce change in this country where "respect for tradition" is the answer given by most people when asked why they have their daughters excised and where literacy is very low, especially in rural areas, among women.

Despite the financial problems that plague the national campaign, there is the conviction among more and more people and the leadership that FGM must be eradicated because of the health damage the operations cause and the danger they represent for the lives of girls and women. Another major conference was held February 14-18, 1992, in Ouagadougou on Traditional Practices Affecting the Health of Women and Children, specifically excision. The Secretary of State of Action Sociale and the president of the National Committee, Mme. Miriam Lamizana, spoke. The central theme was to discuss appropriate strategies to fight against the practice. [20]

At that conference, health and the problems resulting from the mutilations were discussed by a physican, detailing the physical damage and psychological problems. The meeting also covered other damaging practices such as nutritional tabus, the problems of widows and orphans as well as witchcraft, which still persists in some areas. It was again explained to the large audience that FGM is not a religious prescription by Islam. Information on the conference was reported throughout the country by the national publication **SIDWAYA.**

KENYA: MAENDELEO YA WANAWAKE ORGANIZATION (MYWO) INITIATIVE

The Maendeleo Ya Wanawake Organization [21] is the largest and one of the oldest women's organizations in East Africa. Organized in colonial times, it was founded in 1952. Its name literally translated means "women's progress" and it has the largest membership of village women of any women's organization in Africa - hence also political clout. Jane Kiano for many years was its president (until the early 1980s) and not only built the organization but also built Maendeleo House - a handsome, multistory office building at the edge of Uhuru Park, near the University of Nairobi - as a symbol of women's power.[22]

The first time I met Jane Kiano in the early 1970s she talked about her dream to build a house and symbol for the organization and she worked for it for many years. It now stands as a proud monument for women's power in Kenya. The organization has its headquarters, offices and meeting rooms on one floor, but most of the building is rented to different businesses as an income-generating venture. At the time of the 1985 UN Decade Forum, which was held on the university campus, Maendeleo House, which adjoins the area, stood out and could be seen by the thousands of women who came from all over the world to this global gathering of women speaking for their rights.

A short time later, the organization, which always had a good deal of political influence due to its large rural membership, was taken over by KANU, the government party. The organization was nationalized - apparently in an attempt by the president of Kenya to consolidate his power. In addition, there were financial scandals and rivalries which led to the government take over. However, that lasted only a few years and then Maendeleo was privatized once more - no doubt due to the strong international influence promoting democratization and privatization.

Throughout all these trials the organization managed to continue and now has become the first organization of Kenya since independence to make a serious attempt at dealing with FGM.

The difficult history of FGM in Kenya is related in the Case History of Kenya. As recent as 1980, at the UN Mid-Decade Conference, Eddah Gachukia, the leader of the Kenyan delegation, claimed in a public meeting at the Forum that she could not speak on the subject as no information was available and no research had ever been done. When a number of women in the audience from European organizations offered to get funding and provide technical assistance for such a study, Gachukia firmly turned them down, seconded by Wangari Maathai, who headed the National Council of Women of Kenya at that time - the umbrella organization designated to deal with all international activities. They both made it entirely clear that they did not want to have anything to do with FGM and that they did not want to know the facts - because then it no longer could be concealed that thousands of girls every year are horribly mutilated and hundreds die of the immediate results, quite aside from fatalities due to childbirth complications.

For years all Kenyan women's organizations, and especially women leaders, covered up this terrible secret that is fatal for so many helpless girls in rural areas - because in that way these women could claim "FGM is no problem" and follow the line of their great leader Kenyatta, who promoted FGM all his life. Kenyatta had the right to appoint a number of MP's, and chose Eddah Gachukia as the women's representative - which secured her leadership position ever after. But to maintain leadership at the price of girls' and women's lives raises some serious questions.

Kenya's women leaders could have done something a long time ago for the unfortunate girls who are mutilated by the thousands every year. The same women leaders persuaded the UN and the dominant male politicians of their country to have the 1985 Women's Decade Conference in Kenya - which was an important international recognition. At the conference Forum, the Inter African Committee (IAC) organized a number of meetings on FGM, and the mutilations were discussed also by French-speaking groups including Awa Thiam. But the Kenyan women ignored these discussions; none of their women leaders spoke on the subject, despite the fact that thousands of mutilated women can be found in Kenyan hospitals. The conference made millions for Kenyan politicians - as hotel prices were doubled after being taken over by the government.

KENYA: MAENDELEO YA WANAWAKE INITIATIVE (continued)

At the 1990 IAC Conference in Addis Ababa, the Kenyan delegation, made up of Maendeleo members, became interested in the FGM issue, as they heard from the delegates from all over Africa what was being done regarding FGM. This led to representatives of the organization making contact with Population Action International (PAI), which was represented as donors of the conference. [23] The PAI Special Projects Fund has supported many initiatives to stop FGM all over Africa and is the only US-based international population organization that has supported initiatives to stop FGM.

Before a viable program can be designed, it is necessary to establish the facts - which in Kenya have been deliberately concealed and hushed up for so many years, though it is known which ethnic groups practice FGM. Medical reports from colonial times detail that in many rural areas the mutilations performed are drastic, with cuts made into the vagina added to the excision of the clitoris in the belief that this makes childbirth easier and prepares girls for a life of constant childbearing (the average even now is eight children per woman, which means at least a dozen pregnancies). The large Somali population of Kenya all practice infibulation. The mutilations continue to be practiced in the United Nations run Somali refugee camps - as was reported by a woman physician who worked in a Somali camp. [24] Large numbers of refugees from Somalia have recently come to Kenya, where camps have been established for them by the UN.

The program outlined by PAI, which is providing funding and technical assistance through PATH (Program for Appropriate Technology in Health) gives an overview of the project which is being implemented in three phases:

> **Phase I: Quantitative Research (July 1991-June 1992).** In order to know more about the knowledge, attitudes and practices of Kenyan women regarding traditional practices affecting the health of women and children, i.e., female circumcision, nutritional tabus, and early marriage, MYWO conducted survey research in four districts of Kenya where these practices are believed to be widely practiced: Meru, Kisii, Narok and Samburu. PATH/Nairobi worked with MYWO, whom they assisted in the development of the quantitative survey and trained enumerators in interpersonal communication and interviewing techniques.
>
> The findings indicate that 90 percent of women in the 4 districts have undergone various types of circumcision, i.e., predominantly sunna in Kisii, excision in Meru and Narok, and infibulation in Samburu. The circumcision operations were performed 65 percent of the time on girls aged 8-13. They are performed by a traditional circumcisor in the village or bush 93 percent of the time. A circumcision blade was used by 63 percent of the circumcisors for the operation, while another 25 percent used a traditional knife. It was found that 80 percent of the circumcisions were done in a group setting, with 71 percent of the circumcisors using the same instrument for many girls without cleaning in between procedures. After the ceremony, 56 percent of the circumcised girls were left in the care of their mothers and 29 percent in the care of a grandmother.

The majority of the women interviewed (65 percent) wanted the practice to continue, claiming that changes would be difficult to bring about and stating that FGM was a sign of maturity.

From this short summary it is also evident that the operations provide a perfect opportunity for the transmission of AIDS - as the same instrument is used on all girls without cleaning. But even cleaning is not enough - the instrument would have to be sterilized, a procedure that is unknown in rural areas. And AIDS is now rampant in Kenya, with more and more people dying of the disease.

> **Phase II: Qualitative Research (July 1992-April 1993).** MYWO realized that any interventions cannot succeed without more in-depth knowledge about the extent and nature of harmful traditions practiced in Kenya. With technical assistance from PATH, MYWO enhanced the qualitative research capabilities of its staff; identified target groups in each district; created a database of in-depth qualitative information about beliefs and practices; disseminated research results and identified potential sources of funding for the next phase.

KENYA: MAENDELEO YA WANAWAKE INITIATIVE (continued)

The findings are no surprise - that is, the opinions and ideas of those questioned in the four different areas in Kenya are quite similar to those professed by people in other areas of Africa. The practice is considered to be a rite of passage from childhood to adulthood and is a community celebration to recognize the position of each girl as an adult member, enhancing her marriage opportunities. Indeed in some areas uncircumcised girls can't find a husband and the bride-price of a girl who is operated on is higher - that is, she is considered to be a virgin if she is circumcised. The operations are claimed to prevent promiscuity - it is said that this saves men from worrying about their wives.

It is also believed that the mutilations make childbirth easier and prepare a girl for things to come associated with pain including childbirth and beatings by her husband. Women who are circumcised are submissive and dependent on their husbands - assuring male dominance, while women who are not are independent and unlikely to get married, which is a loss for the parents who are honored by the community if their daughter is circumcised. Also, girls are considered "dirty" if they are not mutilated. In some areas the operation and marriage are combined into one big celebration.

But the data also reveal that many mothers are strongly opposed, and that fathers claim to be opposed to the operations; yet the majority of young boys are not. Many opinions are in conflict but it is generally recognized that the practice is decreasing especially in urban areas and among those who are educated. But, as elsewhere, it is said that FGM is a woman's domain - thus shifting the responsibility on those who have the least opportunity to get an education or make their opinions heard.

It is interesting to learn that a number of people report that the operations are done in local hospitals - though the hospitals charge much more. Apparently not only is the prohibition by President arap Moi of 1982 not enforced - which was sent to all hospitals according to newspaper reports - but that these facilities under the governmental health system openly ignore it: A number of people asked by the survey also recommended that FGM should be done in the hospitals in the future.

Many of the people in two of the less traditional ethnic groups, both women and men, oppose the mutilation and recommend large-scale mass information and education campaigns. This same recommendation was made already in 1979 in Khartoum at the WHO Seminar and innumerable times ever since: But it has yet to be tried anywhere.

> **Phase III: Intervention and Evaluation (May 1993-1995)**. MYWO will work with local communities to implement communication strategies that reflect the findings of both the quantitative and qualitative research. The strategies will use the communities' own perceptions to create awareness about the harmful effects of certain traditional practices (with emphasis on FGM) and develop culturally appropriate responses and alternatives. These strategies will target key groups in the community (for example, leaders, mothers of primary students, secondary boys and girls) who influence decisions about FGM and early marriage. They will use local resources and local institutional networks to train, educate and inform members of the target audience throughout the community. Messages about harmful traditions will be integrated into other health and development programs in the four districts.
>
> Because these four districts are ethnically diverse and representative of a large segment of the Kenyan population, these projects can serve as models for replication and adaptation elsewhere in Kenya. The approach of customizing communication strategies for effective eradication of female genital mutilation can be used in many countries.

It may take two or more years after the interventions until any results are available and evaluated. Only then can conclusions about their effectiveness be made. This means more than five years since the research was begun; then positive results have to be adapted to other regions of Kenya - as the investigation is limited to four specific sample areas of different ethnic groups which are made up of very different people. That means a great deal of time, money and effort will be required before any positive results are achieved, provided the sample interventions are positive. PATH also recommended that additional research needs to be made.

TANZANIA: INITIATIVES FOR PREVENTION OF FGM

In Tanzania FGM is practiced in the North in the areas adjoining Kenya - as the operations typically are ethnic practices and not related to the political boundaries drawn by European powers in the 19th century. Therefore only a small percentage of women are affected, yet the mutilations and where they are practiced are as severe and damaging as those practiced in Kenya, including by the Masai, a nomadic ethnic group that live both in northern Tanzania and Kenya and follow their herds.

In April of 1987, a letter signed "Affected Women" appeared in a major national newspaper. It was a general appeal for help to stop the traditional practice of excision. A baseline study funded by NORAD, the Norwegian Development Agency, in the late 1980's confirmed that practices such as FGM, food tabus, child marriage and a variety of other tribal customs had damaging health consequences. A request to the Inter African Committee (IAC) on Traditional Practices Affecting the Health of Women and Children for assistance to form a national committee which could address these issues led to the organization in 1990 of the National Committee on Traditional Practices (NCTP).[26]

In 1990 the Institute for Development Training (IDT)[27] met several key individuals concerned about FGM. A dialogue began about ways to change attitudes and, ultimately, the practices themselves, especially in smaller communities, in this predominantly rural country. IDT was invited by the National Committee to participate in designing a project which this group of volunteers could implement. In January 1991 a plan emerged which included the NCTP, the Christian Council of Tanzania and the Christian Medical Board of Tanzania.

A research study of the Institute of Adult Education of Dar es Salaam, funded by NORAD, was conducted in Arusha, Dodoma, Kilimanjaro, Mara and Singida. The objectives were:

- to seek expert opinions on the practice of FGM and the gravity of the problem and to attempt to find efforts that are being made toward the eradication of the practice of FGM;
- to seek means for designing methodologies and strategies to combat FGM; and
- to attempt to find out the scale and magnitude of the practice in order to inform policy-makers on the practice with a view towards its total eradication.

The recommendations of the study in summary stated:

- Recognizing that the Party is supreme in Tanzania, and that it has branches at the grass-roots level, we recommend that it assumes, among its other roles, the task of educating the people on the adverse effects of FGM.
- The Parents Association and the Women's Organizations are against the practice of FGM. It is recommended that youth are conscientized on the magnitude of the problem of FGM so as to make effective contribution toward the eradication of the practice.
- Since the practice of FGM encroaches on women's rights and freedoms, it is imperative that both central and local governments, as well as parastatals, have a duty to give priority to searching for solutions to this problem. Both women and men should be educated and conscientized.
- The schools should incorporate elements related to FGM and other gender issues in order to build positive attitudes that will eventually lead to the total eradication of FGM.

The study arrived at the following conclusions which in summary are:

- In retrospect, the traditional rationale for the practice of FGM is a ritual that initiates females into adulthood. FGM is still cherished by traditionalists. Mysticism in certain instances seems to force some nonconformists of tribal practices to adhere to this norm. Some quarters still nurse the idea that an uncircumcised woman is impure,is not adult and may bring a curse to a household; FGM is still widely practiced in traditional enclaves.

TANZANIA: INITIATIVES FOR PREVENTION OF FGM (continued)

- The Party, the government and some religious bodies are promulgating total eradication of the practice. Dangerous diseases associated with FGM, such as tetanus and AIDS, have served as deterrents in some areas.
- A number of barriers presented themselves: It is not easy for uncircumcised people to be accepted. In the face of mounting pressure from Party and Government quarters, people who practice FGM tend to go underground. There are allegations that even educated people engage in it. Parents are worried about the size of dowry and marriageability. Some older women and older men defend the practice; others are ready to part with it as long as it is the consensus of the tribes.
- In certain areas FGM is promoted as a cure of some mysterious disease known as "lawa lawa."

The Gender Health Risks project is the name of the program funded by Population Action International [28] which was developed and implemented by IDT and was launched on schedule in June 1991. IDT had been invited to design a project that could be implemented by a group of volunteers and designed this strategy based on a pilot approach to the health problems resulting from FGM. There was general enthusiasm and a commitment to move ahead rapidly among key leaders from all three participating organizations: the National Committee, the Christian Council, and the Christian Medical Board.

Within the first five months there were major achievements: First drafts of community education materials were ready, and workshops for leaders were conducted in two of the four project regions. During 1992 further development of the educational materials - five booklets, a leader's guide and a flip chart - culminated in the printing of thousands of copies of each. Two more workshops for leaders completed training in all four regions. Although the community discussion group phase fell behind its 1992 schedule, all preparations for moving into villages were completed by the end of the year.

There was abiding interest by a few determined women to carry through to a successful conclusion. The Christian Council staff remained very pleased with the project. Letters were received from workshop participants expressing gratitude that such topics were openly discussed. Fifteen focus group sessions in five villages, with men and women stratified into three age groups, were conducted in March by a team representing all organizations. After discussions with all parties, a six-month activities schedule was agreed to, on the assumption that full funding would be available. Fund-raising from many sources was organized by IDT in order to print and test the teaching materials and implement the program. Some of the activities projected include:

- Print and field-test all materials; design T-shirts and get bids for production; analyze focus group results and revise materials.
- Print up to 5,000 copies of each of five booklets, 300 flip charts and 300 leaders' guides.
- Conduct two regional workshops and screen applicants for field team person; hire and train (if funds available).
- Publicize project via radio and newspaper; promote the project in mass media and with government and NGO bodies.
- Launch community discussion groups and solicit support from local politicians and party leders.
- Design questionnaire for medical providers to follow up mailings and develop materials and schedules for evaluation research.
- Monitor community implementation and, if needed, revise strategy; finalize evaluation plans.

The program is being implemented now - the work will have to continue for years before measurable results are achieved. It is especially difficult to get attention and support for programs if the people seeking help are a relatively small group in a very poor country and especially if they are women. Therefore it is very encouraging that this initiative started due to an appeal by women and is being implemented mostly by determined women volunteers.

THE WESTERN WORLD: INITIATIVES TO STOP FGM

It is of course ironic that the former colonial countries of Africa that have failed to effectively address the ongoing female genital mutilations are now faced with the problem on their own home front. Immigrants and refugees fom Africa and the Middle East are spreading the mutilations all over the world. This has forced especially European governments to confront the issue, because health services are provided at taxpayers' expense and most hospitals are under government control. For instance Britain or France had to deal with the issue at home, and so have all other countries that accept refugees. The United States is the only exception to date.

Health care is not only a private service in the US, but privacy between patient and doctor is still an absolute rule. Therefore anything goes - that is, performing any kind of surgery is left up to the individual physician, and the fee the client or patient is willing to pay. To date not a single case of FGM performed in the US on African immigrant girls has been medically documented - that is through gynecological examination. [29]

In the chapter on the Western World, the situation regarding immigrants and refugees is outlined; therefore, it will not be repeated here. But recent reports show that the number of refugees is rapidly escalating all over the world [30] and those who are able to afford it - that is, the educated, the wealthy and often the ousted political leadership - try to find a place to live in the Western World, though many countries including the US also accept penniless refugees with little or no skills because they are persecuted and fear for their lives. That does not mean that there is not also an enormous influx of illegal refugees.

The political discussions of the refugee issue continue all over the world. The terrible plight of women refugees has recently been taken up by some women's organization, including in the political arena, to protect women refugees who are most often doubly victimized. But all this is beyond the scope of this report, though it forms the background of the initiatives to stop FGM among immigrants which is outlined below.

It is unfortunate but the US, though it is the aim of refugees from all over the world including from Africa, has at this writing no organization that has made any effort to prevent FGM among immigrant families. In the absence of any scandals - such as press reports about girls dead due to FGM splashed all over the newspapers as in France - there has been no preventive action or education for refugee families. A law to criminalize FGM has been discussed and introduced in the summer of 1993 and was then made part of the omnibus health bill for women, [31] which also includes statements about the introduction of preventive education to be sponsored by the federal government.

Despite many attempts on my part to persuade women's organizations including NOW (National Organization for Women) to deal with FGM on the grass-roots level by initiating preventive education involving women of immigrant communities, nothing has been done. Experience shows that the most effective way is to work with immigrant communities locally and directly, and I have developed a simple program proposal about how this could be accomplished at very little cost.

To organize conferences, film showings and all kinds of TV and press publicity unfortunately never reaches the people who need education and help on the grass-roots level. Developing health education with and for African immigrants is a difficult, painstaking and unglamorous job. But our experience in Africa with the **Childbirth Picture Books (CBPB)** shows that it can be done, and there are ways to do it with the cooperation of the existing health and family planning system and community groups.

The simple program I proposed that I tried to introduce to the NOW leadership to be carried out by affiliates who volunteer to do so on the local level in areas where immigrants live was of no interest to them. The objective of the pilot program is to train women leaders from immigrant countries to become informal family health advisors among their own groups with the help of the **Childbirth Picture Books** which use graphics to explain reproductive health and the damage done by FGM. Only women from each immigrant community know the customs and can communicate with the people most effectively at their own level. I spoke on FGM at the National NOW Conference in 1990, but to date no one has come forward. [32] But I am ready to take this up with anyone interested in helping by organizing such a grass-roots initiative.

THE WESTERN WORLD: INITIATIVES TO STOP FGM (continued)

Such necessary community efforts do not attract press coverage and so it has been ignored by those who are now beginning to use the issue of FGM to sell books and attract attention to themselves. Unfortunately experience shows that all the media splash in the US does not reach those who need help in Africa or African refugees - they do not even know about it; and after a short time the press finds something new and more exicting.

If the law prohibiting FGM is passed in the US, which may take a long time, the federal government is supposed to organize some preventive initiatives. Therefore it would be important to develop some local initiatives now to gain some experience of what to do and how. In Britain, for instance, FORWARD (see below) was organized and funded by the British government at the Africa Center in London to develop educational programs to prevent FGM for immigrants and also teach social workers who work in areas where African immigrants live about the problem.

But while it is essential to stop the spread of FGM in the West and especially to resist all ongoing efforts to medicalize the mutilations, which the medical establishment unfortunately often promotes - (see The Western World) - it must be clear that the most important issue is to stop FGM at its source, that is in Africa and the Middle East. Unfortunately experience shows returning expatriates don't change the customs at home. Even though a person - most often a man during his university studies in Europe or America - seemingly absorbs Western customs, once he returns home the traditional environment takes over. One person or a family, even by trying hard, cannot change the customs that have prevailed for centuries in many communities.

But what is happening now as a result of Western influences, is that the educated leaders in Africa have their daughters mutilated the medical way and that must be resisted in every way and everywhere. This is the greatest threat for women now because the patriarchal medical system to make money supports medicalization. [33] For the most part very small children are mutilated who may not even know for 15 or more years what has been done to them or by whom: To initiate a malpractice suit after so many years is often impossible. Yes, I have heard from American women who have been circumcised in the US and there have been some malpractice suits. But these isolated cases have no social impact.

Finally it must be understood that all the activities in Europe, for instance in Britain or France, and recently in Canada, to protect refugee children have had little or no influence on what is happening in Africa. To effectively work on prevention of FGM, Africans must be involved first of all. The Inter African Committee under the leadership of Berhane Ras-Work and its many local affiliates (see above), after working against FGM since 1984, have more experience than anyone else. They must be consulted and participate in integrating prevention in all internationally funded health and family planning programs in Africa. This is a political priority and can begin immediately in the population programs by the US Agency for International Development (see below).

In Canada, which has recently accepted many thousands of Somali immigrants, the government funded health services are using the Somali translation of the **Childbirth Picture Books** and have distributed 2,000 in summer 1993 with the help of local health and women's groups. [34] Existing laws, as an investigation shows, make FGM a criminal offense in Canada, [35] therefore, no special legislation needs to be passed. The College of Physicians and Surgeons of the Canadian province of Ontario, where most of the Somali refugees are settling, already two years ago issued a prohibition to its members to perform this surgery and provided information on how to help infibulated women in childbirth. [36] In Australia the issue has also been discussed in connection with immigrants but as in the US no documented case of FGM has been found, (see The Western World).

The summaries given below of the initiatives in Britain and France provide examples of different ways of dealing with FGM, but this does not mean these are the only activities to prevent FGM in European countries, but this is not the priority of this report. However, in **WIN NEWS** a continuing section on FGM is featured in every issue since the summer 1975 where all facts on FGM are reported from all over the world as they become known. I am always grateful for any information: Women's International Network depends on receiving information by, for and about women.

FORWARD -

FOUNDATION FOR WOMEN'S HEALTH RESEARCH AND DEVELOPMENT[37]

FORWARD was organized following the enactment of the Prohibition of Female Circumcision Law in 1985. [38] The British Parliament had debated this law for two years before it was finally passed (see The Western World). The act prohibits surgery on the female genitalia including by physicians except in cases of disease (such as cancer). FORWARD was organized and funded by the British government to support the implementation of this legislation among African immigrants in the United Kingdom.

Stella Efua Graham-Dorkenoo originally from Ghana who has lived in London for many years organized the African Mother and Child Health Campaign at the London Africa Center with the purpose: "to promote good health among African women and their families in the UK supported by the Department of Health, the Manpower Services Commission and from private donors." The organization's objectives as initially outlined are to provide "advisory services to African women, conduct workshops and provide speakers, conduct research and inform the caring professions about the special needs of African women and their families and pioneer health-care strategies."

Over the years FORWARD has developed many different activities and initiatives involving African immigrants to the UK from different African countries. These initiatives have become a model for some other European countries faced with similar problems of African immigrants who are seeking to continue their traditions including the mutilation of their female children even though most of these customs have lost all meaning and usefulness in their new environment (see The Western World).

FORWARD works exclusively with immigrants to the UK and has never organized any programs anywhere in Africa. Among the many programs FORWARD has developed are health education and training programs both for African immigrant families as well as British government social service and health workers teaching and serving the African community in London and the UK. Many community meetings, discussions, plays and celebrations have been organized over the years to attract Africans to the Center. [39]

In February 1989 the First National Conference on FGM in the UK was held by FORWARD. "The main purpose of the conference was to provide a forum for social, community and medical workers to explore social, ethical and legal issues arising from FGM in the UK and to assist professionals to make informed decisions within the framework of the 1985 legislation. . ." The role of the social workers, including school nurses, health visitors, general practitioners and midwifes, was discussed as they are responsible for protecting children from FGM and passing on information on any findings regarding the operations or children at risk.

A manual for educators and group facilitators was published by FORWARD to introduce new ways to discuss FGM by social workers and other community professionals in relevant ways and to share the experience gained by FORWARD working in the community-health field. One of the imaginative ways to reach the larger immigrant community organized by FORWARD is to stage plays with the participation of community members to dramatize the issue and to bring out the concerns involved that often are ignored or covered up.

A play written by the director of FORWARD, Efua Darkenoo, and performed at the Africa Center's Mother and Child Health Campaign exposing the sociocultural dynamics of FGM was a great hit in the African community in the UK, which includes many families from Somalia who are particularly reluctant to give up their tradition of infibulating all girls. The **Childbirth Picture Books** have also been used by FORWARD especially with Somali immigrants. [40]

In July of 1992 FORWARD organized the First Study Conference on FGM in Europe to develop "a coordinated unified approach to the abolition of the practice in Europe and other Western countries." [41] The problems experienced in the UK with African immigrants are not unique; rather immigrants bring along their customs wherever they go and many are reluctant to change, though they and their children's future depends on their willingness to adapt to their new environment.

FORWARD (continued)

As described in the chapter "The Western World", most European governments who accept African refugees had to confront FGM, as it is against the law to mutilate a child, by giving instructions to all health services and hospitals, especially those that serve immigrant families. Health care is publicly funded and available free to immigrants, some of whom request health service providers to mutilate their daughters, according to their customs. African families from urban areas evidently had access to such services at home, which confirms that FGM is being medicalized in Africa. It also shows that African immigrants are not warned that FGM is a criminal offense in the Western world.

In the United Kingdom due to the fact that special legislation was enacted, the issue was far more extensively discussed than in other countries. For the government to support the development of an organization such as FORWARD to work on prevention sets an example. The UK as the largest former colonial power has been the goal of many immigrants from all over the world.

Different European countries have dealt with the issue of preventing FGM in different ways. But FORWARD, due to its support by the British government over the past seven years, has by now much experience. The study conference in 1992 brought together a number of groups working on this issue including those from France, the Netherlands, some Scandinavian representatives and visitors from the US and Canada, in addition to many people from all over the UK as well as many African immigrants. The Conference urged that:

- national groups and individuals should promote a legal framework for action;
- governments and health authorities should stand firm against any attempt to medicalize genital mutilation or genital injury to the girl child.

FORWARD has continuously worked against the medicalization of FGM as the UK law against FGM requires. One reason why it took more than two years to pass this law and why the debate in the House of Lords continued over such a long time was because the organized medical profession at first objected, claiming this was interference in their professional territory. But in the end they agreed. However, the danger of introducing FGM or rather transferring the practice into modern medicine is constant and ubiquitous.

A short time after the FORWARD Conference, the medicalization of FGM created an uproar in the Netherlands when the Health Ministry was misled into suggesting that a mild or so-called "nonmutilating" form of FGM should be permitted to be introduced into the health system which in the Netherlands - much as in most of the rest of Europe - is publicly funded. (See The Western World.) The idea was to accommodate demands by some of the Somali refugees who had been accepted in large numbers after the revolution and civil war in Somalia. After a public uproar and debates carried on in the newspaper, and even in the streets, the Netherland government finally announced that all forms of FGM were prohibited in the Netherlands. [42]

The medicalization of FGM only makes the problem worse by financially rewarding the mutilation of little girls who are never consulted: This fact must be emphasized again and again. Once such mutilations become paid medical procedures they are next to impossible to stop. WHO already in 1982 had released a statement that the introduction of FGM into health care is totally unacceptable (see Appendix). This very same issue has been discussed over and over in Africa for instance in Sudan at the WHO Seminar and was categorically rejected by all African health delegations as well as by WHO.

Looked at from a rational view the very idea to have trained health professionals perform medieval African mutilations in Western hospitals on the genitalia of healthy female infants living in Europe clearly is absurd. Yet the medicalization of FGM comes up again and again: It was again discussed and rejected by all at the FORWARD Conference.

Since then FORWARD has assisted the participants with information on how to develop prevention programs among African immigrants. More and more African immigrants are arriving in Europe and all over the world, fleeing from the constant civil wars all over Africa. Therefore it is especially important now to develop coordinated policies against FGM that also have to be implemented in all internationally run refugee camps.

G.A.M.S. - GROUPE FEMMES POUR L'ABOLITION DES MUTILATIONS SEXUELLES [43]

G.A.M.S. is a private French women's Group for Abolishment of Sexual Mutilations which was organized after the newspapers reported the deaths of several small daughters of African immigrants due to excision. It appears that FGM is practiced in the Paris region where most Africans live: after the press reports the facts could no longer be ignored. Dr. Marie Helene Franjou, a pediatrician runs a group of "Well Baby Clinics" for the French governmental health system She has headed this organization from the start, whose officers and members are from the African immigrant community in Paris.

French health services require every mother who gives birth in France or who has small children to come regularly for checkups and for immunizations to a clinic in her area. It was through these checkups that the extent of the ongoing practice of FGM among Africans in the Paris region was established, quite aside from the girls who died. The clinics where Dr. Franjou works and where G.A.M.S. operates are in the area where many immigrants from the former French African colonies have settled.

G.A.M.S., as a nonprofit organization organized in 1982, affiliated in 1990 with the Inter-African Committee, and considers sexual mutilations an attack on women and their fundamental rights. G.A.M.S. also denounces the medicalization of FGM and works for the eradication of sexual mutilations and other practices that damage the health of women and children. Among the activities of G.A.M.S. is the distribution of information by making contact with and educating African immigrants in France about health.

Since it was set up, G.A.M.S. has worked with the African women - many of them from Mali - who come to the Mother and Child Health clinics, by providing education about the damage done by FGM, which is classified as criminal child abuse in France and against the law. Health professionals teach about reproduction, about the human body, about sexuality about pregnancy and more. This education provides the opportunity to show that sexual mutilations are dangerous for girls and women. This education takes place with the help of African women who translate the information and instructions. The African women from G.A.M.S. serve as interpreters and also use for these meetings the French translation of **the Universal Childbirth Picture Book** with the Additions on Excision published by **WIN NEWS** and the birth model of the Inter African Committee.

G.A.M.S. collaborated with the Ministry of Women's Rights participating in the working group on sexual mutilations. G.A.M.S. members developed the statistics and estimates of how many girls are at risk among the African immigrants. Most of the African families live near Paris; therefore the number of children at risk could be established. This survey was included by the Ministry of Women's Rights in its publication **Les Mutilations du Sex des Femmes Aujourd'hui en France** (Female Sexual Mutilations in France Today),[44] which was launched at a public meeting in November 1984 organized by the Socialist party with many African and French speakers including the Minister of Women's Rights.

Recently, due to the economic downtrend in Europe including in France, many Africans lost their jobs and returned to Africa; fewer immigrants are now arriving due to lack of employment. Therefore, the problem is not as pressing as a few years ago. However, despite all the teaching and educational work by G.A.M.S., especially at the clinics, and despite an information campaign that the operations are prohibited in France, there have been numerous criminal cases. Parents and excisors have been indicted by criminal courts when it was discovered that African girls were still being mutilated.

Until recently despite more court proceedings, some of which dragged on for years, no one went to jail, even though several girls died and though some indicted families had lived in France for years. In one case a father cut up the genitalia of his baby daughter himself with a pen knife. The child died; the father's sentence was suspended! So far no man has ever gone to jail. Yet in almost all cases the fathers organized and/or paid for the mutilations as many of the traditional African women in France are illiterate. [45] However in early 1993 when it was found that a Gambian woman had her two baby daughters excised - they were badly infected and had to be taken to the hospital - the mother was sentenced to five years and jailed for one year. But none of the men responsible for the deaths of several girls ever went to jail.

G.A.M.S. - FRANCE (continued)

Instead of preventive measures, the French government has embarked on a policy of indicting African immigrants for FGM performed in Paris and is now beginning to put them in jail: this, however, only results in African families sending their daughters back to Africa for the mutilations and accomplishes nothing for the girls whose lives are at stake. G.A.M.S., made up of volunteers cannot alone deal with this issue which requires government support - such as FORWARD receives in the UK. Putting African women in jail, especially when they are mothers of small children as the woman from Gambia (see above), will not persuade African families to stop FGM.

The Ministry of Women's Rights was abolished after the socialist government lost the elections. It spoke for women, including immigrant women, and supported a number of initiatives concerning FGM (see The Western World). Since then the French government has become entirely silent regarding FGM.

France during colonial times never sponsored any research on FGM in Africa and they do not now. Basic facts on the practices in Francophone Africa are lacking. Yet France sponsors experts and technical advisers for all Francophone African countries including some who work in maternity hospitals and with women's organizations. There have been more discussions, meetings and debates on FGM by professionals and intellectuals in Paris than anywhere else. But very little action on the grass-roots level, where it is needed most, has resulted from all the talk, least of all in Francophone Africa.

The French government has extensive economic, educational, cultural and technical exchange programs of all kinds in Africa, but almost nothing has been done to teach about women's health and prevent FGM. The issue is entirely and deliberately ignored. For instance, I tried to provide free copies of the **Childbirth Picture Books** in French to the Cooperation - the French development agency of the government - but neither correspondence nor my visits in Paris resulted in any response. All attempts to set up meetings after a translation of **The Hosken Report** was published in 1983 in France [46] were turned down. Francophone West Africa has the highest maternal mortality rates in the world as well as the highest female illiteracy. It is a pity that French women's organizations - except for G.A.M.S. - to date are entirely silent on the subject of FGM.

C.A.M.S. - Comission Internationale pour l'Abolition des Mutilations Sexuelles (International Commission to Abolish Sexual Mutilations) which Awa Thiam from Senegal organized in the early 1980s, held a number of conferences in Paris and one in Dakar. But C.A.M.S. never started any programs to prevent FGM and their former post office Box in Dakar has been discontinued. (See the Western World.)

PROGRAMS / METHODS TO ERADICATE FGM: SUMMARY AND OUTLOOK

The very different initiatives and programs outlined above are based on different methods and ideas of confronting the problem of FGM. All progress depends first of all on the people directly involved and their environment. There is no one way of approaching the eradication of FGM and it is much too soon to evaluate any results.

To be sure, coordination is always an essential requirement - such as the IAC has organized. For any of the actions to be effective, they will have to continue for years. For instance the program in Kenya, following the Family Planning Program model, already has taken several years and the prevention part is only just starting in a few pilot areas. Results will not be known for some time and then the rest of the country must be involved.

Most of the programs outlined here need much more money - including the one in Burkina Faso - initiated and supported by the government. The activities in Somalia used the most comprehensive approach, and this example, now destroyed, may be useful elsewhere. The Egyptian initiatives are a model for countries with extensive health systems. But one question needs to be raised: Is the organization of new, separate programs financed by raising new money the only way? There are already health and population programs in place all over Africa, many of them financed by USAID, which has a very large budget; and there are other sponsors as well: **All of them must be persuaded to integrate FGM prevention in all their current and new programs - for timely and cost-effective results!**

POLITICAL ACTIONS TO STOP FEMALE GENITAL MUTILATION (FGM)

In June 1993, I again presented testimony on Female Genital Mutilation to the US Congress, the Foreign Operations Subcommittee of the Appropriations Committee, chaired by Senator Patrick Leahy. This committee approves all funding for foreign assistance by the the US Agency for International Development (USAID) including health and family planning programs in Africa. A large number of private organizations and contractors are funded by USAID to design and implement the programs in the field in cooperation with the local government ministries and offices.

The funding for family planning and health programs in recent years has averaged about $250 - $300 million and is increasing. But though many multimillion-dollar programs have been implemented in Africa for many years, all of them have ignored the ongoing practice of FGM, even in their own program areas. **In my testimony I stated:**

> The silence about FGM on the part of USAID - now that African leaders have opposed it - is totally irresponsible because **this silence supports the continuation of FGM.** USAID and their contractors have spent millions on family planning, for instance, in Kenya. President arap Moi of Kenya has denounced and prohibited FGM already in 1982; but USAID and their contractors have failed to implement this prohibition in their program areas, showing utter disregard for women's health.
>
> "I pointed out in previous testimony that imported antibiotics and drugs, imported training and medical tools - paid for by US taxpayers including women - are now used by people USAID has trained to mutilate little African girls for money. **USAID is ignoring the modernization and medicalization of FGM** which goes on in all the cities from Bamako to Khartoum. But USAID and its contractors have failed to stop the medicalization of FGM including by those involved in US-funded programs.
>
> There are now active groups in almost all African countries working to stop FGM. For instance, the **Inter African Committee and its affiliates are active in more than 26 countries.** But USAID and their contractors have and continue to ignore them, which is unconscionable. USAID by their failure to support the African initiatives, even where the government is involved, for instance, in Burkina Faso, is condemning thousands of African girls to these permanent mutilations and lifelong terrible suffering and this is utterly reprehensible.
>
> There is no reason why family planning programs should not discourage FGM and speak about the terrible damage done by FGM, which is graphically shown in our **Childbirth Picture Books**. All family planning workers trained by USAID in African countries where FGM is practiced must be taught about the damage done by FGM, urged to stop the mutilations and encouraged to teach against them.
>
> **We urge that USAID and their contractors be required to integrate FGM prevention in all their family planning and health plans and programs in affected countries** in Africa and the Middle East and that every possible support be provided to local groups in Africa, for instance, the affiliates of the IAC, working for the eradication of FGM. All private organizations working for and funded by USAID should do likewise and be required **to provide reports of their actions and document results** of the effectiveness of their teaching.
>
> Similarly, all funding and contributions by the US of family planning organizations, especially UNFPA (United Nations Population Fund) and IPPF (International Planned Parenthood Federation) should be made subject to a requirement to include teaching the prevention of FGM in all family planning programs in all countries where these mutilations are practiced. IPPF, UNFPA and other family planning organizations to which the US contributes, **must be held accountable and show proof of results of their preventive teaching.** We also strongly suggest that all immigrants to the US from FGM-affected countries should be informed that these mutilations are unacceptable and a criminal offense in the USA.

The failure by USAID and all its contractors to prevent FGM in their program areas and to develop preventive teaching as part of their programs on which US taxpayers spend millions annually has resulted in **a steady increase of FGM.**

POLITICAL ACTIONS TO STOP FGM (continued)

Due to population growth FGM now **affects more than 110 million girls and women in continental Africa** (in 1982 this number was estimated at 84 million). Now more girls are mutilated than ever. But **neither USAID nor its contractors have ever done anything to stop FGM.** USAID and its contractors are directly responsible for the deaths and lifelong mutilation of millions of girl children in Africa because they have never included preventive teaching in their health and family planning programs.

As Senator Daniel Inouye, who chaired the same subcommittee at my previous testimony in 1980 said: **"Whether by omission or commission,US AID is responsible,"** he ordered USAID to investigate: but nothing was done.

At present African women are actively involved all over Africa, working and teaching against FGM. Most African heads of state have prohibited FGM. **But USAID and its contractors still refuse to prevent FGM.** This failure is criminal. Some major organizations/people receiving US funding , working in the population / health field are:

- **US Agency for International Development**, Mr. J. Brian Atwood, Administrator, 320 21st St., N.W. Washington, DC 20523
- **IPPF - International Planned Parenthood Federation**, Dr. Halfdan Mahler, Dir., Regent's College, Inner Circle, Regent's Park, London NW1 4NS, UK
- **Pathfinder International**, Mr. Daniel Pellegrom, Director, Suite 217, 9 Galen St., Watertown, MA 02172
- **Family Health International**, Theodore M. King, M.D., Ph.D., President/Chief Operating Officer, P.O. Box 13950, Research Triangle Park, NC 27709
- **INTRAH - International Training in Health**, University of North Carolina Medical School, 208 N. Columbia St., Chapel Hill, NC 27514
- **The Population Council**, Ms. Margaret Catley-Carlson, President, One Dag Hammarskjold Plaza, New York, NY 10017

These organizations have been paid millions by USAID - that is our money as taxpayers - and we have a right to demand that they protect girls and women's health. To claim today that FGM is a "cultural tradition" is a deliberate evasion of responsibility.

FGM is cited as a human rights violation by the Department of State; therefore USAID and the above-listed contractors as well as all others working in health and family planning in Africa must be held responsible for human rights violations. It is ironic that USAID, an agency of the Dpt. of State, is violating its own human rights rules!

We ask you to write and protest to the USAID administrator Mr. Atwood - address above - with a copy to Secr. of State Warren Christopher, Dpt. of State, Washington DC 20520 and Senator Leahy, Chair, Foreign Operations Sub-Committee, US Congress, Washington DC 20510 (copy to your Senator). Please send also a copy to **WIN NEWS**; your help is needed to break this conspiracy of silence.

It is astonishing to learn that all the **"Safe Motherhood"** initiatives have entirely ignored FGM - though all medical facts show that **the highest maternal mortality in the world is in the areas in sub-Saharan Africa where FGM is practiced.** While it is certainly commendable and an important contribution to women's health that at long last the needless deaths of childbearing women in developing countries are recognized and preventive actions are initiated, it is appalling that **FGM is once more deliberately ignored.** These "Safe Motherhood" activities funded by millions of dollars have mainly sponsored international high-level conferences and publicity organized by:

- **Family Care International**, Suite 510, 588 Broadway, New York, NY 10012
- **Safe Motherhood Program**, World Bank, 1818 H St., N.W., Washington, DC 20433
- **John Snow, Inc.** 11th Floor, 1616 N. Fort Myer Dr., Arlington, VA 22209 (for USAID)

The time has come to act: International Population Programs are failing to prevent FGM and to protect women's health; they are directly contributing to the medicalization of FGM. Women and all other taxpayers who contribute to these programs must protest and demand that our right to health is protected. [47]

FGM : A STRATEGY FOR ERADICATION

Dr. Olayinka Koso-Thomas, a gynecologist who worked in the past for the Health Ministry of Sierra Leone and in recent years has run her own clinic for women in Freetown, developed this ground-breaking initiative based on her extensive field experience. This program was published in her book in 1986, [48] in which Dr. Koso-Thomas also included some background information on Sierra Leone as well as a survey of 300 women in Western Sierra Leone analyzing the health problems resulting from FGM, which is practiced in very drastic form throughout Sierra Leone (see Case History: Sierra Leone).

Dr. Koso-Thomas, who as a physician has for years taken care of women, describes in factual terms their health situation and their great suffering resulting from the mutilations. But, she adds, women in the rural areas rarely seek help and the health services are very limited in this very poor country. Dr. Koso-Thomas also points out that in any plan to stop FGM provisions must be made for health care for the unfortunate victims who will suffer for many years to come, even if all the operations are stopped. There are millions of mutilated women who were subjected to these terrible operations as young girls who have health problems for the rest of their lives which often get worse with age. Therefore, the strategy outlined by Dr. Koso Thomas is a two-pronged one: to eradicate the mutilations and to take care of the many health problems of the mutilated women.

The strategies for eradication were originally developed by Dr. Koso-Thomas for her public health thesis at the University of California in Berkeley. While the strategies were developed for Sierra Leone and based on the specific experience in that country, the initiatives are applicable and adaptable wherever FGM is practiced. Therefore they are detailed here as examples, though they have never been implemented. This program uses a comprehensive regional approach yet it works on the grass-roots level, taking a different direction from the national governmental action in Burkina Faso and Somalia.

The thesis of Dr. Koso-Thomas goes into much more detail than the book. In the abstract it is stated that the proposed 20-year program [49]

> ". . . has two main areas of impact: **Health Education**, to increase knowledge of the dangers of circumcision and to correct wrong religious doctrines, and **Health Care**, to provide early diagnosis, treatment, and complete rehabilitation of the victims of circumcision. . . It is anticipated that at the end of the plan period, the mental and physical well-being of the 70 percent of the population who are now at risk will be restored. . . The proposed plan is intended to uproot the practice from its foundations in the traditional communities in the country and effect measures to cure those suffering mentally and physically from past circumcision operations."

Dr. Koso-Thomas, based on her extensive medical practice and on the data of a family planning clinic in Freetown, estimates that between 25-30 percent of women suffer from urinary fistulae due to obstructed labor. This is the result of scarring from the drastic operations by the local excisors, who still enjoy special status in each community. Fistulae make women incontinent and thus such women become outcasts of their communities and families, shunned by everyone: "The practice (FGM) continues as a requirement for marriage in many ethnic groups and is performed with a strong ritualistic flavor."

Excisors called "digbas" are highly respected and feared as they claim to possess magical powers; the belief in supernatural and evil spirits and in all kinds of magic powers is very widespread throughout Sierra Leone and shapes the lives and behavior of most of the people. Therefore education forms the basis of the eradication program which takes a multi-pronged approach over a period of 20 years.

It involves all the leadership of the country, especially the health care sector, since the whole eradication program is developed from the point of view of health. It is designed as a national effort in which a large segment of the population is progressively involved. A **National Committee for the Welfare of Women** is to be formed at the onset, in collaboration with the Ministry of Health, which will be in charge of the direction of the program, assisted by four provincial councils. An organization chart outlines identical educational and health procedures to be followed in each of the four provinces using a similar **Health Education Program** and **Health Care Program**; the latter to take care of the women suffering from the consequences of circumcision.

FGM : A STRATEGY FOR ERADICATION (continued)

A multi-disciplinary research unit will serve both parts of the program and provide educational materials and programs for the former as well as medical procedures and training for the latter. Under the **Health Education** part of the program, a task force will be formed, called the **"fox squad"**, to work directly with and inside the circumcision societies to stop the operations, and change the role of these societies. Instead, other aspects of womanhood training will be strengthened including training in child care and nutrition, thus improving the infant mortality rate.

The **National Committee for the Welfare of Women** will take on the administrative functions, with headquarters in the hospitals and with a staff from the Ministry of Social Welfare and Health. The country will be divided up into four administrative areas, each of which will have similar **Health Education** and **Health Care** programs. The regional programs are planned to be set up in intervals of several years, following the model and experience of the first one, set up in the northern province. A **Community Education Committee** and a **Health Care Committee** will take care of education and health care programs respectively, with specially trained **fox squads** helping with program execution.

Subgroups formed in each of the provincial areas will work on the grass-roots level and will take care of the task of personally contacting specific sectors of the population such as market women, women working in the fields in rural areas; some people will visit homes; others will go to patients in the hospitals; some will go to schools and visit with Imams, the Moslem leaders in the mosques and community leaders: that is, an intensive, educational effort by personal contact is planned - reaching all sectors of the population.

The Health Education Program will depend on special educational materials, booklets and visuals developed by the research group in keeping with local needs. A special education program is planned for the digbas - the woman who perform the operations - and other circumcision society officials.

The Health Care Program, in turn, is designed to help those recently circumcised who are suffering from different complaints as well as those who have sustained birth injuries or fistulae as a delayed result. Both physical as well as emotional support in the form of community groups, is planned. The overall execution of the program is in the hands of the **National Committee for the Welfare of Women**, which in turn is assisted in each of the four regions by a similarly organized Provincial Council. A detailed budget, divided among local contributions and those made by the government or internationally, covers every part and phase of the program.

International assistance is, of course, essential, as the author repeatedly states. The 52-page program includes many tables and a budget that shows a list of local contributions in kind, that is by providing buildings, local supplies, labor, etc., showing that a major part of the work to be done is to be contributed locally. A list of professional/technical advisors, including their qualifications, is given as well as an outline of the organizational structure required to implement the program efficiently and to test all results.

The cost of the program - a budget on an annual basis as well as for the entire 20-year period is provided - is very low especially when compared with the rising health care costs of the mutilations. These so-far hidden costs affect every African country where FGM is practiced, because health care is a governmental responsibility. In rural areas few health care services were available, but this is changing now. (See Health Facts: Overview.)

The budget of the eradication plan projects that the entire cost of the plan may be amortized in a few years after implementation begins. Health care costs will decrease accordingly as fewer girls are excised. This eradication plan, which works on the grass-roots level and involves every community by organizing local people to participate as teams, also divides up the area to be covered among local jurisdictions. Since it is community based, the program can be adopted and adapted in different areas and does not depend on national action. There are many important initiatives detailed in this very comprehensive plan, such as retraining the digbas and organizing a variety of local strategies, that offer many practical solutions that can be used anywhere.

Dr. Koso-Thomas, who works with the IAC, should be consulted and involved in any adaption and implementation of her excellent plan.

MODEL FOR A HEALTHY INITIATION CELEBRATION

Initiation rites, which confirm maturity and entry into the adult community, are practiced by many societies all over the world; most of the practices involve joyful celebrations and teaching the young person her/his responsibilities of adult life. But in large regions of Africa and the Middle East, initiation practices include male circumcision and female genital mutilation (FGM). Infibulation, though it is a requirement for marriage in many Moslem ethnic groups, is usually done on much younger girls and not directly related with coming-of-age ceremonies.

In East Africa, the Kikuyu and many other ethnic groups, in West Africa the Bambara, the Mossi and many others as well as most of the ethnic groups of Sierra Leone and Liberia practice excision as part of initiation.

In the past the girls who survived the group mutilations were separated from their families while their wounds were healing and lived together sometimes for many weeks under the care of the excisor and her helpers in a special area and house of the woman in charge of these activities. The excised girls were taught their responsibilities as adult women, wives and mothers during that time. This was their only sex education and included how to please and serve the husband and to be respectful toward his family and other wives.

The girls are taught that husbands have the right to beat them but they have no right to defend themselves. It was said, for instance in Mali and in Ethiopia, that beatings are a sign of love by the men they must serve. A beaten woman produces good sons it was claimed. The girls - many of them traumatized by the terrible pain of the excision and its aftereffects - were initiated into a life of constant hard work, pain and abuse; and this according to African tradition and custom made them into good wives and mothers. In many rural areas these customs continue to be observed.

But we have learned now, so psychologists who have studied violence confirm, that abuse inflicted routinely and supported by the family and community socializes children for life-long brutality which is practiced without restraint. These violent traditional practices have been ignored or even encouraged under the label of "culture" by the rest of the world at our peril as Somalia demonstrates most vividly; men and boys deliberately starved their own women and children using food to gain power until the rest of the world had to intervene before too many women and children died.

African leaders who care for their people must persuade them to stop the violent initiation traditions that brutalize children and teach lifelong violence. The constant, damaging ruthless civil wars all over sub-Saharan Africa can be correlated in many areas with the violent traditional practices disguised as initiation rites which have no positive function in our present world. Boys especially are socialized to practice violence which by custom and tradition is considered normal behavior for men.

There are better ways to celebrate coming-of-age or the attainment of adulthood than by bloody physical mutilations that result in permanent health damage and excruciating pain. Neither the mutilations nor the traditional teachings by illiterate, uneducated, brutalized old women serve any useful purpose in today's society and world; they certainly do not prepare young people for a productive future in present-day society.

The time has come to close the book on traditional initiation; in fact, it has been stopped in many areas affected by change and with the introduction of schools and by urbanization. But though the traditional rituals have been abandoned in many African towns, the mutilations - that is excision and infibulation - continue to be practiced with no ritual at all and often on babies or very young children. FGM is also done in hospitals or clinics by those who learned Western medicine and do not observe traditions at all but use the operations to make money, perpetuating the physical violence without any embellishments. This demonstrates for everyone what the real objective of FGM is.

The late President Kenyatta of Kenya, who is still greatly admired in Kenya, claimed that initiation was unthinkable without clitoridectomy. He stated that giving up the mutilation of girls would destroy African society. His statements still continue to influence men all over Africa, though they are entirely untrue; many ethnic groups all over Africa, including the Luo in Kenya and many societies all over the world, practice initiation (and always have) without the damaging tortures of genital operations or mutilations of any kind.

MODEL FOR A HEALTHY INITIATION CELEBRATION (continued)

Since initiation is seen as an important landmark in the social life of many communities and families and if Africans wish to preserve these activities of the past which have no real validity in contemporary life, they should be modernized in positive ways, in keeping with new community needs and new aspirations.

Here is an outline of a new approach to confer adult status and recognition on a young person, girl or boy, in assuming the responsibilities of community membership:

A MODERN INITIATION PROGRAM AND AN ADULT STATUS CERTIFICATE

Objectives:

- teaching a young person about her/his adult responsibilities vis-a-vis parents, family members and community. In addition, a period of community service may be added, learning and accomplishing specific tasks;
- teaching a young person about her/his shared responsibilities of married life and the true meaning of marriage partnership;
- participation in and successful completion of a specially designed teaching program on human biology and health, reproduction, sexuality, family planning and childbirth (using the **Childbirth Picture Book** Program) for girls and boys;
- participation in and successful completion of a specially developed teaching program on child care, nutrition, meal preparation, basic household skills and repairs; and learning other desirable community skills that reflect local needs (for example, well digging/irrigation/sanitation/introduction of appropriate technology, etc.). The same program shall be completed by both girls and boys.

Specific sections of the program shall be locally developed according to local needs. These programs shall be designed in ways to make participation possible for literate as well as nonliterate groups.

Certificate of Adult Status (or Maturity):

Any group of young people that has undergone the above training (organized by the village leadership - women and men) shall be awarded a locally designed "Certificate of Adult Status" at an organized, community celebration (much as initiation rituals are now organized). This shall include a formal award ceremony or graduation, where each young person is publicly welcomed into the adult community and promises to contribute her/his service to the community, to make it a better place to live for all community members.

A specially selected panel of respected community members (half women/half men) shall preside over the ceremony, including those who have taught the young people their responsibilities and rights. It is important that women are involved in all the panels and councils in numbers large enough to have a decisive voice. The ceremony itself recognizes the successful completion by the young person of the initiation training and any completed community work: for instance demonstrations of positive results could be included. The certificate formally obligates the young people to uphold community standards and to contribute to their families and community life. Any community service of special merit performed during the initiation training shall be rewarded and cited at this ceremony to provide positive examples.

While it is up to the local communities to decide specifically how to shape their particular celebrations, the national, state or county administrative authority together with local leaders should provide examples by organizing such celebrations and inviting leaders from the region to come, watch and participate. The purpose is to learn how to organize similar initiations in their own communities. That is, actual coming-of-age celebrations should be arranged to set an example, for instance, at regional market towns and/or at places where people from a given area are coming together.

Actual examples of such coming-of-age celebrations where people can see and learn and become involved in such activities are far more effective and persuasive than talking about them. The regional and local political and community leaders should be involved to take up such actions for which regional and national support and financing (depending on the area) should be made available.

MODEL FOR A HEALTHY INITIATION CELEBRATION (continued)

One way to teach change is by organizing new kinds of coming-of-age celebrations in which people from different areas participate as a learning experience. It is much more productive to develop new activities to take the place of damaging customs than to prohibit outright what was done traditionally, no matter how damaging. If the participants enjoy the new activity or celebration, then they will want to repeat it and bring it home. This should be supported by encouraging people to organize their own non traditional coming-of-age celebrations to take the place of what was done before. Women should be involved and join the traditional all-male village or community leadership to plan and organize such activities; since women usually take care of food preparation, which is all important for festivals, they need an equal voice in the other decisions.

Teaching change by example, especially in rural areas where literacy is very low, is the most effective way everywhere, not only in Africa. Involving local people and especially the young themselves, who are the center of all coming-of-age celebrations, provides a good chance for success, that is to replace the physical mutilations. Performing community service is a better way to prove maturity than to subject the young to pain and suffering that may be lifelong. The positive qualities of celebrating coming-of-age should be the focus of this activity.

The success of such an initiative can be established only by its actual implementation which could be organized on a small scale at limited costs with local leadership cooperating. It should be started in several different regions to test this approach in different communities. The whole process should be videotaped as a teaching/learning experience. The videotape can then be shown in different communities all over the region or county and to other areas where initiations traditionally take place.

Rather than prohibiting the mutilations, which has not been successful anywhere as the record shows, the alternative proposed here is to change the contents- stopping the mutilations - while preserving the positive idea. This could be tried out in several countries and proposed to different ethnic groups: It may well establish a positive trend. Different kinds of coming-of-age celebrations can be developed and locally adapted according to local wishes and preferences. Introducing a new kind of maturity celebration provides the local leadership an opportunity to exercise positive guidance and gain prestige since everyone enjoys community festivals, especially the young, who can show off their abilities and worth.

Different versions of such festivals with positive traditional rituals can be designed involving local leadership. These can be proposed and introduced first, supporteded by international grants, to local groups who are interested. This is one approach.

Another is for young people from urban areas, for instance university students or those in higher education, to volunteer to help set up training programs for community work in the rural areas. Such community work would be a new way to gain a certificate of adult status. A new kind of initiation festival will celebrate the completion of the community work by giving a certificate of maturity to the young people - both girls and boys - which will take the place of the traditional initiation. Both male and female students shall be involved. Eventually such rural community service could be required for all university degrees. Volunteers from educational institutions could train young people in the rural areas who do not have the opportunity to go to a university. This will give the young in rural areas the opportunity to learn new skills from their peers to become future community leaders after they gain their adult status certificate.

To organize community services and festivals in rural areas in place of traditional initiations that have lost their relevance in the present-day world may best be done by former members of each rural community who had the opportunity to get higher education; or it might be similar to a domestic Peace Corps. Both female and male students should be required to spend time on such community activities and to work together forming teams as equals, collaborating in teaching the young of each community. By setting an example and demonstrating a new attitude toward each other, they teach the advantages of teamwork and partnership, replacing the traditional mutilations and exploitation of women with cooperation and mutual support.

WOMEN'S INTERNATIONAL NETWORK CAMPAIGN TO STOP FGM:

USING THE UNIVERSAL CHILDBIRTH PICTURE BOOKS

BACKGROUND AND CONTEXT

International actions to stop female genital mutilation (FGM) officially started in 1979 with the World Health Organization Seminar on **Traditional Practices Affecting the Health of Women and Children** in Khartoum, Sudan. The health ministry delegations from the participating African and Middle Eastern countries formulated four recommendations that have served as guidelines ever since. They also have been adopted by the **Inter African Committee** on Traditional Practices Affecting the Health of Women and Children.

These recommendations, besides addressing the countries where FGM is practiced, emphasize education of all people about FGM as well as health training and urge:

> "Intensification of general education of the public, including health education at all levels with special emphasis on the dangers and the undesirability of FGM; and
>
> Intensification of education programmes for traditional birth attendants, midwives, healers and other practitioners of traditional medicine to demonstrate the harmful effects of FGM with a view to enlisting their support to abolish this practice."

THE CHILDBIRTH PICTURE BOOK (CBPB) PROGRAM

The Childbirth Picture Books (CBPBs) were designed to assist with implementation of the WHO Seminar recommendations on the grass-roots level. The **CBPBs** are a picture story of reproduction from a woman's view and provide the basic information on healthy childbirth regardless of language or literacy. **Additions to Prevent Excision and infibulation**, following the same format of the books, are included in all books distributed where FGM is practiced. They graphically show the physical damage done by FGM especially in childbirth and have been very successful in local communities and health centers all over Africa (see letters below).

The full page pictures are accompanied by **a text** to read out loud - as the majority of women in rural areas are illiterate. A **discussion guide** for the presentor is included, also a **picture glossary** of technical terms and a **reading/resource list** of publications.

The books are printed in many languages: In Africa they are used mainly in **English, French** and **Arabic** with the Additions. A **Somali** translation has been added recently, which incorporates the Addition on Infibulation. The books can be readily adapted and translated orally by the presentor according to local needs. The **CBPBs** are designed for local community health workers; the pictures by a medical illustrator are biologically accurate. The experience with the **CBPBs** shows that most people can understand the message that FGM is damaging and harms childbirth (see letters below). **Nutrition supplements, flip charts and color slides** are coordinated with the books.

COMPREHENSION TESTS: Questionnaires have been recently developed to test the knowledge about reproduction and the damage done by FGM of people and families in Africa. Similar questions are asked **before** people are given a CBPB and **after** they have read them to test the effectiveness of the book. This is done to learn if the message **to stop FGM** is understood . At the present time these questionnaires are being used in specific areas in Sierra Leone to try them out. Other countries/areas will be added.

The objective is to develop a testing program to show stastistically the results that are evident from the many letters of usersof the **CBPBs** in many African countries. (See below) Proof of effectiveness is needed to gain support for much larger distribution of the **CBPBs.** Hundreds of letters sent to **WIN NEWS** confirm that the **CBPBs** are wanted and effectively used without any expensive health experts from abroad or sophisticated teaching programs: Most people - as the letters show - are quite able to learn the facts from the pictures by themselves or with the help of local health workers, nurses or midwives.

FGM IS A PUBLIC HEALTH THREAT that affects an estimated 110 million girls and women in continental Africa and this number is still increasing due to population growth - see tabulation of estimates in Health Facts and Overview. FGM also contributes to the spread of AIDS, which is rampant in all areas where FGM is practiced.

WOMEN'S INTERNATIONAL NETWORK CAMPAIGN (continued)

DISTRIBUTION OF CHILDBIRTH PICTURE BOOKS

The **CBPBs** are circulating on the local level in large areas of Africa especially in Sierra Leone, Nigeria, Ghana, Mali, Burkina Faso, Kenya, Ethiopia, Sudan, Egypt and more. They are used in large numbers for health education. The demand for these books on the grass-roots level by local people is continuously growing as shown by the hundreds of letters **WIN NEWS** gets from women and men in the health field, and from teachers, community leaders, nurses, midwives and many others. The books are also distributed in quantity to midwifery schools in several West African countries, including Mali, Burkina Faso, and Cote d'Ivoire. **WIN NEWS** has distributed free books all over Africa since 1982 to all who are asking for them.

The **CBPBs** are also used with the **Additions to Prevent Excision and Infibulation** by many international agencies, including UNICEF, WHO, UNFPA and USAID and by many international health programs in Africa. In the rest of the world the **CBPBs** are used without the additions to teach about healthy childbirth and reproduction, for instance in South and Central America in Spanish; they are also locally printed in India in six Indian languages, in Nepal and the Marshall Islands. There also is a US version used in schools, health and family planning centers.

The **CBPBs** are used with many immigrants and especially with African refugees in Canada and Europe to prevent FGM. In Canada where many Somali refugees have settled, the health ministry has distributed 2000 Somali **CBPBs** in 1993. **WIN NEWS** also sent copies of the Somali translation to the Netherlands, Djibouti and Kenya for refugees. The **CBPBs** have been distributed in all the countries included in this Report.

THE GRASS-ROOTS COMMUNITY CAMPAIGN WITH THE CBPBs

WIN NEWS has been reporting about this campaign at least once a year since the early 1980s - always citing letters from local recipients of the **CBPBs.**

In all books sent in response to a request from areas where FGM is practiced, a message is included asking the recipient to promise that his/her daughters will not be excized and requesting the receivers to spread the message about the dangers and damage resulting from FGM among their families and community. Additional books are offered to all those sending a statement that they will not have their daughters operated.

The positive response to this grass-roots initiative has been very encouraging. **WIN NEWS** continues to get letters from both women and men promising to stop FGM in their families; some also write how they teach and spread the message in their communities. Often letters arrive with many signatures of women and men, promising not to have their daughters operated and asking for **CBPBs.**

Excerpts of some of the letters recently received are printed below. They show the great interest in the subject and the concern of many community people once they know the health facts and the damage done by FGM - which is not known to most people. Some people are so affected that they go to teach their neighbors and in their communities about the damage done by FGM - using the graphic presentations of the books to show the physical problems resulting from the mutilations especially in childbirth. With every mail we get more letters with requests for **CBPBs**, which seem to be circulating in many different communities.

This method of reaching people directly with information they need and want has been very effective: It needs no intermediaries and expensive experts from abroad or eleborate research. The **CBPBs** reach all people personally on a subject that is of great concern - especially in Africa where fertility is so highly prized. Most of all the **CBPBs** are understood by those with limited reading skills. Of course the distribution of the **CBPBs** is not a substitute for organized campaigns, such as the ones described above. But it is the least expensive, most direct way of reaching people with information about reproductive health, that everyone in Africa and around the world urgently needs and that has been mystified, distorted or concealed everywhere, doing great harm especially to women. Sponsorships to distribute more **CBPBs** are welcomed by **WIN NEWS.**

WOMEN'S INTERNATIONAL NETWORK CAMPAIGN (continued)

LETTERS FROM USERS OF THE CHILDBIRTH PICTURE BOOKS (Excerpts)

From Mr. M.N., Kenema, Sierra Leone (July '93)

I was grateful when I received your books because so many people were asking. I have started enlightening them about the harmful effects about women circumcision and what will happen to a women who has been circumcised. . . Because there are not enough for all of us to have one book each, we go to various villages with the books and call on the elderly women who are responsible for the circumcision and first explain to them and later show the pictures. . . We opened a small training centre in that area. . . I am asking you to send me more books to end the harmful effects of this process by training more people. . .

From A.K.F., Kissytown, Kenema, Sierra Leone (July '93)

I have formed a club called "Youth Organization Club" in our village of boys and girls. The purpose of this club is to go around the other villages to tell people about the damage of female circumcision. . . We are succeeding a little bit. A few people have started following our advice. Some have started sending their daughters to our city and larger towns since this is the only way to prevent their girls from being circumcised. As chairman of the above named club, I would appreciate it much to please send us some more of your books.

From S.S., Tamale, Ghana (Nov. '92)

Thank you for the **Childbirth Picture Book**. It arrived intact with the Addition to prevent Excision. At a social gathering the demand for the book cannot be described on this paper. All who saw it will like to read it at home. It is really an education and informative resource book. With a little explanation the pictures in it were all clear to me and everybody. . . About the female circumcision, the practice has died down but it is believed some people may be doing it underground. We the campaigners shall not rest until this is stopped totally. . . My female dependents and daughters will never be circumcised and I shall do my best to educate a lot of people across the country about the dangers of female circumcision. . .

From Ms. F.S., Kenema, Sierra Leone (Feb. '93)

I wish to apply for 20 copies of the **Universal Childbirth Picture Book**. I am a village health worker in one of the remote villages of Sierra Leone. I took a course for Traditional Birth Attendants (TBAs) and recently got my certificate and was sent to a village to teach women on childbirth. I use advice from the **Universal Childbirth Picture Book**. I teach the people to forget about female circumcision - those who bore female children. I would like more books. I am covering over 30 villages on my teaching rounds. I use the books to illustrate why they should change . . . I hereby promise that my daughers will not be circumcised. . . Hoping that you will send these materials on time.

From Mr. A.M., Teacher, Bangui, Central Africa (June '93) - translated

I have received the copy of the **CBPB** you sent which is very useful. First I have learned myself a great deal from this book concerning its use for teaching; it is designed for that purpose and can be readily adapted to make it easy to understand by different students. . . I would like very much to have more copies: This book provides an excellent and concrete means of education and one cannot teach without books. Showing the book to both women and men has resulted in much discussion especially about excision and its damaging results. . .

From Ms. S.O., School of Nursing, Cross River State, Nigeria (Jan. '92)

Thank you very much for your assistance and the books you sent, they are of tremendous importance to me and my colleagues. We use the books in the family health clinic, also prenatal and postnatal clinics. The Excision addition is useful in the labor ward; this we do by showing the pictures of a child delivered by an unexcised mother and then by an excised one. We also use the supplement on nutrition and show foods that have an affordable price to meet the body requirements. . .

WOMEN'S INTERNATIONAL NETWORK CAMPAIGN (continued)
LETTERS FROM USERS OF THE CHILDBIRTH PICTURE BOOKS (Excerpts)

From Mr. M.N., Family Life Education Dakar, Senegal (July '93) - (translated)
I would be grateful if you could send me a copy of the **CBPB** and the Supplement on Excision. I coordinate the training for a program which will introduce family life education in schools. Sex education is an important part of this. I also want to state that my daughter will never be circumcised and I shall tell others about the dangers of female circumcision in order to stop circumcision of all our daughters. I am planning in the framework of the above educational program to carry on the battle against excision through intense consciousness raising.

From Ms. G.A., Workers College, Tamale, Ghana (Nov. '92)
I am a social worker and a campaigner against female circumcision. Please send me a copy of the **Universal Childbirth Picture Book**. I saw a copy with a friend . . .The book was very informative. . . I need a copy of the Addition on Excision. . . I hereby promise that my daughters will never be circumcised. I shall teach others about the dangers of female circumcision. I shall ask them to join me to stop circumcising all girls in our families and families of friends.

From Mr. S.S., Porto Novo, Benin (Aug. '93) (translated)
With this letter we greet you and want to inform you about our efforts to teach people about the process of reproduction. I also promise that my daughters will not be excised and that I shall inform others about the dangers of excision and I am joining with others to put a stop to these practices among our daughters and the children of other families. I would appreciate receiving more books for my teaching program to train medical technicians. I also send you the names of those who work with me and who want books.

From Aigbogun Clinic & Maternity, Abudu, Nigeria (June '93)
The usefulness of the book is that it talks about human life and also teaches of how to keep us away from trouble. I like it because the book deals with practical problems. I show the drawings for more understanding, obviously we need more books for the teaching. Women, families and youth understand the drawings with my explanation. Since you sent me this book there is a great change. When I speak about circumcision of females all of them weep, because the victims of circumcision bleed seriously during labour. 105 candidates in my group promised not to circumcise their daughers.

From A.A., Akim, Oda, Ghana (Dec. '92)
Your booklet is very useful to me. . . It has given me awareness of the evil and the effects of the circumcision of the female genital organ. The illustrations in the booklet have helped me to educate some of our northern tribes who have been practising this. . . I have also been giving talks to women who have been visiting our prenatal and postnatal clinic on the health and the welfare of their new babies. I have established women welfare groups in some of the villages around my clinic to educate them.

From Ms. E.G., Makeni Town, Sierra Leone (Feb. '93)
I wish to appeal to you for your most educative teaching material - the **Childbirth Picture Book**. I introduce myself as a state registered nurse attached to the government Hospital in Makeni. My work in the hospital is to teach families and Junior Health Workers in health care education. Our centre of concentration is on youths, respectively women. The Mobile Clinic comprises other Health Staff from many other Health Centres. . . The staff will in turn teach other people in their various clinics when they return to their various Health Centres. I should therefore ask for fifty (50) copies of the **Childbirth Picture Book** to be distributed among the health workers. The 50 copies will serve as teaching material to educate those in the rural areas not to engage in Female Circumcision citing the dangers to be encountered.

From Nurse K.,Community Health Program, Kono District, Sierra Leone, (Jan '93)
This to inform you that our district has been invaded and we have had to move to Freetown and we have started our work here. . . We are kindly asking you to send the **CBPBs** here; we are strongly continuing our work for health and the people apperciate it. We cannot explain the dangers of excision to the people without the diagrams of the **CBPBs**. . . We thank you for your usual cooperation.

PROGRAM FOR A WOMEN'S HEALTH EDUCATION NETWORK AND SANITARY PRODUCT MANUFACTURING PROJECT

SUMMARY AND OUTLINE:

Health education, specifically information on the biological facts of reproduction and childbirth, is greatly neglected in developing countries. Childbearing, according to the World Health Organization (WHO), is the leading cause of death of women in the poorer, developing countries - especially in Africa.

Many traditional practices related to childbearing are very damaging: Female genital mutilation is the most widespread damaging practice in Africa and the Middle East. Education about reproduction, human biology, nutrition, family planning and child spacing, child care and women's health are needed, especially in societies where women are engaged in frequent childbearing.

The costs of health services are increasing everywhere: Preventive health education could greatly reduce the need for curative care. According to WHO, less than 10 percent of the populations of poor countries have access to modern health care; yet all people can be reached by health education and specifically by the program outlined here.

This health proposal is based on self-support. After the initial introductory period, the costs for the entire education program will be financed from the production of sanitary materials by the project participants, and the expansion of the health education program throughout the region and country will not cost the public or government anything at all.

The need for **independent income** is shared by women all over the world. This project is designed to pay an hourly wage to all working members who participate in the health education sessions. Each network member earns while she learns. To participate in the production work, she will be taught the necessary manual skills and she will also be given the opportunity to take part in the selling of the products. After gaining some experience, she will be invited to take part in the business end of the program including the management and administration of the sanitary material production.

Sanitary napkins are a recurring need for women everywhere. The products available worldwide in the modern sector are expensive and out of reach for a majority of women in developing countries. Rags and other unsanitary materials are often used.

There is a great need for **baby diapers** and for other sanitary cotton products of all kinds related to childbearing and health care. Midwives, birth attendants, maternities, clinics and hospitals use expensive imports or else have to make do with poor substitutes.

The **Sanitary Product Manufacturing Project** is designed to substitute locally made sanitary products for expensive imports and produce high-quality sanitary cotton products from locally grown cotton and materials, using local labor and local initiatives, creating local jobs.

OBJECTIVES:

Health Education: To teach women and girls about the biological facts of reproduction, personal hygiene, childbirth, family planning, nutrition, child care and more, using the **Childbirth Picture Book (CBPB)** as a teaching aid.

Income Generation: To earn an independent income by producing, distributing and selling sanitary cotton products by and for women. The manufacture of sanitary cotton products financially supports the health education as well as generates an income for all participants.

Sanitary Product Manufacture: To produce sanitary napkins and other sanitary cotton products for personal health, childbirth, baby care, etc., including diapers and products needed by birth attendants, midwives, clinics and hospitals.

Health Network Organization and Membership: To develop a self-help education network to promote women's health and stop damaging traditions - especially FGM- by teaching positive health practices, self-help and mutual support by and for women on the grass-roots level. Training in teaching skills and business management to participate in running the product distribution will be available.

PROGRAM FOR
WOMEN'S HEALTH NETWORK AND SANITARY PRODUCT MANUFACTURING
HEALTH EDUCATION: (continued)

USING THE CHILDBIRTH PICTURE BOOK TO LEARN WHILE YOU EARN

Education in personal hygiene and reproduction is not available to most women in developing countries. The Learn While You Earn program makes it possible for women to use their limited time on income-producing activities by joining the Health Network and participating in the production and health education meetings.

The initial meetings of the health production team (limited to 20 women or fewer) will be used to teach the manual skills and to organize the production.

After each participant has learned her manual job, a trained community health worker/ midwife or nurse joins the group as teacher. The room or space where the women work shall be organized in such a way that each woman can easily see the health teacher while she works with her hands. The initial discussion is concerned with the use and care of the sanitary napkins that are being produced - leading to a discussion of menstruation.

The **CBPB** shall be used as a eaching aid to provide an outline for the teaching program. In addition, the flip charts may be used. The health teacher/midwife from the same community or area shall encourage all women to participate in the discussions and questions. To cover the information in the **CBPB** thoroughly will take several months of biweekly meetings. Additional time should be spent on nutrition, child care and family planning and prevention of damaging traditional practices.

Additions on Excision and Infibulation to the **CBPB** are included and to be used where needed, showing the health damage done by the operations. This should be discussed thoroughly, especially in relation to childbirth, after each participant has become familiar with the natural process of childbirth.

After successful completion of each course, participants will receive a **CBPB** of their own and a certificate and become full members of the Health Network. They will be encouraged to set up a group in their own neighborhood and will be offered technical assistance to do so. Alternatively, they may continue on as production team workers and take on more responsibilities as assistants to the teachers, the organizers, etc.

ECONOMIC OUTLINE AND SELF-SUPPORT

The chief raw material used is cotton, locally grown by women farmers. The skills of local women will be enlisted in the production of sanitary materials. A one-time grant will establish a **Rotating Fund** which will be used to set up a network of sanitary production manufacturing centers and to purchase the necessary equipment including sterilizers as needed. Each center, located in village markets or schools, will repay the start-up money over time, from income. Thus, the Rotating Fund will be continuously replenished and be able to finance additional centers.

Each Health Network Center or sanitary material production group is expected to become self-supporting after one to three years and will, in turn, invest in more health/production centers. Local women are enlisted to participate in the network, as production workers for an hourly wage. After they have successfully completed at least one teaching and production cycle (six months to one year), they will be accepted as full health network members and may become distributors or sales agents of the products and/or set up additional health network centers. They also may become organizers, work as teachers, as managers and as administrators locally, regionally and/or nationally.

The network members will have a dual function as health educators and as distributors of sanitary products. The spread of health education will, therefore, be soundly based on economic self-support. All distribution costs are paid from a percentage of sales. Women workers will themselves determine how many hours they wish or are able to work, but teaching sessions must be regularly attended. The income from sales shall be used first to pay wages and salaries; then for raw materials (cotton) and finally to pay back the initial investment/start-up. It is expected that after a year or less there will be enough income to cover current costs and repayment of capital investment can begin. A part of the income shall be set aside to start more Health Network Centers.

PROGRAM FOR
WOMEN'S HEALTH NETWORK AND SANITARY PRODUCT MANUFACTURING (continued)

ORGANIZATION OF PRODUCTION AND DISTRIBUTION

Technical Assistance: The production shall be planned with the technical assistance of an organization like Intermediary Technologies (London), with participation of both rural and urban women and women's organizations and in consultation with the health sector, hospitals and health ministries. The production is expected to consist mainly in manual work with few hand tools and shall be carefully planned step-by-step.

Pilot Program: A group of organizers shall be trained first and gain experience by going through an initial program. These trained organizers will function as Health Network leaders as well as set up the distribution of the products. Several pilot projects shall be set up in villages and urban areas (at least two each) by the initially trained group.

Start-up (Rotating Fund): The Rotating Fund shall finance the training of the organizers (see above), and the start-up costs of the initial pilot projects. It will pay for the materials (cotton) and equipment as needed, as well as the wages of the team workers, the organizers and health teachers, until there is an income. As soon as several centers are fully functioning, women farmers shall be given a contract to supply the cotton.

Distribution: Assistance of women's organizations, especially in the urban areas, shall be enlisted in the distribution. Local women traders and market women shall be shown how to sell the products in local markets. Midwives, local dispensaries and clinics shall be canvased as well as invited to participate in the distribution by being offered a lower rate. Other sales incentives shall be developed according to local needs.

Wages/Earnings: All production workers shall receive a minimum wage per hour. Later, piece-work may be substituted (depending on preference). The health educators, organizers and managers shall earn salaries and receive the necessary **CBPBs**.

RESULTS/EVALUATION

This health education program will have a marked effect on the health of each woman, her family and her community. It will reduce FGM, death in childbirth and infant mortality. Family health and nutrition in households where women are members of the network should markedly improve. The income earned by the network members will benefit especially the children of each family

A formal evaluation should be made of villages that have Health Network Centers compared to **those** that do not, using childbirth, infant and health statistics. Such an evaluation can also be made comparing households, using questionnaires

Community women in both villages and urban areas will learn new skills and have the opportunity to earn a wage while learning how to improve their own and their children's health. Besides engaging in paid production work, they also can increase their income by selling the products they make (house-to-house or in the market). Women who have become full network members will be taught how to organize more Sanitary Product Production Centers and/or to take on various jobs in distribution, management, etc.

There is a great need for products such as sanitary napkins and other cotton-based health materials in all developing countries. A women-for-women production system can make important contributions by substituting imports with locally made sanitary products which cost much less. To make sanitary napkins and other health-related items available locally and inexpensively will also improve the health of many women and children.

The **Health Network and Sanitary Product Manufacturing Program** has a built-in expansion and multiplier factor: It is expected to grow and cover an entire country or region, creating a self-supporting health education system that will become a major factor in improving women's and children's health.

The eradication of damaging traditional practices and customs, especially FGM and other harmful practices related to reproduction and childbirth, can be supported by this program on the grass-roots level and at minimum financial cost. The Health Network also has the potential to create a **modern, women-based health system** that is self-supporting and self-perpetuating.

FOOTNOTES

1. InterAfrican Committee- IAC - on Traditional Practices Affecting the Health of Women and Children, 147, rue de Lausanne, CH-1202 Geneva, Switzerland; President: Berhane Ras-Work. See also **WIN NEWS,** Vol. 10, No. 2, Spring 1984, pp. 35-36.
2. UN Decade Conference FORUM '85 Panel: Traditional Practices Affecting the Health of Women and Children. See **WIN NEWS,** Vol. 11, No. 3, Summer 1985. pp 40-43.
3. Conference Report available from IAC (address above). See also **WIN NEWS** Vol. 17, No. 1, Winter 1991, pp. 38-45.
4. President's Report and Newsletter available from IAC Geneva office, address above. See also **WIN NEWS,** Vol. 18, No. 4, Autumn 1992, p. 35.
5. Organization of African Unity (OAU) Conference on Assistance to African Children, Dakar, Senegal, Nov. 25-27, 1992. See **WIN NEWS,** Vol. 19, No.1,Winter1993, p. 37.
6. Inter African Committee of Nigeria on Traditional Practices Affecting the Health of Women and Children, 5, Tashiu Elias Close, Victoria Island, Nigeria; P.O. Box 6051, Lagos, Nigeria. See **WIN NEWS,** Vol. 17, No. 3, Summer 1991, p. 32.
   Alabi, E.M., Project Coordinator, National Inter African Committee-Nigeria, P.O. Box 10761, G.P.O. Marina, Lagos, Nigeria.
7. Alabi, E.M. "Traditional Methods of Childbirth in Africa - The Nigerian Experience." Published by **Your Task Health Magazine** , The Inter African Committee of Nigeria (address above). See also **WIN NEWS,** Vol. 19, No. 2, Spring 1993, pp. 37-38.
8. Program by National Association of Nigeria Nurses & Midwives (NANNM), P.O. Ikeja, Box 3857, Lagos, Nigeria. Funded by Population Action International (PAI) 1120 19th St., N.W., Suite 550, Washington, DC 20036-3605. See **WIN NEWS,** Vol. 14, No. 2, p. 33.
9. **Women's Health Issues in Nigeria**. Mere N. Kisekka, Editor. Order from Tamaza Publishing Co., Ltd., c/o Elly Engelkes, Makelaarsstraat 26, 1315 JK Almere-Stad, Netherlands. See also **WIN NEWS,** Vol. 19, No. 3, Summer 1993, pp. 43 and 49-50.
10. "Project on the Physical Violation of Young Females". Annual reports are published regularly and available from Cairo Family Planning Association, 50 Goumhouria St., Cairo, Egypt, Aziza Hussein, Director, Aziza Kamel Mahmoud, Project Director. See **WIN NEWS,** Vol. 19, No. 3, Summer 1993, p. 42 and **WIN NEWS,** Vol. 18, No. 4, Autumn 1992, p. 43. **WIN NEWS** has summarized the annual reports every year for the past 10 years usually in the summer or autumn issues.
11. See **WIN NEWS,** Vol. 18, No. 1, Winter 1992, p. 36.
12. BAFROW - Foundation for Research on Women's Health, Productivity and the Environment. 214 Tafsir Demba M'bye Road, Tobacco Road Estate. P.O. Box S.K. 2854, Kanifing, The Gambia.
13. **FEMALE CIRCUMCISION: STRATEGIES TO BRING ABOUT CHANGE - Proceedings of the International Seminar on Female Circumcision, 13-16 June 1988, Mogadishu, Somalia.** AIDoS (Italian Association for Women in Development), Via dei Giubbonari, 30-00186 Rome, Italy See **WIN NEWS,** Vol. 14, No. 3, Summer 1988, pp. 24-33.
14. AIDoS - Associazione italiana donne per lo sviluppo - Address above, Daniela Colombo, Director. AIDoS is engaged in development programs for and with women in many developing countries, especially with programs to eradicate FGM. The teaching materials developed with ILO (International Labor Office) for the SWDO (Somali Women's Democratic Organization) Program are being adapted and used in other African countries in collaboration with the IAC (Inter African Committee) and its affiliates. A videotape of the SWDO conference is available from AIDoS.
15. "AIDoS Information Campaign Program to Eradicate Infibulation in Somalia 1987/88." See **WIN NEWS,** Vol. 13, No. 4, Autumn 1987, pp. 19-21.
16. AIDoS (address above) Training Programs to Eradicate FGM in collaboration with ILO (International Labor Organization), Turin Training Center, Turin, Italy. Includes videotapes and training for trainers, specifically adapted for Ethiopia, Sudan, Nigeria and Gambia. See **WIN NEWS,** Vol. 19, No. 1, Winter 1993, p. 41.

FOOTNOTES (continued)

17. AIDoS (address above) "Training of Trainers - Program to Eradicate FGM." Prototype multimedia/modular training packages adapted for different countries/environments. See **WIN NEWS**, Vol. 18, No. 3, Summer 1992, p. 34.
18. Comite National de Lutte Contre la Pratique de l'Excision (National Committee to Fight Against the Practice of Excision), 01 BP 515, Ouagadougou 01 Burkina Faso, President Mariam Lamizana. See **WIN NEWS**, Vol. 19, No. 3, Summer 1993, pp. 39-41.
19. A 72-minute film, "My Daughter Shall Not Be Excised" ("Ma Fille Ne Sera Pas Excisee"), was made in Burkina Faso by Boureima Nikiema. See **WIN NEWS**, Vol. 16, No. 1, Winter 1990, p. 30.
20. As reported in **SIDWAYS**, a national newspaper of Burkina Faso (in French). See also **WIN NEWS**, Vol. 18, No. 2, Spring 1992, p. 41.
21. Maendeleo Ya Wanawake Organization. P.O. Box 44412, Nairobi, Kenya; Ms. Leah Muuya, Project Director.
22. See **WIN NEWS**, Vol. 3, No. 2, Spring 1977, p. 51.
23. Population Action International (PAI), 1120 19th St., N.W., Washington, DC 20036 - 3605 (called Population Crisis Committee until 1992). PAI is an independent, privately funded research organization and the only donor in the the population field that has funded and assisted programs to eradicate FGM. See also **WIN NEWS**, Vol. 19, No. 2, Spring 1993, p. 44.
24. Paper presented at the National Council for International Health Conference, June 1984, Washington, D.C., by Dr. Sandra Gove, Medical Volunteers International. See also **WIN NEWS**, Vol. 10, No. 3, Summer 1984, p. 38.
25. Program for Appropriate Technology in Health (PATH)/Kenya, P.O. Box 76634, Nairobi, Kenya.
26. The National Committee on Traditional Practices (NCTP), Hon. Jitto Ram, Ministry of Health, P.O. Box 9083, Dar es Salaam, Tanzania.
27. The Institute for Development Training (IDT), 212 E. Rosemary St., Chapel Hill, NC 27514; Ms. Diana L. Altman, Project Coordinator. See also **WIN NEWS** Vol. 19, No. 3, Summer 1993, p. 44.
28. Population Action International (PAI); see footnote 23 above.
29. **American Medical News**, April 27, 1990, "Female Circumcision - Is It Practiced in USA?". See **WIN NEWS**, Vol. 16, No. 3, Summer 1990, pp. 28-30.
30. **The New York Times**, "Stoked by Ethnic Conflict, Refugee Numbers Swell," Nov. 10, 1993 (International Section).
31. Federal Prohibition of Female Genital Mutilation Act of 1993, introduced as part of Women's Health Equity Act: Sec. 262 Title 18 Amendment - 116. Female Genital Mutilation; Sec. 263 Education and Outreach; Sec. 264 Effective Dates. See **WIN NEWS**, Vol. 19, No. 4, Autumn 1993, p. 36.
32. Resolution on FGM passed at National Organization for Women (NOW) Conference. NOW, 1000 16th St., N.W., Suite 700, Washington, DC 20036-5705. See also **WIN NEWS**, Vol. 16, No. 3, Summer 1990, p. 26.
33. See footnote 29 above.
34. "Women's Health in Women's Hands," 344 Dupont St., W., Suite 106, Toronto, Ontario M5R 1V9, Canada. A women's health organization that employs Somali women, including the translators of the **Childbirth Picture Books** into Somali. The Somali translation includes the section on infibulation.
35. From a letter by Ottawa psychologist Dr. Barbara Fulford to **The Globe and Mail**, Aug. 27, 1993. See **WIN NEWS**, Vol. 19, No. 4, Autumn 1993, p. 37.
36. "Canada: College of Physicians and Surgeons of Ontario Prohibits GM." College of Physicians and Surgeons of Ontario, 80 College St., Toronto, Ontario M5G 2E2, Canada. See **WIN NEWS**, Vol. 18, No. 2, Spring 1992, p. 46.

FOOTNOTES (continued)

37. Foundation for Women's Health Research & Development (FORWARD), Africa Centre, 38 King St., Covent Garden, London WC2E 8JT, England, UK.
38. For a copy of the law, see **WIN NEWS**, Vol. 11, No. 3, Summer 1985, p. 44.
39. A newsletter and a number of publications are available from FORWARD as well as teaching programs and guides, reports of meetings, etc. See **WIN NEWS**, Vol. 15, No. 1, Winter 1989, p. 29, and Vol. 15, No. 2, Spring 1989, pp. 38-39, and more.
40. See **WIN NEWS**, Vol. 15, No. 2, Spring 1989, p. 37.
41. The First Study Conference on Genital Mutilation of Girls in Europe, London, July 6-8, 1992. See footnote 37 above for FORWARD address. See also **WIN NEWS**, Vol. 18, No. 4, Autumn 1992.
42. See **WIN NEWS**, Vol. 18, No. 4, Autumn 1992, pp. 30 - 32; Vol. 19, No. 1, Winter 1993, pp. 34-36; and Vol. 19, No. 2, Spring 1993, p. 45.
43. G.A.M.S. - Groupe Femmes pour l'Abolition des Mutilations Sexuelles (Women's Group for the Abolition of Sexual Mutilation), 8, cite Prost, 75011 Paris, France. **WIN NEWS** has regularly reported on G.A.M.S., formed 1983, affiliated with the Inter African Committee 1991.
44. **Les Mutilations du Sexe des Femmes Aujourd'hui en France (Sexual Mutilations in France of Today).** Editions Tierce, 1 rue des Fosses St. Jacques, 75005, Paris, France. Sponsored by the Ministry of Women's Rights. See also **WIN NEWS**, Vol. 11, No. 1, Winter 1985.
45. France - Cases of FGM cited in **WIN NEWS**, Vol. 9, No. 2, Spring 1983, p. 64; Vol. 10, No. 3, Summer 1984, p. 40; Vol. 16, No. 3, Summer 1990, p. 30; Vol. 17, No. 2, Spring 1991, p. 40; Vol. 18, No. 2, Spring 1992, p. 44; Vol. 19, No. 2, Spring 1993, p. 50; and many other issues.
46. Hosken, Fran P. **Les Mutilations Sexuelles Feminines (The Hosken Report** in French). Editions Denoel, 19, rue de L'Universite, 75007 Paris, France. October 1983. Also available from **WIN NEWS.**
47. "Actions to Stop the Spread of FGM" , **WIN NEWS**, Vol. 19, No. 4, Autumn 1993, pp. 33-34.
48. Koso-Thomas, Olayinka, M.D. **The Circumcision of Women: A Strategy for Eradication**. Zed Books Ltd., London, United Kingdom. 1986. See also **WIN NEWS**, Vol. 13, No. 3, Summer 1987, pp. 34-35.
49. See **WIN NEWS**, Vol. 8, No. 2, Summer 1982, pp. 45-58. Thesis in author's files.

BIBLIOGRAPHY

Relevant medical, ethnographic and historic publications.

Index References: (H) Health; (S) Sociology; (B) Background information.

PUBLICATIONS BY FRAN P. HOSKEN

BOOKS/REPORTS (listed by date of publication):

The Hosken Report: Genital and Sexual Mutilation of Females. Second edition (1979). **WIN NEWS**, Lexington, MA 02420, 368 pp. // With Country Case Histories of: Egypt, Sudan, Ethiopia, Somalia, Kenya, Nigeria, Ivory Coast, Burkina Faso (Upper Volta), Mali, Senegal, Sierra Leone, the Arab Peninsula, France and Britain. **(S/H/B)**

Female Sexual Mutilations: The Facts and Proposals for Action - An Action Guide. WIN NEWS, Lexington, MA 02420. May 1980. 102 pp. // A summary of **The Hosken Report** with updates as well as a chapter on "Case Histories: Women Speaking." The key chapter is an Action Guide for international political actions against the spreading mutilations. **(S/H)**

The Hosken Report: Genital and Sexual Mutilation of Females. Third edition (1982). **WIN NEWS**, Lexington, MA 02420. 344 pp. // Update on Country Case Histories (see second edition above) as well as the History of Genital Mutilation; Health Facts and Overview; the WHO Seminar in Khartoum, February 1979; the Politics of Genital Mutilation: A Conspiracy of Silence; Women & Health: Actions for Change; Women and Development; Status of Women. Includes **The Hosken Report Postscript** (1983), 17 pp. **(S/H/B)**

Les Mutilations Sexuelles Feminines. French translation of **The Hosken Report**. Paris: Editions Denoel, October 1983. Copies available from **WIN NEWS**. **(S/H/B)**

RESEARCH ARTICLES (listed by date of publication):

"Genital Mutilation of Women in Africa." MUNGER AFRICANA LIBRARY NOTES , No. 36 (1976). Munger Africana Library, California Institute of Technology, Pasadena, CA 91125. // In booklet form, this is the first article ever published on this subject that provides an overview of the problem, citing East and West African medical sources as well as first-hand information, including an appeal for change. **(S/H)**

"Female Circumcision and Fertility in Africa." WOMEN AND HEALTH, Vol. 1, No. 6 (1976), pp. 3-11. Women and Health, Biological Sciences Program, State University of New York, College at Old Westbury, Old Westbury, NY 11568. // After an introduction providing some background on rural women in Africa, the article relates the medical and health facts from many published medical sources, as well as information from fieldwork in Africa. The last part of the article cites the failure of international organizations to prevent the operations, and makes suggestions for change. **(H)**

> German translation: **"Klitorisbeschneidung: Genitale Verstummelung von Frauen in Afrika."** COURAGE (September 1978).
>
> Italian translation: **"Mutilazioni Sessuali delle Donne Africane."** EFFE, Vol. 4, No. 10/11 (October/November 1978), pp. 3-8. Piazza Campo Marzio 7, Rome, Italy.
>
> French translation and update: **"Les Mutilations Sexuelles en Afrique."** QUESTIONS FEMINISTES, Vol. 8 (May 1980), pp. 43-68. Editions Tierce, 1 rue des Fosses-Saint-Jacques, 75005 Paris, France.

"The Epidemiology of Female Genital Mutilations." TROPICAL DOCTOR, Vol. 8 (1978), pp. 150-56. Royal Society of Medicine, 1 Wimpole St., London W1M 8AE, England. // A survey of genital mutilation from fieldwork, direct interviews and publications from 11 countries in East and West Africa and the Middle East. **(H)**

"Genital Mutilation of Females in Africa - An Urgent Population Policy Issue." KEY ISSUES IN POPULATION POLICY (1978), pp. 255-67. Published by Population Food Fund, Box 255, University Station, Grand Forks, ND 58202. // Proceedings of Capon Springs Public Policy Conference No. 1 of the Population Food Fund, held in fall 1976. **(H)**

"Preventive Care as a Public Health Policy Issue - A Survey of Family Planning and Female Circumcision in East and West Africa." KEY ISSUES IN POPULATION AND FOOD POLICY (1978). Published by Population Food Fund, Box 255, University Station, Grand Forks, ND 58202. // Proceedings of Capon Springs Public Policy Conference No. 2 of the Population Food Fund, held in February 1978. **(H)**

"Women and Health: Genital and Sexual Mutilations of Females." INTERNATIONAL JOURNAL OF WOMEN'S STUDIES, Vol. 3, No. 3 (1980), pp. 300-15. International Journal of Women's Studies, Suite 12, 245 Victoria Ave., Montreal, Quebec, Canada H3Z 2M6. // The importance of the World Health Organization Seminar (Khartoum 1979) to abolish all forms of genital mutilation is discussed, as well as the medical facts. The introduction of sexual mutilation into the modern sector is documented. **(H)**

"Female Circumcision in Africa." VICTIMOLOGY - AN INTERNATIONAL JOURNAL, Vol. 11, Nos. 3/4 (1977-78), pp. 487-98. Emilio Viano, editor. The American University, 3409 Wisconsin Ave., N.W., Washington, DC 20015. // After establishing the medical/health facts, the article provides new information from fieldwork in Kenya and West Africa, as well as previously published research. **(S)**

"Female Circumcision in the World Today: A Global Review." WHO/EMRO TECHNICAL PUBLICATION, Vol. 2, No. 2 (1982), pp. 195-213. Report of World Health Organization Seminar on "Traditional Practices Affecting the Health of Women and Children," Khartoum, Sudan (February 1979). World Health Organization Regional Office, P.O. Box 1517, Alexandria, Egypt. // A worldwide survey of female genital mutilation and outline of methodology to establish the epidemiology. Study to document the spread of female genital mutilation in Africa, the Middle East and Asia. **(H)**

"Female Genital Mutilation in the World Today: A Global Review." INTERNATIONAL JOURNAL OF HEALTH SERVICES, Vol. 11, No. 3 (1981), pp. 415-30. Vicente Navarro, editor in chief. Johns Hopkins Unviersity, Baywood Publishing Co., P.O. Box D, 120 Marine St., Farmingdale, NY 11735. // Based on the research and paper prepared for the World Health Organization Seminar on "Traditional Practices Affecting the Health of Women and Children," with added information from hospital visits in East and West Africa. **(H)**

"Female Genital Mutilations and Human Rights: An Examination of the International Issues and Human Rights Agreements." FEMINIST ISSUES, Vol. 1, No. 3 (1981), pp. 3-23. FEMINIST ISSUES is the English language edition of QUESTIONS FEMINISTES. Transaction Periodicals Consortium, Dept. FI, Rutgers University, New Brunswick, NJ 08903. // This article, after documenting the medical and health results and the spread of the operations into the modern health practice in Africa and the Middle East, raises and examines the human rights questions involved, specifically the right to health and control over one's own body and fertility. **(S)**

GENERAL ARTICLES (listed by date of publication):

"Women and Health in Africa: Genital Mutilation." WOMEN SPEAKING, Vol. 4, No. 15 (1977), pp. 15-18. Women Speaking, 70 Westmount Road, London SE9 IJ3, England. // A summary and documentation of the operations in East and West Africa. **(S)**

"Female Mutilation in Somalia Tests 'Human Rights' Doctrine." POLITICKS & OTHER HUMAN INTERESTS, Vol. 14 (1978), pp. 21-22. Politicks & Other Human Interests, 271 Madison Ave., New York, NY 10016. // Female genital mutilation is a human rights violation, specifically a violation of the right to health and an infringement of the human rights policies of the Carter Administration, and the recently-signed convention of the right to health. **(S)**

"Female Circumcision: Dangerous Rites." SOJOURNER, Vol. 4, No. 7 (March 1979). 143 Albany St., Cambridge, MA 02139. **(S)**

"Genital Mutilation: The Horror the U.S. Ignores." WIN MAGAZINE, Vol. 16, No. 10 (July 1980), pp. 13-16. 326 Livingston St., Brooklyn, NY 11217. **(S)**

"The Politics of Female Genital Mutilation." SCIENCE FOR THE PEOPLE, Vol. 12, No. 6 (November/December 1980), pp. 12-15. 897 Main St., Cambridge, MA 02139. **(S)**

"A World Review of Actions to Abolish Female Circumcision/Genital Mutilation." Proceedings of the International Seminar on Female Circumcision 13-16 June 1988, Mogadishu, Somalia, pp. 15-34. From AIDoS - Italian Association for Women in Development, Via dei Giubbonari 30, 00168 Rome, Italy. **(H/S)**

"Somali Women Organize to End Female Circumcision." DEVELOPMENT FORUM, 19 (March/April 1989). P.O. Box 5850 GCPO, New York, NY 10017. **(S)**

"Female Genital Mutilation: Strategies for Eradication." THE TRUTH SEEKER (July/ August 1989), pp. 22-30. Box 2832, San Diego, CA 92112-9797. **(H)**

"Somalia Campaigns to Eradicate Infibulation." PEOPLE MAGAZINE, Vol. 16, No. 3 (1989). From International Planned Parenthood Federation, P.O. Box 759, Inner Circle, Regent's Park, London NW1 4LQ, England. **(S)**

"Female Genital Mutilation." WOMAN OF POWER (Fall 1990), pp. 42-45. Box 827, Cambridge, MA 02238. **(H)**

"Review of Actions to Abolish Female Genital Mutilation." Presented at the National Council of International Health Conference, 23-26 June 1991, Washington, D.C. **(H/S)**

TESTIMONY IN U.S. CONGRESS CONCERNING FOREIGN ASSISTANCE LEGISLATION

- Foreign Relations Committee (U.S. Senate), April 27, 1981 - Sen. Charles Percy, chair.
- Foreign Affairs Committee (U.S. House of Representatives), March 13, 1981 - Rep. Clement J. Zablocki, chair.
- Appropriations Committee, Subcommittee on Foreign Operations (U.S. Senate):

  April 1, 1980 - Sen. Daniel Inouye, chair.

  May 14, 1981 - Sen. Robert W. Kasten Jr., chair.

  June 8, 1982 - Sen. Robert W. Kasten Jr., chair.

  June 15, 1993 - Sen. Patrick Leahy, chair. (See Editorial, **WIN NEWS**, Vol. 19, No. 3, Summer 1993).

TEACHING MATERIALS TO PREVENT FGM

WIN NEWS publishes The **Universal Childbirth Picture Books (CBPB's)** with Additions on Excision and Infibulation; available in Arabic/English/French. // The **Somali CBPB** includes Infibulation. // Color slides of **CBPB** with Addition on Excision. (**CBPB's** are also available without Additions in many other languages.)

> The **CBPBs** are flexible, adaptable multi-ethnic teaching aids using pictures to explain reproductive health, regardless of language or literacy. They include a Text for each picture, a Discussion Guide, Glossary and an international Reading/ Resource List. Thousands of **CBPB's** are successfully used for prevention of FGM on the grass-roots level. They can be readily adapted and translated. **WIN NEWS** offers technical help and permission to print for educational purposes under its copyright.

THE INTER AFRICAN COMMITTEE provides teaching materials, including three-dimensional models and flannograph flipcharts as well as other training materials and a videotape of their work. 147, rue de Lausanne, CH-1202 Geneva, Switzerland.

AIDoS - Italian Association for Women in Development makes available training materials as well as educational videotapes - Via dei Giubbonari 30, 00168 Rome, Italy.

IDT - Institute for Development Training - Training Course in Women's Health: Module on Female Genital Mutilation. 212 East Rosemary Str., Chapel Hill, NC 27514. USA.

MEDICAL AND ETHNOGRAPHIC PUBLICATIONS

In alphabetical order by author with emphasis on publications of the past 30 years. Index References: (H) Health; (S) Sociology; (B) Background information. NOTE: Books are boldfaced and underlined; articles and reports are underlined; publications and periodicals are boldfaced.

Accad, Evelyne. (Lebanon/sociologist) **Veil of Shame: The Role of Women in Contemporary Fiction of North Africa and the Arab World.** "The Social Position of Women in North Africa and the Arab World," pp. 19-31. Quebec: Editions Naama, 1978. // Summary of the status of women in the Arab world, specifically in the family. **(S/B)**

Adelaja Sr., Dr. O.A., M.D. (Nigeria/Consultant, Medical Statistics, Federal Ministry of Health.) "Final Report on Position of Female Circumcision in Nigeria." Lagos, Nigeria, March 1981. **(H)**

AIDoS (Italian Association for Women in Development). "Female Circumcision - Strategies to Bring About Change." Proceedings of the International Seminar on Female Circumcision, June 13-16, 1988, Mogadishu, Somalia. Also includes "A World Review of Actions to Abolish Female Circumcision/Genital Mutilation," by Fran P. Hosken (see Publications by Fran P. Hosken, above). Report available from AIDoS, via dei Giubbonari, 30 int. 6, 00186 Rome, Italy. **(S)**

Assad, Marie B. (Egypt/sociologist) "Female Circumcision in Egypt: Social Implications, Current Research, and Prospects for Change." **Studies in Family Planning**, Vol. 2, No. 1 (1980), pp. 3-16. // The article examines the social implications of female circumcision in Egypt, also the legal status of the practice and its relation to Islam, including a survey (and analysis) of 54 women at the family planning clinics. **(S)**

Baasher, T.A. (Sudan/Regional Advisor on Mental Health, World Health Organization/ EMRO) "Psychological Aspects of Female Circumcision." Report for the Seminar on Traditional Practices Affecting the Health of Women and Children. **WHO/EMRO Technical Publication**, No. 2 (1979), pp. 71-105. // Examines the psychological aspects including the language, the anxiety of the children and other social factors involved. A survey of 70 adult females living in Alexandria (most of them Sudanese) is included, based on a questionnaire, with an analysis of the data. **(H/S)**

________. "Psycho-Social Aspects of Female Circumcision." Report for the Seminar on Traditional Practices Affecting the Health of Women and Children. **WHO/EMRO Technical Publication,** Vol. 2, No. 2 (1982), pp. 162-80. // The social questions raised in the study are concerned with the origin of the practice as well as the reasons why it is practiced in some communities and not in others. The rituals connected with the operations, especially in the Sudan, are discussed. **(S)**

Barker-Benfield, C.J. (USA) **The Horrors of the Half Known Life: Male Attitudes Towards Women and Sexuality in 19th-Century America.** Harper Colophon Books, 1977. // Background of modern American gynecology and how it deals with women. **(B/S)**

________. "A Historical Perspective on Women's Health Care - Female Circumcision." **Women and Health: Issues in Women's Health Care**, Vol. 1, No. 1 (1976), pp. 13-15, 18-20. // Female circumcision practiced in the U.S. by the Orificial Surgery Society. **(H)**

Bayoumi, Ahmed. (Sudan) "The Training and Activity of Village Midwives in the Sudan." **Tropical Doctor,** Vol. 6, No. 3 (July 1976), pp. 118-25. **(S)**

Bazin-Tardieu, Danielle. (Mali) **Femmes du Mali.** Ottawa, Canada: Editions Lemeac, Inc., 1975. **(B)**

Beasley, Ina M. (UK) "Female Circumcision." **Women Speaking** (July-Sept. 1976), pp. 210-23. **(S/H)**

Beck, Ann. (UK) **A History of the British Medical Administration of East Africa, 1900-1950.** Cambridge: Harvard University Press, 1970. **(H)**

Boserup, Ester. (Denmark) **Woman's Role in Economic Development.** New York: St. Martin's Press, Inc., 1970. **(B)**

Bowesman, Charles, M.D. (UK) **Surgery and Clinical Pathology in the Tropics.** "Ritual Circumcision of Females," pp. 542-57. Edinburgh and London: Livingstone Ltd., 1960. // Dr. Bowesman practiced in Gambia and Ghana. This chapter explains the types of operations and gives the reasons why they are practiced. **(H)**

Bruce-Chwatt, Leonard. (UK) "Female Circumcision and Politics." **World Medicine**, Vol. 2, No. 7 (1976), pp. 44-47. // The politics of the circumcision controversy of the 1920's and 1930's in Kenya, including the support of the operations by President Jomo Kenyatta. **(S/H)**

Cloudsley, Anne. (UK) **Women of Omdurman: Victims of Circumcision.** London: Anne Cloudsley, 1981. // An account of the personal experiences of the author in Sudanese society in the 1950's. **(B/S)**

Commonwealth Expert Group. (UK) **"Engendering Adjustment for the 1990's."** Report of Effect on Women by Structural Adjustment Policies of the World Bank. Commonwealth Secretariat, Marlborough House, Pall Mall, London SW1Y 5BX, England. **(B)**

Cook, R., M.D. (UK/Regional MCH/NUT Advisor, WHO/EMRO) "Damage to Physical Health from Pharaonic Circumcision (Infibulation) of Females: A Review of the Medical Literature." WHO Regional Office of the Eastern Mediterranean, Alexandria, Egypt: 1976. // This review summarizes the health problems from all major medical articles published between 1935 and 1975. Dr. Cook concludes: "The sum total of suffering and disability consequent upon Pharaonic circumcision is therefore considerable." **(H)**

Diallo, Assitan. (Mali) L'excision en Milieu Bambare. Thesis of the Ecole Normale Superieure de Bamako, Mali (1977-78). In French. **(S)**

Duffy, John. (U.S.A.) "Masturbation and Clitoridectomy: A 19th-Century View." **Journal of the American Medical Association**, Vol. 186 (1963), pp. 245-248. // Clitoridectomy performed in order to discourage masturbation in 19th-century America. **(S)**

El Dareer, Asma Abdel Rahim, M.D. (Sudan) **An Epidemiological Study of Female Circumcision in the Sudan.** Thesis submitted for M.Sc. degree in community medicine, Department of Community Medicine, University of Khartoum, Sudan (1980-81). **(H/S)**

________. **Woman, Why Do You Weep? Circumcision and Its Consequences.** London: Zed Press, 1983. See above. **(H/S)**

Epelboin, Sylvie, M.D., and Alain Epelboin, M.D. (France) "L'excision, tradition mutilante ou valeur culturelle? Enfants et jeunes au sahel" (Excision: Mutilating Tradition or a Cultural Value? The Children and the Young in the Sahel). Vol. 4, Nos. 2, 3, 4 (1980), pp. 177-88. Available from ENDA, B.P. 3370, Dakar, Senegal, West Africa. Printed in collaboration with UNICEF. // A survey of excision as practiced by West African ethnic groups including the Bambara. A discussion of the medical aspects and some case histories from Mali, as well as a discussion of West African tradition. **(H)**

Gervis, P. (France) **C'Est Arrive Dans la Sierra Leone.** Paris: Albin Michel, 1957. **(S)**

Ghadially, Dr. Rehana. (India) "The Practice of Female Circumcision Among the Bohra Muslims of India." Department of Humanities, Indian Institute of Technology, Bombay 76, India. **(S)**

Gove, Sandra, M.D., M.P.H., and Laura Diamondstone, R.N., Ph.N. (USA/Volunteers with Medical Volunteers International.) "Medical Team Interaction with Female Circumcision in a Refugee Camp, Bo', Somalia." // Paper presented at the Annual Conference of the National Council for International Health, Washington, D.C., June 1984. **(H)**

Groult, Benoite. (France) "Les Mutilations Sexuelles." **F. Magazine**, No. 14 (1979), pp. 50-56. // An outline of sexual mutilations practiced in Africa and French attitudes about this practice, including a report on the Khartoum Seminar on "Traditional Practices Affecting the Health of Women and Children." **(S)**

________. "Mutilations Sexuelles: Le Scandale Continue." **F. Mazagine**, No. 31 (1980), pp. 70-75. // Report on the operations in Djibouti including in the hospitals and their practice by French immigrants in the Paris area. **(H/S)**

Hansen, Henny Harald. (Denmark) "Clitoridectomy: Female Circumcision in Egypt." **Folk,** Vol. 14-15 (1972/73). Available from Folk Ethnografisk Samling, National Museum, Vester Gade 10, Copenhagen, Denmark. // Dr. Hansen's investigation in Egypt of the practice is described, including several interviews, one with the Grand Mufti (the highest Moslem authority of Egypt). The reasons given for the operations are discussed. **(S)**

Hathout, H.M., M.D. (UK) "Some Aspects of Female Circumcision: With a Case Report of a Rare Complication." **Journal of Obstetrics and Gynecology,** Vol. 79 (1963), pp. 505-07. // A description of the operations and a case history; Dr. Hathout practiced in Egypt. **(H)**

Hoffer, Carol P. (Canada) "Mende and Sherbro Women in High Office." **Canadian Journal of African Studies,** Vol. 6, No. 2 (1972), pp. 151-64. **(B/S)**

Huber, Alfons, M.D. (Austria) "Weibliche Zirkumzision und Infibulation in Athiopien." (A Survey of Female Circumcision and Infibulation in Ethiopia). **Acta Tropica,** Vol. 23, No. 1 (1966), pp. 87-91. In German. // A report on the practices of excision and infibulation as encountered by the author in his 10 years working in Ethiopia for Austrian Development Assistance, including a review of the ethnic groups engaged in these practices. **(H)**

________. "Die Weibliche Beschneidung." **Journal der Tropen Medizin & Parasitologie,** Vol. 20, No. 1 (1969), pp. 1-10. In German. // An overview of female genital operations with emphasis on Ethiopia, including the historic background of the Catholic Church's approval of the operations by a medical mission sent by the Pope in Rome in the 17th century. Also a description of the operations and their distribution. **(H/S)**

________. "Genitalverletzungen Afrikanischer Madchen durch rituelle Eingriffe." Kommission Helmut Bake Verlag Hamburg. Edited by Arbeitsgemeinschaft Ethnomedizin, Vol. 1, No. 1 (1971), p. 79. In German. // A recent survey of female genital mutilations all over Africa discussing the results on women's health and quoting from many sources. Bibliography. **(H)**

________. "Die rituelle Beschneidung der Frau - Sinn und Verbreitung" (The Ritual Circumcision of Women - Its Meaning and Distribution). **Mitteilungen Anthropologischer Gessellschaft Wien,** Vol. 101 (1976), pp. 76-82. In German. // A report on the ritual circumcision practiced in Ethiopia including the historic background of the practice in that country. **(H)**

Imperato, James Pascal, M.D. (USA) **African Folk Medicine: Practices and Beliefs of the Bambara and Other Peoples.** "Traditional Surgery: Circumcision and Excision," pp. 185-90. Baltimore: York Press, 1977. // Dr. Imperato worked extensively in East and West Africa, including on the WHO smallpox eradication campaign. This chapter deals with a description of the traditional circumcision operations, both male and female, and the accompanying rituals of the Bambara. **(H)**

Inter-African Committee (IAC). Conference Report, Second Regional Conference, Addis Ababa, Nov. 19-24, 1990. Inter African Committee, 147 rue de Lausanne, CH 1202, Geneva, Switzerland; or c/o ECA/ATRCW, P.O. Box 3001, Addis Ababa, Ethiopia. **(H)**

Kamara, A.M. "Traditions and Superstitions Among the Themnes and Mendes, and the Effect of Western Type of Education Upon Them." Department of Education Thesis No. 97, Fourah Bay College, Freetown, 1964. **(S)**

Karim, Mahmoud, M.D., and **Roshdi Ammar, M.D.** (Egypt) "Female Circumcision and Sexual Desire." Cairo: Ain Shams University Press, 1965. // A study of 331 circumcised women and the effects of their genital operations on sexual response. A description of the operations and tabulations of the questionnaires. Available from the Department of Obstetrics/Gynecology, Ain Shams University, Faculty of Medicine, Abbassiah, Cairo, Egypt. **(H)**

Kennedy, John G. (USA) "Circumcision and Excision in Egyptian Nubia." **Man: The Journal of Royal Anthropology Institute,** Vol. 5, No. 2 (1970), pp. 1975-91. // Description of the practices in Upper Egypt (Nubia) including a comparison between male and female rituals accompanying circumcision. A description of the rituals and the reasons given (infibulation). **(S)**

Kenyatta, Jomo. (Kenya) Facing Mount Kenya. "Initiation of Boys and Girls," pp. 125-48. New York: Vintage Books, 1965. // This book by Kenya's first president is based on the thesis prepared by Jomo Kenyatta while studying under Malinowski at the London School of Economics; it was first published in the 1930's. An overview of the Kikuyu society and customs, including strong advocacy of clitoridectomy. **(S)**

Koso-Thomas, Olayinka, M.D., M.P.H. The Circumcision of Women: A Strategy for Eradication. London: Zed Books, Ltd., 1987. **(H/S)**

_______. "Proposal for the Eradication of the Practice of Female Circumcision in Sierra Leone," dated March 16, 1981. M.P.H. Thesis, University of California, Berkeley. **(H/S)**

Lantier, Jacques. (France/pseudonym) La Cite Magique et Magie en Afrique Noire. Paris: Librarie Fayard, 1972. In French. (Paperback available from Fayard Press, 75 rue des Saintes Peres, 75278 Paris, Cedex, France.) // Lantier spent many years in West Africa working for the French administration and later for the United Nations. See especially chapters on "Circumcision and Initiation" and "The Mutilation of Women." The book provides important background information for the belief structure that underlies many African customs, including mutilation of female children. **(S)**

Lenzi, Eugenio, M.D.. (Italy) "Damage Caused by Infibulation and Infertility." **Acta Europa Fertilitatis**, Vol. 2, No. 47 (1970), pp. 47-58. // A discussion of the results of genital mutilation on women's health and fertility including four case histories. The author says that "20 to 25 percent of infertility in the Sudan is caused by female circumcision." **(H)**

Little, Kenneth. (UK) African Women in Towns: An Aspect of Africa's Social Revolution. Cambridge: Cambridge University Press, 1973. **(S/B)**

Longo, Lawrence D., M.D. (USA/Worked in Nigeria in Ibadan and Ile Ife.) "Sociocultural Practices Relating to Obstetrics and Gynaecology in a Community of West Africa." **American Journal of Obstetrics and Gynecology,** Vol. 89, No. 4 (1964), pp. 470-75. // A description of practices relating to fertility and birth at the Yoruba in West Nigeria (illustrations/bibliography). **(H)**

________. "Obstetrics and Gynaecology in a West African Community." **Medical Arts and Sciences,** Vol. 18 (1964), pp. 116-24. Loma Linda University. // The results of genital operations, including obstructed labor, are described. **(H)**

________. "Post-Obstetric Genito-Urinary Tract Fistula." **Obstetrics and Gynecology,** Vol. 23 No. 5 (1964), pp. 768-73. // A description and tabulation of fistula operations and their occurrence, most of them resulting from obstructed labor due to excision. **(H)**

Loutfi, Martha F. A New International Order Begins at Home - Rural Women: Unequal Partners in Development. Geneva: International Labour Office, 1980. **(B)**

Minces, Juliette. (France) The House of Obedience: Women in Arab Society. Paris: Editions Mazarine, 1980. Translated and reprinted by Zed Press, London, 1982. // Overview of the status of women in Arab Moslem societies, specifically family life, and the legal and social status of women. **(B)**

Ministry of Women's Rights, France. Les Mutilations du Sexe des Femmes Aujourd'hui en France **(Sexual Mutilation of Women in France Today).** Paris: Editions Tierce, 1984. In French. **(S)**

Minority Rights Group. (UK) Scilla McLean, editor. "Female Circumcision, Excision and Infibulation: The Facts and Proposals for Change," Report No. 47 (1980). New edition 1992. Available from Minority Rights Group, Benjamin Franklin House, 36 Craven St., London WC2N 5NG, England. // A summary of information previously published in other articles and books - no new research. The map on the cover of the first edition was correlated with political boundaries which is incorrect as FGM is an ethnic practice; this was corrected later. **(S)**

Modawi, Suliman, M.D. (Sudan/Senior Consultant, University of Khartoum, Obstetrics/ Gynecology.) "The Impact of Social and Economic Changes in Female Circumcision." Proceedings of the Third Congress of Obstetrics/Gynecology (1973), pp. 242-54. Sudan Medical Association, Khartoum University Press, 1974. // The records of 3,000 case histories analyzed to document sociological changes between 1955-70. Tables and bibliography. **(S/H)**

Murray, Jocelyn Margaret. (UK) **The Kikuyu Female Circumcision Controversy, with Special Reference to the Church Missionary Society's 'Sphere of Influence.'** University of California, Los Angeles, Ph.D. thesis (1974). Available from Silverpoint Order Entry, University Microfilms, a Xerox Company, 300 N. Zeeb Road, Ann Arbor, MI 48106. // The controversies surrounding prohibition of circumcision in Kenya by the British. A 1972 survey of several hundred schoolgirls is included, showing present status of genital mutilation in the same area. **(S)**

Mustafa, Asim Zaki, M.D. (Sudan) "Female Circumcision and Infibulation." **Journal of Obstetrics and Gynaecology**. British Commonwealth, April 1966, p. 302. **(H)**

Nichol, Guy. (USA) "The Clitoris Martyr." **World Medicine**, Vol. 4, No. 16 (1969), pp. 59, 63-65. // The background of the story of Dr. Isaac Baker Brown and his advocacy of female circumcision as a cure for mania and other diseases. **(H/B)**

Ogunmodede, Esther. (Nigeria) "Circumcision: How Much Longer Will We Allow Our Girls to Be Brutalized in This Barbaric Way?" **The Drum** (Nov. 1977), pp. 15-16. **(S)**

Oldfield-Hayes, Rose. (USA/Taught in Khartoum for two years.) "Female Genital Mutilation, Fertility Control, Women's Roles, and the Patrilineage in Modern Sudan: A Functional Analysis." **American Ethnologist**, Vol. 2, No. 4 (1975), pp. 617-33. // A research paper linking social and economic incentives with the ongoing practice of pharaonic circumcision in the Sudan. A field study and analysis is included. **(S)**

Omar, Dr. Roziah. (Malaysia) "Female Circumcision and Malay Women." Department of Anthropology and Sociology, University of Malay, Kuala Lumpur, Malaysia. **(S)**

Pieters, G., M.D. (Belgium/Worked for many years in Somalia in the late 1960's.) "Gynecologie au Pays des Femmes Cousues" (Gynecology in the Country of the Sewn Women). **Acta Chirurgica Belgica**, Vol. 71, No. 3 (1972), pp. 173-93. In French. // A summary of the practice of infibulation and its distribution in Africa (with a map). Description of the traditional operation and of the operations performed in the Mogadishu Common Market Hospital by specially-trained male nurses. **(H)**

________ and **Albert B. Lowenfels**. "Infibulation in the Horn of Africa." **New York State Journal of Medicine** (1977), pp. 729-31. // A short summary of the article by Dr. Pieters, translated into English. **(H)**

Pratiknya, Ahmad Watik, M.D. (Indonesia) "Female Circumcision in Indonesia: A Synthesis Profile of Cultural, Religious and Health Values," pp. 51-56. Proceedings of the Seminar on Female Circumcision, June 13-16, 1988, Mogadishu, Somalia. Published by AIDoS (Italian Association for Women in Development), via dei Giubbonari, 30 int. 6 - 00186 Rome, Italy. **(S)**

Ramali, Dr. Ahmad, M.D. (Indonesia) **Guidelines of Health Care According to Islamic Law.** Jakarta: Dinas Penerbitan Balai Pustaka, 1956. Translated from Indonesian. **(H)**

Rogers, Barbara. (USA) **The Domestication of Women: Discrimination in Developing Societies.** London: Kogan Page Ltd., 1980. **(B)**

Salah, Mrs. Mehani. (Yemen/Maternal and Child Health Supervisor of the Ministry of Health.) "The Health of Women and Children in Democratic Yemen." Report for the Seminar on Traditional Practices Affecting the Health of Women and Children. **WHO/ EMRO Technical Publication**, Vol. 2, No. 2 (1979), pp. 1-6. **(H/S)**

Sanderson, Lilian Passmore. (UK) **Against the Mutilation of Women: The Struggle Against Unnecessary Suffering**. London: Ithaca Press, 1981. // Summary of the medical problems is included in this social study of the conditions in the Sudan. The author was headmistress of a secondary girls' school in the Sudan and Egypt in the 1950's and 1960's. **(S/B)**

Saurel, Renee. (France) "L'Enterree Vive." **Les Temps Modernes** (26 rue de Conde, Paris 6, France), Jean-Paul Sartre, editor. A series of nine articles published in 1979/80. Subsequently published in book form: **L'Enteree Vive (The Buried Live: An Essay About Female Sexual Mutilation).** Preface by Simone de Beauvoir. Paris: Editions Slatkine, 1981. In French. **(S)**

________. **Bouches Cousues: Les Mutilations Sexuelles Feminines et Le Milieu Medical (Mouths Sewn Up: Female Sexual Mutilations and the Medical Establishment).** Paris: Editions Tierce, 1985. In French. **(S)**

Selassie, Alasebu Gebere. (Ethiopia/UN Principal Researcher and Coordinator, Addis Ababa.) "Harmful Traditional Practices Affecting the Health of Women and Children in Ethiopia." UNICEF/AAO, P.O. Box 1169, Addis Ababa, Ethiopia. **(H)**

Shandall, A. Abu-El-Futuh, M.D. (Sudan) "Circumcision and Infibulation of Females: A General Consideration of the Problem and a Clinical Study of the Complications in Sudanese Women." **Sudan Medical Journal**, Vol. 5 (1967), pp. 178-212. // Complete tabulation of various disabilities resulting from the mutilations (4,024 female patients at the Khartoum Hospital). Surveys of the daughters of the patients were made, as well as a number of the husbands. The author also provides information on the historic and religious background in the Sudan and outlines methods to eradicate the practice. This is the only study that provides exact data from clinical studies on the morbidity resulting from the operations. (International epidemiology is outdated.) **(H)**

Silberstein, A.J., M.D. (Belgium) "Circoncision Feminine en Cote d'Ivoire" (Female Circumcision in Ivory Coast). **Ann. Soc. Belg. Med. Trop.**, Vol. 57, No. 3 (1977), pp. 129-35. Available from Institute de Medicine Tropicale Prince Leopolde, Nationale Estraat 155, B-2000 Antwerpen, Belgium. In French.// Dr. Silberstein practiced in the hospital of Odienne in the northwest of the Ivory Coast and he describes the information he collected from direct observation in this area, where practically all women are excised. **(H)**

Steady, Dr. Filomena. (Sierra Leone) "Female Power in African Politics: The National Congress in Sierra Leone." **Africana Library Notes**, Vol. 6, No. 31 (1975-76). **(B)**

Sullerot, Evelyne. (France) **Woman Society and Change.** New York: World University Library, McGraw Hill Book Co., 1973. **(B)**

Taba, A.H. (Iran/Former director of WHO/EMRO) "Female Circumcision." **World Health** (May 1979), pp. 8-9. Available from WHO, 1211 Geneva 27, Switzerland. Reprinted in **Tropical Doctor**, Vol. 10 (1980), pp. 21-23. // The operations and their historic background are described as well as the WHO Seminar on "Traditional Practices Affecting the Health of Women and Children," and its Recommendations. **(H)**

Taoko, Jean G., M.D. (Burkina Faso) "L'excision: Base de la Stabilite Familiale ou Rite Cruel?" (Excision: Basis of Family Stability or a Cruel Rite?). **Famille et Developpement**, No. 2 (Spring 1975). In French. Famille et Developpement is published by ASAFED, B.P. 3907 Lome, Togo, West Africa. // The operations are described as well as health results. Extensive background informationon the traditional customs and practices as well as the reasons given for the operations in West Africa among various ethnic groups. **(S/H)**

Thaddeus, Sereen. (Netherlands) "The Prevalence of Female Circumcision in Yemen/A Compilation of Facts." Submitted to the Royal Netherlands Embassy, Sana'a, December 1992. Ministerie Van Buitenlandse Saken/The Netherlands Ministry of Foreign Affairs, Postbus 20061, 2500 EB S'Gravenhage, The Netherlands. **(S/H)**

Thiam, Awa. (Senegal) **La Parole aux Negresses.** "La Clitoridectomie et l'Infibulation," pp. 77-118. Paris: Denoel/Gonthier, 1978. // A survey of genital mutilation practiced especially in West Africa with case histories as related by women themselves and an outline of the historic background of the operations. **(S/B)**

Tinker, Irene. (USA) **Persistent Inequalities - Women and World Development.** Oxford: Oxford University Press, 1990. **(B)**

Verzin, J.A., M.D. (UK) "Sequelae of Female Circumcision." **Tropical Doctor**, Vol. 5 (1975), pp. 163-69. // A description of the operations and a discusssion of medical and health results. Bibliography included. (Epidemiology is outdated.) **(H)**

VIVA. "The Silence Over Female Circumcision in Kenya." August 1978, pp. 6-15, 72-73. Available from VIVA, P.O. Box 46319, Nairobi, Kenya. // A discussion of female circumcision in Kenya by the women's magazine of Kenya, providing the historic background as well as current social pressures for and against circumcision. **(S)**

Widstrand, Carl Gosta. (Sweden) "Female Infibulation." **Studia Ethnographica Upsaliensa,** Vol. 20 (1964). // The most thorough study of infibulation worldwide from historical, anthropological and social sources. **(S)**

World Health Organization. "**Traditional Practices Affecting the Health of Women and Children: Report of a Seminar**" (Khartoum 1979). **WHO/EMRO Technical Publication,** No. 2 (1979). Available from WHO/EMRO, P.O. Box 1517, Alexandria, Egypt. **(H)**

World Health Organization. **Background Papers to the WHO Seminar on "Traditional Practices Affecting the Health of Women and Children."** **WHO/EMRO Technical Publication,** Vol. 2, No. 2 (1982). Available from the above. **(H)**

HISTORIC PUBLICATIONS

Editor's Note: Many of the medical authors whose articles are listed above used the ethnographic research of Ploss/Bartels (see citation below) - usually some later English editions - as reference. But the information on where the operations are practiced is from the 1885 first edition of **Das Weib,** from "travelers' reports" with no medical or more recent confirmation. The same reports from 1885 are included in all subsequent editions of Ploss/ Bartels as well as in the English translation of this work, edited by Eric Dingwall, **Women: A Historical Gynecological and Anthropological Compendium (1935).** This English translation of Ploss/Bartels still is available and cited, though the facts were never checked and are obsolete. For an updated, current epidemiology, see "Female Genital Mutilation in the World Today: A Global Review," **International Journal of Health Sciences,** and the research paper by Fran P. Hosken included in the Seminar Report on "Traditional Practices Affecting the Health of Women and Children," by WHO/EMRO Technical Publication, Vol. 2, No. 2. See also **WIN NEWS,** Vol. 18, No. 4, p. 29, or contact the Inter African Committee, 147, rue de Lausanne, CH-1202, Geneva, Switzerland.

Beck, Ann. (UK) **A History of the British Medical Administration of East Africa, 1900-1950.** Cambridge: Harvard University Press, 1970.

Burton, Richard Francis. **First Footsteps in East Africa, or an Exploration of Harar.** London: Tylston & Edwards, 1894.

__________. **Personal Narrative of a Pilgrimage to Al-Medinah and Meccah.** London: George Bell and Sons, 1898.

Dingwall, Eric J. **Women: An Historical, Gynecological and Anthropological Compendium.** London: Wm. Heinemann Ltd., 1935. // English translation of Ploss's **Das Weib**.

__________. **The Girdle of Chastity.** London: Routledge, 1931.

__________. **Femina, Libido Sexualis, Compendium of the Psychology, Anthropology and Anatomy of the Sexual Characteristics of the Woman**. New York: Medical Press of New York, 1965. // A summary of the sections concerned with reproduction and sexuality from Ploss with little or no additional information. (Available only in medical/ historical libraries.)

Duden, Barbara and Isabelle Schatten. "Die Gebarmutter das Hungrige Tier" (The Uterus, the Hungry Animal: History of Hysteria). **Courage** (March 3, 1978) p. 20. In German.

Duffy, John. (USA) "Masturbation and Clitoridectomy: A 19th-Century View." **Journal of the American Medical Association,** Vol. 186 (1963), pp. 245-248. // Clitoridectomy performed in order to discourage masturbation in 19th-century America.

Fleming, J.G. (UK) "Clitoridectomy: The Disastrous Downfall of Isaac Baker Brown, F.R.C.S. (1867)." **Journal of Gynecology of the British Empire,** Vol. 67, No. 6 (1960), pp. 1017-34. // The story of Dr. Isaac Baker Brown who in 1867 advocated female circumcision in the UK to prevent a series of diseases including mania.

King, Major J.S. (Bombay Staff Corps.) "On the Practice of Female Circumcision and Infibulation Among the Somal and Other Nations of North East Africa." **Anthropological Society of Bombay,** No. 2 (1890), pp. 2-6.

Memorandum Prepared by the Mission Council of the Church of Scotland. "Female Circumcision: Section I, Medical Aspects of Male and Female Circumcision and Clitoridectomy" (signed by four physicians), 1931. Available from African Library, Boston University.

Montagu, Ashley. "Infibulation and Defibulation in the Old and New Worlds." **The American Anthropologist.** Brief Communications N.S. 47, (1945), p. 465.

Ploss, Heinrich and Max Bartels. Das Weib. First edition (1885). In German. Available in major medical research libraries. // Female circumcision is discussed in the first edition and in all subsequent editions. Dr. Ploss died shortly after the book came out. The second (1886) and all subsequent editions were edited by Bartels, based on Ploss's research. After some 30 editions (which included all the same information on female circumcision with very few additions) the book was translated into English (see Dingwall).

Pridie, E.D., M.D., A.E. Lorenzen, M.D., A. Cruickshank, M.D., J.O. Hovell, M.D., and **D.R. MacDonald, M.D.** (UK) "Female Circumcision in the Anglo-Egyptian Sudan." Sudan Medical Service, Khartoum, Jan. 3, 1945. // A report prepared by the Sudan Medical Service, Khartoum, and signed by: Drs. Ali Bedri, Abdel Halim Mohd, Abdulla Omer Abu Shamma, El Tigani Homd, El Maki, E.D. Pridie, J.S. Hovell, A.E. Lorenzen, D.R. MacDonald and A. Cruickshank. Includes a Foreword by His Excellency the Governor General, Major Gen. Sir Hubert Huddleston, KCMG, CB, DSOMC; a Foreword by Sheik Ahmed El Taher, and a Foreword by El Sayed Sir Abdel Rahman El Madi Pasha.

Remondino, P.C. **History of Circumcision from the Earliest Times to the Present.** Philadelphia and London: F.A. Davis Publishers, 1891.

deVilleneuve, Anne. "Etude sur une Coutume Somalie: Les Femmes Cousues." **Journal de la Societe des Africanistes.** Vol. 6 (1937), pp. 15-32. In French. // Eyewitness description of infibulation operations performed on two sisters in Djibouti including a description of women's lives.

Young, E. Hills. (U.K./In charge of nurses' education in the Sudan in the 1940's.) "Female Circumcision in the Sudan." **Nursing Mirror** (March 1949), pp. 377-78. // An eyewitness report of a traditional operation on two children is presented, as well as health and background facts of the Sudan. After witnessing this operation, the author took steps to prohibit the performance of these operations by their staff midwives.

Zaborowski, M. **La Circonsion ses Origines et sa Reparation en Afrique et a Madagascar (The Circumcision: Its Origin and Spread in Africa and Madagascar).** Anthropologie Paris, 1896.

SERIAL PUBLICATIONS

Cairo Family Planning Association - 50 Goumhouria St., Cairo, Egypt. Publishes an annual progress report and summary of their activities.

FORWARD (Foundation for Women's Health Research & Development) - 38 King St., Covent Garden, London WC2E 8JT, U.K. Newsletter and various training and educational publications available, including a report on the "First Study Conference on FGM in Europe."

WIN NEWS (Women's International Network News). (Quarterly) Fran P. Hosken, publisher/editor; 187 Grant St., Lexington, MA 02420. Continuing section in every issue on "Female Circumcision: Genital and Sexual Mutilation," starting with Vol. 1, No. 3, 1975. The FGM section reports all published information and activities as well as first-hand research reports from Africa. New information in each issue, references and bibliographies.

ETHNIC GROUPS PRACTICING FEMALE GENITAL MUTILATION

CONTINENTAL AFRICA

BENIN - Zugu, Basida, Dandaghie.

BURKINA FASO - Busanga, Mossi; 70 percent of female population

CHAD - Shuwa.

COTE D'IVOIRE - Malinke, Dioula, Guere, Guro, Baule, Mwan, area of Odienne, Lobi.

DJIBOUTI - Entire female population infibulated.

EASTERN AFRICA - Somali, Meru, Embu, Chuka, Kikuyu, Rangi, Nandi, Masai, Kamasia, Pokot, Elgeyo, Njemps, Dorobo, Sebei, Digo, Taita, Giriama, Kisii, Kamba, Swahili, Chaga, Pare, Gogo, Arusha, Tatoga, Turu, Bena, Hehe, Watusi, Xhosa, Suba, Wasembeti, Nilo-Hamitic ethnic groups.

ETHIOPIA - Amhara, Kafitscho, Oromo (Galla), Danakil, Tigre, Ometo, Hamitic Kufa, Babea, Sidamo, Kushite; Somali (Harrar area) infibulation. **ERITREA** - infibulation .

EGYPT - All ethnic groups (Muslim and Copt) except for educated, urban upper class.

GAMBIA - All ethnic groups except Jolloff.

GHANA - Hausa, Yoruba, Kassina, Nankani, North Ghanaian groups, Bolga, Navorongo, Bawku, Lawra, Tumu, Wa, Kussasi, Frafra, Bussauri, Manprusie, Kantansi, Wala, Sissala, Grunshia, Dargati, Lobi, Dagaaba, Kasim, Gonga, Dagomba.

GUINEA - Twenty-four ethnic groups including Foulah, Peul, Malinke (Mandingo), Soussou, Bambara, Kasonke, Serer, Wolof, Conakry area.

KENYA - Masai, Kuria, Kisii, Nandi, Kipsigis, Kamba, Kikuyu, Digo, Taita, Giriama, Dorobo, Samburu, Kamasia, Elgeyo, Pokot (Suk), Embu, Meru, Terik, Marakwet, Chagga, Kavirondo, Watende, Wakamba, Kitosh, Lumbwa, Somali.

LIBERIA - Lorma, Belle, Kissi, Bassa, Kpelle, Gola, Mano, Gio, Vai, Dei, Mende, Krahn, Gbandi.

MALI - Bambara, Dogon, Mossi, Malinke, Saracole, Songhoi, Peul, Wanagara; all ethnic groups except northernmost areas.

MAURITANIA - Black ethnic groups adjoining Senegal and Mali.

NIGER - Peul, southern part of country

NIGERIA - Yoruba, Ibo, Igbo, Fulani, Hausa, Efik, Shuwa and most ethnic groups except Itsekiri; inhabitants of Cross River State.(majority of population)

SENEGAL - Malinke (Mandingo/Wangara), Eulani, Toucouleur, Peul (Fulani), Soce (Casama); all ethnic groups except Wolofs (Dakar area).

SIERRA LEONE - All ethnic groups except Creoles, including Temne, Mende, Loko, Limba, Kono, Kuranko, Susu, Fullah, Mandingo.

SOMALIA - All ethnic groups practice infibulation including Harrar, Afar, Danakil, Galla

SUDAN - Beja, Hadandana, Beni Amir, Kababish, Baggara, Danagla, Shaygia, Gaaliyeen, Rubatab, Amarar, Fallata, Bushairiya, Rashyda, Dongola, Hassanie, Bisharin, Ababde, Mensa, Hababa, Bund Burun, Abn Haraz, Musalam Iye, Awlad Kahil Hassanie, Singa, Sinnar and more; Gezir and Khartoum province; Omdurman area, Nubia; Red Sea Coast, Wad Medani, Humor of West Sudan.

TANZANIA - Masai, Basembeti-Suba, Bakuria, Komaki, Chaga, Pare, Shambala, Gogo, Rangi, Turu, Bena, Hehe, Nilo-Hamitic ethnic groups.

UGANDA - Sebei.

ZAIRE - M'Bwake, Banda, northern area and along Congo River.

SOUTHERN ARAB PENINSULA :OMAN - Most ethnic groups . **YEMEN, BAHRAIN, UNITED ARAB EMIRATES** (some ethnic groups, decreasing)

ASIA: INDONESIA: some Moslem Groups.of Java; **MALAYSIA** : Malays (Moslem)

LIST OF ACRONYMS:

UN	United Nations
UNICEF	United Nations Children Fund
UNDP	United Nations Development Program
UNESCO	United Nations Educational Scientific and Cultural Organization
UNFPA	United Nations Population Fund
UNHCR	United Nations High Commission for Refugees
UNHRC	United Nations Human Rights Center
UNESCO	United Nations Educational Scientific and Cultural Organization
ECOSOC	Economic and Social Council of the United Nations
WB	World Bank
IMF	International Monetary Fund
WHO	World Health Organization
ILO	International Labor Organization
FAO	Food and Agfriculture Organization
ECA	Economic Commission of Africa
OAU	Organization of African Unity
US AID	United States Agency for International Development
FGM	Female Genital Mutilation
IAC	Inter African Committee
CEDAW	Convention on the Elimination of Discrimination Against Women
WIN	Women's International Network
WIN NEWS	Women's International Network NEWS
CBPB	Childbirth Picture Book

WORLD HEALTH ORGANIZATION STATEMENT OF WHO POSITION / JUNE 1982

"WHO has consistently and unequivocally advised that female circumcision should not be practiced by any health professionals in any setting - including in hospitals or other health establishements."

FEDERAL PROHIBITION OF FEMALE GENITAL MUTILATION ACT OF 1993

INTRODUCED AS PART OF WOMEN'S HEALTH EQUITY ACT

by **Congresswoman Patricia Schroeder**

SEC. 262 TITLE 18 AMENDMENT:

(a) IN GENERAL - Chapter 7 of title 18. United States Code, is amended by adding at the end the following new section:

- 116. FEMALE GENITAL MUTILATION

(a) Except as provided in subsection (b), whoever knowingly circumcises, excises, or infibulates the whole or any part of the labia majora or labia minora or clitoris of another person who has not attained the age of 18 years shall be fined under this title or imprisoned not more than 5 years, or both.

(b) A surgical operation is not a violation of this section if the operation is-

"(1) necessary to the health of the person on whom it is performed, and is performed by aperson licensed in the place of its performance as a medical practitioner; or

(2) performed on a person in labor or who has just given birth and is performed for medical purposes connected with that labor or birth by a person licensed in the place it is performed as a medical practitioner, midwife, or person in training to become such a practitioner or midwife.

(c) In applying subsection (b) (1), no account shall be taken of the effect on the person on whom the operation is to be performed of any belief on the part of that or any other person that the operation is required as a matter of custom or ritual.

(d) Whoever knowingly denies to any person medical care or services or otherwise discriminates against any person in the provision of medical care or services, because-

(1) that person has undergone female circumcision, excision, or infibulation; or

(2) that person has requested that female circumcision, excision, or infibulation be performedon any person;

shall be fined under this title or imprisoned not more than one year, or both.

(b) CLERICAL AMENDMENT - The table of sections at the beginning of Chapter 7 of title 18, United States Code, is amended by adding at the end the following new item:

116. Female genital mutilation.

SEC. 263. EDUCATION AND OUTREACH

The Secretary of Health and Human Services shall carry out appropriate education, preventive, and outreach activities in communities that traditionally practice female circumcision, excision, or infibulation, to inform people in those communities about the health risks and emotional trauma inflicted by those practices, and to inform them and the medical community about the provisions of section 262.

SEC. 264 EFFECTIVE DATES

Section 263 shall take effect immediately, and the Secretary of Health and Human Services shall commence carrying out not later than 90 days after the date of the enactment of this Act. Section 262 shall take effect 180 days after the date of the enactment of this Act.

THE UNIVERSAL CHILDBIRTH PICTURE BOOK - (CBPB)

ENGLISH / FRENCH / SPANISH / ARABIC / SOMALI

The drawings by **MARCIA L. WILLIAMS**, a medical illustrator, provide biologically correct information. The CBPBs were circulated world-wide for two years to midwives, physicians and health workers world-wide for comments before printing.

Addressed to the Community Health Worker/Educator worldwide, the CBPBs are a flexible, adaptable multi-ethnic teaching aid, with **34 full-page drawings, a text** with each picture to read out loud, and **a discussion guide** for group meetings The **Glossary** explains technical terms. **An International Reading/Resource List** provides health contacts and information.

FLIP CHARTS (4 X size of book), same pictures, text and discussion guide

COLOR SLIDES are coordinated with the CBPB, text and discussion guide

NUTRITION SUPPLEMENT: English / French / Spanish

EXCISION AND INFIBULATION ADDITIONS: English / French / Arabic

The SOMALI CBPB includes the Addition on Infibulation

The CBPB's have been successfully used worldwide on the grass-roots level, regardless of language or literacy; they can be readily adapted and translated. More than 70.000 books are currently in circulation world-wide.

WIN NEWS offers technical help with adaption and free permission to print for educational purposes under the copyright.

The **CBPBs** are adapted/printed in India by **CHETNA** (Centre for Health Education, Training and Nutrition Awareness) in Hindi and other Indian languages.
Contact: **CHETNA**, Lilavatiben Lalbhai's Bunglow Civil, Camp road, Shahibaug Ahmedabad-380 004, INDIA.
The **CBPBs** are also printed in **Nepal, the Marshall Islands and Senegal**.

Free sample books are available to health programs in developing countries.
For more information and prices / shipping instructions please contact:
WIN NEWS, Fran P. Hosken, 187 Grant St. Lexington MA 02173 USA.

The information in this Report is continuously being updated in **WIN NEWS** which is published four times a year and has a continuing section on FGM. providing new information in every issue, including contacts (names and addresses), reviews of new publications, information on conferences and reports on new developments in Africa..

ABOUT THE AUTHOR

Fran P. Hosken is editor and publisher of Women's International Network - **WIN NEWS** - an "open participatory worldwide quarterly journal by, for and about women" which she started in 1975, International Women's Year.

Before starting **WIN NEWS,** Fran P. Hosken has written for many newspapers and magazines especially on housing, urban development and as architectural critic as well as on women's development worldwide. She has published many hundreds of articles in leading papers and magazines in the US and abroad and was correspondent-at-large for the **Architectural Forum**. She is an architect/urban planner by profession with a Masters Degree in Architecture from Harvard and did several years of postgraduate studies in urban planning at M.I.T. after briefly working in architectural offices.

She has published a number of books and reports, including **The Language of Cities** (published by Macmillan), **The Functions of Cities** (published by Schenkman and as a tape program by McGraw Hill) and **The Kathmandu Valley Towns** (published by Weatherhill). The previous editions of **The Hosken Report** and **The Childbirth Picture Book (CBPB)** / Program are published by **WIN NEWS**. By now the **CBPBs** are available with the Additions to prevent Excision and Infibulation in English, French, Arabic and Somali; a Spanish translation is also available. The **CBPBs** are printed in India by CHETNA in six Indian languages and in Nepal as well as the Marshall Islands. Nutrition supplements, flip charts and color slides are coordinated. More than 80,000 copies of the CBPBs are in use worldwide and more are continuously printed and distributed, translated and adapted in order to enable women everywhere to take charge of their lives and health.

Fran P. Hosken has taught urban studies at college level and has developed some experimental urban teaching programs for children and high school students. She has one of the largest worldwide collections of color slides of buildings and cities which are used for teaching purposes and which she photographed on her many travels all over the world. She is fluent in three languages and reads six. Her early education was in Europe, (Vienna, Austria) and she continued her education at Smith College (B.A.), before getting a professional degree at Harvard. She served as officer in the US Coast Guard/Navy at the end of the war. She has three grown children and lives in Lexington, Massachusetts.

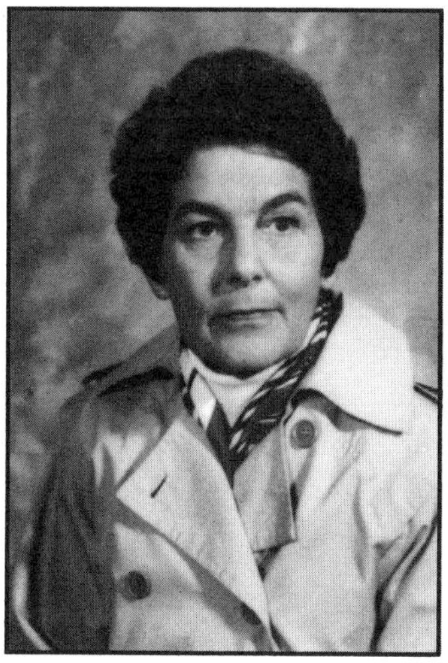

Fran P. Hosken has been accredited as journalist to all three United Nations Women's Conferences as well as to the UN Environment, HABITAT, and Population Conferences and she will cover the 1995 UN Women's Conference in China. **WIN NEWS** reports on "all the news that is fit to print by, for and about women" from all over the world, covering women's organizations, activties, meetings and women's media world-wide, and includes a regular section on FGM. **WIN NEWS** was established to facilitate global networking and to enable women to directly communicate worldwide. Asia and Pacific, Africa and the Middle East, Europe and the Americas are covered in every issue.

Fran P. Hosken has lectured all over the world and led women's tours to China and India and Nepal.

WOMEN'S INTERNATIONAL NETWORK is incorporated as a non-profit organization in Massachusetts and has 501(c)3 status: Contributions are tax-deductible in the USA